ALLE ZEIT WACH
1842

Biological and Psychological Factors in Cardiovascular Disease

Edited by
T. H. Schmidt   T. M. Dembroski   G. Blümchen

Foreword by
M. J. Halhuber

With 153 Figures and 85 Tables

Springer-Verlag Berlin Heidelberg New York
London Paris Tokyo

Dr. med. THOMAS H. SCHMIDT

Abteilung Epidemiologie und Sozialmedizin
Medizinische Hochschule Hannover
Konstanty-Gutschow-Straße
3000 Hannover 61, FRG

Prof. Dr. THEODORE M. DEMBROSKI

Department of Psychology
University of Maryland
Baltimore County
Cantonsville, MD 21228, USA

Prof. Dr. GERHARD BLÜMCHEN

Klinik Roderbirken
5653 Leichlingen/Rhld. 1, FRG

ISBN-13:978-3-642-71236-4 e-ISBN-13:978-3-642-71234-0
DOI: 10.1007/978-3-642-71234-0

Library of Congress Cataloging in Publication Data. Biological and Psychological Factors in Cardiovascular Disease. Based on a conference held in June 1984 at Winterscheid, West Germany. Includes bibliographies and index. 1. Coronary heart disease - Psychological aspects - Congresses. 2. Type A behavior - Congresses. 3. Stress (Psychology) - Congresses. I. Schmidt, Thomas H. II. Dembroski, Theodore M. III. Blümchen, Gerhard. [DNLM: 1. Behavior - physiology - congresses. 2. Coronary Disease - congresses. WG 300 B6147 1984] RC685.C6B53 1986 616.1'2071 86-10105
ISBN-13:978-3-642-71236-4 (U.S.)

Softcover reprint of the hardcover 1st edition 1986

2125/3130-543210

To Hazel, Stans, and Anne

Foreword

An opening address should ask the right questions, which we expect to answer during the coming years. A good opening address should formulate hypotheses for falsification during the conference or in the near future. After Dr. Groen's excellent lecture yesterday, I feel better about my task, because I feel I am not alone in asking the ten questions in my abstract.

It is an honor for me to give this short paper largely based on my experiences during 15 years as medical director of a rehabilitation center in Bavaria, as a teacher at two medical schools in Munich and Innsbruck, and as an old-fashioned holistic cardiologist. However, it also is a difficult task for me because the subject of this conference concerning biobehavioral factors in coronary heart disease is controversial, not only in the medical society, but in my own mind as well.

When I organized one of the first conferences on stress and coronary heart disease in West Germany in 1976, followed by conferences in 1979 and 1980, the semantic problems between physicians and psychologists were very significant. However, communication has improved in this area during the last decade. The most encouraging event in this field was a symposium in May 1984 in Rotenburg/Fulda on the topic "Return to Work after Bypass Surgery", organized by a cardiac surgeon, Dr. Walter. For two days, cardiologists and psychologists were able to talk to one another in a common language reflecting a very high scientific level of sophistication (Walter 1985).

Dr. Ray H. Rosenman and I have just returned from a symposium, organized by the Scientific Council on Rehabilitation of Cardiac Patients of the International Society and Federation of Cardiology, that took place in Santiago de Compostela, Spain (8-9 June, 1984). There, we realized the difficulties of integrating new concepts in medicine into different sociocultural settings for practice, education, and research. That is one reason why I hope that this conference in Winterscheid will help us to understand better the psychosocial aspects of coronary heart disease and to contribute to better preventive cardiology, by which I mean: truly *comprehensive coronary care* under different conditions.

In my abstract, I proposed 10 provocative theses or hypotheses to stimulate an interdisciplinary discussion. These are theses formulated by an elderly physician who spent decades of his life improving cardiac rehabilitation in theory and practice. This practice, I confess, is also of personal significance, as I happened to experience myocardial infarction some time ago.

Let me now explain and comment on some of my theses:

1. *The concept of type A coronary-prone behavior is being adapted into the more differentiated notion of a strategy for mastering chronic social risk situations.*

The type A concept of coronary-prone behavior seems to me to be evolving from the notion of a simple and stable personality trait to that of a coping strategy. If you compare definitions 20 years ago with the recent definition of type A pattern by Rosenman, you realize the difference: The notion of coronary-prone behavior as an interactional concept related to specific social contexts is a very precise definition that outstrips the earlier notion of type A as a simple and stable personality trait. I quote:

> Type A behavior pattern is a set of behaviors that is correlated with enhanced adrenergic response to the daily environment. It includes behavioral dispositions such as ambitiousness, aggressiveness, competitiveness, and impatience; specific behaviors such as muscle tenseness, alertness, rapid and emphatic voice style and the pace of most activities; and emotional responses such as irritability and increased potential for hostility and anger ... It is a characteristic style of coping response to environmental stressors. Type A individuals perceive too many things as a threat to their control over the environment (Rosenman 1984).

2. *The interaction of chronic social risk situations, subacute life events, and coronary-prone behavior,* about which I have learned from my friend J. Siegrist, *seems to me important not only for interdisciplinary research, but also for practice and education.* There is a gap between practice and research at this very moment.
3. *The differences between type A and B are less qualitative than quantitative (continuum). For purposes of intervention and education this view of type A as a continuum is more practicable. It is easier for patients to change their life style when they only have to reduce, rather than transform, a learned and socially accepted attitude.*

If the path from the type A to type B behavior pattern is a continuum, it means more quantitative than qualitative differences in the "need for control". The task of modifying such behavior is thus easier to accomplish. The possibilities for modifying type A behavior and the results of intervention programs are today either the most important obstacles or the most important tools in convincing skeptical cardiologists of the importance of considering psychosocial factors in medical practice.

I believe in *the lifestyle concept* of the WHO! At this moment, however, it is only a belief. We need more intervention studies with a new methodology to avoid some of the pitfalls of the MRFIT study.

4. *After an acute myocardial infarction, coronary-prone behavior has a different meaning than before:* do type A patients show better compliance (for example in exercise therapy) and more denial, overmotivation, and the like?
5. *A better understanding of the advantages and disadvantages of denial is needed for the education of the myocardial infarction patient.*

The fourth and fifth theses are seen as questions or hypotheses to be proven in the near future. I would like to direct the attention of responsible leaders of interdisciplinary research teams to the *interaction* of *coronary-*

prone behavior after myocardial infarction and *compliance* (e.g., in exercise therapy). And what of *denial?* What are the advantages of denial as a coping strategy for MI patients? What are its disadvantages (e.g., as it relates to overmotivation during exercise and training)? What is the relationship between denial and coronary-prone behavior? MI patients probably need some "denial," but not too much.

6. *"After a heart attack, there are more problems in the mind than in the heart!"* (Weeda, personal communication). Have all the consequences of this state of affairs been considered?

It was the Dutch cardiologist and member of the scientific council H. Weeda, not a psychologist or psychiatrist or other "outsider," who summarized his experience in the sentence I have just quoted. Even cardiac surgeons discussing the reasons for no or a late return to work for the bypass patient have realized the importance of the psychosocial aspects of coronary heart disease, the consequences of which we are only now beginning to explore.

7. *The following five goals of cardiac rehabilitation for the patient and his familiy, proposed by R. S. Eliot in 1979 are very helpful in the practice of comprehensive coronary care:*
   1. Acceptance of the disease
   2. Knowledge of the disease, thereby permitting the patient to make better decisions for his future
   3. Emotional support
   4. Sustained adherence to recommendations for therapy
   5. Reaching the optimal functional level

Each of Eliot's five goals of cardiac rehabilitation for the patient *and* his family also includes biobehavioral factors. I would like to direct your attention to the order of these five goals, for to achieve good results for the fifth goal, we first need to achieve the four others.

8. *The implications of points 1–7 for practice, education, and research* – (convincing intervention studies that are lacking at the moment) – *can only be realized through an interdisciplinary approach.*

I hope to avoid misunderstandings by using the phrase "therapeutic team," which involves the following kinds of professionals: physicians, nurses, dieticians, physiotherapists, social workers, psychologists, psychiatrists, and the clergy. Moreover, the patient and his family are also integrated into the "therapeutic community."

9. *The efficiency and effectiveness of interdisciplinary management of the psychosocial aspects of coronary heart disease in primary and secondary prevention depend on the intensity of training and education of all members of the therapeutic team.* Moreover, real integration of the contributions of the psychiatrist, psychologist, nurse, and social worker in addition to the others involved is critical to a successfull outcome.

At this moment, the obstacles of real interdisciplinary cooperation in the framework of rehabilitation and management of biobehavioral factors in coronary heart disease are discouraging. Therefore, these obstacles should be systematically discussed, but not by the members of the medical profession alone. I was impressed at the end of the symposium organized by the

Scientific Council on Rehabilitation of Cardiac Patients in Santiago, 1984, by the number of misunderstandings existing presently. Some reasons for these misunderstandings are listed here. They should be examined and discussed at specially designed conferences:

a) Lack of personal experience and special training in the field of biobehavioral factors in coronary heart disease
b) Semantic problems caused by the specialized scientific languages of different disciplines, especially medicine, psychology, and sociology
c) Diverging philosophies of medicine in various sociocultural and economic settings, for example, the USA and central Europe, resulting in often hidden differences
d) The emotional difficulties doctors experience in accepting a new kind of partnership between coronary patients and their therapists (not only physicians?), for example, the acceptance of self-help groups and similar movements or collaboration with psychologists
e) The fear of expensive "overmedication" and "manipulation" of the patient; in this regard, I remember the comment of an American doctor: "Sickness is not rewarded in the United States."
f) A "nihilistic attitude" towards behavior therapy that requires investigation

I hope the results of this conference, translated into a language comprehensible to the skeptical medical profession, will help to diminish its widespread doubts and augment the possibilities for interdisciplinary cooperation and understanding.

If we use the four levels of scientific acceptance of regimens proposed by Samuel Fox (proven, prudent action, promising, possible), then it seems possible to make the following statement:

10. *A holistic, ecological concept of comprehensive coronary care is justified in 1985 by substantial, although incomplete, data and an acceptably low level of risk.*

At the same time, one is always well advised in finishing an address of this kind with the remark: More research is needed!

M. J. Halhuber

References

Eliot RS (1979) Stress and the major cardiovascular disorders. Futura, Mount Kisco, New York

Rosenman RH (1984) Modification of the coronary-prone (Type A) behavior pattern in the frame of cardiac rehabilitation. International Society and Federation of Cardiology, Scientific Council on Cardiac Rehabilitation, Santiago de Compostella, Spain, June 7-10, 1984

Walter PJ ed (1985) Return to work after coronary bypass surgery. Springer, Berlin Heidelberg New York Tokyo

Preface

The possible role of the interaction of biological and psychological factors in cardiovascular-related diseases, hypertension, and sudden cardiac death has received steadily increasing scientific interest, especially during the past few decades. Behaviors capturing attention as potential coronary-prone tendencies have generally fallen into two categories. The first category includes primarily consummatory behaviors that have been targeted for alteration in an effort to reduce traditional risk factors for coronary heart disease (CHD) in a clinically significant fashion. To this end, enormous international resources derived from both private and public agencies have been devoted to modifying dietary practices, reducing or eliminating the cigarette-smoking habit, initiating and maintaining hypotensive interventions, increasing physical exercise, and the like.

Behaviors in the second category of coronary-prone tendencies have been related to the concept of "stress" in the sense that particular psychosocial attributes are thought to be associated with either chronic or acute physiological processes which excite pathophysiological mechanisms. In this connection, epidemiological studies have attempted to associate prospectively and retrospectively a variety of psychosocial phenomena with clinical manifestations of CHD and the severity of underlying coronary atherosclerosis. The leading example here is the considerable research that has been conducted to examine the links between the Type A coronary-prone behavior pattern and CHD end points. Parallel research has attempted to identify physiological processes associated with the Type A pattern that may be related to pathophysiological mechanisms, which translate Type A attributes into clinical CHD. Similarly, laboratory-based research has addressed comparable issues regarding the role of behavioral factors in the development of essential hypertension. Both lines of inquiry have involved both human and animal subjects.

Despite large amounts of research devoted to both categories of coronary-prone tendencies, CHD remains a mysterious disease. Attempts to establish unequivocally the validity of coronary-prone tendencies that can be generalized to all, or even most, international populations have yielded, at best, mixed positive and negative findings. It would be comforting if the situation were otherwise, but such is not the case. Nevertheless, over the years periodic national and international conferences have convened to assess progress and determine the state of the art in research aimed at the prevention, control, and understanding of cardiovascular disorders. We last organized an international conference concerning biological and psychological factors in CHD in June 1981 at Altenberg, Federal Republic of

Germany. The proceedings of that conference were edited and published in book form.[1] The present volume, like its predecessor, is an outgrowth of a conference, this one held in June 1984 at Winterscheid, Federal Republic of Germany. A quick glance at the list of contributors will reveal an extensive international assemblage of scientists. Although few definitive statements can be made that qualify as generalizable "truths," exciting and promising new findings offered fresh perspectives on behavioral factors in CHD, hypertension, and sudden cardiac death. Indeed, if negative findings were sufficient cause for abandonment of scientific inquiry, little progress would be made in any scientific discipline. Rather, contradictory findings provide the stimulus for more refined questions concerning particular coronary-prone tendencies and related pathophysiological mechanisms. In fact, the latter was one of the main purposes of the conference.

The conference from which the present volume emerged was both financially and technically supported by Ciba-Geigy, Federal Republic of Germany. All the authors join us in extending our deepest gratitude to Ciba-Geigy for its notable generosity, heart-warming hospitality, and exceptional technical support, which made the conference so successful and memorable. Here we particularly thank Dr. László Bethlen for his considerable personal initiative in organizing this conference. We should additionally like to express our warm thanks to Schwarz GmbH, Monheim, Federal Republic of Germany, for financially supporting this publication. Preparation of this volume was greatly facilitated by the patient and skillful work of Stans Dembroski and Hazel Schmidt. Finally we thank Dr. Thomas Thiekötter, Pamela Salomon, and Willi Bischoff, Springer-Verlag, for their experienced editorial assistance during publication.

THOMAS H. SCHMIDT
THEODORE M. DEMBROSKI
GERHARD BLÜMCHEN

---

1 Dembroski T, Schmidt T, Blümchen G (eds) (1983) Biobehavioral bases of coronary heart disease. Karger, New York

Contents

II. Cardiovascular Psychophysiology

III. Pathophysiology

IV. Animal Models

V. Prevention and Control

List of Contributors

Allen MT 406
Anderson DE 500
Appels A 56
Bierck G 447
Billings J 41
Black GW 568
Blümchen G 447
Bohus B 517
Borcherding H 127
Borhani NO 41
Brodner G 127
Bühler FR 287
Chesney MA 568
Clarkson TB 459
Costa Jr PT 85
Dembroski TM 246
De Silva RA 155
de Wit B 355
Dimsdale JE 343
Dittmann KH 104
Eiff AW von 584
Engel BT 96
Eschweiler J 187
Fentrop Th 447
Fokkema DS 517, 527
Frantik E 315
Fredrikson M 418
Gerace TA 41
Groen JJ 3
Halhuber MJ V
Herd JA 389
Hollmann W 614
Holst D von 476
Horvath M 315
Hulley SB 41
Jacobs D 41
Jenkins CD 56
Johnston DW 550
Kaplan JR 459
Kittel F 63
Koepke JP 406
Koolhaas JM 517, 527
Langer AW 406
Langewitz W 584
Langosch W 127
Lasser N 41
Light KC 406
Lulofs R 302
MacDougall JM 246
Mancia G 379
Manuck SB 459
Matthews KA 228
Matschinger H 104
Mittlemark M 41
Mulder P 56
Müller FB 287
Neaton JD 41
Nelesen R 258
Neus H 584
Neus J 584
Obrist PA 406
Otten H 584
Parati G 379
Patel C 533
Payne RL 323
Perini C 287
Pogash RM 139
Pomidossi G 379
Rakaczky CJ 228
Rick JT 323
Riedel W 302
Rosenman RH 15
Rüddel H 584
Schmieder R 584
Schmidt TH 187
Schneiderman N 258
Settels JJ 355
Shekelle RB 41
Sherwood A 406
Siegrist J 104
Siegrist K 104
Slaby A 315
Stamler J 41
Stöhr W 491
Streufert S 139
Tammen A-T 447
Tan F 56
Thierse H 187
Tischenkel N 258
van Houtem J 56
van't Hof M 56
van Oortmerssen GA 517
Waltz M 594
Wesseling KH 355

Introduction

The present volume has arisen from an international conference held in Winterscheid in 1984. As a result, in part, of the mixed positive and negative findings that have emerged since the Altenberg conference in 1981, debate at the conference in Winterscheid was lively, open, and intriguing. In large measure this debate served to focus the emphasis of the contributions now included; they are presented in five sections, described below:

Section I: Psychosocial Factors and CHD

The first section is largely devoted to examination of the association between psychosocial factors and CHD. A particularly interesting perspective in this section concerns the question of which of the many attributes of the multidimensional Type A behavior pattern are likely candidates for coronary-prone status and which are simply benign correlates of the globally defined Type A pattern. Here, the possibility cannot yet be ruled out that some attributes may even confer protective effects. However, once the "toxic" components of Type A are isolated in epidemiological research, the behavioral and physiological properties of these components can be more profitably investigated in both laboratory and natural settings. Work is progressing in this regard in efforts to assess the various dimensions of the Type A pattern separately so that each component can be examined for possible association with CHD end points. Once this is accomplished, investigators can avoid fruitless exercises in research on non-coronary-prone tendencies and better focus efforts on examination of psychosocial attributes that have been firmly linked to CHD. In this connection, other characteristics that are not presently included in the Type A domain may be established as coronary-prone tendencies through sound and rigorous epidemiological research. Likewise, investigations may also reveal that other psychosocial characteristics may be pseudo-coronary-prone tendencies by virtue of their relationship to subjective rather than objective indices of CHD. These and other similarly intriguing issues are explored in Section I.

Section II: Cardiovascular Psychophysiology

As mentioned above, investigation of physiological correlates of behaviors thought to reflect coronary-prone tendencies is currently a major methodology used in attempts to identify pathophysiological mechanisms whereby behavior may be translated into CHD, hypertension, and sudden cardiac death. Such approaches fall in the domain of cardiovascular psychophysiology, which is the major focus of Section II. Although correlates of challenge-induced physiological reactivity have been established for some apparently coronary-prone tendencies, the realm of cardiovascular psychophysiology in its own right also offers much promise for uncovering basic pathophysiological mechanisms in cardiovascular-related disorders. Indeed, the challenge-provoked level of physiological responsivity is stable over time and thus qualifies as a legitimate individual difference variable independent of any behavioral correlates; in fact, it is likely to be a coronary-prone and/or hypertensive tendency that can be reliably assessed using physiological response as the unit of observation. With this technique it is thus possible to transcend the purely behavioral approach by systematically exploring the predictive value of challenge-induced physiological responsivity in prospective and retrospective epidemiological studies. Exploration of related neuroendocrine and mechanical processes associated with cardiovascular reactivity are already yielding valuable leads concerning possible pathophysiological mechanisms responsible for relationships that have been and may be uncovered in epidemiological studies. In this connection, promising new data have emerged suggesting that both a variety of consummatory behaviors and stress can interact to produce both additive and synergistic effects on cardiovascular reactivity that may operate to intensify risk beyond what stress alone or a particular consummatory behavior alone would engender. Such findings suggest that the two categories of coronary-prone tendencies are not as separate as was previously thought. Finally, exciting and innovative methods for assessing physiological reactivity are also considered in Section II.

Section III: Pathophysiology

This section follows naturally from Section II. In Section III a variety of pathophysiological mechanisms that may be related to cardiovascular reactivity are discussed. Behavior-physiological response is considered in relation to pathophysiological mechanisms in hypertension, atherosclerosis, and sudden cardiac death.

Section IV: Animal Models

In Section IV a variety of animal models are described that were designed to parallel, as closely as possible, some of the coronary-prone tendencies thought to exist at the human level. Such attributes as dominance, submissiveness, aggression, and social stress are examined in relation to physiological responsivity and disease end points, including associations with severity of coronary artery disease. A fascinating finding in this line of work is that challenge-induced physiological reactivity is a stable individual difference variable in at least some species of animals. If such is the case, a tremendous amount of research is made possible to explore the implications of physiological reactivity in a variety of paradigms designed to mimic the human situation, including the interaction effects of stress and consummatory behaviors on the disease process. Very exciting and promising preliminary findings in this connection are discussed.

Section V: Prevention and Control

The major focus of the final section is on interventions designed to reduce the risk of CHD. Consideration is given to behavioral, pharmacological, and traditional intervention programs. In addition to the presentation of promising findings in this area, discussion is also directed at possible pathways through which interventions exert effects.

From Clinical Experience to Tested Hypothesis: The Role of Psychosocial Factors in Coronary Heart Disease

J. J. GROEN[1]

Introduction

The influence of psychosocial factors in the development of coronary heart disease has been suspected for many years by family practitioners and physicians like William Osler. The clinical impression that myocardial infarction preferably strikes a certain type of person and frequently occurs after a shattering life event was supported by more systematic clinical observations made from 1935 to 1955, although these observations lacked the support of control groups (Arlow 1945; Dunbar 1943; Dreyfuss 1959; Gildea 1949; Russek and Zohman 1958; Raab 1964). Our first systematic studies took place between 1956 and 1965 and were based on long biographies of 24 successive male, married patients (Groen et al. 1965; 1968 a) who were admitted to the Wilhelmina Gasthuis in Amsterdam. Psychosocial factors were found to precede the onset of disease in all of the patients. Based on these systematic clinical observations, we formulated the hypothesis (Van der Valk et al. 1967) that myocardial infarction seems to occur as a result of a constellation of *three* factors:

1. Certain *personality* characteristics determined by heredity, maturation, and previous experiences), which seem to *predispose* certain individuals more than others to become involved in
2. a certain type of *interhuman conflict situation,* which serves as a more immediately precipitating "stressor"
3. certain types of *behavior* through which the individual, because of his personality, responds to this conflict.

Independent of the Amsterdam study, Friedman and Rosenman (surveyed in 9) in San Francisco, Minc in Perth (Minc 1960; 1963; 1967), and Wolf and co-workers (Wolf 1966; 1969; 1971) in Oklahoma proposed similar, although not quite identically worded, hypotheses.

Personality (Behavior Patterns)

The main feature of the type of personality associated with coronary heart disease may be described as an exaggeration of certain otherwise rather normal behavior patterns found in modern day Western culture. There is a *quantitative* difference in behaviour between these patients and other males. The former are more active, and their aggression finds its main outlet in working activity.

1 Hebrew University, Jerusalem, Israel, and University of Leiden, Department KNO, Academic Hospital, Leiden, The Netherlands

Biological and Psychological Factors
in Cardiovascular Disease
Ed. by T. H. Schmidt, T. M. Dembroski, and G. Blümchen

Work Situation

Coronary heart disease seems to occur with greater frequency in individuals who tend to work harder and longer hours than others. The proportion of time during which a coronary-prone person works, compared with the time during which he relaxes, sleeps, eats, or pursues hobbies, is higher than for other individuals, and he often performs a greater amount of work.

Dedication to and a sense of responsibility toward the work seems to be more intense in these individuals than in others. Work seems to be very deeply ingrained in the patient's sense of duty and conscience. Very striking is this person's tendency to accept challenges, e. g., to assume more tasks than can easily be fulfilled or to accept deadlines and then feel responsible for meeting them on time. These persons sacrifice their leisure and family life in order to fulfill an almost compulsive urge to work more and more and better and better. One might call them *work addicts*. Work is also the principal means by which these persons attempt to climb the social ladder. Many of them achieve higher social positions than their parents (who gave them an example for dutifulness), a consequence they attribute to their hard and conscientious work.

In their work relationships, these individuals demonstrate another characteristic behavior pattern in their tendency to dominate others. They strive toward or fight for power and leadership. A desire to assume responsibility can also be seen as an expression of this striving for dominance. They channel their aggression into hard work more than others, especially during middle age.

Family Situation

The striving for power also demonstrates itself in the family setting as a tendency to dominate spouse and children. The subject's sense of responsible leadership in the family is another marked motivation. Through hard work, these persons expect to improve their financial and social position, which will allow them to provide better for their family. They expect their spouse and children to submit to them, to respect them, and to give them the love to which they are entitled in compensation for their hard work and care. Actually, underlying this tendency for "patriarchal domination" is a great need for family love, although these people rarely admit to it. They seem to tolerate feelings of dependence as poorly as they do feeling of inactivity.

Several of our patients became promiscuous when their wives did not give them the submissive love they needed. In others, promiscuity was an aspect of their urge for masculine achievement. The desire to provide for one's family and climb the social ladder, coupled with an acceptance of challengers, drives many of these people into financial ventures which are beyond their capacities. Others become involved in career rivalries.

Community Situation

These individuals are more often found in certain professions, where climbing the social ladder of our mobile society has become possible through hard, responsible work. They are found in smaller numbers amoung stable rural agricultural and lower class industrial workers. Such persons seem to take a more active part in the social life of the community, smoke more cigarettes, drive expensive cars, and are more socially "involved." Also, in these social activities, they tend to exaggerate or "show off" more than others. Many are drawn to these community activities by the same conscientiousness and sense of responsibility that drive them to work hard for their family.

In their hobbies, which are seldom relaxing, we find the same exaggerated tendencies. Some participate intensely in sports to show that they can still compete with younger people. In their sex life as well, they have to prove to themselves and others that they are active and vigorous, but in so doing, they often tax themselves too much.

These individuals do not like to appeal to others for help in difficult situations and often believe that in modern society every man has to fight for his own position. They have less contact with their extended family, so that in difficult times they receive less support than others would from relatives and friends.

On the whole, they strive for "male" achievements; their ideal is to be strong, admired, and invincible. Their greatest fear is to appear weak, old, dependent, feminine or fearful. Passive wishes are unacceptable and therefore repressed, although these persons do voice such wishes to a doctor when they are given an opportunity to unburden themselves. *Actually, these men are greatly in need of love, and much of their striving is devoted to obtaining power as a substitute for love.* As one of them puts it: "I am a big fellow with a small heart."

Interhuman Conflicts

Myocardial infarction seems to occur following an interpersonal conflict, that is sometimes acute and severe, but that, in many cases, is one of a series of at first seemingly trivial irritations having special meaning for the affected person. The essence of this conflict situation is *frustration* arising from the desire to dominate at work, in the family, or sometimes in the community situation, coupled with frustration of this desire for admiration and social recognition. These frustrations are sometimes caused by a failure (real of imagined) to climb the social ladder, a setback in salary or job position, disobedience or lack of submission by wife or children, chronic or recurrent financial worries, or a real or threatening financial catastrophe. All this occurs *despite* the subject's hard work, which, in his view, should have called for reward rather than frustration. Most of these individuals react to such frustrations as they do to any other challenge, by working even harder. They sometimes feel as though they were fighting with their back to the wall, "like Sisyphus" (Wolf 1969). Their frustrations seem most acute if the very person whom the individual expects to submit to or appreciate him, puts him in a position in which he is the one who has to submit, as, for example, a wife who refuses intercourse or who dominates, criticizes, interrupts or "corrects" the husband in the presence of others, a son who is too independent a domineering business partner or boss or a rival who gains the upper hand by unfair competition. An especially important feature seems to be repeated frustration caused by the "coldness" of a "detached" wife who does not show enough affection.

Reactive Behavior to Conflicts

The frustration stemming from their conflicts does not cause these men to engage in openly aggressive behavior such as fighting, swearing, or other verbal outbursts of anger. Nor do they react in a passive manner, such as crying, complaining to others, engaging in drinking bouts, or openly showing depression. In spite of the conflict, they attempt to "carry on," keep an optimistic attitude, pretend to be indifferent, or deny their inner feelings of tension. Often, they work harder, trying to overcome the difficulties, while continuing to remain cheerful. In general, these men tend to inhibit emotional discharges more than others. This is in contrast to what they report about their youth, many of them describing themselves as quick-tempered and prone to fights or frequent outbursts of rage. There is a marked absence of freely expressed anxiety, fear, or depression in their behavior, even in situations which would "naturally" call for such a reaction. Only after the occurence of their heart attack is it possible for them to express these feelings in outbursts but, even then, they often try to hide their anxiety by telling a joke or denying their feelings.

In several patients, the onset of illness *coincided with several factors related to chronic, recurrent, or acute conflicts,* such as (a) lack of success, i.e., real or threatened failure or defeat in the work situation; (b) lack of love and submission or a revolt against the patient's authority by wife and/or children; (c) no possibility for relaxation, abreaction, or substituted gratification through other successful activities.

It should be pointed out that psychosomatic etiology, as outlined by theory, is specific in three ways. People with a personality structure like that described above will not develop myocardial infarction if their exaggerated striving for dominance is rewarded by success in work and gratification in the family situation. A conflict in the family and/or work situation by itself does not necessarily lead to coronary heart disease when the person can freely discharge his feelings. Only when the *three* causal factors of personality, conflict, and inhibited behavior *combine* does this specific *constellation* lead to disease.

Testing the Hypothesis

Almost immediately after publication of the hypothesis, different methods were applied to test it. At first, these clinical tests concerned *relatively small groups of patients,* either hospitalized or ambulatory, during their recovery from a myocardial infarction. In a later stage, psychological tests and sociological questionnaires became integrated into *epidemiologic prevalence and autopsy studies* (Groen and Drory 1967; Groen et al. 1968b; Medalie et al. 1968). During recent years, these methods have been extended to *incidence (prospective) studies* (Groen et al. 1968c; Medalie et al. 1973a; 1973b). As a result of this work, the hypothesis that psychosocial factors play an important role in the multifactorial etiology of ischemic heart disease is now supported by a considerable body of objective evidence.

Friedman and Rosenman presented the results of their impressive prospective studies, which were later supplemented by the equally impressive predictive value of psychological questionnaires by Jenkins, Bortner, and others (for a review, see Groen 1976). In Israel, Medallie, Groen, and their co-workers were also able to support their previous clinical and prevalence studies by longitudinal (incidence) observations (Groen et al. 1968c; Medalie et al. 1973a; 1973b). This paper gives the results of their incidence study investigating the role of psychosocial factors in the development of coronary heart disease. For measurements of the so-called organic risk factors, the reader is referred to the original publications.

The *psychosocial questionnaire* contained simple questions such as: Have you had any financial problems in the past?; Do you have any financial problems at present?; Have you had any family problems in the past?; Do you have any family problems now?; Have you had any problems with your work (job) in the past?; Do you have any work problems now?; Have you had any problems with your co-workers in the past?; Do you have any problems with your co-workers now?; Have you had any problems with your superiors in the past?; Do you have any problems with your superiors now?; Have you had any problems in attaining the standard of living you desire?

Another set of questions concerned the attitude of the family: Have you had any problems (conflicts) with your family (wife and children) in the past?; Do you have any problems (conflicts) with your family at present? How does it affect you when your wife or children do not listen to you or even oppose you?; Does your wife show you her love? Other questions asked, concerned relationships in the work situation with supervisors and co-workers. From the answers, we computed scores for each separate problem area as well as a total problem score.

The personality score used in this questionnaire consisted of a very simple "anxiety" index, which equalled the number of positive answers (scores of 0, 1, 2, or 3) to the following questions: Do you consider yourself a tense person?; Do you generally or frequently suffer from anxiety?; Do you generally have sleeping problems?

The answers were correlated to the incidence of angina pectoris or myocardial infarction 5 years after the individual had answered the questionnaire. The tables contain only results which were significant beyond the $P<0.01$ level (Tables 1-12).

Space does not permit discussion of these results at length; suffice it to say that the data gave significant support to the hypothesis, which originated from clinical impressions and research, as well as prevalence and autopsy studies. Our hypothesis is similar in some respects, but not identical to the now famous hypothesis concerning the predisposing type A behavior pattern that was so brilliantly developed by Friedman and Rosenman and supported first by their own prospective Western Collaborative Group study and later by several others. The main difference is that we have not used their original structured interview technique, but a more conven-

Table 1. Relation of 5-year incidence of angina pectoris to severity score of psychosocial problems experienced in 1963

Problems (*n*)	Subjects (*n*)	Cases (*n*)	Rate per 1000
0	557	9	16
0+1	1717	42	25
2+3	2242	76	35
4+5	1975	78	39
5	1457	61	43

Table 2. Five-year incidence of angina pectoris (myocardial infarction excluded) as related to anxiety index and wife's love/support

Anxiety score	Wife's love score	Rate per 1000	Significance
0-1	3+	21	not significant
	2+	28	
	+	24	
	–	25	
2-3	3+	52	
	2+	45	
	+	73	0.01 <
	–	93	$P < 0.05$

Table 3. Relation of 5-year incidence of angina pectoris (1963-1968) to financial problems experienced in 1963

	Subjects *(n)*	Cases *(n)*	Rate per 1000 (age-area adjusted)
No financial problems	3884	113	29
Some financial problems	2421	104	43
Many financial problems	1147	38	36
Very many financial problems	1076	45	46

Table 4. Relation of 5-year incidence of angina pectoris (rate per 1000) to anxiety score, psychosocial problems, serum cholesterol, and systolic blood pressure

Anxiety index	Psychosocial problem score	Serum cholesterol and systolic blood pressure			Total
		cholesterol < 207 mg% systolic blood pressure < 133 mmHg	cholesterol > 207 mg% systolic blood pressure < 133 mmHg	cholesterol > 207 mg% systolic blood pressure > 133 mmHg	
0-1	< 10	12	11	39	22
	> 10	17	30	36	26
2-3	< 10	21	32	91	44
	> 10	51	68	97	64
Total *(n)*		19	26	48	29

tional psychosocial questionnaire, developed along the lines of Gutman (Groen et al. 1968b). Another difference is that, in the Dutch-Israeli study, not only is personality regarded as a predisposing factor, *but also the life situation,* in which the problems associated with financial circumstances, work, family, and especially attitude and behavior of the subject's wife are considered. These aspects are of special im-

Table 5. Relation of 5-year incidence of angina pectoris experienced between 1963 and 1968 (rate per 1000) to anxiety index, psychosocial problems, and ECG in 1963 (nonspecific T waves or ischemia)

Anxiety index	Psychosocial problems score	ECG in 1963				Total	
		Normal		Nonspecific T waves or myocardial ischemia			
0-1	<10	20	22	43	44	22	24
	>10	25		44		26	
2-3	<10	32	54	(185)[a]	96	44	57
	>10	63		(66)[a]		63	
Total		27		53		29	

[a] not statistically significant

Table 6. Correlation of appreciation shown by superiors in the work situation and incidence of myocardial infarction over 5 years

Superiors' appreciation (1963)	High	Moderate	Little or none
Subjects *(n)*	4965	3126	1522
Incidence (rate per 1000 from 1963 to 1968)	40	46	56

Table 7. Correlation of problems encountered with superiors in the work situation and incidence of myocardial infarction over the subsequent 5 years

Problems with superiors (1963)	None	Not serious	Serious and very serious	Very serious
Subjects *(n)*	4283	2749	2627	1032
Adjusted incidence rate per 1000 (1963-1968)	40	44	51	55

portance for *preventive studies* - which I sincerely hope will be launched in the near future - in which not only diet, smoking, and other habits are taken into consideration, but also the individual's interactions within his social group.

Finally, it should be recalled that many of the so-called classic "risk factors" are in one way or another connected to psychocultural behavior. Cigarette smoking is a cultural habit in Western Society, to which certain individuals, because of their personality structure and interpersonal life situation, seem to be especially addicted. Consuming a diet rich in saturated fat and cholesterol is also a cultural pattern, in which some individuals, driven by personal desires and social circumstances, indulge more than others. Some individuals by virtue of their personalities and life sit-

Table 8. Number of psychosocial problems and experience of wife's love and support in 1963 correlated with incidence of myocardial infarction over the subsequent 5 years

Number of problems (1963)	Incidence of myocardial infarction between 1963 and 1968 (rate per 1000)	
	Wife's love and support	
	None or little	Much or very much
0	49	34
0-1	48	41
2-3	58	47
4-5	?[a]	40

[a] Too few subjects to determine incidence

Table 9. Incidence of new cases of ischemic heart disease over 5-year period (1963-1968) among 10059 male Israeli civil servants 40-60 years of age as related to synagogue attendance (rate per 1000)

Synagogue attendance	Incidence
Daily	29
Sometimes	37
Rarely or never	56

Table 10. Incidence of angina pectoris (1963-1968) as related to complaints of anxiety in 1963 (10000 government employees in Israel)

	Subjects *(n)*	Cases *(n)*	Case rate per 1000
Never anxious	4734	134	30
Sometimes anxious	2400	81	34
Often anxious	1065	65	60
Very often anxious	319	20	66
Total employees alive in 1968 who had filled in this item in 1963	8518	300	38

Table 11. Incidence of angina pectoris (1963-1968) as related to work problems experienced in 1963 (10000 government employees in Israel)

	Subjects *(n)*	Cases *(n)*	Case rate per 1000
No work problems	4289	125	31
Some work problems	3036	134	44
Many work problems	1262	58	46
Total employees alive and followed until 1968	8587	317	37

uations are more prone than others to the sedentary way of life that is a part of modern industrial society. The same holds true for hypertension, diabetes, and obesity, each of which are pathologic conditions strongly correlated with both personality and psychosocial environmental influences. Age and sex are biologically deter-

Table 12. Incidence of angina pectoris (1963–1968) as related to family problems experienced in 1963 (10000 government employees in Israel)

	Subjects (*n*)	Cases (*n*)	Case rate per 1000
No family problems	1653	54	33
Few family problems	3997	133	34
Some family problems	1345	70	38
Many family problems	371	42	50
Very many family problems	221	18	95
Total employees alive and followed until 1968	8587	317	37

mined, but also influenced by and linked to the sociocultural milieu and the interpersonal communication and activities of the individual in his immediate social group. *Thus, it appears that most of the "organic" risk factors that have been shown to play a role in the multifactorial causation of coronary heart disease are related both to the social habits in "Western" society in general and to certain personality and situational characteristics that make these "Western" psychosocial behavior patterns more risky for some individuals than for others. Coronary heart disease is a classic example of the biosocial paradigm out of which chronic disease evolves.* For a survey of publications in which studies of the author and his co-workers from the Netherlands and Israel are reviewed, the reader is referred to Groen (1976).

References

Arlow JA (1945) Identification mechanisms in coronary occlusion. Psychosom Med 7: 195

Dreyfuss F (1959) Role of emotional stress preceding coronary occlusion. Am J Cardiol 3: 590

Dunbar F (1943) Psychosomatic Diagnosis. Hoeber, New York

Gildea A (1949) Special features of personality which are common to certain psychosomatic disorders. Psychosom Med 11: 273

Raab W (ed) (1964) Prevention of ischaemic heart disease. Thomas, Springfield, Ill.

Russek HI, Zohman BL (1958) Relative significance of heredity, diet and occupational stress in coronary heart disease of young adults. Am J Med Sci 235: 266

Groen JJ (1976) Psychosomatic aspects of ischaemic (coronary) heart disease. In: Hill OW (ed) Modern trends in psychosomatic medicine, vol 3. Butterworths, London, pp 288

Groen JJ, Drory S (1967) Influence of psychosocial factors on coronary heart disease: a comparison of autopsy findings with the results of a sociological questionnaire. Pathol Microbiol 30: 779

Groen JJ, van der Valk JM, Treurniet N, Kits van Heyningen H, Pelser HE, Wilde GJS (1965) Het acute myocardinfarct, een psychosomatische studie. Bohn, Haarlem

Groen JJ, van der Valk JM, Treurniet N, Kits van Heyningen H, Pelser HE, Wilde GJS (1968 a) Psychological factors in the causation of myocardial infarction. In: Psychotropic drugs in internal medicine: an international symposium. Excerpta Medica, Amsterdam, p 199

Groen JJ, Dreyfuss F, Gutman L (1968 b) Epidemiological, nutritional and sociological studies of atherosclerotic (coronary) heart disease among different ethnic groups in Israel, In: Miras CJ, Howard AN, Paoletti R (eds) Progress in Biochemical Pharmacology: Recent Advances in Atherosclerosis, vol 4, p 230

Groen JJ, Medalie JH, Neufeld H, Riss E (1968 c) An epidemiological investigation of hypertension and ischaemic heart disease in Israel. Isr J Med Sci 4: 775

Medalie JH, Kahn HA, Groen JJ et al. (1968) The prevalence of ischaemic heart disease in relation to selected variables. Isr J Med Sci 4: 789

Medalie JH, Kahn HA, Neufeld HN, Riss E, Groen JJ, Goldbourt U (1973 a) Five-year myocardial infarction incidence: associations of single variables to age and birthplace. J Chronic Dis 26: 329

Medalie JH, Snijder M, Groen JJ, Neufeld H, Ris E, Goldbourt U (1973 b) Angina pectoris among 10000 men, 5-year incidence and univariate analysis. Am J Med 55: 583

Minc S (1960) The civilized pattern of human activity and coronary heart disease. Med J Aus 2: 87

Minc S (1963) Some psychological factors in coronary heart disease. Psychosom Med 25: 133

Minc S (1967) Emotions and ischaemic heart disease. Am Heart J 73: 713

Van der Valk JM, Groen JJ (1967) Personality structure and conflict situations in patients with myocardial infarction. J Psychosom Res 11: 41

Wolf S (1966) Mortality from myocardial infarction in Roseto. JAMA 195: 142

Wolf S (1969) Psychosocial forces in myocardial infarction and sudden death. Circulation 39-40 [Suppl 4]: 74

Wolf S (ed) (1971) The artery and the process of arteriosclerosis. Plenum, New York

I. Psychosocial Factors and CHD

Current and Past History of Type A Behavior Pattern

R. H. Rosenman[1]

The early 1950s witnessed an explosion of interest in the roles of the diet, physical activity, and risk factors such as serum total cholesterol, blood pressure, and cigarette smoking in the twentieth-century incidence of coronary heart disease (CHD). Interest in a causal role of the diet was stimulated early by correlations of CHD mortality rates in selected countries with their dietary fat intakes (Keys 1953). However, the latter were obtained from imprecise data, and the inclusion of a larger number of countries by Yudkin (1957) appeared to lead to an opposite conclusion. A causal role of physical activity was suggested by the results of a study of London doubledeck transport workers (Morris et al. 1953), although a different conclusion could be reached from an alternative reassessment of the same data (Rosenman and Friedman 1958, 1959a). A causal role of the classic risk factors was indicated by findings from prospective studies of population groups (Epstein 1965), the validity of which was established by numerous epidemiological, clinical, and laboratory investigations.

However, in his last paper, White (1974) pointed out that CHD was infrequent until well into the twentieth century, and that its subsequent sharp increase in western societies could not be ascribed to any sudden change of hereditary factors, to a larger population of older individuals, or to either better physicians or improved technology. It also seems clear that the relative immunity of prior generations cannot per se be ascribed to a lower intake of dietary fats, higher level of physical activity, or an absence of the risk factors, despite their importance in the pathogenesis of CHD. Thus, CHD was infrequent among a large population of middle- and upper-class males who habitually ingested a high caloric-fat diet, who engaged in little significant aerobic exercise, whose hypertension remained untreated, and whose serum lipids were, in all probability, similar to ours (Michaels 1966).

Such factors, therefore, do not appear to explain historical changes in rates of CHD and similarly appear unable to explain more than a fraction of present geographical differences of such rates (Werko 1976). For example, in the United States in 1950, age-adjusted CHD mortality rates were significantly higher in the northeastern states than elsewhere (Enterline and Stewart 1959). In view of the considerable evidence that links CHD rates with urbanization and industrialization (Lipowski 1975; Marmot 1982; Sigler 1959), it is not surprising that two decades later a marked increase of CHD occurred in the southeastern states, along with a parallel increase of industrialization and population density (Mason et al 1981). However, the latter have not been associated with such a parallel increase of CHD in Japan, a society which differs from most western groups by replacing individual competi-

1 Department of Behavioral Medicine, SRI International, Menlo Park, California, USA

Biological and Psychological Factors
in Cardiovascular Disease
Ed. by T. H. Schmidt, T. M. Dembroski, and G. Blümchen

tiveness with an emphasis on group cooperation and social network support in its rapid industrialization (Cohen 1978; Matsumoto 1970).

Other geographical differences of CHD rates also do not appear to be explained by differences of diet or risk factors (Djordenic et al. 1972). The striking effects of different environmental milieus on the rates of CHD that occur in association with the risk factors can be seen in prospective studies comparing Framingham, Massachusetts with areas where we seek holiday respites because of their far more relaxed ambience. After full adjustment for differences of risk factors, the rate of CHD in males is much higher in Framingham, for example, than in Yugoslavia (Kozarevic et al. 1976), Puerto Rico, and Hawaii (Gordon et al. 1974). The CHD incidence in Framingham males is three times as high as in Parisian males (Ducimetière et al. 1980), despite the latter's well-known high saturated-fat.diet, relative lack of aerobic exercise, and prevalence of cigarette smoking, alcohol ingestion, and other risk factors. Parisian men are probably far more devoted to leisure activities and to an appreciation of aesthetics than are most men in industrialized American cities.

Whether CHD rates are high or low, the incidence of CHD in such population groups nevertheless remains associated with levels of the risk factors. However, it seems clear that these associations are with a relative rather than an absolute risk of CHD, nor do such factors provide individual specificity of risk. It has been repeatedly claimed by some that the risk factors confer on CHD prediction a mathematical precision that is expected to prevail for any population. The fallacy of such a presumption is shown by the cited geographical differences, by the significantly higher rates in males in the United States compared with European males, after adjustment for differences in risk factors (Keys et al. 1972), as well as by results of such recent studies as the Multiple Risk Factor Intervention trial (MRFIT 1982, Stallones 1983), in which the observed rate of CHD during follow-up was much less than that predicted from such risk equations.

The discerning observer cannot fail to note that the rate of CHD that occurs in association with risk factors is significantly influenced by the ambient situation in which an individual lives and works, as well as by other factors that distinguish one individual from another. It now appears prudent to pay increased attention to the individual who possesses a risk factor, and not merely to the risk factor per se. The validity of this belief is supported by the finding that, when full account is taken of the risk factors in prospective studies, they account for only about one-third of the observed numerical incidence of CHD (Keys 1972; Rosenman et al. 1976a). Indeed, a large number of studies have shown that in subjects undergoing repeat coronary angiography over time, but without intervening surgery, the risk factors that are related in epidemiological studies of the incidence of CHD do not appear to be related to the rate of progression of their basic coronary atherosclerosis (Kramer et al. 1983).

M. Friedman and I were not aware of these findings when we began our studies of cholesterol metabolism in animals in 1950. These studies helped us to understand the mechanisms that control the serum cholesterol level (Friedman and Rosenman 1955), as well as to explain its derangement in thyroid dysfunction (Rosenman et al. 1952) and nephrosis (Rosenman et al. 1956). Since we had the advantage of working both in the experimental laboratory and in clinical practice, we also were able to determine serum cholesterol levels repetitively in a large number of patients, both clinically healthy and with CHD. The animal and clinical studies taught us that the serum cholesterol level is controlled primarily by its rate of egress from, rather than input into, the plasma (Friedman et al. 1967). It also became apparent to us that subjects with high and low serum cholesterol levels did not exhibit such differences because of dietary factors (Friedman and Rosenman 1957), and that many subjects exhibit significant fluctuations of their serum cholesterol that cannot be ascribed to alterations of diet.

Although reported later, the results prospective studies showed that subjects who developed CHD during follow-up had not exhibited any prospective differences of diet (Paul et al. 1963; Kannel 1970). We were also aware that most individuals with classic risk factors still remain free of CHD over time, and that CHD can occur in many subjects without elevated levels of risk factors (Bruhn and Wolf 1970).

We had observed (Friedman and Rosenman 1957; Rosenman and Friedman 1959) that:

1. Coronary morbidity had markedly increased in the middle-aged American male during the past five decades, while his diet, long characterized by an overabundance of calories, animals fats, and proteins, had not undergone parallel change (Trulson 1959).
2. Although the presence of elevated serum lipids enhances proneness to CHD, considered as a group, subjects with CHD exhibit relatively small differences from control subjects.
3. It is not possible to incriminate a change in biological inheritance to account for the relatively rapid twentieth-century increase in incidence of CHD.
4. Various groups such as Haitian and Jamaican Negroes, who ingest low-fat diets and have low serum lipid levels, exhibit as much aortic atherosclerosis as do their American counterparts but have a strikingly lower incidence of CHD (Groom et al. 1959; Robertson 1959).
5. The increasing coronary morbidity in middle-aged American males had not been accompanied by a parallel increse in the frequency, extent, or severity of coronary atherosclerosis *per se* (Morris 1951; Saphir et al. 1956), or by any demonstrated increase in lipid levels.
6. Many groups ingesting a diet high in animal fat still have markedly less CHD than do other groups on a comparable diet (Rosenman and Friedman 1959b).
7. Critical surveys (Yudkin 1957) had disproved any close relationship between national dietary fat ingestion and relative coronary mortality.
8. The immunity of the premenopausal American woman to clinical CHD could not be ascribed to lesser intake of dietary fats or to lower serum lipid levels (Friedman and Rosenman 1957) compared with her male counterpart.

It was in the middle 1950s that we therefore began seriously to question the role of the traditional and already popularized factors in the pathogenesis of the increase of CHD that had occurred in western societies during the prior five decades. Although it was already clear that the incidence of CHD was associated with twentieth-century urbanization and industrialization, we were surprised to find from our own surveys (Friedman and Rosenman 1955, 1957; Rosenman and Friedman 1959) that available epidemiological studies of CHD had almost entirely failed to assess the possible influence of socioeconomic and other psychosocial factors in the populations that were variously being investigated. This finding was even more surprising in view of the fact that as good or even better correlations could be obtained between the presence of certain socioeconomic stresses and the incidence of CHD than between the latter and, for example, a high-fat dietary intake (Yater et al. 1948; Gover and Pennell 1950; Brock and Bronte-Stewart 1955a; Gertler and White 1954; Bronte-Stewart et al. 1955b; Sigler 1959).

In particular, we wondered whether the rising incidence of CHD in western societies might stem from some emotional interplay induced by new stresses imposed by our industrialized civilization, acting in conjunction with the diet, physical inactivity, and the risk factors. This suspicion was strengthened by the finding in epidemiological surveys that populations without such socioeconomic stresses were largely free of CHD, regardless of their habits of diet, exercise,, or other risk factors. Our most noted historians were pointing out that western societies were fraught with stresses that were not only restricted to their industrialized populations but also were uniquely new, having never been witnessed in any prior historical period. A prominent new factor was the more rapid pace of life. Toynbee (1961) emphasized this when he wrote that "at the earliest moment at which we catch our first glimpse of man on earth, we find him not only on the move but already moving at an accelerating pace. This crescendo of acceleration is continuing today. In our generation, it is perhaps the most difficult and dangerous of all the current problems of the human race."

We began to survey our own patients with CHD, observing facets of what later was termed Type A behavior pattern (TABP). In view of their frequent if not invariable exhibition of serum cholesterol levels that were higher than those in subjects without CHD, taken as a group, but in the absence of dietary differences, the question arose whether their pace of life might be a factor in elevating serum cholesterol. We therefore considered it important to ascertain what might happen when a group of tax accountants were faced with a situational incident, such as the 15 April tax deadline, which clearly imposed an acute sense of time urgency on most of the subjects. The men were bled every 2 weeks for more than 5 months for serum cholesterol and blood clotting determinations and were closely questioned at each visit to the laboratory concerning their sense of time urgency. We were not entirely surprised to find that fluctuations of considerable degree occurred in the serum cholesterol levels of many of the subjects. However, when the stimulus of work deadlines occurred and imparted a sense of acute time pressure, a significant rise of serum cholesterol and acceleration of blood clotting was frequently observed. Moreover, these changes could not be ascribed to alterations of diet, weight, or exercise patterns, since these were closely controlled (Friedman and Rosenman 1959). The results of this study were soon confirmed (Thomas and Murphy 1958; Dreyfuss and Czazckes 1959; Grundy and Griffin 1959; Hammarsten et al. 1957; Groen et al. 1962; Wertlake et al. 1968; Jenkins et al. 1969; Rahe et al. 1971, 1974; Rosenman and Friedman 1974, Dimsdale and Herd 1982). The rise of serum cholesterol level appears to occur in response to a stress which an individual perceives as requiring a sustained increase in either physical or mental performance (Clark et al. 1975). The early belief that TABP might relate to CHD by reason of A/B differences of serum cholesterol (Rosenman and Friedman 1963), was later discarded with the finding that the association of TABP with incidence of CHD was independent of other risk factors (Rosenman et al. 1975).

In view of the observed responses of accountants to an environmental stimulus imparting an acute sense of time urgency, it was considered important to study groups of subjects who habitually exhibited a chronic sense of time urgency because of their immersion in vocational as well as avocational pursuits. However, by this time, we had observed that this behavior was frequently accompanied by certain other behaviors, comprising a syndrome that we had found to be quite characteristic of younger and middle-aged patients with CHD, and that was exhibited far less frequently by subjects without CHD, regardless of their risk factors. For descriptive purposes, the former pattern was termed Type A and the latter Type B, and we observed that most individuals exhibited one or the other to a greater or lesser extent (i.e., the fully or incompletely developed Type A or Type B behavior patterns).

At this juncture we described TABP as characterized by (1) an intense, sustained drive to achieve self-selected but usually poorly defined goals; (2) profound inclination and eagerness to compete; (3) persistent desire for recognition and advancement; (4) continuous involvement in multiple and diverse functions constantly subject to time restrictions or deadlines; (5) habitual propensity to accelerate the rate of execution of many physical or mental functions; and (6) extraordinary mental and physical alertness. Type B behavior pattern was regarded as mainly the converse of Type A, with relative absence of drive, ambition, sense of time urgency, desire to compete, and involvement with deadlines. The respective behavior pattern were described to a small group of laymen from several corporations and newspaper organizations, and they were asked to select 30- to 60-year-old associates who most closely fitted the respective patterns. Over 96% of those selected subsequently agreed to participate in the study of 83 Type A and 83 Type B men. An additional group of 46 unemployed men who had been blind since birth or an early age were also studied, in the belief that they would exhibit a state of emotional anxiety. The lay selectors were specifically requested to exclude subjects that they knew had heart disease. It was found that the subjects with TABP exhibited significantly higher average serum cholesterol, more rapid blood clotting, and greater prevalence of corneal arcus and clinical CHD than did the other two groups of subjects; these differences were not found to be due to any differences of stature, diet, smoking, or exercise habits (Friedman and Rosenman 1959).

A similar prevalence study was then done in a female population (Rosenman and Friedman 1961). A small group of lay selectors again chose for us two groups of subjects based on their exhibition of the respective behavior patterns. The 125 subjects with TABP were employed in positions imparting chronic deadline and time pressure, while the 132 subjects with the Type B pattern were housewives who were either not otherwise employed or who occupied only clerical positions. In order to eliminate the possible effects of diet, smoking, and alcohol ingestion, two groups of nuns were selected by the Mothers Superior of their orders, again based solely on their exhibition of the Type A or B pattern. As with the study in males, the women with TABP were found to exhibit higher average serum cholesterol levels and higher prevalence of hypertension, corneal arcus, and evidence of CHD. The differences found were not ascribable to any differences in stature, diet, smoking, or exercise. The same differences prevailed in the groups of nuns.

Although the results of these two studies seemed to be significant, they could not be accepted as epidemiologically valid. A later finding of interest was made by Brozek et al. (1966), who had administered certain psychological tests at intake in a prospective study of Minnesota businessmen. They found that, compared with men who remained clinically healthy during 14 years of follow-up, those who suffered CHD had exhibited, at statistically significant levels, a higher activity drive and were more likely to "be on the go" and to "speak, walk, write, drive, work, and eat fast even when they did not have to do so," a characteristic description of a major aspect of TABP. In fact, the scales of the Thurstone Temperament Schedule used in the study were subsequently found in several studies to correlate significantly with TABP (Rosenman et al. 1976a; Chesney et al. 1981).

By the late 1950s it was believed important to do a prospective study of CHD in a sufficiently large population to test the hypothesis that TABP was associated with the incidence of CHD. In the described prevalence studies, the behaviors of the subjects were able to be studied by the investigators themselves. However, the scope of the proposed study required training others to administer an interview which would be tape-recorded for later audition and scoring by Rosenman et al. (1964) to assess the behavior patterns. Experience gained in the two prevalence studies helped us to develop this interview. After attempting to delineate the two behavior patterns by a number of standard and other questionnaires, we found that self-report bias and lack of self-insight by many subjects made their use invalid. We believed that a structured interview would be the method of choice since it allowed a trained interviewer to observe the important motor activities of a subject and to observe and assess the quality and intensity of emotional changes and overtones accompanying the responses to structured questions; it also gave interviewers the flexibility to vary their approach to a subject and, when appropriate, to add challenging questions that purposely served to interrupt the subject's answers. The concept of TABP was based primarily on observation of the behaviors of younger and middle-aged subjects with CHD, including what C. D. Jenkins later termed their "stylistics." We emphasized (Rosenman et al. 1964) that the correct assessment of a subject's behavior pattern depended far more on the motor and behavioral qualities accompanying the person's response to questions that on the actual content of the answers. Thus, interviewers were taught to observe the subject's degree of mental and physical alertness, speed of movement, physical restlessness, facial grimaces such as scowling and teeth and jaw clenching, and the nature of vigorous gestures such as first clenching and desk pounding.

In conceptualizing TABP and designing an interview for its assessment in the late 1950s, Friedman and I were not aware that others had previously recognized many of its facets in patients with CHD. The historical findings in this regard are rather sparse, but of great interest because of their consistency. A German physician, Von Dusch (1868), cogently observed that persons with loud vocal stylistics and excessive work involvement were predisposed to development of CHD. Over a period of two decades, Osler (1910) strongly implicated stress and hard-driving behavior, and wrote that "I believe that the high pressure at which men live, and the habit of working the machine to its maximum capacity are responsible for [arterial degeneration] rather than excesses in eating and drinking ..." Osler went on to describe that his typical patient with CHD was „not the delicate, neurotic person ... but the robust, the vigorous in mind and body, *the keen and ambitious man, the indicator of whose engine is always at 'full speed ahead'.* There is indeed a frame and facies suggestive of angina - the well 'set' man from 45-55 years of age, with military bearing, iron-gray hair and florid complexion" (emphasis added), which is indeed an accurate, albeit terse, description of Type A behavior. Many years were to pass before several psychiatrists studied patients with CHD. The Menningers (1936) were apparently the first, observing in 1936 that their patients with CHD exhibited strongly aggressive tendencies. Dunbar (1943) found them to be hard-driving and goal-directed individuals. Kemple (1945) was particularly perceptive in recognizing that CHD patients were very ambitious and compulsively striving to achieve goals that incorporated power and prestige, but that they lacked subtle adaptive responses and sensitivity to nuances in their environment, and constantly depended on achievements in daily living because of their inability to indulge in creative thought. Arlow (1945) and Gildea (1949) had also observed the ambitious, hard-driving characteristics of their CHD patients.

These early investigators portrayed a remarkably similar psychological facade in describing their patients with CHD. However, little attention was given to their findings, perhaps in part because they failed to pursue their studies and in part because they presented their findings mainly in psychiatric parlance, writing in psychiatric journals rarely read by cardiologists. We also believed that more cognizance was not taken of their findings because most had failed to consider the role of the environmental milieu in the genesis of the personality facade that they found to be characteristic of their patients with CHD, despite the dramatic and uniquely new aspects of the milieu associated with the rapid increase of CHD (Toynbee 1961; Lipowski 1975). However, Stewart (1950) did correlate the conditions of modern stress with an increased rate of CHD in the United Kingdom.

On the other hand, little causal relevance was given to the hard-driving and goal-directed activities that had been observed in the group of young patients with CHD that were studied by Gertler and White (1954). The psychologists and psychiatrists (Miles et al. 1954) who also studied these subjects had concluded that they showed no psychological differences from control subjects, which was all the more surprising since the CHD patients also exhibited work patterns that were excessively long, and had fewer vacations than found in their control subjects (Bronte-Stewart et al. 1955).

It therefore appears important to emphasize that Type A refers to a pattern of behaviors, rather than to personality per se. Miles et al. (1954) had sought and failed to find evidence for a coronary-prone personality and based their conclusions on subjective rather than objective interpretation of the contrasting behaviors of their subjects with and without CHD. Mordkoff and Parsons (1967) later appeared to have committed a similar error in their unsuccessful search for a coronary-prone personality (Rosenman et al. 1968). Among other things, they cited the conclusions drawn by Keith et al. (1965) as having failed to find an association of TABP with CHD in the group of patients that they studied. However, in a reassessment of their findings, Cassel (see Keith et al. 1965) pointed out that Keith et al. had failed to grasp the epidemiological necessity of comparing the distribution of behavior types among the coronary and noncoronary groups of their own subjects. Indeed, when this was done, Cassel pointed out that their own data actually provided a converse conclusion from that of Keith et al., namely, one in support of the relationship between CHD and TABP. Keith et al. had drawn a negative conclusion, despite their own findings that, if all of their noncoronary cases "are combined into a noncoronary category, and the results tested, interview ratings do significantly discriminate coronary patients from noncoronary."

It also should be emphasized that TABP probably often results from the interaction of individuals with their specific environment, a milieu that provides an individual with the challenges that evoke specific Type A behaviors. The presence or absence of TABP must be assessed in the individual's specifically challenging environment. Pattern A is concerned with enhanced aggressivenes, ambitiousness, drive, competitiveness, and time urgency. Such behavioral characteristics cannot be expected to be present, for example, in a man hospitalized for acute myocardial infarction; indeed, perhaps nothing might temporarily eliminate such attributes more effectively. It seemed unfortunate (Roseman et al. 1968) that Keith et al. (1965) studied a population of which a substantial number were hospitalized with acute myocardial infarction at the time they were interviewed. This recurring error of formulation is pointed up in their own assessment of subjects with angina pectoris, most of whom were not hospitalized at the time of study, and in 75% of whom they judged TABP to be present.

The discussion of studies by Mordkoff and Parsons (1967) and by Keith et al. (1965) may appear to be a digression. However, it is important to point out that their criticisms reflected the considerable resistance to the concept of TABP and its relationship to CHD that was forthcoming from both cardiologists and psychiatrists, and that was exemplified at the Timberline Conference on Psychophysiological Aspects of Cardiovascular Disease (1964). Moreover, earlier criticisms such as these had served to help us formulate the structrued interview (SI) (Rosenman et al. 1964; Rosenman 1978b) that was developed for use in the Western Collaborative Group Study (WCGS). Thus, the SI was designed not to seek out a coronary-prone personality, but merely to assess the presence or absence of the Type A behaviors that result from the interaction of individuals with their specific environmental milieu.

We considered TABP to be a particular action-emotion complex that is exhibited by an individual who is engaged in a relatively *chronic* and excessive struggle to obtain a usually unlimited number of things from his or her environment in the shortest period of time or against the opposing efforts of other things or persons in this same environment. This chronic struggle may consist of attempts to achieve or do more and more in less and less time, or of a *chronic* conflict with one person or a group of persons. In either case, however, the person with this behavior pattern never despairs (despite the intensity or duration of the conflict) of winning the struggle, thus differing from the subject with a classic anxiety state who, finding or believing challenges or afflictions to be overwhelming, seeks therapeutic reassurance from a physician, psychiatrist, or interested friends. The Type A person usually advances confidently to grapple with challenges, while the subject with anxiety neurosis often retreats.

We believed that the contemporary western environment had encouraged the increasing prevalence of TABP because it appeared to offer special rewards to those who can think, perform, communicate, and, in general, live more rapidly and aggressively than their peers. Also, with the increasing urbanization and technological progress fostered by western society, a continual densification of population and an ever more urgent necessity for finely timed synchronization of interdependent human services presented challenges not really experienced by earlier generations. Thus, we believed that TABP did not stem primarily from an individual's personality, but emerged when certain challenges or conditions of the milieu arose that elicited a particular response or complex of responses in susceptible individuals. This inclusion of the milieu as a necessary part of TABP, of course, implied that if the challenges or conflicts of the milieu were severe enough, any subject, regardless of basic personality, might so react to these phenomena that TABP would emerge. This same concept also implied that, if the challenges or conflicts of the milieu were removed, an already present TABP might diminish. As can be seen, unlike the cited psychiatrists, we considered that there frquently is a sociological or socioeconomic as well as an intrinsic psychological component underlying TABP.

TABP may be a characteristic style of response to environmental stressors that threaten an individual's sense of control over his or her environment (Glass 1977). Thus, TABP appears to be an enhanced performance to assert and maintain control over the environment whenever this control is challenged or threatened. The high drive and pace of Type A persons reflect their need for mastery over their environment. Such persons are often deeply committed to their vocation, relatively neglecting other aspects of their lives in favor of an impatient, competitive, and hostile drive to achieve ever-expanding but often poorly defined goals.

TABP appears to be an overt behavioral style of living that is neither a personality trait nor a standard reaction to challenge, but rather is the reaction of a characterologically predisposed person to a situation which is perceived as a threat or challenge. It is characterized by enhanced degrees or even extremes of competitiveness, striving for achievement, aggressiveness, impatience, restlessness, hyperalertness, tenseness of facial musculature, explosive speech stylistics, and a chronic sense of time urgency that leads to the acceleration of thought and of most actions. Type A persons tend to have characteristic values, thoughts, and approaches to interpersonal relationships, as well as characteristic emphatic gestures, taut facial expressions, upper thoracic respiratory movements, rapid motor activity, accelerated pace, vigorous stylistics of speech, and other typical mannerisms.

Persons without such enhanced behavioral traits are called Type B, with an overt behavior pattern that is far more relaxed, easygoing, satisfied, and unhurried. Type B persons are rarely beset by desires to participate in an ever-growing number of events. Thus, the Type B behavior pattern is not merely the absence of the excessive drive, ambition, aggressiveness, and impatience that characterize the Type A person, but is a different style of response to the environmental milieu that is infrequently associated with the need to compete and to rush the pace of activities, or with the response of hostilitiy/anger dimensions that are exhibited by Type A persons.

It is important to distinguish TABP from the concept of "stress," since it is neither a stressor situation nor a distressed response, but rather is a style of overt behavior with which Type A persons confront life situations, whether pleasant or troubling, but particularly when the situation provides an element of perceived challenge. As such, it must be sharply differentiated from simple neurosis.

The SI (Rosenman et al. 1964) was designed to allow an interviewer to assess the relative presence of characteristic motor signs and stylistics of speech, and other Type A behaviors; the degree of drive and ambition; the degree of past and present competitiveness, aggressiveness, and hostility; and the degree of impatience and sense of time urgency. A larger number of questions than were used in the final SI were initially formulated, the interview being designed to assess the various Type A behaviors by questions that relate to most aspects of everyday life and the individual's environment, and his or her response to perceived milieu challenges. Over a period of several years, these questions were asked of subjects who obviously exhibited TABP, many of whom had developed clinical CHD. This experience allowed us to select those questions which most readily evoked Type A responses for the final version of the SI that was used in the WCGS (Rosenman 1978 b). Shortly after the WCGS was begun, the hostility/anger dimensions of TABP, which we had emphasized as important (Rosenman et al. 1964), were reinforced by the addition of two questions at the end of the interview that were specifically designed to question subjects directly about their frequency and intensity of anger/hostility as well as the method of expressing it. The interviewers were thaught to challenge the subject repeatedly during the interview and to be flexible enough in its administration to be able to vary the interview by sudden interruptions and other irritations designed to elicit impatience, hostility, and other Type A behaviors in the susceptible individual, and particularly in the many subjects in whom such behaviors might be covert.

A significant part of the assessment of the behavior pattern from the SI is based on observation of the subject's stylistics (Rosenman 1978 b). We had long observed that these were a prominent characteristic of Type A subjects, usually reflecting their drive, impatience, and hostility. This belief was reinforced by the results of a specially designed voice analysis test that readily appeared to engender TABP in the susceptible person (Friedman et al. 1969). The value of the speech stylistics for assessment of TABP in the SI was strongly supported by the studies of Scherwitz et al. (1977) and Schucker and Jacobs (1977).

A number of other studies have shown that TABP has substantial stability over time (Jenkins et al. 1967 a; Gerace and Smith 1984), and that the SI has high levels of interrater agreement among well-trained interviewers (Caffrey 1968; Jenkins et al. 1968; MRFIT 1979).

The SI requires training and should have ongoing validation for its administration and assessment. This has understandably led to a search for simpler methods of assessment of TABP and particularly for its coronary-prone behaviors. Researchers have administered an array of psychometric questionnaires, such as the Adjective Checklist of Gough and Heilbrun, Thurstone Temperament Schedule, Eysenck Personality Inventory, SCL-90-R, State-Trait Anxiety Inventory (STAI), Work Environment Scale, California Psychological Inventory, Cattell 16-Personality Factors Test, and Barratt Impulsiveness Scale. The Activity Scale of the Thurstone Temperament Schedule was found to correlate significantly with TABP in several studies (Rosenman et al. 1976 a; Chesney et al. 1981). This result was also found for a group of items from the Adjective Checklist (Rosenman et al 1976 a; Chesney et al. 1981), a finding recently confirmed by others (Herman et al. 1981).

The SI was used initially in the WCGS. During its progress, it also was used in a study of Benedictine and Trappist monks and brothers by Caffrey, who had spent considerable time with us to learn its administration and to observe normal persons as well as CHD patients who exhibited Type A or Type B behavior patterns during the interview. In his large "double blind" study, a significantly higher prevalence of CHD was observed in subjects who were independently assessed as exhibiting TABP (Caffrey 1969).

The various psychometric questionnaires and scales have provided strong construct validity for the concept of TABP, but their results are influenced by the validity of a subject's insight and by a response bias that may often provide inaccuracy of self-reports. Moreover, a number of studies have shown that these scales appear largely to measure attitudes rather than the behaviors observed and assessed by the SI (Matthews et al. 1982). Although the Jenkins Activity Survey (JAS) and the Bortner Questionnaire continue to show relatively lo specificity for TABP (Meininger and Zyzanski 1983), they appear to measure similar behavioral characteristics and to achieve significant test-retest reliability (Johnston and Shaper 1983).

During the course of the WCGS, three other psychologists became independently interested in TABP. Bortner and Rosenman (1967) developed a scale for assessment of TABP that was later shortened by Bortner (1969) and found to classify correctly 75% of Belgian subjects (Kittel et al. 1978). The best-studied questionnaire, was developed by Jenkins et al. (1967b). It provides a composite Type A scale and three subscales that have variably been found to correlate with TABP. Appels (1972) was concerned with the relationships of various cultural aspects of TABP and their associations with CHD. With his coworkers, he developed the Maastricht Questionnaire for studying the relationship of occupational and emotional deprivation that can lead to a "vital exhaustion" that is predictive of imminent coronary events (Nixon 1976, 1984; Appels 1982; Falger 1982).

The past decade has witnessed considerable interest in TABP by a large number of other psychologists whose work, among other things, has provided further construct validity to the concept of TABP and its initially observed behavioral facade. Because of space limitations, the reader is referred to several reviews (Matthews 1982; Rosenman and Chesney 1980, 1982) for the many references. These studies have found that Type A persons are orderly and well-planned, self-controlled and self-confident; are self-involved and extreme in striving for achievement with an orientation that leads to denial of fatigue, symptoms of illness, and even CHD; are deeply involved with vocation and often suffer from work overload and inability to relax away from work; prefer to work alone and are not easily distracted by peripheral events considered to be irrelevant to such tasks; are hyperalert, outgoing, fast-paced, tense, unrelaxed, aggressive, competitive, time-conscious, and impatient; have an enhanced desire to control their environment and an increased frequency and intensity of job conflicts and dissatisfactions; and exhibit an often suppressed hostility that is more overt when frustrations are perceived.

The relationship of TABP to CHD has been studied by a number of investigators in the United States, Europe, and elsewhere, who have confirmed the original observations (Friedman and Rosenman 1959; Rosenman and Friedman 1961) of a significant association of TABP with the prevalence of CHD that is independent of other risk factors (see Jenkins et al. 1976, 1979; Feinleib et al 1978; Rosenman and Chesney 1980, 1982).

The association between TABP and CHD has also received major confirmation in prospective studies. The first was the WCGS. This was a prospective epidemiological study of 3154 initially well men, aged 39-59 years at intake in 1960-1961, who were employed by 10 participating Californian companies. Subjects were comprehensively studied for all risk factors. The population and methodology are described elsewhere (Rosenman et al. 1964), as are findings at follow-up (Rosenman et al. 1975).

The 8.5-year follow-up found that CHD had occurred in 257 men. Final results showed that men classified as Type A at intake were 2.37 times as likely to develop CHD over the follow-up period as were Type B subjects. When multivariate statistical adjustment for other risk factors was made, the relative Type A/B risk of CHD decreased to 1.97, the small difference (0.40) between adjusted and nonadjusted relative risk being the amount of risk conferred by other standard risk factors, which showed small correlations with TABP (Brand et al. 1976; Rosenman et al. 1976b). The significant adjusted remainder (1.97) represented the relative risk for TABP that was independent of other risk factors. These findings indicated a synergistic pattern for CHD risk in which TABP operates with nearly a constant multiplicative effect applied to whatever background level results from other risk factors. Thus, TABP appeared to double the risk of CHD at all levels of other risk factors in a relationship that did not diminish with age. The observed associations could not be attributed to chance fluctuation since both adjusted and nonadjusted relative risk ratios achieved high statistical significance (*P*0.001) and were close (Brand et al. 1976) to those found at Framingham (Kannel and Gordon 1974; Haynes et al. 1980).

In the WCGS, the association of TABP with CHD incidence prevailed for initial myocardial infarction, whether symptomatic or silent, as well as for angina pectoris (Rosenman et al. 1975). Although significant CHD incidence occurred in Type A men, even at low risk factor levels, Type B subjects at similar levels exhibited relative CHD immunity (Rosenman et al. 1966a). TABP was also strongly associated with recurring and fatal CHD events in the WCGS (Rosenman et al. 1976b; Jenkins et al. 1971, 1976).

Other investigators have confirmed the relationship between TABP and CHD incidence. As part of the study of CHD among Japanese men in Japan, Hawaii, and California, 2437 men in Hawaii completed the JAS in 1967-1968. Despite the small number classified as Type A, CHD rates were found to be associated with hard-driving and competitive behavior. Japanese men in Hawai who had undergone cultural change were more prone to CHD, and those who were both culturally mobile and Type A had two to three times greater CHD risk than other subjects during follow-up (Cohen 1978). These results supported the original TABP construct as being an interaction between an individual and the environment that challenges the susceptible person and thereby evokes TABP.

Major confirmation was also obtained in the Framingham Study (Haynes et al. 1980, Haynes and Feinleib 1982). A cohort of 1822 subjects was administered an extensive psychosocial questionnaire in 1965-1967 that provided measures of behavior, situational stress, sociocultural mobility, and somatic strain. Among these items, the Framingham Type A Scale (FTAS) was significantly correlated with daily stress, emotional lability, tension, anger symptoms, and ambitiousness. The FTAS was significantly correlated with CHD prevalence in both sexes, after controlling for other risk factors. Subjects aged 40–74 years and free of CHD ($n = 1674$) were then followed for 8 years in a prospective manner.

During this follow-up, Type A men were found to be more than twice as likely as Type B men to develop angina and myocardial infarction, with stronger associations in white- than in blue-collar workers. The respective incidence of angina and infarction was also 3.32 and 2.14 times higher in Type A than in Type B women. All such associations prevailed after controlling statistically for other risk factors (Haynes et al. 1980). At the 10-year follow-up, these differential CHD rates for Type A and B subjects continued to prevail (Haynes and Feinleib 1982), and it was stated that "Finally, the results from the Framingham Study confirm the findings reported by the WCGS, and, as such, support the notion that Type A behavior is an important risk factor for coronary heart disease among both men and women."

It should be noted that the FTAS (Haynes et al. 1978) is a self-report inventory that consists of 10 questions designed to assess TABP. These questions were included in a pool of 300 items that were administered to participants in the Framingham Heart Study. As with the JAS, the FTAS questionnaire contains items largely relevant to the hard-driving and impatience aspects of TABP, but is weak with regard to the anger/hostility dimensions. Although found to be internally consistent, it is a questionnaire that lacks the normative data required to make it a valid psychometric scale for mesurement of TABP.

The Bortner Scale (1969) was used to assess TABP in the French-Belgian Cooperative Group prospective study (1982) of 2699 men, aged 40–60 years at intake. It also confirmed a strong and independent association of TABP with the subsequent incidence of CHD over a 5- to 8-year period of follow-up.

In WCGS subjects who died during the period of follow-up, Type A compared with Type B subjects were also observed to exhibit significantly greater severity of coronary atherosclerosis (Friedman et al. 1968). Other investigators used coronary angiographic data to confirm this association in both sexes, again finding it independent of other risk factors (Krantz et al. 1978; Zyzanski et al. 1976; Blumenthal et al. 1978; Frank et al. 1978).

In these studies of the relationships of TABP to the prevalence and incidence of CHD and to the severity of coronary atherosclerosis, the SI was found to be a significantly stronger predictor than were questionnaires such as the JAS (Blumenthal et al. 1978; Brand, to be published). This difference is presumably due to the fact that TABP is directly observed during the SI, but only approximated by the content of answers given in the questionnaires.

Several studies failed to confirm these relationships. Thus, a relationship between TABP and the extent of angiographic coronary atherosclerosis was not found by Dimsdale et al. (1978). Although the SI was used for assessment, they provided no data to demonstrate the competence of either the interviewers or the apparently different persons who assessed their interviews. Similarly, a relationship between TABP assessed both by SI and the JAS was not found in the MRFIT study (see this volume, Shekelle et al.) The reasons for this result are unclear, but it may in part be ascribed to a brief period of training that was provided for the naive interviewers, who were selected by others, and the failure of adequate follow-up tutelage during the intake of subjects in this study. In the WCGS, the carefully chosen interviewers were trained over a period of several months, during which time they were frequently provided with the opportunity for observing and conversing with CHD patients and for administering the SI under direct tutelage to CHD patients, as well as to clinically healthy subjects with well-delineated Type A or B behavior patterns. Moreover, throughout the 18-month period of intake in the WCGS, Rosenman regularly sat in during interviews and met with the interviewers several times each month to audit and comment on their interview technique. This ongoing procedure was believed essential to reinforce their interview technique and alertness to the behaviors they were assessing. Unfortunately, no such procedures were permitted by the methodology used in the MRFIT Study.

Other factors also may have played an important role in the negative correlations between TABP and CHD incidence in the MRFIT Study (1982). The subjects already were at highest predicted risk by reason of other risk factors that included hypercholesteremia, hypertension, and heavy cigarette consumption. It also may be questioned whether coronary-prone Type A subjects would have volunteered to participate in a long-term study that sought immediate cessation of smoking, marked alteration of diet, and frequent appearance at the study sites. Indeed, the markedly lower than predicted incidence of CHD that was observed to occur in this study during follow-up strongly suggests that the participants were biased by health consciousness and other factors that, despite high levels of the classic risk factors, were associated with a much lower incidence of CHD.

A current reassessment of the SIs given to these subjects at intake into the study may well find that the subjects who exhibited global Type A behaviors were nevertheless relatively low on the specific coronary-prone Type A behaviors that are associated with the incidence of CHD.

Some investigators have also failed to find an association of TABP with prevalence of CHD. However, a review of such studies indicated that these investigators usually had little personal familiarity with TABP and assessed TABP in their subjects with questionnaires whose validity for such purposes has been questioned repeatedly.

During the course of the WCGS, Friedman and Rosenman attempted to delineate mechanisms that might explain the associations of TABP with CHD. An early belief that an effect of TABP on elevating serum cholesterol levels (Rosenman and Friedman 1963) might be partly responsible was discarded when the relationship of TABP to CHD incidence in the WCGS was found to be independent of other risk factors (Rosenman et al. 1966b). Many hormonal factors were studied and the findings have been summarized elsewhere (Rosenman and Friedman 1974; Rosenman and Chesney 1980, 1982).

Catecholamines probably play an important role in mediating relationships between TABP and both coronary atherosclerosis and CHD incidence. An increased incidence of CHD is a twentieth-century phenomenon associated with the accelerated pace and pressure of life in industrialized societies. Raab (1953) early emphasized the role of catecholamines in twentieth-century western life, and he recognized that adrenergic responses were enhanced in individuals with TABP, compared with more relaxed persons (Raab and Gigee 1954). Levi and Anderson (1975) pointed out dramatic changes in our environment that have not been accompanied by suitable modification of man's genetically determined, but now obsolete, psychobiological reaction pattern, and they noted that the stress reactions that promoted survival for Stone Age man when confronting a wolf pack are inappropriate for modern man when confronting a traffic jam or many other forms of stress. Nixon (1976) emphasized the tendency of Type A persons, in particular, to show these reactions and exceed their homeostatic mechanisms, a pattern well described by Osler (1910) and Raab (1953).

It has been found that subjects with CHD exhibit enhanced catecholamine discharge in response to emotional stress and during physical exertion (Nestel et al. 1967, Voudoukis 1971). Such enhanced discharge is associated with aggressiveness, competitive drive, anger, and time urgency (Elmadjian et al. 1958), which are major TABP facets. Thus, it is not surprising that increased norepinephrine excretion by Type A subjects was found in work settings (Friedman et al. 1960) and in competitive situations (Friedman et al. 1975). Associated challenge-induced cardiovascular responsivity and TABP was later confirmed by others (Dembroski et al. 1978; Simpson et al. 1974). Enhanced norepinephrine discharge is a phasic phenomenon during exposure to the invironment that induces TABP in predisposed individuals who have the desire or need to perform at maximum capacity in response to external challenges and threats. The Minnesota prospective study of Minnesota businessmen pointed to the importance of catecholamines, finding that the cold pressor test, which reflects adrenergic responsiveness, was strongly predictive of CHD incidence (Keys et al. 1971). This same study also found that an accelerated pace of motor activity was similarly associated with CHD incidence (Brozek et al. 1966).

TABP results from an interplay between an individual and the environment, and its overt manifestations, represent characterological responses of Type A persons to a milieu perceived as a challenge. Enhanced discharge of norepinephrine occurs when challenges perceived as relevant require rapid and competitive responses by such persons (Simpson et al. 1974; Friedman et al. 1975; Ward et al. 1985). Therefore, autonomic arousal is better studied in dynamic response than by static measurements. Static measurements have shown no Type A/B differences in heart rate or blood pressure (Rosenman et al. 1964; Shekelle et al. 1976). However, differences are often, albeit not invariably, observed during exposure to laboratory stressors. Specifically, Type A compared with Type B subjects generally have been found to exhibit a greater rise of heart rate, systolic and/or diastolic blood pressure, and catecholamine secretion along with increased peripheral vasoconstriction during the SI, reaction-time tasks, cognitive puzzle solving, exposure to noise and to uncontrollable aversive factors, psychomotor performance tests, and the cold pressor test (Friedman et al. 1960, 1975; Dembroski et al. 1978). In general, the enhanced cardiovascular (CV) response of Type A subjects is greater in males than in females (Dembroski et al. 1978; Sime and Parker 1978) and when the challenge is of high rather than low order. Responses tend to be greatest in Type A subjects who exhibit the most competitiveness, impatience, and hostility, the attributes that particularly characterize relationships between TABP and CHD incidence (Matthews et al. 1977) an between TABP and severity of coronary atherosclerosis (Williams et al. 1980).

The results of a large number of studies of CV responses of adults to mental stressors have not invariably found differences in Type A and B subjects. However, wherever such differences have been observed, greater responsiveness of heart rate and blood pressure was noted in Type A subjects. Similar enhanced CV responsiveness has been observed in Type A compared with Type B children (Lawler et al. 1981; Siegel et al. 1983; Matthews and Jennings 1984), although not found in all studies (Blake et al. 1984). Others have questioned whether the methods used to assess TABP in children are actually selecting hyperactive and problem children as exhibiting Type A behavior (Hunter et al. 1984).

It is important to point out that, although Type A persons tend to exhibit enhanced CV responses to laboratory challenges compared with Type B persons, such enhanced responses are highly selective. Thus, they occur during tasks that are perceived as challenges, and that involve time urgency to perform cognitive processing in the form of decision making or problem solving (Ward et al. 1985). They do not occur in response to challenges of a physical nature (Ward et al. 1985), suggesting that there is little genetic basis for enhanced CV responses in Type A persons. The selective nature of CV responses again supports the conceptualization of TABP as an interaction between individuals and their environmental milieu. An enhanced secretion of norepinephrine in Type A compared with Type B subjects (Friedman et al. 1960, 1975) of course underlies their exaggerated CV responses to salient stressors (Ward et al. 1985). However, the catecholamine response to stressors is a normal one that merely appears to be greater in Type A than in Type B subjects. This enhanced Type A response does not appear to reflect a postulated (Dembroski et al. 1978) difference in CV "reactivity" *per se,* but rather appears to be an increased "responsiveness" engendered by a differential A/B cognitive perception of the milieu stressor. Thus, the enhanced Type A noradrenergic response occurs only to stressors that are perceived to be salient challenges.

Considerable attention has been given to CV reactivity as a marker for hypertension. Although younger persons with labile blood pressure, particularly those with a family history of hypertension, do tend to exhibit exaggerated CV responses to various stressors, the majority of such persons do not progress to sustained hypertension. Moreover, despite their tendency to exhibit similar hyperresponsiveness, Type A persons do not exhibit greater prevalence of hypertension (Roseman et al. 1964; Shekelle et al. 1976). Thus, it would appear that other factors determine which subjects with labile blood pressure and CV hyperresponsiveness develop sustained hypertension.

CV reactivity has also been considered to be a marker for CHD and has been considered by some (Dembroski et al. 1978) to provide the link between TABP and CHD. Eliot has popularized the "hot reactor" in the lay media as marking the future victim of CHD. However, it should be noted that no scientific data have appeared to support this hypothesis. The original studies found that Type A subjects exhibit enhanced noradrenergic responses only to laboratory and milieu stressors that are cognitively perceived as challenges (Friedman et al. 1960, 1975). This, of course, is responsible for the observed greater CV responses by Type A subjects, but this is another dimension from differential CV reactivity due to inherent constitutional differences between Type A and B subjects. It is the author's opinion that it is not the *magnitude* of the CV responses of Type A persons but more *frequent* responses throughout their environmental milieu that is causally linked with their increased incidence of CHD.

The relationship between central and peripheral mechanisms has been emphasized to be one with bidirectional influences (Krantz and Durel 1983; Rosenman 1978a, c, 1983). TABP may reflect an excessive sympathetic nervous system response to environmental stressors acting in one direction and an underlying biological or psychobiological factor perhaps affecting the expression of TABP in the other direction.

Aside from differences of catecholamine responses to cognitively perceived challenges, Type A males appear to secrete more testosterone (Zumoff et al. 1978), a finding confirmed by Williams et al. (1982). This finding, of course, is consistent with the fact that testosterone correlates with aggressive behavior.

Some attention has been given to genetic (Rosenman et al. 1976; Horn et al. 1976; Eaker 1984) and developmental antecedents of TABP (Matthews 1978). Although a discussion of this subject is beyond the present scope, the evidence suggests that TABP is mainly a learned syndrome of associated behaviors, despite an observed familial similarity (Bortner et al. 1970). Nevertheless, it is likely that it is superimposed on a substrate that is partly influenced by genetically determined factors. It also is beyond the scope of the present paper to discuss the considerable attention that has been given to the interaction of TABP with the work setting (Waldron et al. 1977, Chesney et al. 1980, 1983; Waldron 1978).

One milestone in the history of TABP resulted from the December 1978 meeting of a group of distinguished scientists who were assembled by the National Heart, Lung, and Blood Institute to study the association of TABP with CHD. They concluded that this association is a valid one that is largely independent of other risk factors and is of the same order of magnitude as that associated with recognized risk factors for CHD (Cooper et al. 1981).

The results of this conference, as well as of ongoing studies, stimulated interest in two orther aspects of TABP. One is the delineation of those components of TABP which are more causally related than others to the incidence of CHD. The second is the modification of TABP for primary and secondary prevention of CHD. Thus, a reduced incidence of CHD was hypothesized from WCGS data to be associated with effective modification of TABP (Brand et al. 1976).

TABP includes a cluster of associated behavioral dispositions, specific behaviors, and emotional responses (Rosenman et al. 1964, Rosenman 1978b; Rosenman and Chesney 1980, 1982). Scoring the SI by its components is not new. Indeed, the very conceptualization of the SI in the late 1950s delineated specific components of TABP, and these were assessed and scored in this manner in the WCGS (Rosenman et al. 1964). Other investigators later also used this methodology. Although reported follow-up in the WCGS was based mainly on global behaviors (Rosenman et al. 1975, 1976b), a study of the intake SI responses was done early in 25 men who participated in the WCGS but who were excluded from prospective follow-up because their intake ECGs showed that they had previously suffered a "silent" myocardial infarction. These subjects were compared with matched control subjects, and it was found that the *hostility* component of TABP was significantly higher in the men with "silent" myocardial infarction (Jenkins et al. 1966). It was therefore believed important to examine the SI components in a larger sample of WCGS subjects at approximately the midpoint of its follow-up. In this study, Dr. Bortner was asked to do a blind rating of the SI responses of the first 62 men who suffered CHD between

1961 and 1965, comparing them with the SI responses of two control subjects matched by age and occupation to each subject who had incurred CHD during this period. His untimely death prevented him from seeing the results of his component analysis. To avoid any bias by the author, another psychologist was later asked to correlate his assessments with the occurence of CHD. This analysis of Bortner's component scoring (Matthews et al. 1977) showed that, among the specific components of TABP, it was those that related to competitive drive, impatience, and potential for hostility that particularly identified the subject as coronary-prone. A current analysis of the same data by Spielberger and Rosenman (to be published) reveals that the anger/hostility dimensions of TABP are dominant behaviors of coronary-prone subjects in the WCGS. This finding is consonant with the original conceptualization of TABP (Rosenman et al. 1964). Later investigators have confirmed the relationship of Type A hostility/anger dimensions to CHD (Haynes et al. 1980; Williams et al. 1980).

Although psychometric measures have only limited success for assessment of TABP (Rosenman and Chesney 1980, 1982), it is significant that hostility/anger items and scales of such measures are found to discriminate the Type A/B behavior patterns (Rosenman et al. 1976a; Chesney et al. 1981), as well as to correlate with enhanced Type A cardiovascular responsiveness (Diamond et al. 1982). It is also significant that other psychometric measures, regarded by some as measurements of Type A hostility/anger dimensions, are correlated with CHD incidence occurring in several populations (Barefoot et al. 1983; Shekelle et al. 1983) and with the severity of basic coronary atherosclerosis in subjects studied by coronary angiography (Williams et al. 1980).

The relationship of anger/hostility dimensions to CHD is an important one (Rosenman 1984a) that has led to some recent confusion in the lay media. Although TABP was found and confirmed to be a risk factor for CHD, there is strong evidence that the Type A anger/hostility dimensions may be one of its major components that confers coronary-proneness (Jenkins et al. 1966; Matthews et al. 1977). This Type A component was also found to be related to the incidence of CHD in the Framingham Study (Haynes et al. 1980), but only spuriously apart from TABP, since the Framingham Type A questionnaire was directed primarily at the impatience and accelerated pace of activities of TABP, and a separate scale was used to assess their anger/hostility dimensions. Several studies used a purported hostility scale of the MMPI (Minnesota Multiphasic Personality Inventory) and found it to be associated with the incidence of CHD (Barefoot et al. 1983; Shekelle et al. 1983). The issue has been confused by inference from such studies that the hostility/anger dimensions relate to CHD apart from TABP, apparently failing to recognize the well-established fact that such dimensions are dominant Type A behaviors (Rosenman et al. 1964; Rosenman and Chesney 1980, 1982). It is the author's opinion that a high level of competitive and aggressive drive may be the dominant Type A behavior that, in turn, leads to accelerated pace of activities and enhanced hostility/anger dimensions, but that the various components of TABP cannot be regarded as being isolated from their associated behaviors.

One problem that is relevant for future studies is to determine whether MMPI scales that were used in reported studies are appropriate measures for assessment of hostility/anger dimensions. Although there appears to be some correlation (Spielberger et al. 1983), it has been pointed out by Megargee (1984) that the interpretation given to these MMPI scales has not been supported by construct validation for the belief that they measure hostility/anger dimensions, with much evidence to the contrary. One interpretation is that they measure cynicism (P.T. Costa 1984, personal communication); another is that they assess the quality and quantity of social supports (Barefoot et al. 1983; Shekelle et al. 1983). Further confusion is introduced by the finding that the scales are related not only to the incidence of CHD, but also to mortality from cancer and all causes (Barefoot et al. 1983; Shekelle et al. 1983).

It is again beyond the present scope to discuss the problems that relate to modification of TABP. However, it should be understood that modification does not imply changing a Type A into a Type B individual, but only acting to diminish those Type A behaviors that appear to have adverse effects on the rate of progression of coronary atherosclerosis and/or that relate to the incidence of CHD, including the precipitation of acute coronary events. Various methodologies have been described (Rosenman and Friedman 1977; Roskies 1978; Roskies et al. 1978). The results of various studies suggest that a cognitive strategy (Jenni and Wollersheim 1979) is superior to anxiety management (Suinn and Bloom 1978), but that modification is best approached with a strategy that integrates cognitive, physiological, and behavioral methods (Rosenman and Friedman 1977; Rosenman and Chesney 1984). There is evidence that such an approach may be effective for reduction of recurring coronary events in postinfarction patients (Rahe et al. 1979; Friedman et al. 1982; Thoresen et al. 1982). In the Recurrent Coronary Prevention Project (Friedman et al. 1982), Thoresen (C. Thoresen 1984, personal communication) will soon report that at the 3-year follow-up, effective modification of TABP was associated with a fivefold lower rate of recurring fatal and nonfatal coronary events, compared with subjects who either did not participate in the modification program or showed little evidence of behavior pattern change during the treatment period.

Pharmacological modification of TABP has been observed clinically for many years (Rosenman 1978a, 1978c, 1983; Rosenman and Chesney 1981) and recently has been found by others to diminish coronary-prone Type A behaviors (Krantz et al. 1982; Schmieder et al. 1983). Such pharmacological effects appear to be induced by agents such as clonidine, which diminishes central noradrenergic secretion, and beta-adrenergic blockers that inhibit the peripheral effects of catecholamine. Various aspects of their use are described elsewhere (Rosenman 1984b; Rosenman and Chesney 1984).

This contribution has attempted to describe some of the thoughts and observations that led to the conceptualization of TABP as resulting from an interaction of individuals with their environmental milieu, and to describe some of the findings that related TABP to CHD. The limitations of space prevented inclusion of many valuable contributions. With some exceptions, later studies by many researchers have provided strong validation of the TABP construct, have confirmed its relationship to CHD, and have helped to clarify those Type A behaviors which appear particularly to confer coronary-proneness. Innovative research is needed in the future to clarify rather than confuse the relevant issues. Such newer approaches might enhance the knowledge required for purposes of primary as well as secondary prevention of CHD.

References

Arlow J (1945) Identification of mechanisms in coronary occlusion. Psychosom Med 7: 195-209
Appels A (1972) Het hartinfarc een cultuurziekte? Tijdsch Soc Geenesk 50: 446-448
Appels A (1982) The psychological setting of imminent myocardial infarction. Act Nerv Super [Suppl] 3: 144-150
Barefoot JC, Dahlstrom WG, Williams RB (1983) Hostility, CHD incidence and total mortality: 25-year followup study of 255 physicians. Psychosom Med 45: 59-63
Blake S, Murray D, Prineas R, Gillum R (1984) Cardiovascular reactivity in Type A children during a cognitive challenge. CVD Epidemiol Newsletter 35: 18
Blumenthal J, William R, Kong Y, Schanberg S, Thompson L (1978) Type A behavior and angiographically documented coronary disease. Circulation 58: 634-639
Bortner R (1969) A short rating scale as a potential measure of Pattern A Behavior. J Chronic Dis 22: 87-91
Bortner R, Rosenman R (1967) The measurement of Pattern A behavior. J Chronic Dis 20: 525-533
Bortner R, Rosenman R, Friedman M (1970) Familial similarity in Pattern A behavior: father and sons. J Chronic Dis 23: 39-43
Brand R, Rosenman R, Sholtz R, Friedman M (1976) Multivariate prediction of coronary heart disease in the Western Collaborative Group Study compared to the findings of the Framingham Study. Circulation 53: 348-355
Brock J, Bronte-Stewart B (1955) Arteriosclerosis in African populations. Symposium on arteriosclerosis of the Minnesota Heart Association p 102
Bronte-Stewart B, Keys A, Brock J (1955) Serum cholesterol, diet and coronary heart disease: an inter-racial survey in the Cape Peninsula. Lancet 2: 1103-1108
Brozek J, Keys A, Blackburn H (1966) Personality differences between potential coronary and noncoronary subjects. Ann N Y Acad Sci 134: 1057-1064
Bruhn JG, Wolf S (1970) Studies reporting "low rates" of ischemic heart disease: a critical review. Am J Public Health 60: 1477-1495
Caffrey B (1968) Reliability and validity of personality and behavioral measures in a study of coronary heart disease. J Chronic Dis 21: 191-204
Caffrey B (1969) Behavior patterns and personality characteristics related to prevalence rates of coronary heart disease in American monks. J Chronic Dis 22: 93-103
Cassel J (1966) Letter to the edior. Psychosom Med 28: 282-284
Chesney M, Rosenman R (1980) Type A behavior in the work setting. In: Cooper C, Payne R (eds) Current concerns in occupational stress. Wiley, New York
Chesney MA, Rosenman RH (1983) Specificity in stress models: examples drawn from Type A behavior. In: Cooper CL (ed) Stress research: issues for the eighties. Wiley, London
Chesney M, Black G, Chadwick J, Rosenman R (1981) Psychological correlates of the coronary-prone behavior pattern. J Behav Med 4: 217-220
Clark D, Arnold E, Foulds E, Brown D, Eastmead D, Parry E (1975) Serum urate and cholesterol levels in Air Force Academy cadets. Aviat Space Environ Med 46: 1044-1050
Cohen J (1978) The influence of culture on coronary prone behavior. In: Dembroski T, Weiss S, Shields J, Haynes S, Feinleib M (eds) Coronary-prone behavior. Springer Berlin Heidelberg New York
Cooper T, Detre T, Weiss S (eds) (1981) Coronary-prone behavior and coronary heart disease. A critical review. Report of the Coronary-Prone Behavior Review Panel. Circulation 13: 1199-1215
Dembroski T, MacDougall J, Shields J, Petitto J, Lushene R (1978) Components of the Type A coronary-prone behavior pattern and cardiovascular responses to psychomotor performance challenge. J Behav Med 1: 159-176
Diamond E, Schneiderman N, Schwarta D, Smith J, Vorp R, Pasin R (1984) Harassment, hostility and Type A as determinants of cardiovascular reactivity during competition. Society of Behavioral Medicine, Abst. E 104, Philadelphia
Dimsdale J, Herd J (1982) Variability in plasma lipids in response to emotional arousal. Psychosom Med 44: 413-430
Dimsdale J, Hackett T, Hutter A Jr, Block P, Catanzo D (1978) Type A personality and extent of coronary atherosclerosis. Am J Cardiol 42: 583-586

Djordjenic B, Fidanza F, Karvonen M, Menotti A, Puddu V, Taylor H (1972) Probability of middle-aged men developing coronary heart disease in 5 years. Circulation 45: 815-828

Dreyfuss F, Czazckes J (1959) Blood cholesterol and uric acid of healthy medical students under the stress of an examination. Arch Int Med 103: 708-711

Ducimetière P, Cambien F, Richard J, Rakotovao R, Claude J (1980) Coronary heart disease in middle-aged Frenchmen. Lancet 1: 1346-1349

Dunbar H (1943) Psychosomatic diagnosis. Hoeber, New York

Eaker E (1984) Behavioral phenotynes. In: Rao DC et al. (eds) Genetic epidemiology of coronary heart disease. Liss, New York

Elmadjian F, Hope J, Lamson E (1958) Excretion of epinephrine and norepinephrine under stress. Recent Prog Horm Res 14: 513-518

Enterline P, Stewart W (1959) Geographic patterns in deaths from coronary disease. Public Health Rep 71: 849-857

Epstein F (1965) The epidemiology of coronary heart disease: a review. J Chronic Dis 18: 735-774

Falger P (1982) Factors contributing tc the development of vital exhaustion and depression in male myocardial infarction patients. Act Nerv Super [Suppl] 3: 151-156

Feinleib M, Brand R, Remington R, Zyzanski S (1978) Association of the coronary-prone behavior pattern and coronary heart disease. In: Dembroski T, Weiss S, Shields J, Haynes S, Feinleib M (eds) Coronary-prone behavior. Springer Berlin Heidelberg New York

Frank K, Heller S, Kornfeld D, Sporn A, Weiss M (1978) Type A behavior and coronary heart disease: angiographic confirmation. JAMA 240: 761-763

French-Belgian Collaborative Group (1982) Ischemic heart disease and psychological patterns. Prevalence and incidence studies in Belgium and France. In: Denolin H (ed) Psychological problems before and after myocardial infarction. Karger, Basel

Friedman M, Rosenman R (1955) Deranged cholesterol metabolism and its possible relationship to atherosclerosis: a review. J Gerontol 10: 60-83

Friedman M, Rosenman R (1957) Comparison of fat intake of American men and women; possible relationship to incidence of clinical coronary artery disease. Circulation 16: 339-347

Friedman M, Rosenman R (1959) Association of specific overt behavior pattern with blood and cardiovascular findings. J Am Med Assoc 169: 1286-1296

Friedman M, Rosenman R, Carroll V (1958) Changes in the serum cholesterol and blood-clotting time in men subjected to cyclic variation of occupational stress. Circulation 17: 852-861

Friedman M, St. George S, Byers S, Rosenman R (1960) Excretion of catecholamines, 17-ketosteroids, 17-hydroxycorticoids, and 5-hydroxyindole in men exhibiting a particular behavior pattern (A) associated with high incidence of clinical coronary artery disease. J Clin Invest 39: 758-764

Friedman M, Byers S, Rosenman R (1967) Factors controlling serum lipid and lipoprotein levels and their significance in the etiology of atherosclerosis. In: Blumenthal H (ed) Cowdry's arteriosclerosis, (2nd ed). Thomas, Springfield

Friedman M, Rosenman R, Straus R, Wurm M, Kositchek R (1968) The relationship of behavior pattern A to the state of coronary vasculature. Am J Med 44: 525-537

Friedman M, Brown A, Rosenman R (1969) Voice analysis test for detection of behavior pattern: responses of normal men and coronary patients. JAMA 208: 828-836

Friedman M, Byers S, Diamant J, Rosenman R (1975) Plasma catecholamine response of coronary-prone subjects (Type A) to a specific challenge. Metabolism 4: 205-210

Friedman M, Thoresen C, Gill J (1982) Feasibility of altering Type A behavior pattern after myocardial infarction. Recurrent coronary prevention project study: methods, baseline results, and preliminary findings. Circulation 66: 83-92

Gerace T, Smith J (1984) Stability of Type A behavior in young males. Cardiovasc Dis Newsletter 35

Gertler M, White P (1954) Coronary disease in young adults: a multi-disciplinary study. Harvard University Press, Cambridge

Gildea E (1949) Special features of personality which are common to certain psychosomatic disorders. Psychosom Med 11: 273-277

Glass D (1977) Behavior patterns, stress and coronary disease. Erlbaum, Hillsdale

Glass D, Snyder M, Hollis J (1974) Time urgency and the Type A coronary-prone behavior pattern. Appl Soc Psychol 4: 125-140

Gordon T, Garcia-Palmieri M, Kagan A, Kannel W, Schiffman J (1974) Differences in coronary heart disease in Framingham, Honolulu and Puerto Rico. J Chronic Dis 27: 329-337

Gover M, Pennell M (1950) Statistical studies of heart disease; mortality from eight specific forms of heart disease among white persons. Public Health Rep 65: 819-824

Groen J, Tjiong B, Kamminger C, Willebrands A (1962) The influence of nutrition, individuality and some other factors, including various forms of stress on the serum cholesterol: an experiment of nine months duration in 60 normal human volunteers. Voeding 13: 556-563

Groom D, McKee E, Webb C (1959) A comparative study of coronary disease in Kaitian and American Negroes. South Med J 52: 504-510

Grundy S, Griffin A (1959) Effects of periodic mental stress on serum cholesterol levels. Circulation 19: 496-498

Hammersten J, Cathey C, Redmond R, Wolf S (1957) Serum cholesterol, diet and stress in patients with coronary artery disease. J Clin Invest 36: 897 (abstract)

Haynes S, Feinleib M (1982) Type A behavior and the incidence of coronary heart disease in the Framingham heart study. In: Denolin H (ed) Psychological problems before and after myocardial infarction. Karger, Basel

Haynes S, Levine S, Scotch N, Feinleib M, Kannel W (1978) The relationship of psychological factors to coronary heart disease in the Framingham study: I. methods and risk factors. Am J Epidemiol 107: 362-383

Haynes S, Feinleib M, Kannel W (1980) The relationship of psychosocial factors to coronary heart disease in the Framingham study: III. 8 year incidence of CHD. Am J Epidemiol 111: 37-58

Herman S, Blumenthal J, Black G, Chesney M (1981) Self-ratings of Type A (coronary prone) adults: do type as know they are type as? Psychosom Med 43: 405-413

Horn J, Plomin R, Rosenman R (1976) Heritability of personality traits in adult male twins. Behav Genet 6: 17-30

Hunter S, Parker F, Williamson G, Webber L, Berenson G (1984) Measurement assessment of Type A coronary-prone behavior pattern and hyperactivity/problem behaviors in children: are they related? The Bogalusa heart study. CVD Epidemiol Newsletter 35

Jenkins C (1976) Recent evidence supporting psychologic and social risk factors for coronary disease. N Engl J Med 294: 987-994, 1033-1038

Jenkins CD, Rosenman RH, Friedman M (1966) Components of the coronary-prone behavior pattern: their relation to silent myocardial infarction and blood lipids. J Chronic Dis 19: 599-6

Jenkins C, Rosenman R, Friedman M (1967a) Reproducibility in rating the coronary prone behavior pattern. J Chronic Dis 20: 371-379

Jenkins C, Rosenman R, Friedman M (1967b) Development of an objective psychological test for the determination of the coronary-prone behavior pattern in employed men. J Chronic Dis 20: 371-379

Jenkins C, Rosenman R, Friedman M (1968) Replicability of rating the coronary-prone behavior pattern. Br J Prev Soc Med 22: 16-22

Jenkins C, Hames C, Zyzanski S, Rosenman R, Friedman M (1969) Psychological traits and serum lipids. I. Findings from the California Psychological Inventory. Psychosom Med 31: 115-128

Jenkins C, Zyzanski S, Rosenman R, Cleveland G (1971) Association of coronary-prone behavior pattern scores with recurrence of coronary heart disease. J Chronic Dis 24: 601-611

Jenkins C, Zyzanski S, Rosenman R (1976) Risk of new myocardial infarction in middle-aged men with manifest coronary heart disease. Circulation 53: 342-347

Jenkins C, Rosenman R, Zyzanski S (1979) Jenkins activity survey. Psychological Corporation New York

Jenni M, Wollersheim J (1979) Cognitive therapy, stress management training and the Type A behavior pattern. Cognitive Ther Res 3: 61-73

Johnston D, Shaper A (1983) Type A behavior in British men: reliability and intercorrelation of two measures. J Chronic Dis 2: 203-207

Kannel W (1970) The Framingham study - an epidemiological investigation of cardiovascular disease - section 24 - the Framingham diet study: diet and the regulation of serum cholesterol: National Heart and Lung Institute, Dept Health, Education and Welfare, Washington DC

Kannel W, Gordon T (eds) 1974) The Framingham study, DHEW publication (NIH) 74-599. US Government Printing Office, Washington DC

Keith R, Lown B, Stare F (1965) Coronary heart disease and behavior patterns: An examination of method. Psychosom Med 27: 424-434

Kemple C (1945) Rorschach method and psychosomatic diagnosis: personality traits of patients

with rheumatic disease, hypertension, cardiovascular disease, coronary occlusion, and fracture. Psychosom Med 7: 85-89
Keys A (1953) Atherosclerosis: a problem in newer public health. J Mt. Sinai Hospital 20: 118-125
Keys A (1972) Presented at the annual conference on CV disease epidemiology of the american heart association, Tampa, Florida 28 February
Keys A, Taylor H, Blackburn H, Brozek J, Anderson J (1971) Mortality and coronary heart disease among men studied for 23 years. Ann Intern Med 128: 201-205
Keys A, Aravanis C, Blackburn H, Vanbuchem F, Buzina R, Djordjenic B, Fidanza F, Karvonen M, Menotti A, Puddu V, Taylor H (1972) Probability of middle-aged men developing coronary heart disease in 5 years. Circulation 45: 815-828
Kittel F, Kornitzer M, Zyzanski S, Jenkins C, Rustin R, Degre C (1978) Two methods of assessing the Type A coronary-prone behavior pattern in Belgium. J Chronic Dis 31: 147-155
Kozarevic D, Pirc B, Ravic Z, Dawber T, Gordon T, Zukel W (1976) The Yugoslavia cardiovascular disease study - II. Factors in the incidence of coronary heart disease. Am J Epidemiol 104: 133-140
Kramer J, Kitzaume H, Proudfit W, Matsuda Y, Williams G, Sones F, Jr (1983) Progression and regression of coronary atherosclerosis: Relation to risk factors. Am Heart J 105: 134-144
Krantz D, Durel L (1983) Psychobiolcgical substrates of the Type A behavior pattern. Health Psychol 2: 393-411
Krantz D, Sanmarco M, Selvester R, Mathers K (1978) Psychological correlates of progression of atherosclerosis in man. Psychosom Med 41: 467-475
Krantz D, Durel L, Davia J, Shaffer R, Arabian J, Dembroski T, MacDougall J (1982) Propranolol medication among coronary patients: relationship of Type A behavior and cardiovascular response. J Hum Stress 8: 4-13
Lawler K, Allen M, Critcher E, Standard B (1981) The relationship of physiological responses to the coronary-prone behavior pattern in children. J Behav Med 4: 203-216
Levi L, Andersson L (1975) Psychosocial stress: population, environment, and quality of life. Spectrum, New York
Lipowski Z (1975) Sensory and information inputs overload: behavioural effects. Compr Psychiatry 16: 199-221
Marmot M (1982) Socio-economic and cultural factors in ischemic heart disease. In: Denolin H (eds) Psychological problems before and after myocardial infarction. Karger, Basel
Mason T, Fraumeni J Jr, Hoover R, Blot W (1981) An atlas of mortality from selected diseases, NIH publication 81-2397. Department of health and human services. US Government Printing Office (NIH), Washington DC
Matsumoto Y (1970) Social stress and coronary heart disease in Japan. A hypothesis. Milbank Mem Fund Q 48: 9-36
Matthews K (1978) Assessment and developmental antecedents of the coronary-prone behavior pattern in children. In: Dembroski T, Weiss S, Shields J, Haynes S, Feinleib M (eds) Coronary-prone behavior. Springer, Berlin Heidelberg New York
Matthews K (1982) Psychological perspectives on the Type A behavior pattern. Psychol Bull 91: 293-323
Matthews K, Jennings J (1984) Cardiovascular responses of boys exhibiting the Type A behavior pattern. Psychosom Med 46: 484-497
Matthews K, Glass D, Rosenman R, Bortner R (1977) Competitive drive, pattern A, and coronary heart disease: a further analysis of some data from the Western collaborative group study. J Chronic Dis 30: 489-498
Matthews K, Krantz D, Dembroski T, MacDougall J (1982) The unique and common variance in the structured interview and the Jenkins Activity Survey measures of the Type A behavior pattern. J Personal Soc Psychol 42: 303-313
Megargee EI (1984) The dynamics of aggression and their application to cardiovascular disorders. Chesney M, Rosenman R, Goldston W (eds) Anger and hostility in behavioral medicine McGraw Hill, New York
Meininger J, Zyzanski S (1983) The validity of Type A behavior scales for employed women. Am J Epidemiol 118: 424
Menninger K, Menninger W (1936) Psychoanalytic observation in cardiac disorders. Am Heart J 11: 10-26

Michaels L (1966) Etiology of coronary artery disease: an historical approach. Br Heart J 28: 258-264
Miles H, Waldfogel S, Barbabee E, Cobb S (1954) Psychosomatic study of 46 young men with coronary artery disease. Psychosom Med 16: 455-477
Mordkoff A, Parsons O (1967) The coronary personality: a critique. Psychosom Med 29: 1-14
MRFIT behavior pattern study (1979) - I. Study design, procedures, and reproducibility of behavior pattern judgments. J Chronic Dis 32: 293-305
MRFIT (1982) Risk factor changes and mortality results. JAMA 248: 1465-1477
Morris J (1951) Recent history of coronary disease. Lancet 1: 1-7
Morris J, Heady J, Raffle P, Roberts V Parks J (1953) Coronary heart disease and physical activity of work. Lancet 2: 1053-1057, 1111-1120
Nestel PJ, Verghese A, Lovell RRH (1967) Catecholamine secretion and sympathetic nervous responses to emotion in men with and without angina pectoris Am Heart J 73: 227-234
Nixon P (1976) The human function curve. Practitioner 217: 765-769, 935-944
Nixon P (1984) Stress, life, style, and cardiovascular disease. A cardiological odyssey. Br J Holistic Med 1: 20-29
Osler W (1910) The Lumleian Lectures on angina pectoris. Lancet 1: 839-844
Paul O, Lepper M, Phelan W, Dupertuis G, MacMillan A, McKean H, Park H (1963) A longitudinal study of coronary heart disease. Circulation 28: 20-28
Raab W (1953) Hormonal and neurogenic disorders. Wilkins and Wilkins, Baltimore
Raab W, Gigee W (1954) Total urinary catechol excretion in cardiovascular and other diseased conditions. Circulation 9: 592-598
Rahe R, Rubin R, Gunderson E, Arthur R (1971) Psychologic correlates of serum cholesterol level in man. Psychosom Med 33: 399-410
Rahe R, Rubin R, Arthur R (1974) Three investigators study serum uric acid, cholesterol and cortisol variability during stess of everyday life. Psychosom Med 36: 258-268
Rahe R, Ward H, Hayes V (1979) Brief group therapy in myocardial infarction rehabilitation: Three to four-year follow-up of a controlled trial. Psychosom Med 41: 229-242
Robertson W (1959) Atherosclerosis and ischaemic heart disease; observations in Jamaica. Lancet 1: 444-446
Rosenman R (1978a) The role of the Type A behavior pattern in ischemic heart disease: modification of its effects by beta-blocking agents. Br J Clin Pract [Suppl 1] 32: 58-65
Rosenman R (1978b) The interview method of assessment of the coronary prone behavior pattern. In: Dembroski T, Wiess S, Shields J, Haynes S, Feinleib M (eds) Coronary-prone behavior. Springer, Berlin Heidelberg New York
Rosenman R (1978c) Role of Type A behavior pattern in the pathogenesis of ischemic heart disease, and modfication for prevention. Proceedings of PAAVO NURMI conference, Helsinki, Finland, September, 1977. Adv Cardiol 25: 1-12
Rosenman R (1983) Coronary-prone behavior pattern and coronary heart disease. Implications for the use of beta-blockers for primary prevention. In: Rosenman R (ed) Psychosomatic risk factors and coronary heart disease: indications for specific preventive therapy. Huber, Bern
Rosenman R (1984a) Health consequences of anger and implications for treatment. In: Chesney M, Rosenman R, Goldston W (eds) Anger and hostility in behavioral medicine. McGraw Hill, New York
Rosenman RH (1984b) Modification of the coronary-prone (Type A) behavior pattern in the frame of cardiac rehabilitation. Proceedings of the symposium of the scientific council on rehabilitation of cardiac patients, International society and federation of cardiology, held at Santiago de Compostela, Spain, 8-9 June, 1984
Rosenman R, Chesney M (1980) The relationship of Type A behavior pattern to coronary heart disease. Act Nerv Super (Praha) 22: 1-45
Rosenman RH, Chesney MA (1981) Psychological profiles and coronary heart disease. In: Kielholz W, Siegenthaler P, Taggart A, Zanchetti P (eds) Psychosomatic cardiovascular disorders - when and how to treat. Huber, Bern
Rosenman R, Chesney M (1982) Stress, Type A behavior, and coronary disease. In: Goldberger L, Breznitz S (eds) Handbook of stress. Macmillan, New York
Rosenman RH, Chesney MA (1984) Type A behavior pattern: its relationship to coronary heart disease and its modification by behavioral and pharmacological approaches. In: Zales MR (ed) Stress and Health and Disease, Brunner-Mazel, New York

Rosenman R, Friedman M (1958) The possible relationship of occupational stress to clinical coronary heart disease. California Med 89: 169-174, and 1959, 90, 168-171

Rosenman R, Friedman M (1959) The possible relationship of the emotions to clinical coronary heart disease. In: Pincus G (ed) Hormones and atherosclerosis. Academic New York

Rosenman R, Friedman M (1961) Association of specific behavior pattern in women with blood and cardiovascular findings. JAMA 24: 1173-1184

Rosenman R, Friedman M (1963) Behavior patterns, blood lipids, and coronary heart disease. JAMA 184: 934-938

Rosenman R, Friedman M (1974) Neurogenic factors in pathogenesis of coronary heart disease. Med Clin North Am 58: 269-279

Rosenman R, Friedman M (1977) Modifying type A behavior pattern. J Psychosom Res 21: 323-331

Rosenman R, Byers S, Friedman M (1952) The mechanism responsible for the altered blood cholesterol content in deranged thyroid states. J Clin Endocrinol 12: 1287-1299

Rosenman R, Friedman M, Byers S (1956) The causal role of plasma albumin deficiency in experimental nephrotic hyperlipemia and hypercholesteremia. J Clin Invest 35: 522-532

Rosenman R, Friedman M, Straus R, Wurm M, Kositchek R, Hahn W, Wethessen N (1964) A predictive study of coronary heart disease. The Western collaborative group study. JAMA 189: 15-22

Rosenman R, Friedman M, Jenkins C, Straus R, Wurm M, Kositchek R (1966a) The prediction of immunity to coronary heart disease. JAMA 198: 1159-1162

Rosenman R, Friedman M, Straus R, Wurm M, Jenkins C, Messinger H, Kositchek R (1966b) Western collaborative group study: a follow-up experience of two years. JAMA 195: 86-92

Rosenman R, Friedman M, Jenkins C, Straus R, Wurm M, Kositchek R (1967a) Clinically unrecognized myocardial infarction in the Western Collaborative Group Study. Am J Cardiol 19: 776-782

Rosenman R, Friedman M, Jenkins C, Straus R, Wurm M, Kositchek R (1967b) Recurring and fatal myocardial infarction in the Western Collaborative Group Study. Am J Cardiol 19: 771-775

Rosenman R, Friedman M, Jenkins C, Bortner R (1968) Is there a coronary-prone personality? Int J Psychiatry 5: 427-429

Rosenman R, Brand R, Jenkins C, Friedman M, Straus R, Wurm M (1975) Coronary heart disease in the Western Collaborative Group Study: final follow-up of 8.5 years. JAMA 233: 872-877

Rosenman R, Rahe R, Borhani N, Feinleib M (1976a) Heritability of personality and behavior. Proceedings of the first international congress of twin studies, Rome, Italy, November 1974. Acta Genet Med Gemellol 25: 221-224

Rosenman R, Brand R, Sholtz R, Friedman M (1976b) Multivariate prediction of coronary heart disease during 8.5 year follow-up in the Western Collaborative Group Study. Am J Cardiol 37: 903-910

Roskies E (1978) Considerations in developing a treatment program for the coronary-prone (Type A) behavior pattern. In: Davidson P (ed) Behavioral medicine: changing health life styles. Brunner Mazel, New York

Roskies E, Spevack M, Surkis A, Cohen C, Gilman S (1978) Changing the coronary-prone (Type A) behavior pattern in a nonclinical population. J Behav Med 1: 201-216

Saphir O, Ohringer L, Silverstone H (1956) Coronary arteriosclerotic heart disease in younger age groups: its greater frequency in this group among increasingly older necropsy population. Am J Med Sci 231: 494-501

Scherwitz L, Berton K, Leventhal H (1977) Type A assessment and interaction in the bevhavior pattern interview. Psychosom Med 39: 229-240

Schucker B, Jacobs D (1977) Assessment of behavioral risks for coronary disease by voice characteristics. Psychosom Med 39: 219-228

Schmieder F, Friedrich G, Neus H, Rudel H, von Eiff W (1985) The influence of beta-blockers on cardiovascular reactivity and Type A behavior pattern in hypertensives. Psychosom Med 45: 417-432

Shekelle R, Schoenberger J, Stamler J (1976) Correlates of the JAS Type A behavior score. J Chronic Dis 29: 381-394

Shekelle RB, Gale M, Ostfeld AM, Paul O (1983) Hostility, risk of CHD, and mortality. Psychosom Med 45: 109-114

Siegel J, Matthews K, Leitch C (1983) Blood pressure variability and the Type A behavior pattern in adolescents. J Psychosom Res 27: 265-272

Sigler L (1959) The mortality from arteriosclerotic and hypertensive heart diseases in the United States. I. Possible relation to distribution of population and economic status. Am J Cardiol 1: 605-611

Sime W, Parker C (1978) Physiological arousal in male and female students with either Type A or B behavior patterns. Med Sci Sports 10: 51-53

Simpson M, Olewine D, Jenkins C, Ramsey F, Zyzanski S, Thomas G, James C (1974) Exercise-induced catecholamines and platelet aggregation in the coronary-prone behavior pattern. Psychosom Med 36: 476-487

Spielberger CD, Jacobs GA, Russell S, Crane RS (1983) Assessment of Anger: The State-Trait Anger Scale. In: Butcher JN, Seielberger CD (eds) Advances in personality assessment, vol 2. Erlbaum, Hillsdale

Stallones R (1983) Mortality and the multiple risk factor intervention trial. Am J Epidemiol 117: 647-650

Stewart I (1950) Coronary disease and modern stress. Lancet 2: 867-878

Suinn R, Bloom L (1978) Anxiety management training for pattern A behavior. J Behav Med 1: 25-35

Thomas C, Murphey E (1958) Further studies on cholesterol levels in the Johns Hopkins medical students: the effect of stress at examination. J Chronic Dis 8: 661-670

Thoresen C, Friedman M, Gill J, Ulmer D (1982) The recurrent coronary prevention project: Some preliminary findings. Acta Med Scand 660: 172-192

Timberline Conference on Psychophysiologic Aspects of Cardiovascular Disease (1964) Psychosom Med 36: Part 2

Toynbee A (1961) A study of history. Oxford University Press, London

Trulson M (1959) The American diet: past and present. Am J Clin Nutr 7: 91-97

Von Dusch T (1868) Lehrbuch der Herzkrankheiten. Engelman, Leipzig

Voudoukis I (1971) Exaggerated cold-pressor response in patients with atherosclerotic vascular disease. Angiography 22: 57-62

Waldron I (1978) The coronary-prone behavior pattern, blood pressure, employment and socioeconomic status in women. J Psychosom Res 22: 79-87

Waldron I, Zyzanski S, Shekelle R, Jenkins C, Tennebaum S (1977) The coronary-prone behavior pattern in employed men and women. J Human Stress 3: 2-18

Ward M, Chesney M, Swan G, Black G, Parker S, Rosenman R (1985) Cardiovascular responses in Type A and Type B men to a series of stressors. J Behav Med (to be published)

Werko L (1976) Risk factors and coronary heart disease - fact or fancy? Am Heart J 91: 87-98

Wertlake P, Wilcox A, Haley M, Peterson J (1968) Relationship of mental and emotional stress to serum cholesterol levels. Proc Soc Exp Biol Med 97: 163-165

White P (1974) The historical background of angina pectoris. Mod. Concept Cardiovasc Dis 43: 109-112

Williams R Jr, Haney T, Lee K, Yong Y, Blumenthal J, Whalen R (1980) Type A behavior, hostility, and coronary atherosclerosis. Psychosom Med 42: 539-549

Williams R Jr, Lane J, Kuhn C, Melosh W, White A, Schanberg S (1982) Type A behavior and elevated physiological and neuroendocrine responses to cognitive tasks. Science 218: 483-485

Yater W, Traum A, Brown W, Fitzgerald R, Geisler M, Wilcox B (1948) Coronary artery disease in men eighteen to thirty-nine years of age. Am Heart J 36: 334-340, 683-690

Yudkin J (1957) Diet and coronary thrombosis, hypothesis and fact. Lancet 2: 155-162

Zumoff B, Rosenfeld R, Friedman M, Byers S, Rosenman R, Hellman L (1978) Comparison of plasma and urinary steroids in men with Type A and Type B behavior patterns. Conference proceedings no. 231. Prospective medicine opportunities in aerospace medicine. Advisory Group for Aerospace Research and Development, NATO

Zyzanski S, Jenkins C, Ryan T, Flessas A, Everist M (1976) Psychological correlates of coronary angiographic findings. Arch Int Med 136: 1234-1237

Type A Behavior and Risk of Coronary Heart Disease in the Multiple Risk Factor Intervention Trial

R. B. Shekelle, S. B. Hulley, J. D. Neaton, J. Billings, N. O. Borhani, T. A. Gerace, D. Jacobs, N. Lasser, M. Mittlemark, and J. Stamler[1]

In 1972, when the Multiple Risk Factor Intervention Trial (MRFIT) was being organized, the only prospective epidemiological evidence linking the Type A behavior pattern to increased risk of coronary heart disease (CHD) came from the Western Collaborative Group Study (WCGS), which found that men characterized as Type A by means of a structured interview had twice the risk of CHD in comparison to those characterized as Type B, and that this higher level of risk persisted after adjustment for age, blood pressure, cigarette smoking, and serum cholesterol level (Rosenman et al. 1964, 1975, 1976).

In addition, Dr. Jenkins and Dr. Zyzanski, working with Dr. Rosenman, had developed a self-administered, objectively scored questionnaire - the Jenkins Activity Survey (JAS) - for assessing behavior pattern (Jenkins et al. 1967, 1971; Jenkins 1978). This questionnaire was administered to participants in WCGS about midway through the course of the study. Results showed that the JAS Type A score was positively and significantly associated with incidence of CHD (Jenkins et al. 1974).

Given the potential importance of these findings, and the need to determine their consistency in a variety of populations, particularly by prospective investigations, MRFIT decided to conduct a substudy - the MRFIT Behavior Pattern Study - which would investigate the Type A hypothesis.

Methods of Procedure

MRFIT was a randomized primary prevention trial designed to evaluate the effects of multifactor intervention on risk of death from CHD. Participants were men who, at entry, were 35-57 years of age and had no evidence of angina pectoris or myocardial infarction as determined by history and ECG. However, their levels of cigarette

1 For the Multiple Risk Factor Intervention Trial Research Group. School of Public Health, University of Texas Health Science Center at Houston; Department of Epidemiology and International Health, University of California School of Medicine, San Francisco; Division of Biometry, School of Public Health, University of Minnesota, Minneapolis; Medical Research Institute, San Francisco; Department of Community Health, University of California School of Medicine, Davis; Department of Epidemiology and Public Health, University of Miami School of Medicine, Miami; Division of Epidemiology, School of Public Health, University of Minnesota, Minneapolis; New Jersey Medical School, Newar; and the Department of Community Health and Preventive Medicine, Northwestern University School of Medicine. Most of this work was done while Dr. Shekelle was with the Department of Preventive Medicine, Rush-Presbyterian-St. Luke's Medical Center, Chicago, USA. (Correspondence should be addressed to Dr. R. B. Shekelle, School of Public Health, University of Texas Health Science Center at Houston, P.O. Box 20186, Houston, TX 77225, USA).

Biological and Psychological Factors
in Cardiovascular Disease
Ed. by T. H. Schmidt, T. M. Dembroski, and G. Blümchen

smoking, serum cholesterol, and diastolic blood pressure, as determined at an initial screening visit, were sufficiently high to place them in the upper portion - initially the upper 15%, later the upper 10% - of the distribution of a risk score derived from the Framingham Heart Study. Men were ineligible for MRFIT when serum cholesterol was 350 mg/dl or higher, diastolic blood pressure was 115 mmHg or higher, body weight was greater than or equal to 150% of desirable weight, and illnesses or disabilities likely to impair full participation in the trial were present. Various recruitment procedures were used, but the most common was voluntary screening of industrial and governmental employee groups. Men accepted into MRFIT were randomly assigned to Special Intervention (SI) - a program comprising treatment for hypertension, counseling for cessation of cigarette smoking, and dietary advice for lowering blood cholesterol levels - or to Usual Care (UC), i.e., referral to usual sources of health care. Details of the trial have been published (Benfari and Sherwin 1981; Multiple Risk Factor Intervention Trial Research Group 1982).

Both the structured interview (Rosenman 1978; Multiple Risk Factor Intervention Trial Group 1979) and Form B of the JAS (Jenkins 1978) were used to assess behavior pattern at entry. The JAS was administered to all participants at all 22 clinical centers as part of a larger take-home questionnaire given between the second and third screeening visits. The Type A score, calculated at the MRFIT Coordinating Center according to directions provided by Dr. Jenkins and Dr. Zyzanski, had been standardized to distribute in the WCGS population with a mean of zero and standard deviation of ten points. Positive scores indicated Type A behavior, while negative scores indicated Type B.

In view of its cost and the problems involved in standardizing interviews at multiple centers, we decided to use the structured interview at a limited number of clinics. Ultimately, interviews were conducted at eight centers: four in Chicago, and one each in San Francisco, Minneapolis, Newark, and Davis, California. Since assessment of behavior pattern by the structured interview involves subjective judgement, establishing procedures that would enhance comparability among the MRFIT centers and with WCGS was a very important part of our planning. For this purpose, we developed a detailed written protocol with the assistance of Dr. Ray H. Rosenman, who served as a consultant to the Behavior Pattern Study. In this capacity, he advised on all matters relating to the behavior assessment interview, assisted in selecting interviewers, conducted training programs for the interviewers, assessed and reviewed each interviewer's technique and adequacy, and assessed ratings assigned to participants as the study progressed.

The procedures by which interviewers were selected, trained, and certified, and by which the interview assessments of behavior pattern were made and reviewed, have been published in detail (Multiple Risk Factor Intervention Trial Group 1979), and are summarized below:

1. Candidates for training as interviewers were required to demonstrate in a pretest the ability to discriminate Type A1 from Type B patterns on prerecorded interviews, after reading a description of these patterns.
2. Interviewers were trained centrally by Dr. Rosenman and his staff. The training sessions generally lasted for 5 days and comprised lectures and demonstrations, practice with prerecorded materials, and interviews with volunteers.

3. Interviewers were required to meet predetermined standards of performance prior to conducting interviews for the study. This involved judging a set of 100 prerecorded interviews which Dr. Rosenman had previously assessed, and also performing interviews with 16–20 pilot subjects, which were subsequently audited by Dr. Rosenman. Certification required at least 75% agreement with Dr. Rosenman in judging major category - that is, Type A1-A2 vs. Type X-B - and a rating of "good" or better in performing the interview. Ultimately, 12 persons from a field of 23 candidates were selected for training in the interview technique, and 6 met the criteria for certification. In addition, two auditors from Dr. Rosenman's staff also met these criteria for certification.
4. The interviews were recorded, and the recordings - together with the interviewer's behavior checklist and judgement of behavior pattern - were mailed daily to the MRFIT Coordinating Center in Minneapolis. No information about behavior pattern was retained at the clinical center. The recordings were copied at the Coordinating Center, and the originals forwarded to the San Francisco MRFIT clinical center. Two auditors were employed there, and one or the other listened to each interview, reviewed the behavior checklist, and recorded her own assessment of behavior pattern without knowledge of the interviewer's previous assessment.
5. The auditor's assessments were returned to the Coordinating Center, where they were compared with those made initially by the local interviewer. All cases where the interviewer and auditor disagreed in major category - that is, one said A1 or A2 while the other said X or B - were referred to Dr. Rosenman, who adjudicated the discrepancy and returned his judgement to the Coordinating Center.
6. A continuous, three-stage quality control procedure was designed and administered by the Coordinating Center to ensure that the frequency of agreement in major category between interviewers and auditors did not fall below 80%. In addition, a random sample of all interviews was selected continuously throughout the period of recruitment for assessment by Dr. Rosenman.
7. Interviewers were site-visited once by Dr. Rosenman and once by one of the auditors.

Behavior pattern was judged on a four-point scale: A1, A2, X, and B. A1 indicated participants who exhibited all or most of the Type A characteristics; A2, X, and B indicated decreasing levels of similarity to that pattern (Rosenman 1978). Since we had at least two, and often three, assessments of behavior pattern for each participant, the protocol specified that the assessment to be used for investigating the association between behavior pattern and risk of CHD would be Dr. Rosenman's or, when that was not available, the auditor's.

All participants were followed through 28 February 1982, a period of 6–8 years (mean = 7.1 years). Deaths were systematically ascertained by clinic staff, and cause of death was assigned by a three-member panel of cardiologists not associated with any MRFIT center. Neither this panel nor clinic staff had access to assessments of behavior pattern.

Resting 12-lead ECGs were obtained according to a standard protocol at entry and at each annual re-examination. ECGs were analyzed according to Minnesota coding criteria (Prineas et al. 1982) by visual procedures and, independently, by computer. Disagreements for major Q-waves were adjudicated by two cardiologists.

Cases that met specified criteria for clinically significant change from the baseline ECG were classified as definite nonfatal myocardial infarction (MI). These judgements were based solely on the ECGs, without other knowledge of participants.

The major purpose for the MRFIT Behavior Pattern Study was to investigate the hypothesis that men assessed as Type A (A1-A2) would have a higher incidence of first major coronary events, i.e., coronary death and definite nonfatal MI, in comparison to those assessed as types X and B. The hypothesis was formulated in this way - A1-A2 vs. X-B - because it was most comparable to the procedure used previously in MCGS. In order to guard against the possibility that the association of behavior pattern with risk of CHD might differ between UC and SI, i.e., there might be a significant association in one group but not in the other, the protocol specified that the critical test would be in UC since men in that group did not participate in a systematic intervention program and, therefore, would presumably be more comparable to men participating in a strictly observational study.

After MRFIT began but prior to its termination and analysis of data, Haynes and colleagues published their results indicating that the Framingham Type A score was associated prospectively with risk of CHD among men employed in nonclerical white-collar occupations but not among men employed in clerical or blue-collar occupations (Haynes et al. 1980). In view of this result and the observation that less than 11% of participants in WCGS were classified as laborers (Rosenman et al. 1964), we formulated the following subgroup hypothesis: in men employed full-time in managerial, professional, and technical occupations, i.e., U.S. Census Bureau occupational codes 1-245 (US Bureau of the Census 1971), those assessed as A1-A2 would have a higher incidence of first major coronary events than those assessed as X-B.

The two null hypotheses were tested by calculating the chi-square statistic from a fourfold contingency table. The critical value for rejecting the null hypothesis was set at the one-sided 5% level of statistical significance.

Log-linear models (Bishop et al. 1975) were used to determine whether the association between behavior pattern and risk of CHD differed among clinics or between SI and UC. Proportional hazards (Cox-type) regression models (Kalbfleisch and Prentice 1978) were used to investigate the association of Type A behavior to risk of first major coronary event after adjustment for age at entry, diastolic blood pressure, serum cholesterol level, number of cigarettes smoked per day, number of alcoholic drinks consumed per day, and educational attainment. When comparing A1-A2 vs. X-B, assessments of behavior pattern were represented in the multivariate model by a single dichotomous variable, Type A, which was coded O for patterns X-B and 1 for patterns A1-A2. In other multivariate analyses, interview assessments of behavior pattern were represented by three dichotomous variables - X, A2, and A1 - with each coded 0 if absent or 1 if present. The regression coefficients were used to estimate the risk associated with the corresponding behavior pattern relative to the risk for pattern B.

In analyses of the JAS, the distribution of Type A scores was divided approximately into quintiles in order to examine trends in morbidity and mortality. Univariate tests for linear trends were performed using a procedure described by Wood (1978). The JAS Type A score was entered as a continuous variable in multivariate analyses.

Table 1. Frequency distribution by interviewer's and auditor's ratings

Auditor's rating	Interviewer's rating				Total
	A1	A2	X	B	
A1	786	319	8	13	1126
A2	352	708	61	89	1210
X	24	95	54	44	217
B	28	133	57	339	557
Total	1190	1255	180	485	3110

4-point agreement = 61%; 2-point agreement = 85%

Table 2. Frequency distribution by interviewer's and Rosenman's ratings. Random sample of 413 men

Rosenman's rating	Interviewer's rating				Total
	A1	A2	X	B	
A1	113	36	0	0	149
A2	35	106	8	4	153
X	6	16	11	10	43
B	2	16	7	43	68
Total	156	174	26	57	413

4-point agreement = 66%; 2-point agreement = 87%

Results

Interview Assessments of Behavior Pattern

Behavior pattern was assessed by interview at entry at eight clinical centers for 3110 men: 1103 (35.5%) Type A1, 1211 (38.9%) Type A2, 269 (8.7%) Type X, and 527 (16.9%) Type B. Of these, 1550 were randomly assigned to UC, and 1560 were assigned to SI.

Reliability

Table 1 shows the frequency distribution of these 3110 participants according to the interviewer's assessment and the auditor's assessment of behavior pattern. Of 1190 men judged Type A1 by the interviewer, the auditor agreed in 66% of cases, judged 30% as A2, 2% as X, and 2% as B. Of 1255 men judged Type A2 by the interviewer, the auditor agreed in 56% of cases, judged 25% as A1, 8% as X, and 11% as B. Of 180 men judged as Type X by the interviewer, the auditor judged 4% as Type A1, and divided the remainder rather evenly into the other three categories: 34% as A2, 30% as X, and 32% as B. Of 485 men assessed Type B by the interviewer, the auditor agreed in 70% of cases, judged 9% as X, 18% as A2, and 3% as A1. For all 3110 men, agreement was 85% on the two-point scale (A1-A2 vs. X-B) and 61% on the four-point scale.

Table 3. Frequency distribution by auditor's and Rosenman's ratings. Random sample of 413 men

Rosenman's rating	Auditor's rating				Total
	A1	A2	X	B	
A1	123	25	1	0	149
A2	36	102	10	5	153
X	2	17	15	9	43
B	2	3	4	59	68
Total	163	147	30	73	413

4-point agreement = 72%; 2-point agreement = 90%

Table 2 shows the frequency distribution of a random sample of 413 participants according to the interviewer's assessment and Dr. Rosenman's assessment. For 113 men judged Type A1 by the interviewer, Dr. Rosenman agreed in 72%, judged 23% as Type A2, and 5% as either X or B. At the other end of the scale, of 57 men judged Type B by the interviewers, Dr. Rosenman judged 7% as A2, 18% as X, and agreed in 75%. Overall agreement was 87% on the two-point scale (A1-A2 vs. X-B), and 66% on the four-point scale.

Table 3 shows the frequency distribution of the same random sample of 413 men according to the auditor's assessment and Dr. Rosenman's assessment. Results were similar to those described above, except the percentage agreement was somewhat higher: 90% on the two-point scale, and 72% on the four-point scale.

Behavior Pattern and Risk of CHD

Analysis by log-linear models yielded no evidence that the association between behavior pattern and risk of first major coronary events differed among clinics (chi-square = 2.81, $df = 7$, $P = 0.90$) or between UC and SI (chi-square = 0.66, $df = 1$, $P = 0.42$). Therefore, detailed results have been presented in Fig. 1 for UC and SI combined and for the eight clinics combined. Variation among the four groups in risk of first major coronary event was small (chi-square = 3.85, $df = 3$, $P = 0.29$) and showed no clear evidence for a graded association. Type A2 had the lowest crude risk, 3.30%, while Types B, X, and A1 were similar in crude risks (4.36%, 4.46%, and 4.90%, respectively). These results were not changed substantially after adjustment by Cox-type regression analysis for age, diastolic blood pressure, serum cholesterol level, cigarette smoking, consumption of alcohol, and educational attainment; in comparison to Type B, the adjusted relative risks for Types X, A2, and A1 were 0.95, 0.73, and 0.99, respectively.

Comparing A1-A2 with X-B, the crude relative risk was 0.92 (4.06%/4.40%), and the adjusted relative risk (as calculated from the partial Cox regression coefficient of −0.1368 with standard error of 0.2001) was 0.87, with 95% confidence interval (C. I.) of 0.59-1.29. (In UC, the crude and relative risks were 1.08 and 0.99, respectively, while in SI they were 0.82 and 0.81.) In the multivariate regression analysis, risk of first major coronary event was positively and significantly associated with age at randomization ($P < 0.001$) and with first screen measurements of dia-

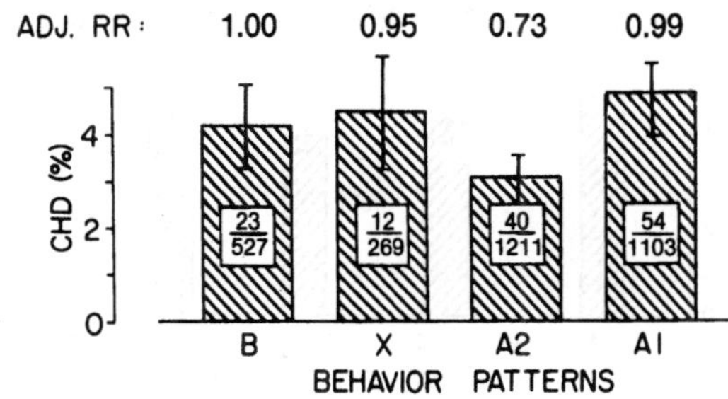

Fig. 1. Risk of first major coronary event (CHD death and definite nonfatal MI by annual ECG) according to behavior pattern. UC and SI groups combined at eight clinical centers combined. Mean follow-up of 7.1 years. *Adj. RR* indicates relative risks adjusted by Cox-type regression analysis for age, diastolic blood pressure, serum cholesterol level, cigarette smoking, consumption of alcoholic beverages, and educational attainment

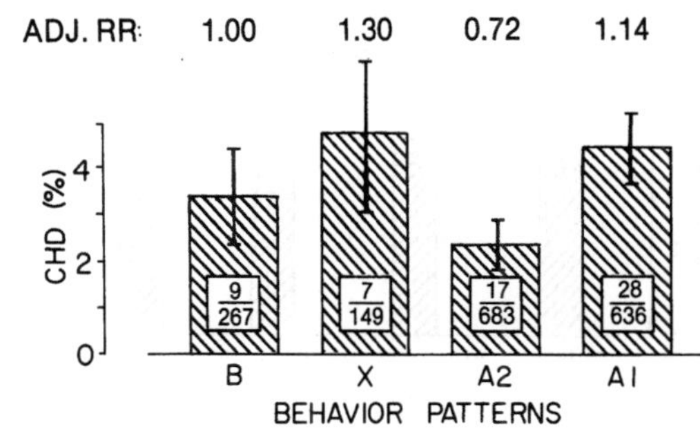

Fig. 2. Risk of first major coronary event (CHD death and definite nonfatal MI by annual ECG) according to behavior pattern in men employed full-time in professional, technical, and managerial occupations. UC and SI groups combined at eight clinical centers combined. *Adj. RR* indicates relative risks adjusted by Cox-type regression analysis for age, diastolic blood pressure, serum cholesterol level, cigarette smoking, and consumption of alcoholic beverages

stolic blood pressure ($P = 0.027$), serum cholesterol level ($P < 0.001$), and number of cigarettes smoked per day ($P < 0.001$).

Since use of beta-blocking agents may modify the expression of Type A behavior, analyses were repeated omitting 519 men for whom propranolol had been prescribed for treatment of hypertension. The results were similar to those shown in Fig. 1; risks of first major coronary events for Types B, X, A2, and A1 were 4.67%, 5.00%, 3.23%, and 4.79%, respectively.

Figure 2 shows results for the subgroup of 1735 men who were employed full-time in professional, technical, and managerial positions. These results do not differ substantially from those shown in Fig. 1, except that the sampling error is somewhat larger because of the reduced sample size. Incidence of first major coronary events was 3.41% in 1319 men judged A1-A2 and 3.85% in 416 men judged X-B. The relative risks were 0.89 unadjusted, and 0.84 (95% C.I. of 0.47–1.49) after adjustment by Cox-type regression analysis for the previously listed variables.

Assessments of behavior pattern were not significantly associated with risk of CHD death or with total mortality in UC or SI, separately or combined (results not

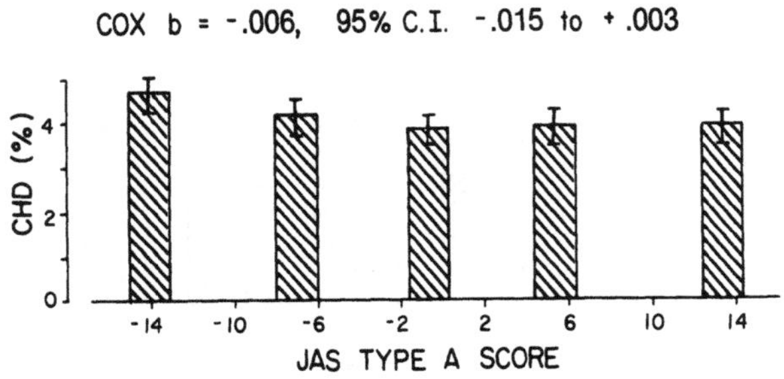

Fig. 3. Risk of first major coronary event (CHD death and definite nonfatal MI by annual ECG) according to quintile of the distribution of the JAS Type A scores. UC and SI groups combined at 22 clinical centers combined ($n = 12772$). *b* indicates the partial Cox regression coefficient adjusted for age, diastolic blood pressure, serum cholesterol level, cigarette smoking, consumption of alcohol, and educational attainment. *C. I.* indicates the 95% confidence interval for the regression coefficient

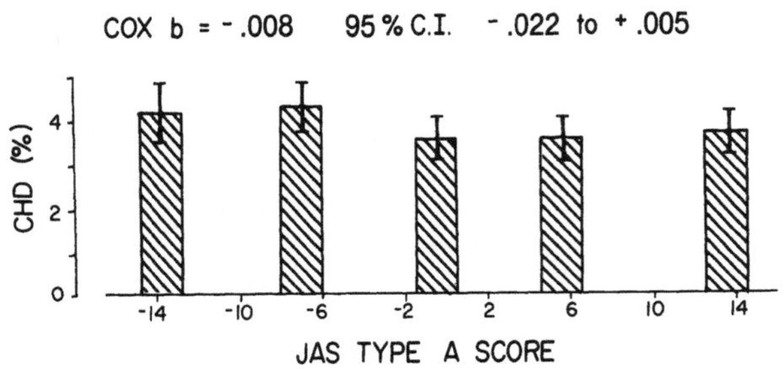

Fig. 4. Risk of first major coronary event (CHD death and definite nonfatal MI by annual ECG) according to quintile of the distribution of the JAS Type A scores in men employed full-time in professional, technical, and managerial occupations. UC and SI groups combined at 22 clinical centers combined ($n = 6504$). *b* indicates the partial Cox regression coefficient adjusted for age, diastolic blood pressure, serum cholesterol level, cigarette smoking, and consumption of alcoholic beverages

shown). Although angina pectoris was not an end point in MRFIT, information about chest pain was obtained by the Rose questionnaire (Rose and Blackburn 1968) at baseline and at each annual re-examination. In addition, the examining physician's opinion was systematically recorded as to whether or not angina pectoris had occurred. Analysis of these data (results not shown) also showed no significant associations with behavior patterns. Using the examining physician's diagnosis, crude relative risks of angina pectoris for A1-A2 compared with X-B were 1.09 in SI, 1.01 in UC, and 1.05 overall.

JAS Type A Scores

A total of 12772 participants (99.3% of all 12866 participants) completed the JAS between the second and third screening visits prior to randomization in sufficient detail for Type A scores to be calculated. The scores distributed approximately normally with mean of -0.9 and standard deviation of 9.6 points. (As mentioned earlier, the mean and standard deviation in the WCGS population were 0 and 10, respectively.)

The JAS Type A score was not significantly associated with risk of first major coronary events in either UC or SI (the partial Cox regression coefficients were −0.010 in UC and −0.003 in SI), and detailed results have been presented in Fig. 3 only for both groups combined. The incidence of first major coronary events was slightly higher in the lower two quintiles than in the upper three quintiles of the distribution of JAS Type A scores, but the trend was not statistically significant in either univariate or multivariate analyses. After adjustment for age, diastolic blood pressure, serum cholesterol level, cigarette smoking, consumption of alcohol, and educational attainment, the adjusted Cox regression coefficient was negative in sign, −0.006, but its 95% C.I. included zero (−0.015-0.003). Similar results were obtained when the analysis was restricted to the 6504 men employed in professional, technical, and managerial occupations (see Fig. 4). In both univariate and multivariate analyses of CHD death and of total mortality (results not shown), the JAS Type A score had small negative coefficients in UC and in SI, but the 95% C.I.s included zero in every instance.

Discussion

These results have led us to conclude that assessments of behavior pattern were not associated with risk of CHD in MRFIT. The adjusted relative risk of a first major CHD event for Type A men (A1-A2 vs. X-B) was 0.87 with 95% C.I. of 0.59 to 1.29. The precision of this estimate, as indicated by the C.I. indicates that the relative risk in the population was less than 1.3. In contrast, Brand (1978) found that the adjusted relative odds of CHD for Type A men in WCGS was 1.97 with 95% C.I. of 1.49-2.62. Since WCGS and MRFIT are the only propective studies with results based on assessments made by the structured interview, and since random sampling error is an unlikely explanation for the difference in results, review of the two studies has led us to consider the following questions. Could the difference in outcome have been due to differences in the prevalence of coronary risk factors; to differences in the procedures by which participants were recruited and selected; to differences in the procedures for assessing behavior pattern; or to differences in the procedures for detecting and defining endpoints?

First, evidence from WCGS and the Framingham Heart Study indicates that the higher prevalence of coronary risk factors in MRFIT should have enhanced, not diminished, the opportunity to detect a difference in risk between Type A and Type B men. Rosenman et al. (1975) showed that Type A men in WCGS had higher risk of CHD than Type B men regardless of the presence or absence of other coronary risk factors. Moreover, Brand (1978) concluded that the WCGS data were consistent with the hypothesis that Type A behavior approximately doubled the risk conferred by age, blood pressure, serum cholesterol, and cigarette smoking. His Fig. 1.2A clearly shows that the difference in risk between Types A and B was larger among men with three or four risk factors than among those with none or only one. Analysis of the 10-year incidence data from the Framingham Heart Study by Haynes et al. (1983) indicated that the difference between Type A and Type B men in risk of CHD increased with increasing levels of other coronary risk factors.

With regard to the second question, i.e., whether the absence of an association in MRFIT could be due to a selection bias, Criqui (1974) has shown that "pure risk factor bias", e. g., a bias of selection that changed the prevalence of Type A from 50% to 74%, could not by itself have biased the relative risk. Therefore, the higher prevalence of Type A behavior in MRFIT as compared with WCGS cannot account for the absence of an association between behavior pattern and risk of CHD.

The MRFIT population was highly selected - 3.6% of 361662 men initially screened were enrolled in the trial - and it seems reasonable to believe that persons who participate in a clinical trial might differ in various ways from persons who participate in long-term observational studies such as WCGS and the Framingham Heart Study. For example, a bias of selection could have occurred if the positive association between Type A and risk of CHD were mediated by some third factor, e. g., hostility, and if Type A men who had this factor were less likely to volunteer for a clinical trial than Type A men who did not have this characteristc. This hypothesis may be a promising area for further investigation. Recent studies have indicated that hostility is associated with severity of coronary artery disease in patients undergoing diagnostic coronary a angiography (Williams et al. 1980) and with incidence and mortality from CHD and other diseases (Barefoot et al. 1983; Shekelle et al. 1983). High scores on the hostility scale used by Williams et al. (1980), Barefoot et al. (1983), and Shekelle et al. (1983) are achieved by endorsing items which indicate that one has little confidence in his fellow man, and sees people as dishonest, immoral, ugly, and mean. Although we are unaware of evidence bearing directly on this point, it seems reasonable to hypothesize that persons with such attitudes would be less likely than others to participate in research involving intervention.

As noted earlier, prevalence of Type A was substantially higher in MRFIT than WCGS. Although this could not have biased the relative risk by itself, it is possible that the higher prevalence was due to changes in the procedure for assessment which resulted in some men who would have been classified as Type B in WCGS being classified as Type A in MRFIT. Such misclassification would be most likely to occur between adjacent categories, e. g., A2 to A1, or B to X or A2, and would have little effect on comparisons of A1 with B. Since the adjusted relative risk of a first major coronary event for A1 vs. B was 0.99 (see Fig. 1), such misclassification is an unlikely explanation for the difference in results between MRFIT and WCGS.

Inter-judge reliability was apparently similar in both studies (Rosenman 1978; Multiple Risk Factor Intervention Trial Group 1979). However, the training of interviewers was much briefer in MRFIT than WCGS, and the opportunity for direct supervision was much more limited. Therefore, it is possible that the interviewers in MRFIT were, as a group, less skilled that the interviewers in WCGS, and that the recorded materials on which the auditors and Dr. Rosenman relied were consequently less adequate. Data to evaluate this possibility are not presently available. However, if this explanation were correct, it would imply that formidable problems exist in ensuring validity of global assessments of behavior pattern, and that procedures for making valid assessments may not be generally accessible to other investigators. How does one determine *a priori* whether or not assessments are being made in a valid manner? This question deserves serious attention.

Bias due to misclassification could also have occurred if men who were correctly classified as Type A at entry subsequently changed both their behavior pattern and their risk of CHD. This seems an unlikely explanation for the absence of an association in MRFIT. Measurements of serum cholesterol level, diastolic blood pressure, and cigarette smoking at the first screening visit were positively and significantly associated with risk of first major coronary events in MRFIT despite the attention that was focused on changing these risk factors. In contrast, no systematic attempt was made to change Type A behavior.

Finally, with regard to end points, the crude relative risks associated with Type A behavior in WCGS were 2.12 for all CHD, 2.16 for symptomatic MI, 2.12 for clinically unrecognized MI, 2.97 for angina pectoris, and 2.21 for CHD death (Rosenman et al. 1975, 1976). The fact that behavior pattern was uniformly associated in WCGS with these various categories of end points, and the absence of an association in MRFIT between behavior pattern and CHD death, make differences in procedures for detecting and classifying endpoints an unlikely explanation for the difference in outcome.

Clearly, many questions remain to be answered, and it would be unwarranted to conclude that the Type A behavior pattern, or some aspects of it, have no association with risk of CHD. On the contrary, the French-Belgian Collaborative Group (1982) has recently reported a positive association prospectively between Type A as assessed by the Bortner scale and risk of CHD. These new findings add to the body of evidence that has been reviewed elsewhere (Dembroski et al. 1978; Review Panel on Coronary-Prone Behavior and Coronary Heart Disease 1981; Stamler 1980; Matthews 1982). However, failure to confirm the earlier findings of WCGS, despite use of the structured interview and the JAS, a detailed protocol, and a high level of quality control, raises questions about the generalizability of the Type A hypothesis in its present form, and about the predictive validity of the procedures currently used to assess behavior pattern. Until these questions are resolved by further research, it is our judgement that the status of Type A as a risk factor for CHD is uncertain.

Acknowledgments. The authors express deep appreciation to the interviewers and auditors: Dorothy Amundsen, Joyce Graham, Susan Grube, Victoria Perez, Beth Shucker, Audrey Simberkoff, and Dorothy White; to Steven Broste, formerly at the MRFIT Coordinating Center, for overseeing management of data; to Dr Ray H. Rosenman for his important contributions in all matters relating to the assessment of behavior pattern; to Dr. C. David Jenkins and Dr. Stephen J. Zyzanski for providing the procedure for scoring the JAS; and to the participants for their cooperation. This project was supported by funds from the National Heart, Lung, and Blood Institute under several contracts, including NHLBI NO1-HV-22971.

Credit Roster

The principal investigators and senior staff of the clinical, coordinating and support centers, the NHLBI, and members of the MRFIT Policy Advisory Board and Mortality Review Committee are as follows

Steering Committee
- O. Paul, MD (chairperson)

American Health Foundation, Mahoney Institute for Health Maintenance, New York
- C. B. Arnold, MD, MPH (principal investigator)
- R. Mandriota, MS, MEd
- R. P. Ames, MD
- J. Ruff Eisenbach, RN
- E. Bohm

Boston University, Boston
- H. E. Thomas, Jr. MD (principal investigator)
- W. B. Kannel, MD (co-principal investigator)
- R. Rotondo, MA
- J. Connors, RD
- F. N. Brand, MD
- L. K. Smith, MD
- M. T. Prisco, RN
- P. Greene, MA

Cox Heart Institute, Kettering, Ohio
- P. Kezdi, MD (principal investigator)

E. L. Stanley, MD (co-principal investigator)
W. L. Black, MD
F. A. Ernst, PhD
E. J. Case, RN, MS
V. Bentley
D. Covert, MS
M. Lucius, RD, MEd
F. Paris
R. Semmett
L. Skotko

Dade County Department of Public Health, Miami
G. Christakis, MD, MPH (principal investigator)
J. M. Burr, MD (co-principal investigator)
T. A. Gerace, PhD (co-principal investigator)
M. E. Wilcox, RD, MEd
D. Bramson, RD, MS
J. Benezra, MEd
J. Weddle
J. Kaye, MEd
M. Padron

Dalhousie University (MRFIT ECG Center), Halifax, Nova Scotia, Canada
P. M. Rautaharju, MD, PhD (principal investigator)
H. Wolf, PhD

Harvard University, Boston
R. C. Benfari, PhD (principal investigator)
K. M. McIntyre, MD, JD (co-principal investigator)
O. Paul, MD (co-principal investigator)
E. Danielson, MA
J. Ockene, PhD
D. Kousch-Howard, RN
A. D. Baldwin, MD

Kaiser Foundation Research Institute, Portland, Ore
J. B. Wild, MD (principal investigator)
M. Greenlick, PhD (co-principal investigator)
J. Grover, MD (co-principal investigator)
S. Lamb
J. Bailey
J. Dyer, MPH
B. Brokop, RN
V. Stevens, PhD
G. Bailey, RN

Lankenau Hospital, Philadelphia
W. Holmes, PhD (principal investigator)
J. E. Pickering, MD (co-principal investigator)
J. Allaire, MEd
E. L. Duffy, RD
D. Fellon, RN
B. Feinstein, MSA
D. Hutchins, MD
G. Rubel, RD

National Center for Disease Control, Atlanta
G. R. Cooper, RhD, MD (principal investigator)
D. D. Bayse, PhD
D. T. Miller, PhD
A. Hainline, Jr, PhD
M. Kuchmak, PhD
D. A. Wiebe, PhD
C. L. Winn
L. Taylor
B. L. Botero
J. B. Gill, Jr

New Jersey Medical School, Newark
N. L. Lasser, MD, PhD (principal investigator)
N. Hymowitz, PhD (co-principal investigator)
K. C. Mezey, MD
B. Munves, PhD
E. Parell, RD
S. Burgio, MS, RD
V. Lasser, MA, RD
B. Johnson
S. Jeffrey
E. Rice

Northwestern University, Chicago
J. Stamler, MD (principal investigator)
D. Moss, MS
V. Persky, MD
E. Robinson, MS
L. Van Horn, MA, RD
K. Shannon, MA
D. Meyers, MD

University of Chicago
L. Cohen, MD (principal investigator)
J. Morgan, RhD (co-principal investigator)
G. Grundmann, MS, RD
T. D. Vestal, PA
B. Huang

St Joseph's Hospital Chicago
D. M. Berkson, MD (principal investigator)
G. Lauger, MS
S. Grujic, MD
D. Obradovic, MD
E. Pardo
S. Dua, MS
S. McGowan

Institutes of Medical Sciences-University of California, San Francisco and Berkeley
J. Billings, PhD, MPH (principal investigator)
S. B. Hulley, MD, MPH (co-principal investigator)
W. M. Smith, MD, MPH (co-principal investigator)

S. L. Syme, PhD (co-principal investigator)
R. Cohen, MS
L. Dzvonik, MA, RD
L. Roos
M. Kahn, RN
Institutes of Medical Sciences, San Francisco
Central Laboratory, San Francisco
G. M. Widdowson, PhD (co-principal investigator)
G. Z. Williams, MD (co-principal investigator)
S. B. Hulley, MD, MPH (co-principal investigator)
M. L. Kuehneman (laboratory manager)
Rush-Presbyterian-St Luke's Medical Center, Chicago
J. A. Schoenberger, MD (principal investigator)
J. C. Schoenenberger, PhD
R. B. Shekelle, PhD
G. S. Neri, MD
T. Dolecek, MS, RD
E. Betz, RD
L. Skweres, RD
F. Oppenheimer, RD
N. Gernhofer, MS, RD
G. G. Hardy
E. McGill, RN
Y. Hall, MS
Rutgers Medical School, Piscataway, NJ
N. H. Wright, MD, MPH (principal investigator)
S. A. Kopel, PhD (co-principal investigator)
K. R. Suckerman, PhD
M. Schorin, MPH, RD
St Louis Heart Association, St Louis
N. Simon, MD (principal investigator)
J. D. Cohen, MD (co-principal investigator)
E. Bunkers, RD
B. Ronchetto, RN
E. Grodsky
A. Fressola
J. Daniel-Gentry, MS, RN
R. Treiman, MD
W. Sullivan, MD
University of Alabama in Birmingham
H. W. Schnaper, MD (principal investigator)
G. H. Hughes, PhD (co-principal investigator)
A. Oberman, MD
C. C. Hill, PhD
R. Allen, PA
C. Bragg, RD
S. Stokes, RD
P. Johnson
University of California, Davis
N. O. Borhani, MD (principal investigator)
C. Sugars, RD
K. Kirkpatrick
M. Lee, MD
S. DeBourelando, MPH, RD
F. LaBaw, RN
J. Turner-Tucker
University of Maryland, Baltimore
R. W. Sherwin, MB, BChir (principal investigator)
M. S. Sexton, PhD, MPH (co-principal investigator)
N. E. Cusack, RD
Q. T. F. de Barros, MS
P. C. Dischinger, PhD
J. Fox Spizler, MS
J. D. Heiner, MD
M. B. Pilkington, RN, MSN
B. L. Scanlon, MA
University of Minnesota, Minneapolis
R. H. Grimm, Jr, MD, MPH (principal investigator)
M. Mittelmark, PhD (co-principal investigator)
R. S. Crow, MD (co-principal investigator)
H. Blackburn, MD (co-principal investigator)
D. Jacobs, PhD (co-investigator)
D. Rains, MS
M. McDonald, RN, MS
K. Lenz
University of Minnesota ECG Coding Center, Minneapolis
R. J. Prineas, MB, PhD (director)
R. C. Crow, MD (associate director)
University of Minnesota, Nutrition Coding Center, Minneapolis
I. M. Buzzard, PhD (director)
P. V. Grambach (former director)
J. Wenz, MS (associate director)
University of Minnesota Coordinating Center, Minneapolis
M. O. Kjelsberg, PhD (principal investigator)
G. E. Bartsch, ScD (co-principal investigator)
J. D. Neaton, MS (co-principal investigator)
B. M. Aus
J. Bendickson
S. K. Broste, MS
J. E. Connett, PhD
A. G. DuChene
D. A. Durkin
D. L. Gorder, MS
P. V. Grambach
G. A. Grandits, MS
D. H. Hultgren
A. Knickerbocker
W. L. Rasmussen
K. H. Svendsen, MS
L. Wille

University of Pittsburgh
- L. H. Kuller, MD, DPH (principal investigator)
- R. McDonald, MD (co-principal investigator)
- A. Caggiula, PhD (co-principal investigator)
- L. Falvo-Gerard, MN, MPH (co-principal investigator)
- E. Meilahn, MPH
- N. C. Milas, RD, MS
- R. Russell, RD, DPH
- J. Horbiak, RD, MPH
- M. Alman, RN
- K. Southwick, ASCP
- R. Moyer
- E. Gahagan

University of South Carolina, Columbia
- W. K. Giese, PhD (principal investigator)
- J. F. Martin, MD (co-principal investigator)
- J. A. Keith, PhD (co-principal investigator)
- H. H. Harrison, RN
- D. E. Mathis, MAT
- C. K. Brown

University of Southern California, Los Angeles
- E. Fishman, MD (principal investigator)
- L. Wampler, PhD
- G. Newmark, MA, RD
- F. Rosenfield, MPH
- S. Siddiqui, MD
- W. Savage, MS, RD
- A. Bradford, MS, RD

Policy Advisory Board
- W. Insull, Jr, MD (chairperson)
- J. W. Farquhar, MD
- C. D. Jenkins, PhD
- E. Papaport, MD
- D. J. Thompson, PhD
- H. A. Tyroler, MD
- P. W. Willis III, MD
- W. T. Friedewald, MD
- W. Zukel, MD

Mortality Review Committee
- J. T. Doyle, MD (chairman)
- H. B. Burchell, MD
- P. N. Yu, MD
- P. W. Willis III, MD (former member)

National Heart, Lung, and Blood Institute Staff, Bethesda, Md
- W. T. Friedewald, MD program director)
- C. D. Furberg, MD (project office director)
- J. A. Cutler, MD (scientific project officer)
- W. J. Zukel, MD (former program director)
- E. R. Passamani, MD (former scientific project officer)
- C. T. Kaelber, MD (former scientific project officer)
- M. E. Farrand, RD, MS
- J. L. Tillotson, RD, MA
- J. I. Verter, PhD
- M. C. Wu, PhD
- T. Gordon
- M. Halperin, PhD
- D. L. McGee, PhD
- T. P. Blaszkowski, PhD
- K. A. Eberlein, MPH
- C. E. Harris
- P. L. Dern, MD
- L. M. Friedman, MD
- G. S. May, MB, BChir
- A. J. Vargosko, PhD

References

Barefoot JC, Dahlstrom WG, Williams RB Jr (1983) Hostility, CHD incidence, and total mortality: 25-year follow-up study of 255 physicians. Psychosom Med 45: 59-63

Benfari RC, Sherwin R (eds) (1981) Forum: the Multiple Risk Factor Intervention Trial (MRFIT). The methods and impact of intervention over four years. Prev Med 10: 387-553

Bishop YMM, Fienberg SE, Holland PW (1975) Discrete multivariate analysis: theory and practice MIT Press, Cambridge

Brand RJ (1978) Coronary-prone behavior as an independent risk factor for coronary heart disease. In: Dembroski TM, Weiss SM, Shields JL, et al. (eds) Coronary-prone behavior. Springer, Berlin Heidelberg New York, pp 11-24

Criqui MH (1974) Response bias and risk ratios in epidemiologic studies. Am J Epidemiol 109: 394-399

Dembroski TM, Weiss SM, Shields JL, et al. (eds) (1978) Coronary-prone behavior. Springer, Berlin Heidelberg New York

French-Belgian Collaborative Group (1982) Ischemic heart disease and psychological patterns - prevalence and incidence studies in Belgium and France. Adv Cardiol 29: 25-31

Haynes SG, Feinleib M, Kannel WB (1980) The relationship of psychosocial factors to coronary heart disease in the Framingham Study: III. 8 year incidence of coronary heart disease. Am J Epidemiol 111: 37-58

Haynes SG, Feinleib M, Eaker ED (1983) Type A behaviour and the ten-year incidence of coronary heart disease in the Framingham Heart Study. In: Rosenman RH (ed) Psychosomatic risk factors and coronary heart disease. Huber, Bern, pp 80-92
Jenkins CD (1978) A comparative review of the interview and questionnaire methods in the assessment of the coronary-prone behavior pattern. In: Dembroski TM, Weiss SM, Shields JL, et al. (eds) Coronary-prone behavior. Springer, Berlin Heidelberg New York, pp 71-88
Jenkins CD, Rosenman RH, Friedman M (1967) Development of an objective psychological test for the determination of the coronary-prone behavior pattern in employed men. J Chronic Dis 20: 371-379
Jenkins CD, Zyzanski SJ, Rosenman RH (1971) Progress toward validation of a computer-scored test for the Type A coronary-prone behavior pattern. Psychosom Med 33: 193-202
Jenkins CD, Rosenman RH, Zyzanski SJ (1974) Prediction of clinical coronary heart disease by a test for the coronary-prone behavior pattern. N Engl J Med 290: 1271-1275
Kalbfleisch JD, Prentice RL (1980) The statistical analysis of failure time data. Wiley, New York
Matthews KA (1982) Psychological perspectives on the type A behavior pattern. Psychol Bull 91: 293-323
Multiple Risk Factor Intervention Trial Group (1979) The MRFIT Behavior Pattern Study: I. Study design, procedures, and reproducibility of behavior pattern judgements. J Chronic Dis 32: 293-305
Multiple Risk Factor Intervention Trial Research Group (1982) Multiple Risk Factor Intervention Trial: risk factor changes and mortality results. JAMA 248: 1465-1477
Prineas RJ, Crow RS, Blackburn H (1982) The Minnesota code manual of electrocardiographic findings. Wright, Boston
Review Panel on Coronary-Prone Behavior and Coronary Heart Disease (1981) Coronary-prone behavior and coronary heart disease: a critical review. Circulation 63: 1199-1215
Rose GA, Blackburn H (1968) Cardiovascular survey methods. WHO Monogr Ser, no. 56. World Health Organization, Geneva
Rosenman RH (1978) The interview method of assessment of the coronary-prone behavior pattern. In: Dembroski TM, Weiss SM, Shields JL, et al. (eds) Coronary-prone behavior. Springer, Berlin Heidelberg New York, pp 55-69
Rosenman RH, Friedman M, Straus R, et al. (1964) A predictive study of coronary heart disease: the Western Collaborative Group Study. JAMA 189: 15-22
Rosenman RH, Brand RJ, Jenkins CD, et al. (1975) Coronary heart disease in the Western Collaborative Group Study: final follow-up experience of 8.5 years. JAMA 233: 872-877
Rosenman RH, Brand RJ, Sholtz RI, et al. (1976) Multivariate prediction of coronary heart disease during 8.5 year follow-up in the Western Collaborative Group Study. Am J Cardiol 37: 903-910
Shekelle RB, Gale M, Ostfeld AM, et al. (1983) Hostility, risk of coronary heart disease, and mortality. Psychosom Med 45: 109-114
Stamler J (1980) Type A behavior pattern: an established major risk factor for coronary heart disease? The key life-style trait responsible for the coronary epidemic? In: Rapaport E (ed) Current controversies in cardiovascular disease. Saunders, Philadelphia, pp 76-106
US Bureau of the Census (1971) 1970 Census of population classified index of industries and occupations. US Government Printing Office, Washington DC
Williams RB Jr, Haney TL, Lee KL, et al (1980) Type A behavior, hostility, and coronary atherosclerosis. Psychosom Med 42: 539-549
Wood LL (1978) Comparison of linear trends in binomial proportions. Biometrics 34: 496-504

The Predictive Power of the A/B Typology in Holland: Results of a 9.5-Year Follow-Up Study*

A. Appels,[1] P. Mulder,[2] M. van't Hof,[3] C. D. Jenkins,[4] J. van Houtem,[1] and F. Tan[5]

Introduction

After the establishment of a positive association between type A behavior and the incidence of myocardial infarction in both the Western Collaborative Group Study (WCGS) and the Framingham Study, the question arises whether this behavior pattern has predictive power in other countries besides the U.S.A. Several European case control and cross-sectional studies have confirmed the higher prevalence of the type A behavior pattern (Verhagen et al. 1980; Appels et al. 1982; Falger et al. 1985) among coronary patients. These studies do not however answer the question of whether type A behavior predicts coronary heart disease (CHD). The Kaunas-Rotterdam Intervention Study (KRIS) provided the opportunity of testing the hypothesis that type A behavior is unconfoundedly associated with the incidence of CHD.

The Kaunas-Rotterdam Study

Between 1972 and 1974, a cardiovascular screening program was carried out in Kaunas (Lithuania, SSR) and Rotterdam. The main objective of this feasibility study was to acquire experience in multifactorial intervention (Glasunov et al. 1981). In each city, a sample of 4000 males between 45 and 59 years of age representing various socioeconomic strata of an open urban population was identified, subjected to a baseline survey, and subsequently invited to participate in the screening. In Rotterdam, 3365 males (88%) participated in the screening. The most important reasons for nonparticipation were outright refusal (8%) and no response at all (4%).

The risk factors measured at screening were: blood pressure, cholesterol, glucose, Quetelet Index, ECG, the Reeder Stress Scale, education, occupation, the Jenkins Activity Survey, Rose's Questionnaire to assess angina pectoris, health status, and medical history, and habits relating to smoking, drinking and physical activity. Details of the recruiting and measurement procedures have been described elsewhere (Glasunov et al. 1981).

* This study is supported by grant no. 31 009 from the Dutch Heart Foundation.
1 Department of Medical Psychology, State University of Limburg, Limburg, Holland
2 Department of Epidemiology, Municipal Public Health Services, Rotterdam, Holland
3 Department of Mathematical Statistics, Nijmegen University, Nijmegen, Holland
4 Department of Preventive Medicine University of Texas, Galveston, U.S.A.
5 Department of Statistics, State University of Limburg, Limburg, Holland

Biological and Psychological Factors
in Cardiovascular Disease
Ed. by T. H. Schmidt, T. M. Dembroski, and G. Blümchen

Assessment of Type A Behavior in the KRIS Study

In order to assess type A behavior, the Jenkins Activity Survey (JAS, form B) (Jenkins et al. 1979) was translated into Dutch and its back-translation into English discussed with the author of the test. Some pretests had shown that the Dutch translation needed some minor adaptations, especially with regard to those items that invite the respondent to compare himself with other people. To these items, the response category "the same as others" had to be added.

The JAS was completed by 3171 participants (94%). Noncompletion was mainly due to administration errors. The educational level of 1% of the sample was too low to permit JAS completion.

To study the construct validity of the JAS, a subsample of 243 participants was interviewed by means of the structured interview (SI). This subsample consisted of participants who were invited for a second screening because of possible glucose in tolerance. This sample was chosen because no association between type A behavior and glucose intolerance was expected (and empirically not found in this sample).

JAS scores were computed in two ways. Scores for the overall type A scale and the three subscales of job involvement (J), hard-drivingness (H), and speed and impatience (S) were computed using the weights obtained in the WCGS (5). Furthermore a Dutch adaptation score was calculated because an item analysis had shown that a number of items did not contribute to the replication of the SI by the questionnaire. A latent trait analysis was used for the Dutch adaptation. This analysis resulted in a 36-item form which had a correspondence with the SI of 74% (Appels et al. 1982). During the years between the adaptation of the Dutch form and the follow-up study, this scoring system was found to have a number of practical disadvantages (especially for clinical use). Therefore, a simpler item analysis was performed which resulted in a selection of 24 items, all of which correlated with the SI. These items are dichotomized, resulting in a scale with a minimum score of zero and a maximum score of 24 (Appels 1985).

The internal consistency of this scale is 0.84 (Crombach's alpha). The percentage of correct classifications is 73% for those assessed as type A and 75% for those assessed as type B. In the next paragraphs, we shall report on the 24-item form of the Dutch adaptation only.

Follow-up Study

The KRIS study was designed as a feasibility study and not as a follow-up study. No regular check-ups were made, but after a period of about 9.5 years, an extensive study of the original participants was carried out.

Those who were still alive received a mailed questionnaire asking for any heart troubles they might have experienced in the previous 10 years. If the answers contained the slightest indication that a coronary event could have occurred during the follow-up period, a physician contacted the general practitioner and (in the case of policlinical or clinical contact with a hospital) the cardiologist. The death certificates of those who had died between the initial screening and the end of follow-up were collected and the cause of death noted.

Table 1. Data base of the KRIS follow-up study

	(n)	(%)
Follow-up survey of nonparticipants	232	7
Lost to follow-up (emigration, etc.)	52	2
Deceased	350	10
Respondents	2731	81
	3365	100

Table 2. Classification of former KRIS participants after 9.5 years' follow-up

	(n)
Nonrespondent morbidity questionnaire	232
Lost to follow-up (emigration, etc.)	52
Unknown cause of death	23
Noncardiac cause of death	215
Fatal myocardial infarction	112
Nonfatal myocardial infarction	157
Angina pectoris	54
Bypass operation	21
No coronary heart disease	2499

Table 1 describes the data base of the follow-up study. Of the participants, 10% were no longer alive and 2% lost to follow-up owing to emigration.

The percentage of nonrespondents among those who were still alive was only 8%. However, it was found that the number of heavy smokers among the nonrespondents was disproportionately high.

During the follow-up period, 157 nonfatal and 112 fatal coronary events occurred (Table 2). Soft events (i.e., documented cases of angina pectoris and coronary bypass surgery without prior or subsequent myocardial infarction) were observed in 54 and 21 cases respectively. The number of those suffering from angina pectoris is probably underestimated because the presence of angina pectoris was only noted when it was documented by hospital records. The definitions used to classify the nonfatal cases are included in the Appendix. It should be noted that those who died because of myocardial infarction may have experienced one or more nonfatal events before death. Owing to the design of the follow-up study however, that information is unknown.

Data Analysis

Before data analysis, those groups who might have had CHD at screening were excluded. Criteria for exclusion were (a) the presence of angina pectoris as assessed by the Rose Questionnaire and (b) Minnesotacode I.1-3; IV.1-3; V.1-3; or VII.1. Furthermore, the group with insufficient follow-up data, i.e., nonrespondents, lost to follow-up and those whose cause of death was noncardiac or unknown, were ex-

Table 3. Association of type A (SI) with fatal and nonfatal myocardial infarction during follow-up

	Type A	Type B	Total
Coronary event	7	11	18
No coronary event	92	99	191
Total	99	110	209

Table 4. Association of type A (SI) with fatal events during follow-up

	Type A	Type B	Total
Fatal event	4[a]	0	4
No fatal event	110	129	239
Total	114	129	243

[a] Fischer exact probability $P = 0.04$

Table 5. Mean scores of coronary cases (fatal and nonfatal events) and those who remained free of CHD

	Case	Noncase	*P*
JAS - AB	0.3	0.7	n.s.
Subscale J	-12.5	-12.0	n.s.
Subscale H	9.5	9.4	n.s.
Subscale S	-3.9	-3.9	n.s.
Dutch form	12.11	11.73	n.s.

cluded. The group of noncardiac deaths was excluded because they might have experienced a myocardial infarction prior to death.

Results

Type A Behavior as Assessed by the SI and the Incidence of CHD

Table 3 presents the association between type A behavior and the combined incidence of fatal and nonfatal infarctions for the small group interviewed by the SI. Among the 99 participants assessed as type A, seven coronary events occurred (7%), whereas 10% of the type B participants experienced a coronary event. This difference does not tend to support the hypothesis that type A is predictive of CHD, but is far from significant. When fatal events only are taken into account, the total number of observations increases because those who died of noncardiac causes and living nonrespondents are also included in this analysis. Fatal events either an initial or a recurrent but fatal event, occurred in type A subjects only. The association is significant and tends to support the hypothesis that type A is predictive of CHD (Table 4).

Table 6. Mean scores of those who developed angina pectoris or underwent by-pass surgery (cases) and those who remained free of CHD (noncases)

	Case	Noncase	*F*	*P*
JAS - AB	0.9	0.7	0.05	n.s.
Subscale J	-11.4	-12.0	0.29	n.s.
Subscale H	11.2	9.3	3.66	0.06
Subscale S	-4.2	-3.9	0.03	n.s.
Dutch form	13.3	11.8	4.32	0.03

Type A Behavior as Assessed by the JAS and the Incidence of CHD

It was possible to study the correlation between the JAS and the incidence of CHD in a much larger sample of which the exact size depended on the number of missing values for each subscale. On the average, the analyses are based on a total of 2500 subjects.

Table 5 shows the results of the univariate association between the JAS and the cumulative incidence of nonfatal and fatal myocardial infarction. None of the four scales was found to be associated with the incidence of myocardial infarction.

Table 6 shows the association betwen the JAS and such soft events as angina pectoris and coronary bypass. Both the hard-drivingness scale and the Dutch adaptation of the JAS were found to be associated with the incidence of soft events.

Multivariate Analyses of the JAS

Although no association between any of the JAS scales and somatic risk factors was found at screening, multivariate analyses and analyses of distinct strata were performed. Separate analyses for those with high and low education levels, for the follow-up years 1-5 and 6-10, or for the younger and older halves of the participants did not substantially change the negative correlation described above. Multiple logistic regression analyses also failed to show that the Dutch adaptation of the JAS contributed to the prediction of future coronary events.

Discussion

It is a well known principle that those who want to plague a scientist repeat his study but use a smaller sample and a slightly different method to assess the predictor variable. The group interviewed here was small, and its mean age 5 years over the mean age of those studied in the WCGS. Errors in the assessment of type A behavior are possible. The first author of this study, A. Appels, was trained by Rosenman in 1971. To check the agreement of his assessments with the "golden standard", he assessed 40 interviews from the WCGS in 1972 and classified 85% of these interviews correctly. Given these limitations, the significance of positively replicating the WCGS finding that the incidence of fatal coronary events is associated with Type A behavior pattern should not be underestimated.

The absence of a relation between the JAS and the incidence of myocardial infarction and cardiac death is disappointing. Its prospective association with angina pectoris and coronary bypass surgery, however, indicates that the test has some cardiovascular relevance. Using additive models, the JAS did not contribute to the prediction of the cumulative incidence in multivariate analyses, but moderator effects may show up in interactive models. These analyses are currently being performed.

References

Appels A (1985) Jenkins activity Survey: dutch translation and adaptation. Swets and Leitlinger, Lissboa

Appels A, Jenkins CD, Rosenman RH (1982) Coronary-prone behavior in the Netherlands: a cross-cultural validation study. J Beh Med 5: 83-90

Falger P, Appels A, Bekkers J (1985) Biographische Analyse und Herzinfarkt. Z Gerontol 18 (to be published)

Glasunov I, Dowd J, Baubiniene A, Grabauskas V, Sturmans F, Schuurman J (eds) (1981) The Kaunas-Rotterdam intervention study. Elsevier/North Holland, Amsterdam

Jenkins CD, Zyzanski S, Rosenman R (1979) Jenkins activity survey manual. Psychological Corporation, New York

Verhagen F, Nass C, Appels A, van den Bastelaer A, Winnubst J (1980) Cross-validation of the A/B typology in the Netherlands. Psychoth Psychosom 34: 178-186

Appendix: Definition of Myocardial Infarction used to classify nonfatal cases during follow-up study. Anamnestic, electrocardiographic, and enzymal findings were used to make a classification based on a number of points.

Myocardial Infarction

Anamnestic Data

Chest pain
- sudden appearance of increase
- unrelated to physical effort
- duration longer than 20 min
- pressing or spastic character
- no reaction to nitroglycerine
- radiation

(One characteristic, 1 point; two characteristics, 2 points)

Electrocardiogram

Presence of "injury current"

Minnesota code 1.1 or 1.2 (Q wave deviations) and/or 7.1 (left bundle block; in the case of an initial myocardial infarction

Description by cardiologist of a "typical myocardial infarction" (One of the above characteristics, 2 points)

Minnesota code 1.3 (moderate Q wave deviations) and/or 5.1 or 5.2 (negative T)
Description by the cardiologist of "suspected myocardial infarction" (One of the above characteristics, 1 point)

Enzyme Levels

Both SGOT and CPK levels above values considered to be normal in the hospital (2 points)
Either SGOT levels or CPK levels above those considered normal in the hospital (1 point)
Evolution of enzyme values suggesting a probable diagnosis of myocardial infarction (1 point)

Coding

Cases in which all data are available
- 0-1 point: no myocardial infarction
- 2-3 points: possible myocardial infarction
- 4 points: probable myocardial infarction
- 5-6 points: certain myocardial infarction

Cases in which only two criteria are available
- 0-1 point: no myocardial infarction
- 2 points: possible myocardial infarction
- 3-4 points: probable myocardial infarction

Cases in which only a general clinical diagnosis is available
- probable myocardial infarction

Angina Pectoris (AP)

Possible AP: anamnesis by cardiologist indicative of AP
Probable AP: anamnesis by cardiologist indicative of AP and ECG deviations during pain or during physical excercise testing
Certain AP: anamnesis by cardiologist indicative of AP and occlusions found during catheterization

Type A and Other Psychosocial Factors in Relation to Coronary Heart Disease

F. KITTEL[1]

Five different aspects of the relation of psychosocial factors to coronary heart disease (CHD) will be considered: psychosocial interrelations, the association of psychosocial factors with the prevalence of coronary risk factors and with CHD, and the influence of psychosocial factors on the evolution of coronary risk factors and on the incidence of coronary heart disease.

The present findings were derived from data gathered under the auspices of the Belgian Heart Disease Prevention Project (BHDPP), which is part of an international randomized controlled trial of multifactorial intervention involving 60881 men aged 40–59 years. The whole study has been designated the World Health Organization European Collaborative Group (WHOECG 1974). In the BHDPP, 30 factories were paired off (Fig. 1) and assigned to a control ($n = 10900$) or to an intervention group ($n = 8509$). Prevalence data were obtained for the total intervention group ($n = 7398$) and for 10% of the control group ($n = 901$) (De Backer et al. 1977).

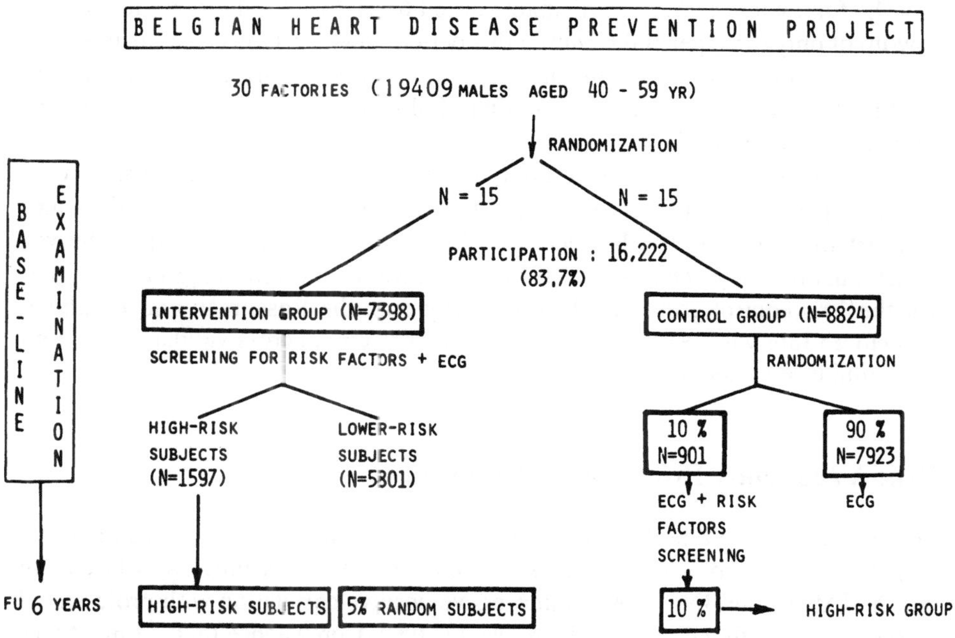

Fig. 1. Organization of the Belgian Heart Disease Prevention Project. *FU*, follow-up

1 Université de Medicine et de Pharmacie, Laboratoire D'Epidemiologie et de Medicine Sociale, Campus Erasme CP. 590/5, 808 route de Lennik, 1070 Bruxelles, Belgium

Biological and Psychological Factors
in Cardiovascular Disease
Ed. by T. H. Schmidt, T. M. Dembroski, and G. Blümchen

Table 1. Type A prevalence (%) by professional status and educational level (10% control group)

Social variable	Category	SI	BNP	JAS-AB	JAS-S	JAS-J	JAS-H
Professional status	Top executives	67	53	58	48	61	48
	Middle manager	61	43	58	43	26	47
	White collar	50	42	54	31	15	34
	Vocational	37	26	48	30	14	35
	Skilled blue collar	33	21	32	21	4	33
	Semi-skilled blue collar	29	16	25	24	0	45
	Unskilled blue collar	15	10	27	15	0	33
	p^a	***	***	***	***	***	NS
Educational level	University	67	49	56	47	62	47
	Graduate school	70	67	62	46	31	39
	Post secondary school	64	30	59	32	23	43
	Normal school	53	36	59	27	24	49
	Senior high school	61	42	55	42	24	42
	Junior high school	46	35	42	31	9	37
	Primary school	27	16	31	21	3	36
	p^a	***	***	***	***	***	NS

[a] *** < 0.001

The follow-up of 16222 participants lasted 6 years with a mortality loss to follow-up of only three per 1000. During this period, low-risk subjects in the intervention group had access to mass media information, while high-risk subjects were given face-to-face counselling. At the final follow-up of the whole sample, the participation rate was 73%.

At baseline examination, in addition to bioclinical measures, social characteristics, and personality trait assessments, similarity to the type A behavioral pattern was determined using the Bortner scale (BNP) and the Jenkins Activity Survey questionnaire (JAS) (Jenkins et al. 1979) for the whole intervention group as well as for the 10% control group. In the latter subgroup, the Rosenman and Friedman Structured Interview (SI) was also used in order to obtain cross-validation for both self-administered questionnaires.

Type A and Other Psychosocial Interrelations

In the BHDPP, the type A behavior pattern and its specific components of speed, impatience, and job involvement, as determined by the Rosenman and Friedman SI, the JAS, or the BNP show an impressive positive correlation with professional status and educational level, with an average type A prevalence that is three times greater in the highest categories. Many earlier studies discovered the same positive relationship between type A and education or profession (Mettlin 1976; Shekelle et al. 1976; Waldron et al. 1977; Haynes et al. 1978a; Jenkins et al. 1979).

The association of type A behavior with educational level and professional status (Table 1) seems to be both independent and synergistic, as shown by bivariate and multivariate analysis (Kittel et al. 1982). Actually, the precocious learning of

Table 2. Comparison of type A among executives and white collar workers 40-54 years in the WCGS and in the BHDPP (10% control group)

Population	Interview					Interview	BNP	JAS-AB
	B4	B3	AB	A2	A1	A2+A1 (%)	⩾196 (%)	⩾0 (%)
WCGS	11	38	1	41	9	50	50	50
BHDPP	1	26	21	45	7	52	38	52

Table 3. Validity, sensibility, and specificity (%) of the Bortner scale (BNP) and JAS (JAS-AB) for total group, group of executives and white collar workers, and group of blue collar workers (10% control group)

Measure	Population	Validity	Sensibility	Specificity
BNP	total	72	48	87
	executives + white collar workers	68	55	82
	blue collar workers	75	40	90
JAS-AB	total	68	61	74
	executives + white collar workers	70	72	68
	blue collar workers	67	47	76

Validity: global agreement
Sensibility: A1 + A2 agreement
Specificity: AB + B3 + B4 agreement

type A behavior, revealed through the education gradient, appears to be further reinforced by a particular professional and family life situation. Cultural differences in the overall prevalence of type A, for instance between the United States (Western Collaborative Group Study, WCGS) and Belgium (BHDPP), could be partially due to socioprofessional differences in the populations studied.

As can be seen from Table 2, when a sample comparable with the WCGS is selected in the BHDPP, namely executives and white collar workers aged 40-54 years, the prevalence of type A is similar in both countries as far as the SI and JAS are concerned, although in Belgium there are fewer extreme and more intermediate examples of type A behavior. Related to the issue of cultural influences, I would like to mention some findings of three outstanding researchers in this field. According to Matthews and Krantz (1976), the environmental influence on type A behavior is confirmed by an absence of genetic determination of this syndrome, with the possible exception of the trait of hard-driving behavior. After studying black and white men and women, Waldron et al. (1977) found that "how type A is expressed in a particular group may depend to a considerable extent on the general norms and values of the group". Furthermore, in an excellent book on the theoretical and conceptual analysis of type A, Price (1982), stated that "the socio-cultural belief that an open economy is good appears to play a major role in encouraging Type A. ... In practice, unlimited upward mobility is applied differently in our society" (pp. 42, 43).

One could conclude that type A is linked to a certain value system and therefore reserved for a particular category of individuals. Looking more closely at the very low prevalence of type A in lower social categories, one could also ask if type A is really less prevalent in those categories or whether the assessment instruments are inadequate. If we still assume the SI to be the "gold standard," then the following answer could be given.

As shown in Table 3, although the validity or global agreement between the SI and the two questionnaires is acceptable even for the blue collar category, agreement of type A classification in the blue collar group is quite low. This could indicate that the questionnaires are less adequate for this group, which, in turn, might partially explain why type A was not predictive for CHD among blue collar workers in the Framingham Study (Haynes et al. 1980).

Moreover, independently of socioprofessional class, overall type A appeared in our studies to be particularly correlated with neuroticism, as measured by the Eysenick Personality Inventory (EPI) (Kittel et al. 1982), and with subjective stress experienced at work (Kittel et al. 1983). This suggests firstly that type A subjects are prone to a certain emotional instability, if we use Eysenick's definition of neuroticism, and secondly that they are given to seeking out stressful situations or to perceiving situations as stressful.

Prevalence of Coronary Risk Factors

In the BHDPP, prevalence data on classic risk factors such as the Body Mass Index (BMI) or the ratio of weight to height^2, cholesterol levels, smoking, and systolic blood pressure were analyzed in relation to psychosocial variables.

A certain number of associations appeared by means of multiple regression analyses. For instance, a low BMI was associated with personality traits, namely more pronounced neuroticism, whereas higher cholesterol levels were linked to sociocultural variables such as being French speaking and of higher professional status. More cigarette smokers were found in the lower classes, and heavy cigarette smoking was more strongly related to psychological dimensions such as overall type A, impatience and a low anality score. Finally, high systolic blood pressure seemed to be associated with various psychosocial dimensions such as isolation, introversion and nonexpressed impatience. However, these findings reflect only tendencies, since the variability of the risk factors explained by these psychosocial dimensions is quite small.

It is perhaps more important to comprehend the association of psychosocial variables with the complete coronary risk profile. This profile has been assessed using the multiple logistic function (MLF) of which the formula is:

$$P = \frac{1}{1 + e^{-(\alpha + \beta_i \cdot x_i)}}$$

where P is the probability of developing a "hard" event (sudden death, fatal or nonfatal myocardial infarction, MI) in 5 years, x_i stands for the risk factors (age, BMI, cholesterol, smoking, and systolic blood pressure), and β_i is the weighting coefficient. The results of the multiple regression analysis are shown in Table 4.

It is obvious that, even if a less favorable risk profile is statistically linked with the status of belonging to the French culture and with a tendency to be more social-

Table 4. Stepwise multiple regression of initial coronary risk profile (MLF) by psychosocial variables ($n = 3974$)

Significant variables		R^2 (%)[a]
Language[b]	+	1.5
Social conformity (L-EPI)	+	1.1
JAS-J	/−/	0.7
Extraversion (E-EPI)	/−/	0.2
JAS-AB	+	0.2

language +, more French; social conformity +, more socially conforming; JAS-J /−/, less job involved; extraversion /−/, less extroverted; JAS-AB +, more type A

[a] R^2: Increment of squared multiple correlation coefficient
[b] Language: 1 Dutch; 2 French

ly conforming, less job involved, more introverted, and more type A, the association is in reality very weak or nonexistent.

The absence of an association between coronary risk profile and social class has been confirmed in two American studies (Shekelle et al. 1976; Haynes et al. 1978a). However in Norway (Holme et al. 1976) and in Great Britain (Marmot et al. 1978), a negative association was found.

The independence of overall type A or its components with the classic risk factors measured at rest has revealed a lack of association between type A and global coronary risk profile. As in the WCGS (Brand et al. 1976), the Western Electric Company Study (Shekelle et al. 1976), and the Framingham Study (Haynes et al. 1978a), the BHDPP also came to this same conclusion.

Concerning the relation of personality traits to coronary risk profile, one study's findings diverge from and another study corroborates our results. In Sweden, it has been shown that subjects at higher coronary risk were more extraverted and neurotic, as measured by the EPI (Floderus 1974). In the Framingham Study, on the other hand, no relationship was found between MLF and repressed or expressed anger or between MLF and tension or anxiety (Haynes et al. 1978a, b).

Prevalence of Coronary Heart Disease

In the intervention group of the BHDPP ($n = 6112$), the prevalence of coronary heart disease was analyzed by comparing healthy subjects (89%, called group A) and pathologic subjects (11%). The pathologic group was further subdivided into four subgroups:

1. Group B: 4% angina without ECG abnormalities
2. Group C: 0.7% angina with ECG abnormalities
3. Group D: 5.4% ECG abnormalities (unknown) without angina
4. Group E: 0.9% ECG abnormalities (known) without angina

Angina was determined by the Rose questionnaire (London School of Hygiene) (Rose and Blackburn 1968) and ECG abnormalities were considered present with Minnesota Code $I_{1\text{-}2\text{-}3}$, $IV_{1\text{-}2\text{-}3}$, or $V_{1\text{-}2\text{-}3}$.

Table 5. Multiple stepwise discriminant analysis applied to prevalence of CHD in the Belgian Heart Disease Prevention Project

Groups	Variables	F
A: free of CHD	age	***
versus	systolic blood pressure	***
B+C+D+E; all CHD cases	JAS-AB	***
	cholesterol	**
A: free of CHD	age	***
versus	JAS-AB	***
B+C: all angina		
A: free of CHD	age	***
versus	socio-occupational class	*
E: ECG abnormalities+	systolic blood pressure	*
no angina (known)	smoking /−/	*
	JAS-AB	*

* $P<0.05$; ** $P<0.01$; *** $P<0.001$

Several discriminant analyses were performed between these various groups and subgroups.

An example of this type of analysis with the JAS-AB is given in Table 5 (Kornitzer et al. 1981). The five classic risk factors were systematically entered. Besides the psychological factors, professional status was introduced as well. The most important results of multivariate analysis comparing subjects free of CHD and pathologic groups can be summarized as follows:

Social Variables. Pathologic subjects belonged more often to the French cultural group, were older, and showed higher systolic blood pressure and cholesterol levels. Being a member of the French cultural group remained a significant discriminator for the whole angina subgroup (B+C) and for the whole abnormal ECG subgroup (D+E), as well as for the subgroup with known abnormal ECG (E). One should note the general failure of professional status, educational level, or marital status to discriminate subjects both with and without CHD.

Psychological Variables. Positively, overall type A (based on JAS-AB and BNP), speed and impatience (JAS-S), and neuroticism (N-EPI) and, negatively, job involvement (JAS-J) appeared to be significant discriminators for all the various pathologic groups. Hard-driving behavior (JAS-H) seemed to be a discriminator only for the angina group. It should be stressed, though, that no psychological score was a discriminator for the nonsymptomatic pathologic state. However, the subject's knowledge of having ECG abnormalities was directly related to professional status.

No consensus has been reached concerning the association of social variables and the prevalence of CHD. In an earlier review of 35 mortality studies and 21 morbidity studies related to social class, an equal number of studies showed either a relation or no relation (Antonovsky 1968). Several reasons can account for those divergent results: different selection bias, definition of outcome, or lack of control for risk factors.

At this time, the evolution of CHD prevalence in our industrialized countries tends to be unfavorable for less educated subjects or subjects of lower professional status (Syme and Berkman 1976). Nonetheless, the independent contributions of social variables to the prevalence of CHD will not be fully understood unless the coronary risk profile is taken into account by means of appropriate multivariate analysis. This holds true for all psychosocial variables investigated.

The association of behavioral variables with the prevalence of CHD has been widely studied. At least 15 American and European studies have dealt with this subject, most of them showing a positive association of type A, measured according to different methods, with the prevalence of CHD. However, only two American and two European studies controlled for the classic risk factors. The first of these four studies revealed a lack of association of type A (JAS-AB) with MI in univariate analysis that became apparent after controlling for the classic risk factors (Shekelle et al. 1976).

The second study showed that type A, as determined by the Framingham scale, was independently and significantly associated with the prevalence of CHD in women under 65 years of age as well as with the prevalence of MI in men of the same age (Haynes 1978).

The third study, which was conducted in Sweden, concluded that the presence of type A, after controlling for classic risk factors, predicted statistically a CHD risk of 2.7 for subjects with CHD compared with subjects without CHD and of 1.6 for subjects with CHD compared with subjects at high risk (Orth-Gomer et al. 1980).

The last study, using multivariate analysis, was unable to show that type A, as measured by the Bortner scale, was associated with CHD (MI and angina) when neuroticism was entered simultaneously (FBCG 1982).

In conclusion, no definite statement can be made concerning the independent association of social class with the prevalence of CHD. The positive association of type A with CHD has probably been overestimated due to a lack of controls for other risk factors or confounders linked to CHD.

Evolution of Risk Factors

The huge amount of information obtained from the BHDPP must also be considered in terms of the evolution of risk factors as a function of psychosocial variables. As described, four risk factors were measured at baseline and at final screening in the 10% control group and in the intervention group, members of which took part in a mass media intervention program (low-risk subjects) or had face-to-face counselling (high-risk subjects).

As the main focus lies on type A in relation to CHD, only the evolution of the coronary risk profile will be considered. A global comparison of the intervention and control groups reveals that the intervention program had a beneficial impact on the final risk profile. This is mainly due to the face-to-face counselling given the high-risk group. An analysis based on the change in MLF (final minus initial value) presents the same picture, though the results are not statistically significant. However, the percentage of net change in the coronary risk profile is about 7% in the total intervention group and 12% in the high-risk subgroup who received individual

Table 6. Analysis of variance/covariance of delta MLF coefficients of the model by multiple regression high-risk subgroup

Sources of variation	delta MLF coefficients
Covariate	
Initial MLF	−0.16766***
Main effects	
group	−0.00291**
JAS-AB	0.00035
JAS-S	0.00045
JAS-J	0.00300
JAS-H	−0.00073
Interactions	
Group × JAS-J	−0.00274*
Constant	0.01588

Group, JAS-AB, JAS-AS, JAS-J, JAS-H: Dummy variables (−1, +1)
* P, 0.05; ** P, 0.01; *** P, 0.001

counselling. The positive association between overall type A or its components and the favorable evolution of the coronary risk profile which is observable through univariate analysis vanishes in variance/covariance analysis.

One exception to this is the job involvement dimension, which has a protective influence on the coronary risk profile in the low-risk group. It is likely that, in the high-risk group, the intensive intervention program neutralizes behavioral differences, as is shown in the variance/covariance analysis (Table 6, Fig. 9).

Very little has been published so far on the evolution of risk factors in the framework of multifactorial intervention trials, especially in relation to psychosocial factors. To my knowledge, only the Multiple Risk Factor Intervention Trial (MRFIT) group has reported on this issue. The first study centered on change in smoking habits (Ockene et al. 1982). Success in smoking cessation appears to be improved by a combination of factors, including high expectation of success, few cigarettes smoked upon entry in the program, ease of prior cessation attempts, long period of prior abstinence preceding the current attempt to stop smoking and a high degree of personal security. The success of the program seems furthermore to lie in its individualization. This confirms the BHDPP finding, where cessation or reduction of cigarette smoking were achieved through face-to-face counselling only. The second study comes from the Harvard center, one of the 22 centers of MRFIT (Eaker et al. 1982). The analyses revealed that no one model can explain changes for the three risk factors of hypercholesterolemia, high blood pressure, and smoking. A reduction in cholesterol levels, when this was the only risk factor of concern, was associated with group sessions, whereas the contrary was observed when all three factors were present to a high degree. Cessation of smoking was more successful when combined with group sessions, an absence of stressful life events, and a sense of personal security for subjects under medication and for younger subjects not under medication. Internal locus of control (i. e., the individual's ability to control his environment rather than be controlled by it) was beneficial with regard to reduction of blood pressure, medication, and weight.

Incidence of CHD

Incidence Results from the BHDPP

The incidence of CHD was determined for the sample as a whole on the basis of fatal and nonfatal events occurring during the follow-up period of 6 years. Diagnoses were made from the records of hospitals, general practitioners, or specialists by one of the BHDPP physicians, who did not know to which group the subjects belonged. Necropsy records were used when available. Morbidity follow-up was continued as long as the subject was at work according to the international protocol. Further information was obtained through ECG and the Rose questionnaire at the final examination.

All the events were classified as either hard or soft events. Hard events were defined as sudden death (SD), fatal MI (FMI), nonfatal MI (NFMI), and Minnesota ECG code $I_{1\text{-}2}$ at final examination indicating a probable MI. Events defined as soft included angina (at follow-up), other ischemic diseases, Minnesota codes I_3, $IV_{1\text{-}2\text{-}3}$, or $V_{1\text{-}2\text{-}3}$ at the final examination (respectively, possible MI, ST segment depression of varying degrees, T wave inversion of variable degree), and anginas in the final Rose questionnaire. However, in this paper, only hard events are considered.

Furthermore, the population analyzed here is restricted to subjects free of CHD at the start of the trial, as defined in the prevalence of CHD section, as well as to subjects who were either still working retired and drop-outs during follow-up. Incidence results of the intervention group and the 10% control group are discussed, as these groups provide complete data in terms of initial bioclinical and psychosocial measurements. Very recently, global incidence and mortality results comparing the total intervention and control groups were published (Kornitzer et al. 1983).

Univariate Analysis

The incidence rates of hard events were studied in relation to initial bioclinical, social, and behavioral variables.

Bioclinical Risk Factors. Risk factor categories are defined as follows:

BMI: <22, <25, <28, >28
Cholesterol: <220, <240, <280, >280
Systolic blood pressure: <110, <140, <160, >160
Diastolic blood pressure: <80, <90, <100, >100
Smoking: smokers, nonsmokers
MLF: <0.0084, <0.0140; <0.0240, >0.0240

Figure 2 displays the six graphs showing the annual hard event rate (per 1000) by risk factor category in both the intervention and 10% control group, as well as the relative risks (RR) calculated between the most extreme categories for each risk factor. In fact, in the intervention group, the comparison of proportions by risk categories shows a statistically significant positive correlation for all factors, except BMI. In contrast, in the 10% control group, significant differences appear only for the MLF categories. One should remember, however, that the 10% control group is ten

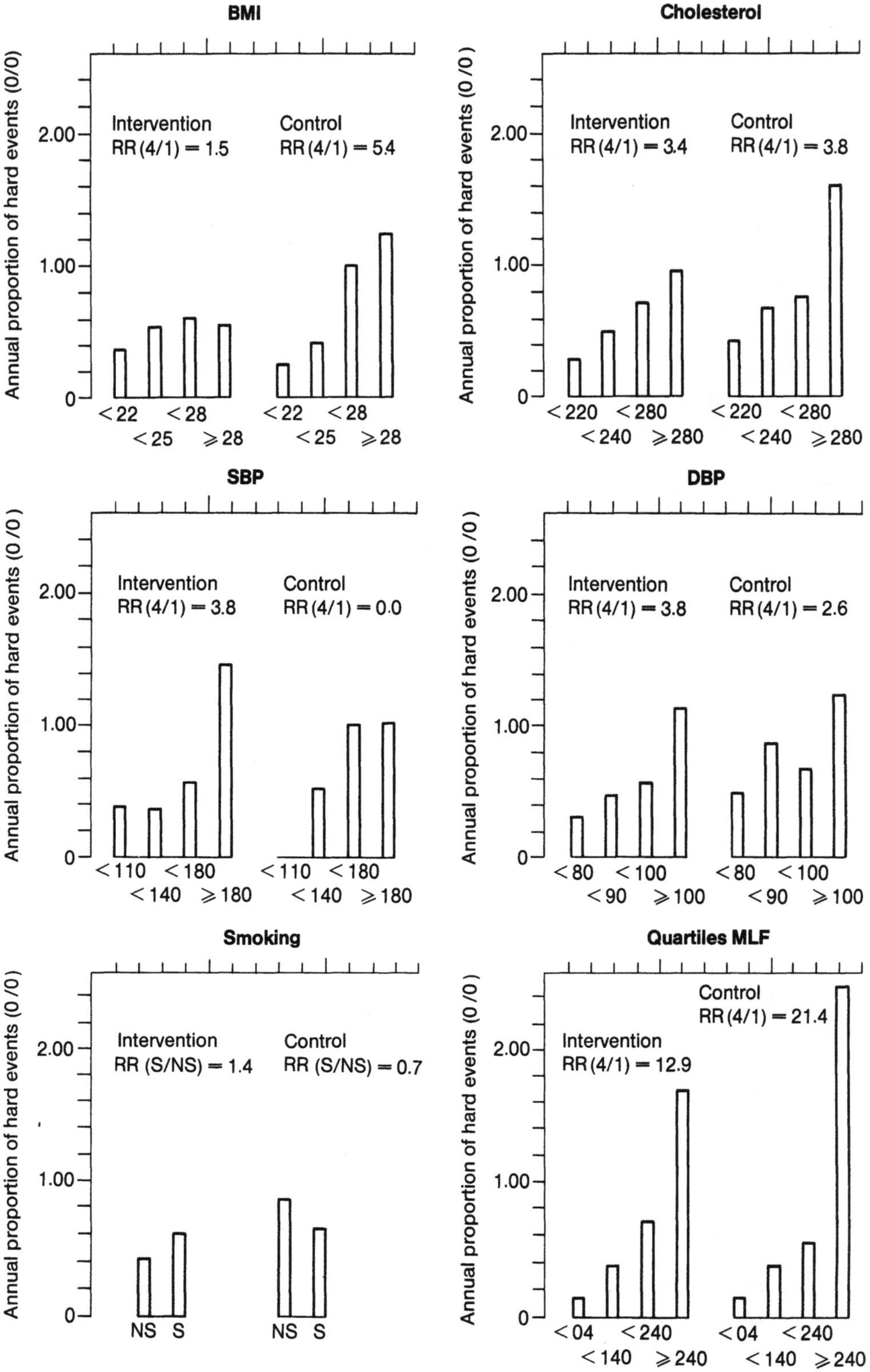

Fig. 2. Incidence of hard events according to categories of risk factors. *BMI,* body mass index; *SBP,* systolic blood pressure; *DBP,* diastolic blood pressure; *MLF,* multiple logistic function; *RR,* relative risk

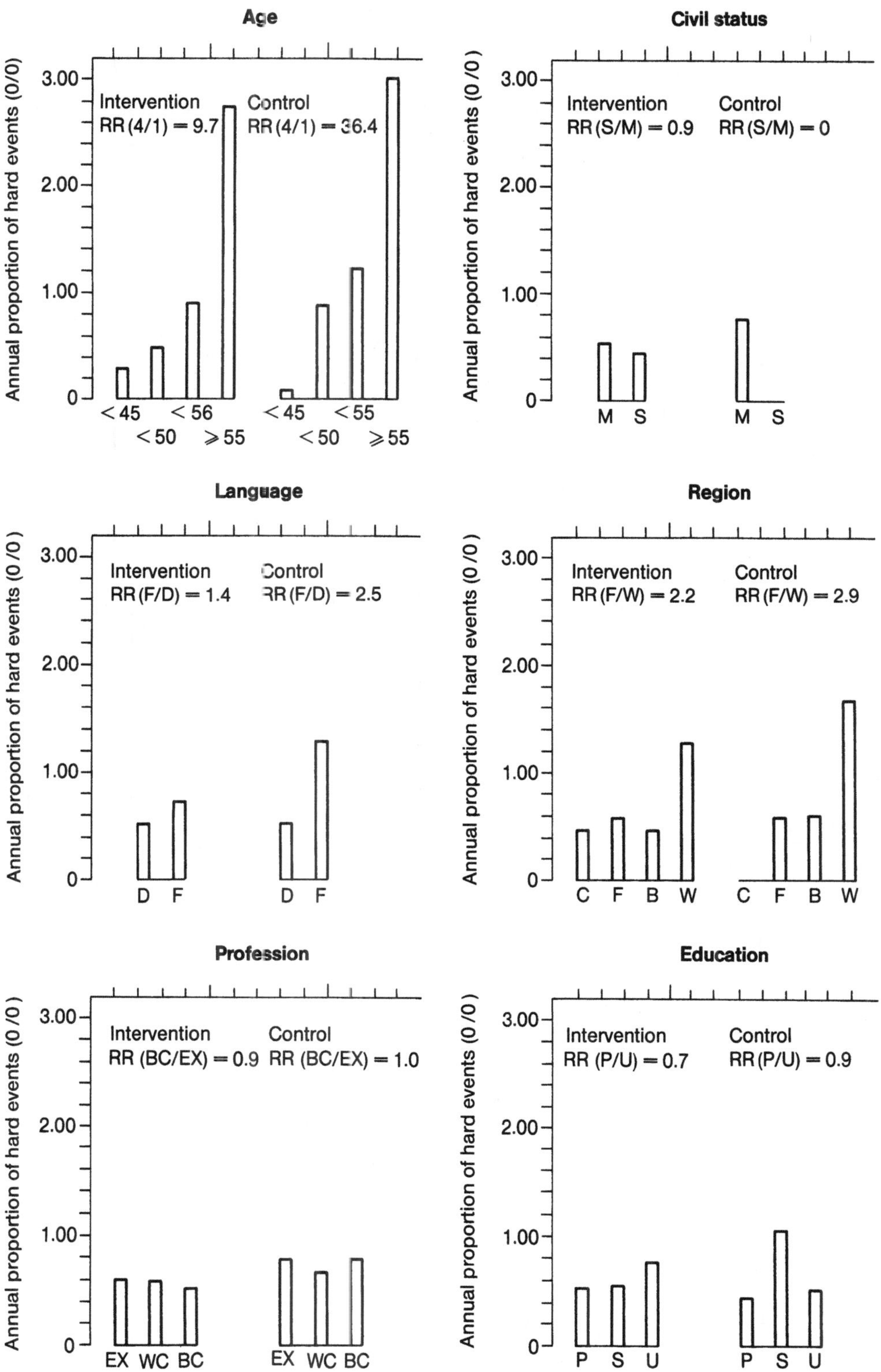

Fig. 3. Incidence of hard events according to categories of social variables. *M*, married; *S*, single; *D*, Dutch; *F*, French; *C*, Campine; *F*, Flanders; *B*, Brussels; *W*, Wallonia; *EX*, executive; *WC*, white collar workers; *BC*, blue collar workers; *P*, primary school; *S*, secondary school; *U*, university; *RR*, relative risk

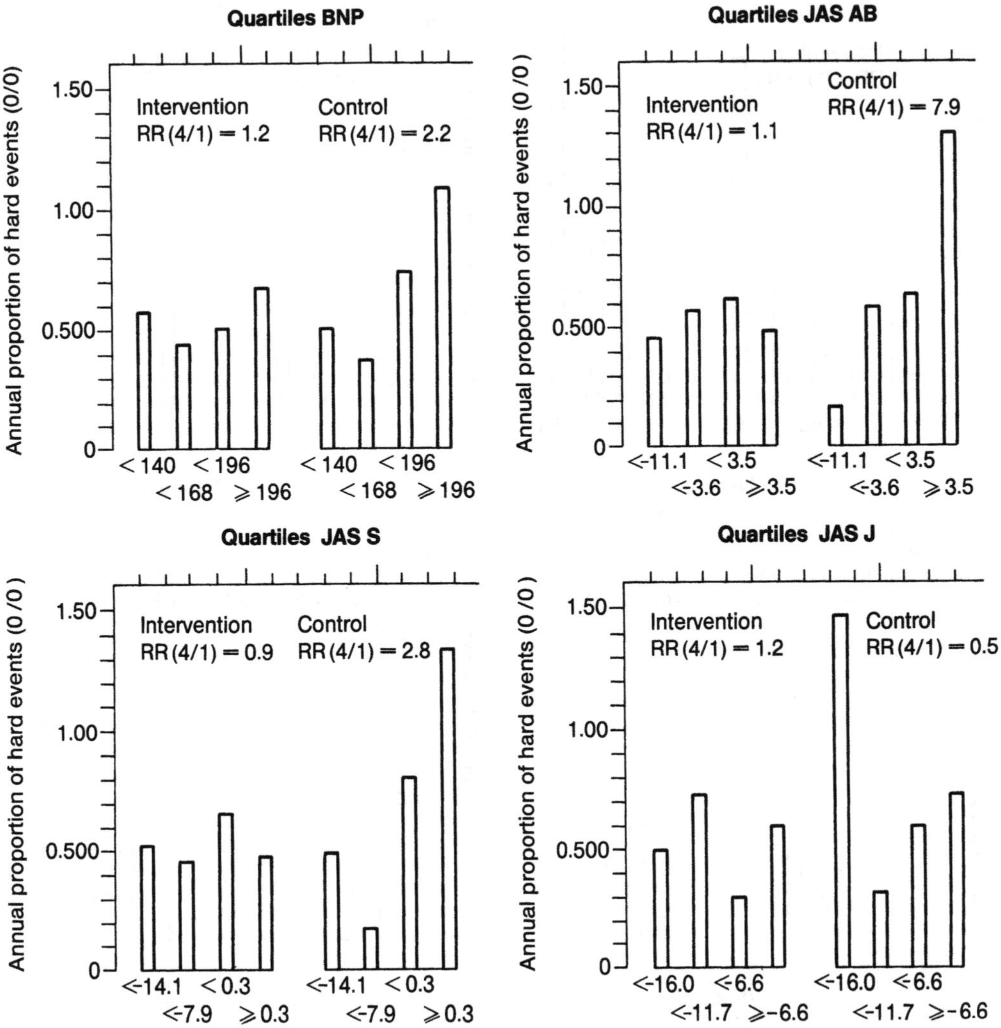

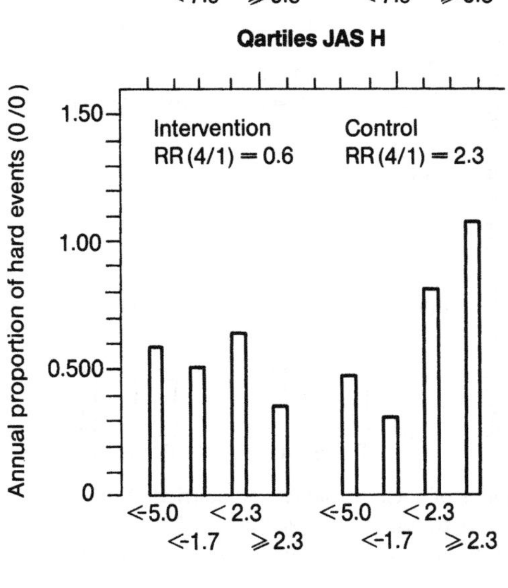

Fig. 4. Incidence of hard events according to quartiles of type A score, as determined by questionnaire. *RR*, relative risk

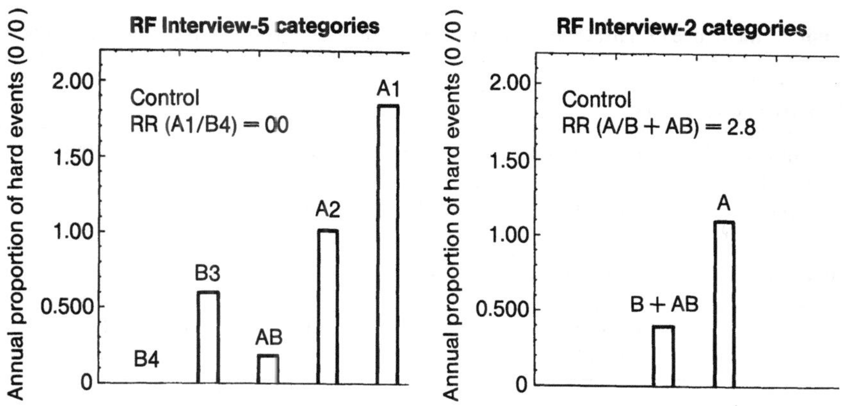

Fig. 5. Incidence of hard events according to type A, as determined by interview. *RR*, relative risk

times smaller than the intervention group, significantly reducing the statistical power of the Chi square test. Nonetheless, the predictive power of the MLF is particularly striking in this untreated group, as shown by the RR of 21.4 between extreme quartiles.

Social Variables. Six social variables divided into the following categories were also studied:

Age: <45, <50, <55, >55
Civil status: married, single
Language: Dutch, French
Region: Campine, Flanders, Brussels, Wallonia
Profession: executives, white collar workers, blue collar workers
Education: primary, secondary, university

The six graphs in Fig. 3 show the annual hard event rate (per 1000) by social factor categories. Only in the intervention group did the differences in the incidence rates for the age and region categories reach statistical significance, though a discernible tendency between language categories was present. In the 10% control group, the same picture appears, but French-speaking subjects manifested statistically higher incidence rates than did Dutch-speaking subjects. In both groups, no differences in the incidence rates between categories relating to profession, education, or marital status were found. Age, which is a hybrid sociobiological factor, obviously appears to be the most predictive factor.

Behavioral Variables. Both the Bortner scores (BNP) and the JAS scores (JAS-AB, JAS-S, JAS-J, and JAS-H) were broken down into quartiles, while the SI was divided into the usual two (A/B) and five categories ($A_1/A_2/X/B_3/B_4$). The incidence rates by quartiles of scores are presented in Fig. 4. In the intervention group, no significant correlation appeared between any of the scores. Relative risks are therefore close to one. Two separate analyses of executives and white collar workers and of blue collar workers produced similar results. In contrast, in the control group, a

Table 7. Incidence of hard events (%) by type A score (JAS-AB) in two professional subgroups

Categories Jenkins' cutting points		1 < −5	2 < 5	3 > 5	*P*	RR 3/1
Executives and white collars workers	intervention ($n = 1085$)	−3.5	3.6	3.7	(0.99)	1.1
	control ($n = 206$)	−3.2	1.4	8.3	(0.11)	2.6
Blue collar workers	intervention ($n = 2060$)	−2.8	3.6	1.8	(0.31)	0.6
	control ($n = 238$)	−2.3	6.1	8.0	(0.24)	3.5

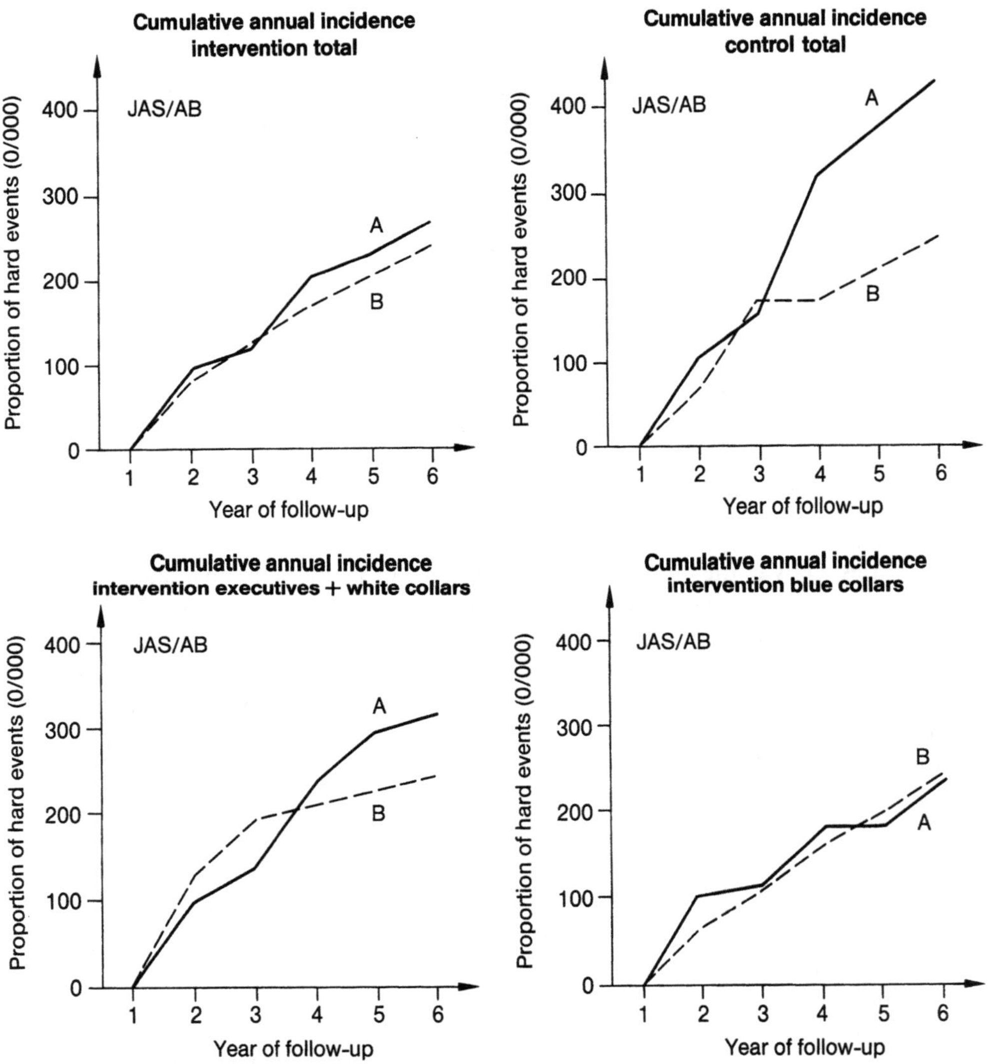

Fig. 6. Cumulative annual incidence of hard events according to occupational status

positive correlation with hard events can be observed for all behavioral scores except for job involvement, where the correlation was negative.

In Fig. 5, the incidence rates by SI categories are shown for the control group only, as no SI was administered in the intervention group. In the first graph, a positive correlation is shown and the relative risk between type A and type B subjects reaches 2.8 ($P \leqslant 0.07$). In the second graph, the positive correlation remains, but is not as strong for the intermediate AB category.

In order to ascertain whether the lack of predictive power of type A in the intervention group was due to the categorization method used, Jenkins' cutting points for JAS-AB in relation to incidence were applied (Jenkins et al. 1974). Furthermore, to exclude a possible confounding effect, socioprofessional status was taken into account as well (Table 7). It seems clear that, even with this method, JAS-AB showed no positive correlation with incidence, nor was the RR between extreme categories, which we found to be close to 1, similar to Jenkins' findings, where the RR was 1.8.

Cumulative annual incidence (per 10000) was calculated by survival methods enlarged to include all hard events for type A and type B subjects as determined by JAS-AB, with the aim of investigating a possible diluting effect of type A over the years. As is apparent from Fig. 6, this appears not to be the case. In fact, an opposite, although weak tendency appeared after the 3rd year in the total 10% control group and in executive and white collar subjects in the intervention group. Performing analyses separately on fatal and nonfatal hard events failed to improve the predictive power of type A.

Multivariate Analyses

Multiple logistic function analysis by the Duncan and Walker method was applied to both the 10% control group and the intervention group. The analysis was performed separately for each behavioral factor, but with systematic inclusion of all risk factors, cultural origin, and professional status. Logistic coefficients, standard deviation of the risk factors, standardized relative risks (approximate), and significance of *t* test are presented for each variable in Tables 8 and 9.

However, as stated by Rosenman et al. (1976) standardized relative risks for dichotomous variables, like the behavioral categories used here, are not particularly appropriate, although they allow risk comparison with the other factors. Table 8 summarizes the results obtained in the control group and Table 9 those of the intervention group. These results obtained by this sophisticated method unfortunately confirm the results and conclusions obtained in the univariate analysis.

In the control group, age is the strongest predictor (RR = 2.7) immediately followed by overall type A, JAS-AB, and hard-driving behavior (RR = 1.9). Belonging to the French cultural group and being impatient has a degree of predictive power as well. Though the relative risk of the SI is of the same order (RR = 1.6), it barely reaches statistical significance.

In the intervention group (Table 9), age is also the best predictor (RR = 1.9). The next best predictors are cholesterol, smoking, and systolic blood pressure (RR = 1.4). However, none of the social or behavioral variables show up as predictors of hard events.

Table 8. Incidence of hard events as shown by multiple logistic coefficients for CHD risk factors over 6-year period according to the method of Duncan and Walker (10% control group)

	Logistic coefficient	Standard deviation risk factor	Standardized relative risk[a]	Significance of probability[b]
Intercept	−23.807			
Age (years)	0.217	4.567	2.7	0.0006
BMI (kg/m^2)	0.134	3.324	1.6	0.06
Systolic blood pressure (mmHg)	0.013	16.969	1.2	0.33
Cholesterol (mg/100 ml)	0.007	38.778	1.3	0.27
Smoking (3-8)	0.036	1.824	1.1	0.80
Language (1, 2)	0.157	0.459	1.7	0.03
Profession (1, 2, 3)	0.126	0.773	1.1	0.70
SI (1, 2)	− 0.898	0.495	1.6	0.11
BNP (0, 1)	0.638	0.455	1.3	0.27
JAS-AB (0, 1)	1.290	0.490	1.9	0.02
JAS-S (0, 1)	1.122	0.439	1.6	0.04
JAS-J (0, 1)	− 0.621	0.345	0.8	0.50
JAS-H (0, 1)	1.303	0.481	1.9	0.02

Smoking: 3 = nonsmokers; 4 = pipe, cigar, <5 cigarettes; 5 = <10 cigarettes; 6 = <20 cigarettes; 7 = <30 cigarettes; 8 = ≥30 cigarettes
Language: 1 = Dutch; 2 = French
Profession: 1 = executives; 2 = white collar workers; 3 = blue collar workers
SI: 1 = A; 2 = B
BNP: 0 = B; 1 = A
JAS: 0 = B; 1 = A

[a] $e(\beta i \cdot SD)$

[b] $t = \frac{\beta i}{SE_{\beta_i}}$

In Fig. 7, the six graphs show the percentage of observed cases by quintiles of calculated MLF in the two groups. In the two bottom graphs, the MLF is calculated using the five classic risk factors. In the middle graphs, the MLF is estimated using the five classic risk factors and the two social variables. At the top, the MLF is computed using the five classic risk factors, the two social variables, and JAS-AB scores. In the control group, it is obvious that type A (JAS-AB) improves the predictive power of the MLF, whereas the contrary occurs in the intervention group.

In Fig. 8, the six graphs compare the number of expected cases with the number of observed cases by deciles or quintiles of MLF calculated as described for the previous graph for the two groups as a kind of accuracy check of the computed MLF. In the control group, the correlation coefficient is increased by adding the two social variables to the risk factors and is further magnified by adding JAS-AB. The slope approaches unity. In the intervention group, the correlation coefficient decreases by adding the social and behavioral variables. The slope even declines from 0.78 to 0.66 and finally to 0.45.

Explanations for those divergences of the predictive power of type A between the two groups are numerous. The first hypothesis that could be formulated is that

Table 9. Multiple logistic coefficients for CHD risk factors for a 6-year period according to Duncan and Walker method (intervention group)

	Logistic coefficient	Standard deviation risk factor	Standardized relative risk[a]	Significance of probability[b]
Intercept	−17.024			
Age (years)	0.154	4.156	1.9	0.0001
BMI (kg/m²)	0.011	3.079	1.0	0.74
Systolic blood pressure (mmHg)	0.019	16.005	1.4	0.001
Cholesterol (mg/100 ml)	0.010	36.475	1.4	0.0002
Smoking (3-8)	0.197	1.761	1.4	0.0002
Language (1, 2)	0.018	0.305	1.0	0.95
Profession (1, 2, 3)	− 0.096	0.710	0.9	0.51
SI (1, 2)		not determined in this group		
BNP (0, 1)	0.329	0.424	1.1	0.18
JAS-AB (0, 1)	0.032	0.470	1.0	0.89
JAS-S (0, 1)	− 0.193	0.422	0.9	0.46
JAS-J (0, 1)	− 0.392	0.294	0.9	0.37
JAS-H (0, 1)	− 0.375	0.476	0.8	0.11

Smoking: 3, nonsmokers; 4, pipe or cigar, <5 cigarettes; 5, <10 cigarettes; 6, < 20 cigarettes; 7, <30 cigarettes; 8, >30 cigarettes
Language: 1, Dutch; 2, French
Profession: 1, executives; 2, white collar workers; 3, blue collar workers
SI: 1, A; 2, B
BNP: 0, B; 1, A
JAS: 0, B; 1, A

[a] $e(\beta i \cdot SD)$

[b] $t = \frac{\beta i}{SE_{\beta_i}}$

there is an interaction between type A and the intervention program. This could happen in two ways. Firstly, type A or its components enhance the effects of the intervention program, but previous results have not supported this promise. Only job involvement has been shown to have a protective effect on coronary risk profile, but this effect is most prominant in the absence of intervention. Secondly, the intervention program might have a positive effect on behavior as well. Because no type A determination took place at the final examination, this influence cannot be ruled out, although preliminary, but negative, results obtained in another prospective study without intervention do not provide evidence in favor of this assumption.

A second reason could be the diluting effect of type A on CHD after several years. Survival analysis of the data, enlarged to include all hard events, did not make it possible to corroborate this hypothesis.

A third solution to be considered does not reject the type A concept as such, but rather the particular type A measures used in the intervention group, namely the Bortner scale and the JAS.

A fourth possibility is that type A by itself, without the classic risk factors, is unable to predict outcome. Other protective factors such as social support network,

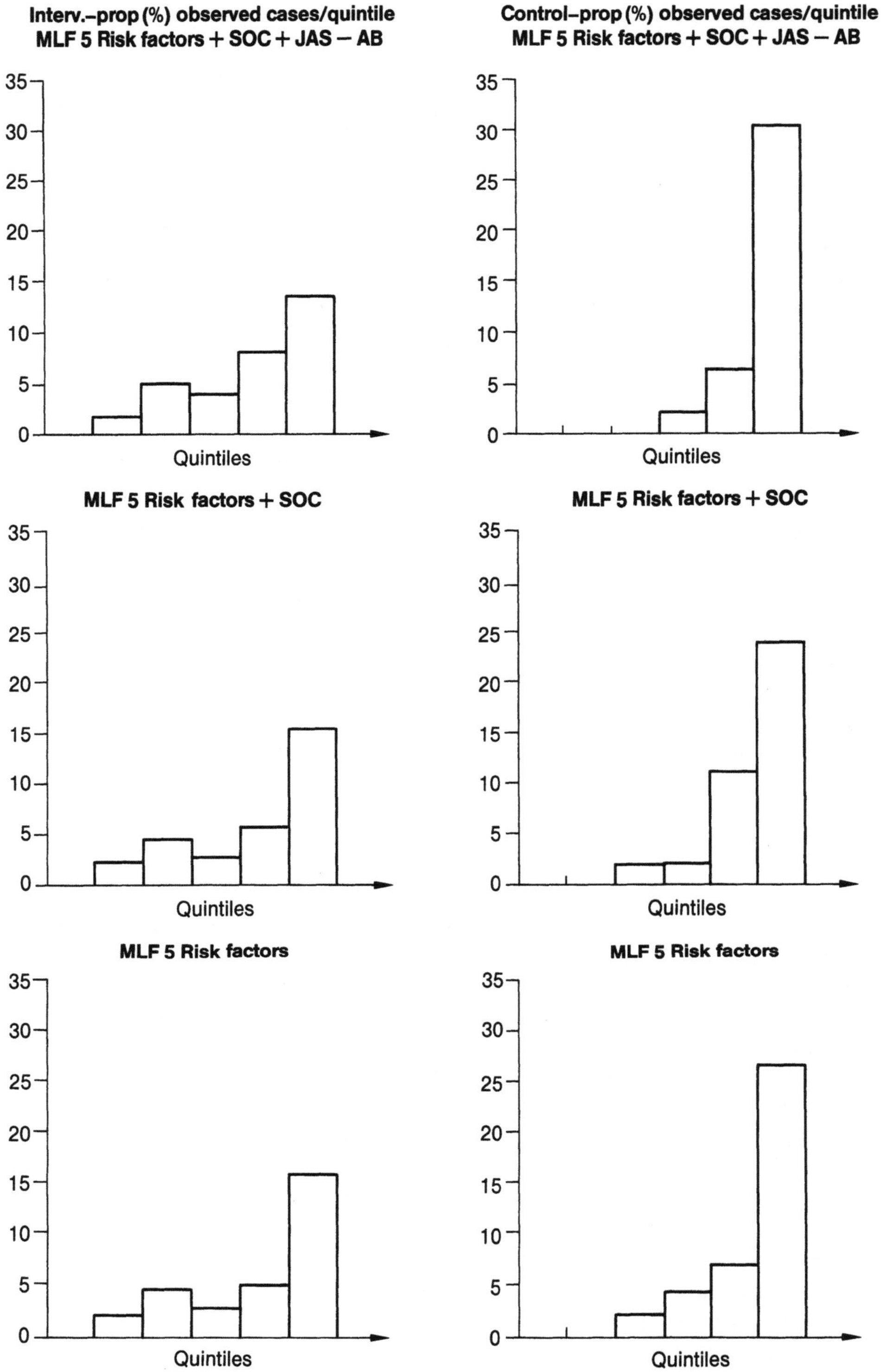

Fig. 7. Incidence of hard events according to quintiles of calculated multiple logistic functions. *MLF*, multiple logistic function; *SOC*, socio-occupational class; *JAS-AB*, type A scores

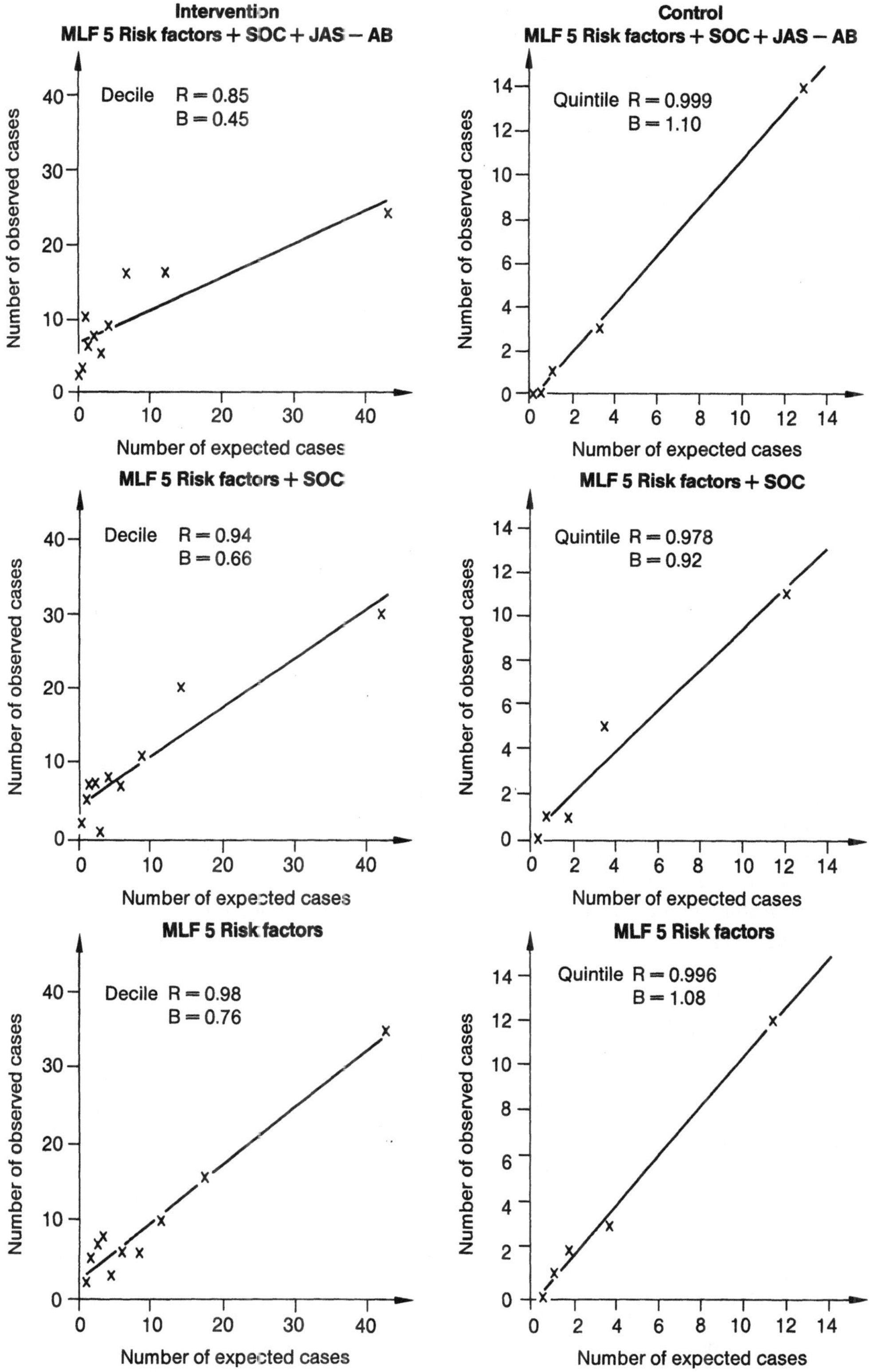

Fig. 8. Incidence of hard events as shown by the relation between observed and expected cases. *R*, correlation coefficient; *B*, slope of regression line; *MLF*, multiple logistic function; *SOC*, socio-occupational class; *JAS-AB* type A score

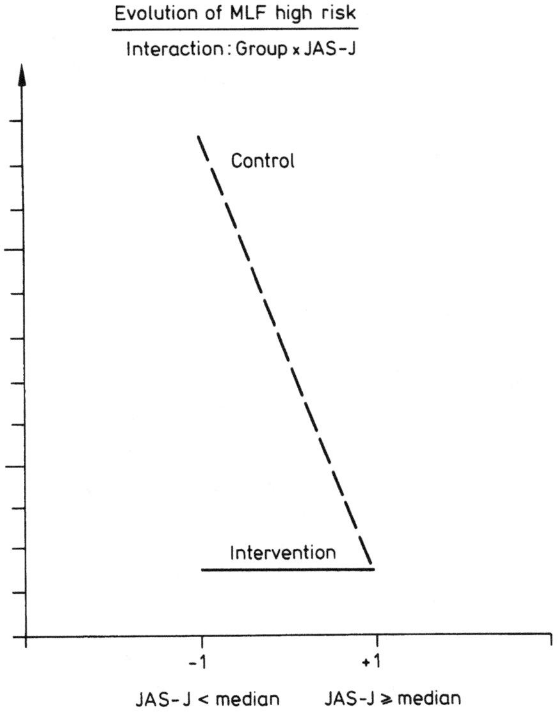

Fig. 9. Evolution risk profile based on data presented in Table 6. —, intervention; - - -, control 10%; JAS-J: *−1*, < median; *+1*, ≥ median

coping mechanisms, as well as other factors contributing to CHD such as hostility, hyperreactivity, and lack of control could interact and weaken or supplant type A influence.

Although an exhaustive and thorough review of the rich literature on the relation of psychosocial factors to the incidence of CHD would be valuable, the references in this chapter are restricted to very recent publications. Concerning social variables related to CHD, two studies from Great Britain (Rose and Marmot 1981) and Finland (Salonen 1982) showed "social class" to be negatively related to the incidence of CHD. In the Whitehall Study of men aged 40–64 years, coronary mortality after 7.5 years was 3.6 times higher in the lowest social class than in the highest. The social class difference was partly explained by the known coronary risk factors, but most of the difference remained unexplained. After controlling for age, smoking, blood pressure, serum cholesterol, and single status (RR = 2.3), the 6-year longitudinal Eastern Finnish Study of 3644 men aged 30–59 years revealed that low educational level (RR = 2.1) and low income (RR = 1.7) were predictive of fatal CHD. Yet, no relation to CHD incidence could be established for two other psychosocial dimensions used in the Honolulu Heart Program: acculturation and social networks (Reed et al. 1982, Reed et al. 1983). Multivariate analyses of the data obtained from 4563 men of Japanese ancestry living in Hawaii showed only a borderline association ($P \leq 0.08$) of one social network scale with nonfatal MI.

Despite the well-known positive findings of many studies (Jenkins et al. 1974; Rosenman et al. 1976; Haynes et al. 1980), some recent studies, including ours, were unable to demonstrate any predictive value of the type A behavior pattern. In the

Honolulu Heart Program, the 8-year incidence among 2187 Japanese men was not significantly related to type A, as measured by JAS (Reed and Cohen 1982). Moreover, autopsy findings of 48 men who died showed no association of type A either with microscopic evidence of MI, or with degree of atherosclerosis in the coronary arteries and aorta. In the MRFIT Study, the SI was administered to 3110 and the JAS to 12772 subjects (Shekelle et al. 1983). It appeared that the RR of CHD death for type A subjects (as assessed by the SI), as compared with type B subjects was 1.03 after adjustment for other risk factors, while JAS-AB scores were inversely related to CHD fatality after adjustment.

In the Finnish Twin Cohort Study, after a 6-year follow-up of 23076 males aged 35-64 years, the short version of the Bortner type A scale was analyzed in terms of CHD incidence (Koskenvuo et al. 1983). For coronary heart disease, it appeared that type A subjects (highest decile) showed a higher mortality than type B subjects (lowest decile), based on expected rates of 0.4 and 0.6 respectively, but the analysis was based on three subjects. Thus, the issue remains unresolved.

References

Antonovsky A (1968) Social class and the major cardiovascular diseases. J Chronic Dis 21: 65-105

Brand RJ, Rosenman RH, Sholtz RI et al (1976) Multivariate prediction of coronary heart disease in the Western Collaborative Group Study compared to the findings of the Framingham Study. Circulation 53: 348-355

De Backer G, Kornitzer M, Thilly C et al (1977) The Belgian multifactor preventive trial in CVD: design and methodology. Hart Bull 8: 143-146

Eaker E, Benfari R, Reed R (1982) Coronary risk factor intervention: Characteristics associated with change. J Clin Psychol 38: 703-717

Floderus B (1974) Psycho-social factors in relation to coronary heart disease and associated risk factors. Nord Hygien Tidskrift Stockholm [Suppl] 6

French-Belgian Collaborative Group (1982) Ischemic heart disease and psychological patterns. Adv Cardiol 29: 25-31

Haynes SG, Levine S, Scotch N et al (1978a) The relationship of psychosocial factors to coronary heart disease in the Framingham Study. I. Methods and risk factors. Am J Epidemiol 107: 362-283

Haynes SG, Feinleib M, Levine S et al (1978b) The relationship of psychosocial factors to coronary heart disease in the Framingham Study. II. Prevalence of coronary heart disease. Am J Epidemiol 107: 384-403

Haynes SG, Feinleib M, Kannel W (1980) The relationship of psychosocial factors to coronary heart disease in the Framingham Study. III. Eight-year incidence of coronary heart disease. Am J Epidemiol 111: 37-58

Holme I, Helgeland A, Hjermann I et al (1976) Coronary risk factors and socio-economic status. Lancet II: 1396-1397

Jenkins CD, Rosenman R, Zyzanski S (1974) Prediction of clinical coronary heart disease by a test for the coronary-prone behavior pattern. N Engl J Med 290: 1271-1275

Jenkins CD, Zyzanski S, Rosenman R (1979) JAS manual. The Psychological Corp, New York

Kittel F, Kornitzer M, de Backer G et al (1982) Metrological study of psychological questionnaires with reference to social variables: the Belgian Heart Disease Prevention Project (BHDPP). J Behav Med 5: 9-35

Kittel F, Kornitzer M, De Backer G et al (1983) Type A in relation to job-stress, social and bioclinical variables: the Belgian Physical Fitness Study. J Human Stress 2: 37-45

Kornitzer M, Kittel F, De Backer G et al (1981) The Belgian Heart Disease Prevention Project: type A behavior pattern and the prevalence of coronary heart disease. Psychosom Med 43: 133-145

Kornitzer M, De Backer G, Dramaix M et al (1983) Belgian Heart Disease Prevention Project: Incidence and mortality results. Lancet I: 1066-1070
Koskenvuo M, Kaprio J, Langinvainio M et al (1983) Mortality in relation to coronary-prone behavior. A six-year follow-up of the Bortner scale in middle-aged Finnish men. CVD Epidemiol N 34: 40 (abstract 5)
Marmot M, Rose G, Shipley M et al (1978) Employment grade and coronary heart disease in British civil servants. J Epidemiol Community Health 32: 244-249
Matthews K, Krantz D (1976) Resemblances of twins and their parents in pattern A behavior. Psychosom Med 38: 140-144
Mettlin C (1976) Occupational careers and the prevention of coronary-prone behavior. Soc Sci Med 10: 367-372
Ockene J, Benfari R, Nuttall R et al (1982) Relationship of psychosocial factors to smoking behavior change in an intervention program. Prev Med 11: 13-28
Orth-Gomer K, Ahlbom A, Theorell T (1980) Impact of pattern A behavior on ischemic heart disease when controlling for conventional risk indicators. J Human Stress 2: 6-13
Price V, Friedman M (1982) Type A behavior pattern: A model for research and practice. Academic, New York
Reed D, Cohen J (1982) Type A behavior and coronary heart disease among Japanese men in Hawaii. Circulation 66 (II): 236 (abstract 945)
Reed D, McGee D, Cohen J et al (1982) Acculturation and coronary heart disease among Japanese men in Hawaii. Am J Epidemiol 115: 894-905
Reed D, McGee D, Yano K et al (1983) Social networks and coronary heart disease among Japanese men in Hawaii. Am J Epidemiol 117: 384-396
Rose G, Blackburn H (1968) Cardiovascular survey methods. World Health Organization, Geneva
Rose G, Marmot M (1981) Social class and coronary heart disease. Br Heart J 45: 13-19
Rosenman R, Brand J, Sholtz R et al (1976) Multivariate prediction of coronary heart disease during 8.5-year follow-up in the Western Collaborative Group Study. Am J Cardiol 37 (i): 903-910
Salonen J (1982) Socio-economic status and risk of cancer, cerebral stroke, and death due to coronary heart disease and any disease: A longitudinal study in Eastern Finland. J Epidemiol Community Health 36: 294-297
Shekelle R, Schoenberger J, Stamler J (1976) Correlates of the JAS type A behavior pattern score. J Chronic Dis 29: 381-394
Shekelle R, Hulley S, Neaton J et al (1983) Type A behavior and risk of coronary heart death in MRFIT. CVD Epidemiol N 33: 34 (abstract 61)
Syme S, Berkman L (1976) Social class, susceptibility and sickness. Am J Epidemiol 104: 1-6
Waldron I, Zyzanski S, Shekelle R et al (1977) The coronary-prone behavior pattern in employed men and women. J Human Stress 3: 2-18
WHO European Collaborative Group (1974) An international controlled trial in the multifactorial prevention of coronary heart disease. Int J Epidemiol 3: 219-224

Is Neuroticism A Risk Factor for CAD? Is Type A a Measure of Neuroticism?

P. T. Costa Jr.[1]

This contribution has two main purposes. The first is to present a brief review of the empirical evidence which demonstrates that the personality dimension of neuroticism (N) is related to increased somatic complaints, including chest pain or angina-like complaints, but is not causally or etiologically related to objective signs or pathophysiological evidence of disease, especially coronary artery disease (CAD). The second purpose is to consider the implications of this empirical generalization for the conceptualization and assessment of the coronary-prone behavior pattern (CPBP) or type A behavior pattern (TABP).

Recent Medical Literature

Most psychologists believe that the two major clinical manifestations of CAD - myocardial infarction (MI) and angina pectoris (AP) - are interchangeable and infallible indicators of coronary artery disease. Most clinical cardiologists, however, regard the former as "hard" and the latter as "soft" signs or indicators of CAD (Costa 1981). They want to distinguish between these two manifestations because they recognize that angina pectoris can lead to misdiagnosis rates that are quite high, often as high as 20%-30% (Kemp et al. 1973).

Traditional medical teachings have emphasized the value of the clinical history in making a diagnosis of CAD. However, current cardiological literature contains several areas of controversy concerning the clinical validity of specific chest pain symptoms predicting angiographic findings. These issues should be of concern to biobehavioral researchers interested in TABP and other behavioral and psychosocial factors in CAD since typical AP is one of the two principal clinical criteria for operationally defining CAD, and misdiagnoses can lead to spurious psychosocial and behavioral predictors.

AP and MI represent two distinct clinical manifestations of coronary heart disease. A patient may have one or the other or both. It is crucial to note, however, that history of MI, like ECG test results, is a relatively objective indicator of coronary heart disease. Chest pain symptoms, although they are frequently good predictors of disease outcomes, are essentially subjective, and potentially biased by psychological factors. As we shall see, failure to distinguish between subjective indicators (e.g., chest pain symptoms) and objective indicators (e.g., sudden death, transmural MI, complete stenosis or occlusion of coronary arteries) is responsible for conflict-

1 Gerontology Research Center (Baltimore), National Institute on Aging, National Institutes of Health, PHS, U.S. Department of Health and Human Services, Bethesda, and the Francis Scott Key Medical Center, Baltimore, MD 21224, USA

Biological and Psychological Factors in Cardiovascular Disease
Ed. by T. H. Schmidt, T. M. Dembroski, and G. Blümchen

ing and confusing research results. This is an unfortunate practice and should be discouraged. The precise operational definition of coronary heart disease is one of the most crucial variables determining the outcome of any study investigating specific psychological risk factors. Researchers interested in identifying psychological risk factors for coronary heart disease should not collapse subjective and objective indicators of disease into a global category of CHD. Rather, discrete diagnostic end points, (e.g., chest pain MI, asymptomatic anatomical disease,) singly and in combination should be employed as criteria.

There is increasing agreement in the literature that the clinical features obtained from a careful history (even when obtained by an experienced physician) routinely used to diagnose CAD are not as valid predictors of CAD as was once thought. These clinical features are derived from the patient's history - especially prior anginal symptoms - and the results of the physical examination and electrocardiographic testing. The advent of angiography, which offers a direct measure of coronary arterial stenosis, permits a distinction to be made between those patients with actual stenosis and those who present with anginal symptoms but no verifiable stenosis or disease. Studies have shown that between 20% and 30% of patients referred for angiography, notwithstanding a history of anginal complaints, have "clean" arteries (Cohn et al. 1972; Day and Sowton 1976).

Because this condition is similar to, but clearly distinct from, the AP associated with actual CAD, Hermann et al. (1973) have suggested that it might more appropriately be called "angina-like chest pain without identifiable cause." Kemp et al. (1973) demonstrated in a 6-year follow-up study of patients with anginal complaints but no verifiable occlusion that patients' conditions do not worsen with time; indeed, their morbidity and mortality experience is similar to those of the population at large. Banks et al. (1971) also failed to find any relationship between length of anginal history and the amount of CAD. Based on this absence of negative outcome, Kemp et al. (1973) suggested that the nature of the condition is benign.

Horwitz (1974) has questioned the validity of diagnosing CAD based solely on clinical observation. In his subjects neither the location nor the frequency of the pain of anginal episodes nor concomitant symptoms (e.g., breathlessness, weakness) distinguished between verified CAD patients and patients with chest pain but no CAD. Similarly, Proudfit et al. (1968) concluded that the pain site is probably not related to the location of coronary stenoses or obstructions. Moreover, Fuster et al. (1975) observed that angiographic patterns in patients with anginal episodes at night or at rest are similar to those of patients who experience exertional and emotional angina. This fact they interpreted as indicating that other, nonanatomical factors play a role in triggering AP.

Comparison across studies is made difficult by the lack of consensus on scoring schemes for rating the severity of luminal narrowing or maximal artery stenosis. However, there seems to be a growing body of evidence which suggests that clinical symptoms associated with chest pain or AP do not necessarily indicate the presence of coronary stenoses. One needs to remember that AP is still a powerful predictor of CAD, but, when AP alone is used as a criterion of CAD, a significant number of false positive results are included from patients who have pseudo-angina.

If these misdiagnoses were the results of random error, their only effect on risk factor studies would be to make it somewhat more difficult to detect true associations. However, there is good reason to think that pseudo-angina is systematically related to psychosocial variables, and is thus a source of possible bias in results.

Neuroticism and CAD: Risk Factor or Pseudo Factor?

There is by now a relatively large body of retrospective studies, reviewed by Jenkins (1971) and Steptoe (1981) which report associations between measures of traits in the domain of neuroticism and CAD. Neuroticism represents a normally distributed dimension of emotional stability vs. maladjustment and comprises anxiety, hostility, depression, poor impulse control, self-consciousness and related traits indicating a propensity to experience negative affect. In reviewing over 45 studies of behavioral risk factors in CAD, Jenkins (1976) concluded that neuroticism was associated with CAD, but he noted that the variables of anxiety and neuroticism were more consistently related to AP than to MI. Jenkins concluded that, along with life dissatisfaction, family problems, and "psychosocial discord," "the anxiety-neuroticism dimension represents one more risk factor that operated differently for angina than for infarction."

In view of recent medical evidence, however, it becomes essential to ask whether N is a risk factor for true angina, or only for pseudo-angina. Even when limited to actual AP, however, retrospective studies do not provide a firm basis for inferring that psychological states or traits have a causal role in the development of CAD. Instead, it is plausible to argue that anxiety or depression may be an outcome of angina. Only prospective studies, in which personality is measured before the development of CAD symptoms or signs, can demonstrate a causal influence of neuroticism, or any other personality variable.

Such a study was done by Ostfeld et al. (1964), but has either been ignored or not fully appreciated. Ostfeld and colleagues prospectively examined 1885 men over a 4½-year period, using the 16PF and the MMPI to investigate personality factors contributing to CAD. They contrasted the personality scores of men who had and those who had not developed CAD, and those who developed only AP and those men who had only developed MI. They found that the HsK and Hy scales from the MMPI along with the Emotional Instability scale from the 16PF (all measures of neuroticism) were elevated in men before the development of AP; whereas men who were to develop MI were not different from those without coronary disease on any of the 26 personality scales.

In their discussion they stated that the AP-only group had a greater tendency prior to the occurrence of the disease to complain about somatic symptoms of all sorts and to be worried about their health in the absence of objective findings. In contrast, the men in the MI-only group "if anything, complained about their health even less than is usual within the noncoronary group." These findings of polysymptom complaints are consistent with a large body of data showing the influence of neuroticism on somatic complaints (Costa and McCrae 1985). Finally, these authors called attention to an important implication of their study that reinforces one of the major arguments of the present paper: "The fact that the men who developed only angina pectoris differed in some aspects of personality from men who had MI indicates that it is an error to study the relevance of psychological factors to CHD without specifying the clinical form of the disease."

Further confirmation of the different personality profiles of AP and MI patients comes from a prospective study of AP among 10000 Israeli men (Medalie et al. 1973; Medalie and Goldbourt 1976) where the incidence of angina complaints was twice as great among men scoring in the top half of the sample on a three-item anxiety index. The anxiety score was not predictive of MI, however.

Jenkins et al. (1978) found that different items on the Jenkins Activity Survey (JAS) distinguished AP from MI patients. Responses indicating reactivity to environmental stimulation and frustration, and proneness to irritation when interrupted distinguished men who later developed AP but not men developing silent and acute MIs. The Framingham Type A scale shows a similar differential relatedness to the development of AP as measured by the Rose questionnaire (Rose 1972) among working women and white-collar men in the Framingham study population (Haynes et al. 1978).

All these studies make a valuable contribution in separating AP from MI as criteria. But a necessary next step is to distinguish true AP from pseudo-angina. This requires objective confirmation of coronary artery status, either by long-term follow-up or by arteriography. Recent studies using both these approaches suggest that N is a risk factor only for the development of pseudo-angina.

Some evidence relevant to this hypothesis is provided by a recent longitudinal retrospective-prospective study of CAD diagnoses in a sample of 123 men followed up for periods of from five to 20 years (Costa et al. 1982). Subjects were divided into four groups:

1. Those with a physician's diagnosis of probable or definite angina, but no resting or exercise stress ECG signs of CAD or history of MI in a follow-up period of from 5 to 11 years after diagnosis
2. Those with both anginal complaints and ECG signs of CAD
3. Those with ECG signs of ischemia, but no anginal complaints
4. An age-matched reference group free from both signs and symptoms of CAD

Using the Guilford-Zimmerman Temperament Survey (GZTS), a standardized, objective personality measure, which was obtained at least 1 year prior to the first appearance of signs or symptoms, we found that the ten GZTS personality variables did not predict the development of CAD, but emotional instability scores and higher somatic complaint scores from the Cornell Medical Index (CMI) were predictive of anginal diagnoses in men who showed no other hard signs of CAD. Even when followed for periods up to 12 years, individuals high in neuroticism and reporting angina but without other evidence of CAD did not have an increased risk of MI.

The Costa et al. (1982) study did not employ coronary angiography to determine disease status or end points. Elias et al. (1982), however, administered several measures of anxiety, depression and somatic complaints to a group of 136 men and women who underwent arteriography. Their results were striking. They found a significant negative or inverse correlation between these measures of neuroticism and maximum percentage of stenosis of the coronary arteries. Schocken et al. (1984), in a sample of 110 patients referred for cardiac catheterization, found a similar negative relation between trait anxiety and presence of diseased arteries, using a criterion of 75% stenosis in one or more major coronary arteries.

Recently, Bass and Wade (1984) reported on a series of 99 English patients with chest pain who underwent angiography and who were assessed blindly with regard to angiography results, using standardized psychiatric and social interviews and the Eysenck Personality Questionnaire (EPQ). They classified patients into three groups: (1) no disease or normal coronary arteries (NCA); (2) slight disease, less than 50% obstruction of any vessel; and (3) significant disease, with lesions causing more than 50% obstruction in one or more vessels. Psychiatric morbidity was higher in the normal and near-normal groups (group 1, 58%; group 2, 67%) than patients with significant coronary artery disease (24%). Even more interesting was their finding that the most frequent diagnosis in the normal or NCA group was anxiety neurosis, while the most common diagnosis in the diseased group was depressive neurosis. While the authors do not comment on the different forms of psychiatric morbidity in the NCA and CAD groups, it is plausible to consider the diagnoses of depressive neurosis in the significant CAD group as a consequence of the patients' condition or as a reaction to the alterations in functioning, activity, and lifestyle caused by their diseased hearts. Patients in the nondiseased group (NCA) had higher EPQ neuroticism scores than patients in either of the other 2 groups. Separate sex analyses revealed that the EPQ N effect was significant only for male patients with NCA.

The NCA patients of both sexes experienced a variety of physical symptoms in addition to chest pain. Most frequent complaints were breathlessness at rest, accompanied by sighs and gasps; episodes of faintness and giddiness; palpitations; excessive sweating; suffocation; smothering; and peripheral paresthesiae. These physical symptoms were reported significantly more frequently than by patients in the significant disease group (3), with near-normal patients in an intermediate position.

Far from being a risk factor for true AP, all these studies find that neuroticism is unrelated or inversely related to actual or real AP and is in fact higher in patients with NCA or pseudo-angina.

Symptom Reports as Mediators

How do high N people without CAD become diagnosed as having AP? We know that neuroticism leads to a wide variety of somatic complaints, including chest pain reports. Such complaints would cause them to be referred for CHD diagnostic evaluation and testing much more frequently than low N individuals without CHD. Recently, my colleagues and I tested this hypothesis in a study of 83 male and female patients who kept detailed chest pain diaries for about 2 weeks prior to undergoing diagnostic coronary cine angiography (Costa et al. 1985; Engel et al. 1985). The results of this relatively small scale study strongly supported the hypothesis. Chest pain reports were uniformly less related to atherosclerotic obstruction of the coronary arteries than they were to the patients' level of neuroticism. Neuroticism influenced chest pain symptom reports, and these chest pain reports were more predictive of the patient's enduring personality than they were of the anatomical lesions in their coronary arteries. The findings are summarized in Table 1.

Table 1. Summary of significant variables predicting angiographic evidence of CAD and neuroticism

Criterion	Chest pain diary variable	Correlation	Significance
CAD	Pain brought on by walking	0.42	$P<0.01$
	Sleeping prior to pain	−0.31	$P<0.05$
	Accompanying symptoms:		
	sighing	−0.25	$P<0.05$
	breathlessness	−0.23	$P<0.05$
	dizziness	−0.25	$P<0.05$
	Resting to cope with pain	−0.36	$P<0.05$
Neuroticism	Severity of chest pain	0.27	$P<0.05$
	Accompanying symptoms:		
	breathlessness	0.30	$P<0.05$
	dizziness	0.34	$P<0.01$
	Affect before pain onset:		
	angry	0.32	$P<0.05$
	annoyed	0.49	$P<0.01$
	tense	0.44	$P<0.01$
	afraid	0.38	$P<0.05$
	worried	0.54	$P<0.001$
	upset	0.50	$P<0.001$
	Sensation of chest pain:		
	stabbing	0.26	$P<0.05$
	Profile of Mood States (POMS)		
	tension	0.55	$P<0.001$
	depression	0.50	$P<0.001$
	anger	0.55	$P<0.001$
	fatigue	0.34	$P<0.01$
	confusion	0.50	$P<0.001$
	Total mood disturbance	0.58	$P<0.001$

The most striking aspect of these results is that there is only one positive predictor of angiographically determined CAD, namely walking as the precipitant of chest pain. That effort-induced chest pain is related to presence and severity of arterial disease is hardly new. William Heberden wrote eloquently of its importance in 1772. What is remarkable is that neither any of the other 40 variables characterizing each chest pain report (including 4 other activity precipitants, 9 mood states, 5 pain sensations, 4 pain locations, 8 pain radiation sites, 5 concomitant physical symptoms, 5 coping reactions), nor the number of chest pain episodes during the observation period, nor the average pain severity from the daily chest pain diaries had any predictive significance.

Four of the chest pain variables in fact showed negative relations to angiographic results. Sleeping prior to chest pain was significantly negatively related to obstructive lesions, as was the presence of sighs and dizziness with the chest pain, and the proportion of times that rest was the coping reaction to deal with the pain.

By contrast, Table 1 shows very clearly the pervasive influence of neuroticism on the reporting and characterization of the chest pain diaries. Three of the five accompanying sensations, breathlessness, dizziness and palpitations, were significantly positively related to N, as was the rated severity of the pain, and a characterization of the pain as stabbing. The largest number of neuroticism correlates (with the correlations of greatest magnitude) centered around affective states prior to the chest pain (reporting feelings of anger, annoyance, tension, worry, fear, and upset). In addition to the diary reports which patients completed after each chest pain episode, they completed a standardized mood measure, the Profile of Mood States (POMS) each day at about the same time in the evening (6 p.m.). When average mood scores were computed, all six of the negative mood scales were significantly related to the neuroticism measure, ranging from 0.34 to 0.55; and the total mood disturbance score correlated 0.58 with the CMI N scores. None of the POMS mean level scores were significantly related to angiographic findings, though several showed negative trends. The neuroticism score showed a significant negative relation ($r = -0.22$, $n = 62$, $P < 0.05$, one-tailed) with the cut-off for significant luminal narrowing of 50% stenosis.

We also obtained physicians' estimates of their patients' typical chest pain, and these data similarly showed meagre predictive relations with angiographic outcomes. The correlations between the physicians' ratings or estimates of patients' typical chest pain episodes gives a picture of how a patient's neuroticism might influence the physician's diagnostic decision-making: Physicians judged patients with high N scores to have more chest pain episodes, precipitated by emotional arousal or stress with accompanying weakness, than low N patients. These ratings reflect the patients' own perceptions, but, as we have seen, they are unrelated to arteriographic lesions. We can posit that the doctor's clinical diagnosis of angina is largely based upon the patient's reports; because N affects self-reports of somatic complaints, the physician's diagnosis is determined chiefly by the patient's neuroticism, not the patient's coronary stenoses.

The work of Timothy Smith and his colleagues at the University of Utah also provides additional support for the view that N influences patients' anginal reports but does not influence the disease process. Smith et al. (1984a) reported results of a study exploring the relations of anger, neuroticism, and Type A with the experience of angina in a sample of 40 men and 10 women referred for diagnostic angiography. They correlated three standardized psychometric inventories - Jenkins Activity Survey (JAS), Spielberger State-Trait Anger Scales (STAS), Eysenck Personality Inventory neuroticism (EPI-N scores) - with four 9-point Likert questions regarding patients' experience of angina. Examined also were the correlations between these measures and angiographic findings of arterial stenosis. Of interest in the present context are the relations between the four anginal questions and the psychometric measures of Type A, anger, neuroticism and CAD. Frequency of angina was significantly related only to the STAS ($r = 0.55$); patients ratings of their anginal severity was unrelated to the JAS, STAS or EPI-N scores. Interference in daily activities caused by angina was significantly correlated with the JAS (0.40), STAS (0.53), and EPI-N (0.46), but avoidance of activities because of angina was significantly related only to the EPI-N scores (0.37). Most importantly, extent of arterial obstruction was unrelated to the four angina questions and to scores on the JAS, STAS, and EPI-N.

With these data in hand, I believe we can confidently reject the hypothesis that neuroticism is a risk factor for CAD. Neuroticism influences patients' reports and physicians' diagnoses, but it does *not* lead to development of coronary artery disease.

Implications for the Conceptualization and Measurement of Type A

Can the same conclusion be applied to Type A? We cannot be sure until the same distinctions are made between AP and MI, and between verified AP and pseudo-angina in Type A research. The possibility that Type A predicts only pseudo-angina is especially great for some of the Type A questionnaires or scales that are strongly related to neuroticism. Haynes and her colleagues (1978) found that the highest correlations for the Framingham Type A Scale (FTAS) were with measures of daily stress (0.47), emotional lability (0.43), and tension (0.42). Chesney et al. (1981) furthermore showed that the FTAS was much more strongly related to various measures of neuroticism - EPI-N scores, $r=0.45$; Spielberger State Trait Anxiety Inventory (STAI), $r=0.42$; Derogatis' SCL-90R Anxiety, $r=0.39$, Depression, $r=0.37$ - than it was to Type A ratings derived from the structured interview (SI, $r=0.20$).

Smith et al. (1983) explored the psychological correlates of the FTAS scale in a sample of 143 college students. They found that for both males and females the FTAS was significantly correlated with several measures of general and specific trait anxiety as well as with several scales and the total score on a measure of irrational beliefs. They concluded that the FTAS's "unique pattern of correlations with anxiety, irrational thinking and (low) self-control must qualify the interpretation of findings obtained with this scale." Further evidence that the FTAS is more a measure of neuroticism than of coronary-prone behavior is given by Smith's findings that FTAS scores correlated 0.50 and 0.41 with the STAS and the EPI-N scores, respectively (Smith 1984). Smith and O'Keefe (1984) have replicated these findings regarding the lack of divergent validity of the FTAS from measures of neuroticism by obtaining significant correlations in a sample of 100 male and 100 female undergraduates with the Beck Depression Inventory (0.28), STAS (0.42), and scales of Frequency (0.38) and Severity (0.40) of Daily Hassles.

If the FTAS is a measure of N, it should not be positively related to CAD. And, in fact, Smith et al. (1984b) found a nonsignificant *negative* tendency ($r[50]=-0.21$, $P<0.15$) for FTAS scores to be associated with angiographically documented CAD. This finding is understandable from the present line of argument, and, especially if replicated on larger samples, further bolsters our claim that measures that tap primarily neuroticism-related traits will not be predictive of CAD.

Recent research with global Type A scores, derived from either the structured interview (SI) or questionnaire measures (cited in Dembroski and MacDougall 1985) have failed to find associations with angiographically documented severity of CAD. Dembroski and MacDougall (1985) have suggested that only certain components of the global Type A construct confer coronary risk. Among the many components of the complex and heterogeneous construct of Type A, attention has been given to (1) nonverbal paralinguistic stylistics of Loud, Explosive, Rapid and Accelerated Speech, and Latency of Answers; (2) factor analytically-derived self-report measures of Time Pressure, Hard-Driving Behavior, Speed of Activity, Competitiveness, and Impatience; and (3) the attitudinal and behavioral dimensions of Potential for Hostility, Anger-In, and Verbal Competitiveness. The present review suggests that components related to N will not be predictive, and that researchers should focus on components related to other psychological constructs.

Much greater attention needs to be given to the psychological interpretation of the hostility component within the global Type A construct. Evidence from studies utilizing component scoring of the SI (Dembroski et al. 1979; Dembroski et al. 1985; MacDougall et al. 1985) as well as psychometric measures (MMPI-HO scale: Cook and Medley 1954) Barefoot et al. 1983; Shekelle et al. 1983a; Williams et al. 1980) indicate the predictive importance of hostility and anger as the "toxic" components of the TABP. Yet most measures of anger or hostility correlate highly with N; indeed, anger or hostility is often considered a facet of neuroticism (cf. McCrae and Costa 1984). The problem is to identify a fundamental dimension of personality that is orthogonal to N but captures the essence of the hostility-component formulations of the Type A construct. One promising candidate can be found in the Agreeable-Antagonistic dimension of the Norman taxonomy, defined by such adjectives as soft-hearted-ruthless, trusting-suspicious, and forgiving-vengeful. Persons who describe themselves or are rated by peers as antagonistic set themselves against others. Cognitively, they are mistrustful and skeptical; affectively, they are callous and unsympathetic; behaviorally, they are uncooperative, stubborn, and rude.

Attempts to identify behavioral predictors of CAD have followed a number of false leads, of which neuroticism is perhaps the clearest example, and there is no guarantee that agreeableness-antagonism may not prove to be another. At present, however, it seems to be a construct well worth pursuing.

Acknowledgments. I wish to thank Stephanie V. Stone for her help in reviewing the angiographic literature and for many stimulating comments. Robert R. McCrae and Alan B. Zonderman deserve my thanks for their helpful critical comments. I also wish to acknowledge the generosity and assistance of Timothy W. Smith for providing me with the results from his ongoing research.

References

Banks DC, Raferty EB, Oram S (1971) Clinical significance of the coronary arteriogram. Br Heart J 33: 863-870

Barefoot JC, Dahlstrom WG, Williams RB (1983) Hostility, CHD incidence and total mortality: a 25-year follow-up study of 255 physicians. Psychosom Med 45: 59-63

Bass C, Wade C (1984) Chest pain with normal coronary arteries: a comparative study of psychiatric and social morbidity. Psychol Med 14: 51-61

Chesney MA, Black GW, Chadwick JH, Rosenman RH (1981) Psychological correlates of the Type A behavior pattern. J Behav Med 4 (2): 217-229

Cohn PF, Vokonas PS, Most AS, Herman MV, Gorlin R (1972) Diagnostic accuracy of two-step post-exercise ECG: results in 305 subjects studied by coronary arteriography. JAMA 202: 501-506

Cook W, Medley D (1954) Proposed hostility and pharisaic-virtue scales for the MMPI. J Appl Psychol 38: 414-418

Costa PT Jr (1981) Neuroticism as a factor in the diagnosis of angina pectoris. Behav Med Up 3: 18-20

Costa PT Jr, McCrae RR (1980) Somatic complaints in males as a function of age and neuroticism: a longitudinal analysis. J Behav Med 38: 668-678

Costa PT Jr, McCrae RR (1985) Hypochondriasis, neuroticism, and aging: when are somatic complaints unfounded? Am Psychol (to be published)

Costa PT Jr, Fleg JL, McCrae RR, Lakatta EG (1982) Neuroticism, coronary artery disease and chest pain complaints: cross-sectional and longitudinal studies. Exp Aging Res 8 (1): 37-44

Costa PT Jr, Zonderman AB, Engel BT, Baile WF, Brimlow DL, Brinker JA (1985) The relation of

chest pain symptoms to angiographic findings of coronary artery stenosis and neuroticism. Psychosom Med 47 (3): 285-293
Day LJ, Sowton E (1976) Clinical features and follow-up of patients with angina and normal coronary arteries. Lancet II: 334-337
Dembroski TM, MacDougall JM (1985) Beyond global Type A: relationships of paralinguistic attributes, hostility and anger-in to coronary heart disease. In: Field T, McCabe P, Schneiderman N (eds) Stress and coping. Erlbaum, Hillsdale
Dembroski TM, MacDougall JM, Lushene R (1979) Interpersonal interaction and cardiovascular response in Type A subjects and coronary patients. J Human Stress 5: 28-36
Dembroski TM, MacDougall JM, Williams RB, Haney TC (1985) Components of Type A, hostility and anger-in: relationships to angiographic findings. Psychosom Med 47 (3): 219-233
Elias MF, Robbins MA, Blow FC, Rice AP, Edgecomb JL (1982) Symptom reporting, anxiety, and depression in arteriographically classified middle-aged chest pain patients. Exp Aging Res 8: 45-51
Engel BT, Baile WF, Costa PT Jr, Brimlow DL, Brinker JA (1985) A behavioral analysis of chest pain patients suspected of having coronary artery disease. Psychosom Med 47: 274-284
Fuster V, Frye RL, Connolly DC, Danielson MA, Elveback LR, Kurland LT (1975) Arteriographic patterns early in the onset of coronary syndrome. Br Heart J 37: 1250-1255
Haynes SG, Levine S, Scotch NA, Feinleib M, Kannel WB (1978) The relationship of psychosocial factors to coronary heart disease in the Framingham Study. I. Methods and risk factors. Am J Epidemiol 107: 362-383
Herman MV, Cohn PF, Gorlin R (1973) Editorial: angina-like chest pain without identifiable cause. Ann Int Med 79 (3): 445-447
Horwitz LD (1974) The diagnostic significance of anginal symptoms. JAMA 29 (9): 1196-1199
Jenkins CD (1971) Psychologic and social precursors of coronary disease. N Engl J Med 284: 244-255, 307-317
Jenkins CD (1976) Recent evidence supporting psychologic and social risk factors for coronary disease. N Engl J Med 987-994, 1033-1038
Jenkins CD, Zyzanski SJ, Rosenman RH (1978) Coronary-prone behavior: one pattern or several? Psychosom. Med 27: 25-43
Kemp HG, Vokonas PS, Cohn PF, Gorlin R (1973) The anginal syndrome associated with normal coronary arteriograms: report of a six-year experience. Am J Med 54: 735-742
Likoff W, Segal BL, Kasparian H (1967) Paradox of normal selective coronary arteriograms in patients considered to have unmistakeable coronary heart disease. N Engl J Med 276: 1063-1066
MacDougall JM, Dembroski TM, Dimsdale JE, Hackett TP (1985) Components of Type A, hostility, and anger-in: further relationships to angiographic findings. Health Psychol 4 (2): 137-152
McCrae RR, Costa PT Jr (1985) Updating Norman's "adequate taxonomy": intelligence and personality dimensions in natural language and in questionnaires. J Pers Soc Psychol 49: 710-721
McCrae RR, Costa PT (1984) Emerging lives, enduring dispositions: personality in adulthood. Little, Brown, Boston
Medalie JH, Goldbourt U (1976) Angina-pectoris among 10000 men. II. Psychosocial and other risk factors as evidenced by a multivariate analysis of a five-year incidence study. Am J Med 60: 910-920
Medalie JH, Synder M, Groen JJ, Neufeld HN, Goldbourt U, Riss E (1973) Angina pectoris among 10000 men: 5 year incidence and univariate analysis. Am J Med 55: 583-594
Ostfeld AM, Lebovits BZ, Shekelle RB, Paul O (1964) A prospective study of the relationship between personality and coronary heart disease. J Chronic Dis 17: 265-276
Proudfit WL, Shirey EK, Sheldon WC, Sones FM Jr (1968) Certain clinical characteristics correlated with extent of obstructive lesions demonstrated by selective cine-coronary arteriography. Circulation 38: 947-951
Rose G (1972) Epidemiology of ischaemic heart disease. Br J Hosp Med 7: 285
Schoken DD, Worden TJ, Harrison EE, Spielberger CD (1984) Anxiety differences in patients with angina pectoris, nonanginal chest pain, and coronary artery disease. Paper presented at the 57th scientific sessions. American Heart Association, Miami Beach, Florida, November 1984
Shekelle RB, Gale M, Ostfeld AM, Paul O (1983 a) Hostility, risk of coronary heart disease and mortality. Psychosom Med 45: 109-114

Shekelle RB, Hulle SB, Neaton J, et al (1983b) The MRFIT Behavior Pattern Study. II: Type A behavior pattern and incidence of coronary heart disease. CVD Epidemiology Newsletter 34

Smith TW (1984) Type A behavior, anger and neuroticism: the discriminant validity of self-reports in a patient sample. Br J Clin Psychol 23: 147-148

Smith TW, O'Keefe JL (1985) The Inequivalence of Self-Reports of Type A Behavior: Differential Relationship of the Jenkins Activity Survey and Framingham Scale with Affect, Stress and Control. Motivation and Emotion 9: 299-311

Smith TW, Houston BK, Zurawski RM (1983) The Framingham Type A scale and anxiety, irrational beliefs, and self-control. J Hum Stress 9 (2): 32-37

Smith TW, Follick ML, Korr KS (1984a) Anger, neuroticism, Type A behavior and the experience of angina. Br J Med Psychol 57: 249-252

Smith TW, Korr KS, Follick MJ, McCartney JR (1984b) The Framingham Type A scale and severity of coronary artery disease. Paper presented at the annual meeting of the American Psychological Association. Toronto

Steptoe A (1981) Psychological factors in cardiovascular disorders. Academic, New York

Williams RB, Haney TL, Lee KL, Kong Y, Blumenthal JA, Whalen RE (1980) Type A behavior, hostility, and coronary atherosclerosis. Psychosom Med 42: 539-549

Type A: Behavior or Trait?

B. T. Engel[1]

Introduction

For years, participants at conferences such as this one have reported that persons characterized as Type A are at higher risk for coronary artery disease (CAD) than are others not so unfortunately endowed. These informants readily acknowledge that the two major tests of Type A, the structured interview (SI), and the Jenkins Activity Survey (JAS), do not correlate well with one another (MacDougall et al. 1979; Chesney et al. 1981; Matthews et al. 1982). However, they argue that that discrepancy is because the two instruments measure different components of Type A. That truism is usually followed by the assertion that the SI is better than the JAS because it is based on behavioral observations that are not possible with the JAS. At the same time, it is acknowledged that the JAS is better for scientific purposes because it yields quantified, scaled scores which provide finer means of relating Type A to other, quantified scores.

Reviewers (e.g., Krantz et al. 1982) tell us that some aspects of Type A predict some aspects of CAD better than others. There are even data which suggest that some aspects of Type A predict different manifestations of CAD; for example, Jenkins et al. (1978) have reported that men who developed myocardial infarctions (MIs) responded differently on the JAS from men who had so-called silent MIs, and both of these groups were different from those who reported symptoms characteristic of angina pectoris. Laboratory studies, purporting to show that Type A persons generally behave differently from Type B persons, use a variety of tasks, most of which could be characterized as diabolical, and certainly as unnatural – for example, it seems unlikely that business executives are likely to own video games, let alone play them against experts who are half their ages. These same reviewers advise us that some investigators believe that Type A is not a set of isolated behaviors; rather, it is a "coping style" which operates "throughout life" (Krantz et al. 1982). Still other theorists are purported to believe that Type A persons manifest an idiosyncratic, attentional style (Krantz et al. 1982). Recently, Williams et al. (1980) proposed that hostility is the pathognomic component of Type A, an interpretation which was supported by Shekelle et al. (1983) on an independent sample of subjects. What is particularly fascinating about the notions of lifelong coping styles or hostility is that both of these factors are usually defined as traits, not behaviors.

This tendency to blur behaviors with traits has pervaded much of the debate about Type A. Most of the investigators of Type A insist that it is behavior, elicited

1 Gerontology Research Center (Baltimore), National Institute on Aging, National Institute of Health, PHS, U.S. Department of Health and Human Services, Bethesda, and Francis Scott Key Medical Center, Baltimore, MD 21224, USA

Biological and Psychological Factors
in Cardiovascular Disease
Ed. by T. H. Schmidt, T. M. Dembroski, and G. Blümchen

Table 1. Indicators of angina pectoris derived from a clinical history

1. Date of onset
2. Date of most recent occurrence
3. Location and radiation of pain
4. Character of pain
5. Severity of pain
6. Relation of pain to effort
7. Relation of pain to emotion, cold weather, or other eliciting events
8. Usual duration of pain
9. Relief of pain with rest or with a vasodilating agent

by certain classes of situations, whereas many of the critics argue that the predictive power of Type A measurements necessarily depends upon its trait qualities. One cannot have it both ways: If Type A is a behavior, it is stimulus specific; if it manifests itself across situations, then it is a trait. I think that much of the confusion among proponents of Type A comes from the fact they do not appreciate that traits are assessed by measuring behaviors. However, the attribute which traits have is that they are not specific to any particular situation such as the SI, but rather are manifest across a number of situations. As a matter of fact, a trait theorist would recognize that a Type A person might even appear to be Type B during a structured interview because of his unique learning background with respect to interviews. In any case, the ingredient missing from this debate is the data! What is needed is a cross-situational assessment of the behaviors seen in the SI which led to the diagnosis, Type A, in the first place. Such data would show clearly whether the SI really is an accurate prediction of a Type A trait or whether it reflects interview-specific behaviors which have limited generality.

Recently, my colleagues and I completed a study which might serve as a model for evaluating Type A in vivo (Engel et al. 1985; Costa et al. 1985). As is well known, the diagnosis of angina pectoris is based almost exclusively on a clinical history which elicits information about nine factors (Table 1). These factors are not greatly different from those Heberden (1802) described almost 200 years ago, and the method for collecting these data certainly has not changed. The critical point to note from the factors in Table 1 is that most of them are symptoms which are supposedly elicited by an imbalance between myocardial oxygen demand and myocardial blood supply, viz., CAD. Thus, the presence of CAD is inferred from responses elicited during a clinical history which focuses on recollections of symptoms which may have occurred during specific events. The main difference between a clinical history of angina and a structured interview is that the SI not only elicits recollections but also is itself considered to be an eliciting event.

Method

Our questions were very simple:

1. To what extent do the retrospective data collected during a clinical history accurately portray the experiences reported by the patient?

Table 2. Self-reported antecedents of chest pain episodes

Antecedent event	Percentage of episodes, event present
A. Activity	
1. Sleeping	15
2. Sitting	30
3. Walking	32
4. Other exercise	22
B. Social context	
1. Alone	35
2. With another person	65
C. Setting	
1. Work	7
2. Home	80
3. Other	13
D. Mood	
1. Content	47
2. Happy	14
3. Laughing	3
4. Annoyed	5
5. Angry	2
6. Worried	6
7. Afraid	1
8. Tense	12
9. Upset	10

Table 3. Self-reported concomitants of chest pain episodes

A. Characteristics	Mean
1. episodes/day	0.6
2. minutes/episode	4.0
3. days studied	16.5
4. pain severity	35.8
Concomitant event	**Percentage of episodes event present**
B. Physical Symptoms	
1. Breathlessness	34
2. Sighs	14
3. Dizziness	7
4. Palpitations	15
5. Weakness	30
C. Pain sensations	
1. Burning	11
2. Pressing	31
3. Squeezing	12
4. Stabbing	9
5. Aching	38

2. To what extent do the experiences, either collected during the history or as they occur, in vivo, correlate with CAD as measured by coronary artery angiography.

To answer these questions we selected a cohort of patients who had been referred to the Johns Hopkins Hospital for evaluation of chest pain and for consideration for coronary artery bypass surgery. Coronary angiography, of course, is one of the final tests given in this assessment.

Patients who volunteered for our study completed a number of questionnaires. One of these was a self-report form about their chest pains which they filled out each time they had a chest pain, and which they mailed to us daily. Thus, we were able to collect data on chest pains as they occurred, in vivo, and we were able to compare these self-reports with physician reports since we asked the referring physicians to complete an appropriate form which best reflected their assessments of their patients' chest pains (see Engel et al. 1985) for examples of the forms completed by the patients and by the physicians). Subsequently, we analyzed the frequencies of occurrence of specific symptoms in relation to specific behavioral categories.

Table 4. Self-reported pain characteristics

Pain characteristic	Number of subjects, reporting event	Percentage of episodes event present
A. Location		
1. Sternum	60	63
2. Left upper chest	36	35
3. Left lower chest[a]	28	36
4. Left arm	18	24
5. Neck or jaw	16	50
6. Right upper chest	14	35
7. Right arm	13	20
8. Right lower chest[a]	9	26
B. Radiation		
1. Left arm	35	49
2. Left upper chest	27	50
3. Right arm	20	40
4. Sternum	18	42
5. Neck or jaw	17	34
Right upper chest	12	27
7. Right lower chest[a]	9	48
8. Left lower chest[a]	8	46
9. None	20	

[a] Includes abdomen.

Results

Table 2 presents a summary of the symptoms which the patients reported as anteceding their chest pains. Among the noteworthy findings are: (1) 55% of the events were related to physical activities; (2) 65% of the events occurred in the presence of another person; (3) 80% of the events occurred at home, perhaps because these patients were awaiting their hospital admissions for angiography; (4) and finally, fully 64% of the events occurred at times when the patient was experiencing positive affects. Please note that positive affects are not even discussed during a clinical history.

Table 3 presents the concomitants of the events. The average patient had fewer than one episode/day which lasted about 4 min and which was rated as about 36 on a pain scale of 0 (none) to 100 (severe). The most common symptoms accompanying a chest pain were breathlessness or weakness. The most common pain sensations were pressing or aching. The primary locations of pain (Table 4) varied considerably from one patient to the next, and from one event to the next in the same patient. Furthermore, there was very little consistency in the nature of the pain radiations (Table 4), and almost 25% of the patients never report radiating pain. Neither the self-reported severity nor the duration of pain correlated significantly with the location or radiation of the pain. Furthermore, the duration of the pain also did not correlate significantly with any of the physical symptoms or any of the pain sensations. However, the self-reported severity did correlate significantly with some of the symptoms and some of the pain sensations.

Table 5. Self-reported consequences of chest pain episodes

Consequent event	Percentage of episodes event present
A. Coping reaction	
1. Nitroglycerin	51
2. Other medication	5
3. Rest	38
4. Other	6
B. Behavioral reaction	
1. Carried on	59
2. Changed activity	41

Table 5 reports the consequences of the anginal events. About half of the events were treated with nitroglycerin, and almost 40% of the events were treated by rest. On most occasions (about 60%), after the event had passed, the patient went back to what he was doing. However, there are some important interactions between antecedents or setting factors and subsequent behavior. Subjects who were asleep tended to go back to sleep. Subjects who were at work tended to return to their ongoing activities; but subjects who were at home were unlikely to return to their ongoing activities. Similarly, subjects who were exercising (other than walking) were likely to change their activity, as were subjects who were alone at the time of the episode.

Table 6 compares the referring physicians' estimates of some of the antecedents or concomitants of chest pain with the patients' self-reports. Among the many noteworthy findings in this table are:

1. The physicians' estimates of the number of episodes and the severity of the episodes were significantly greater than were the patients' estimates, approximately 2.5-fold and 1.5-fold, respectively.
2. It is clear that the physicians attended carefully to the activities that the patients said they were emitting at the time of the event since there is good agreement between the physician estimates and the self-reports on sleep-related events and walking-related events. For example, among the 6 patients for whom the physicians judged sleep-related chest pains to be typical, 58% of episodes occurred during sleep; among the 57 patients for whom the physicians judged sleep-related chest pains to be atypical, only 14% of the pains occurred during sleep.
3. With the exception of dizziness, there is poor agreement between the self-reported symptoms or pain sensations and the physician-estimated symptoms or sensations. For example, among the 29 patients for whom the physicians judged the sensation of pressing to be typical, 42% of the events were so characterized; however, among the 33 patients for whom the physicians judged pressing to be atypical, 44% of the events were reported to have produced the sensation.

Table 6. Comparisons among patients' self-reports and physicians' estimates

Outcome measure	Number of subjects	Physicians' estimates	Patients' self-reports	
A. Episodes/week	57	11.2	4.5	
B. Pain severity	62	47.4	32.5	
	Physicians' characterization of event			
	Typical		Atypical	
	Number of subjects physicians identified	Percentage of episodes event present	Number of subjects physicians identified	Percentage of episodes event present
C. Antecedents				
1. Sleeping	6	58	57	14
2. Resting	17	27	46	37
3. Walking	28	46	35	30
4. Exercising or working	30	28	33	17
5. Emotionally aroused[a]	25	13	38	9
D. Concomitants				
1. Physical symptoms				
a) Breathless	0	-	59	56
b) Sighs	32	23	27	29
c) dizzy	2	67	57	13
d) palpitations	6	45	53	28
e) weakness	13	52	46	57
2. Pain sensations				
a) burning	7	29	55	12
b) pressing	29	42	33	44
c) squeezing	22	25	40	14
d) stabbing	2	0	60	11
e) aching	7	50	55	54

[a] Based on percentage of episodes during which patients were annoyed, angry, worried, afraid, tense, or upset.

Discussion

Finally, there is one irony to all of this. The data I have just cited relate the self-reports of chest pain to the physician estimates of angina pectoris. Since these estimates enter importantly into the decision to carry out coronary artery angiography, they are clinically very significant. The irony has been fully documented elsewhere (Costa, this volume). Almost without exception none of the data reported either by the physicians or by the patients predict CAD; however, many of the data do correlate with neuroticism, a trait which is known to correlate highly with symptom reporting among people with any of a variety of chronic medical disorders (Costa and McCrae 1980). In this sense these data affirm a finding which one sees often in cross-situational studies: Separate domains of behavior are internally very consistent; however, cross-domain correlations frequently are very poor (e.g., Foerster et al. 1983).

It is well-known that retrospective reports of significant events in a person's life are often misreported. For example, Horowitz et al. (1977) have shown that patients who are asked to complete "life stress" questionnaires show a low reliability in reporting events, even when the events were once judged by the patients to have elicited considerable life stresses. With respect to the issue of the assessment of Type A, I have tried to show that it is possible to evaluate elicited responses even under difficult circumstances - in this instance, when the eliciting events are painful and disruptive. It is clear from trait research, and widely accepted by proponents (Epstein 1979, 1980) as well as by critics (Mischel and Peake 1982) of personality theory that the expressions of traits can only be assessed by measuring behavior across many situations and over time. The hallmark of a trait is not that it occurs equally in all situations and at all times but that it has a high probability of occurrence across situations and over time.

All investigators of Type A acknowledge that it is made up of many factors. Among those that have been reported repeatedly to account for a considerable portion of the variance underlying the Type A construct are competitiveness, striving for achievement, aggressiveness, impatience, and a sense of time pressure (Dembroski et al. 1985). However, these indices have been derived from cohorts who were studied in one of another context. Usually, the subjects were selected by the SI or JAS, and the components noted above were extracted from a factor analysis. This method allows the researcher to cross-validate the components across samples. However, it is wholly inadequate for predicting how an individual will behave across situations. Yet that is precisely the aspect of Type A which makes it a putative predictor of CAD. It would be very useful to characterize subjects on the basis of a Type A assessment such as the SI, and *then* to carry out field studies to determine the extent to which a trait measured by the assessment correlates with behavior, in vivo. Do persons who score high on the Type A measure of job involvement show this attitude in the workplace; do persons who appear aggressive or hostile in the interview behave that way in other situations; does impatience during a Type A interview predict impatience while standing in a queue or waiting at a traffic signal? Clearly, field studies using self-report and peer-report assessments could readily reveal how well Type A-like behavior measured in one context predicts Type A-like behavior in other contexts. Unless and until investigators of Type A measure the relevant behaviors across situations and over time, we will never know what the attributes of Type A are which predict various aspects of CAD. We already know that the correlations between components of Type A and components of CAD are too low to tease out the predictors from the coincidental correlates. Increasing the number of persons interviewed will not solve the problem, since that will only lower the variance of the correlations and not increase their magnitudes; designing more diabolical laboratory situations will not solve the problem, since one is still left with the need to validate the laboratory findings against naturally occurring situations; abandoning one component of Type A and replacing it by another - e.g., shifting attention from competition to hostility - will never solve the problem, since various components of Type A share common variance, and since neither component has been evaluated properly in any case; and finally, "physiologizing" about which cognitive processes cause which cardiovascular changes - which, in turn, may not even be antecedents of CAD - will certainly never solve the problem. It seems clear that Type A is a real phenomenon, but its attributes are obscured by measurement deficits which can only be overcome by multiple samples taken across situations and over time.

References

Chesney MA, Black GW, Chadwick JH, Rosenman RH (1981) Psychological correlates of the Type A behavior pattern. J Behav Med 4: 217-229

Costa PT (1985) Chest pain symptoms, coronary stenosis and neuroticism. (to be published)

Costa PT, McCrae RR (1980) Somatic complaints in males as a function of age and neuroticism: a longitudinal analysis. J Behav Med 3: 245-257

Costa RT, Zonderman AB, Engel BT, Baile WF, Brimlow DL, Brinker J (1985) The relation of chest pain symptoms to coronary stenosis and neuroticism in patients suspected of having coronary artery disease. Psychosom Med 47: 285-293

Dembroski TM, MacDougall JM (1985) Beyond global type A: relationships of paralinguistic attributes, hostility and anger-in to coronary heart disease. In: Field T, McCabe P, Schneiderman N (eds) Stress and coping. (to be published)

Engel BT, Baile WF, Costa PT, Brimlow DL, Brinker J (1985) A behavioral analysis of chest pain in patients suspected of having coronary artery disease. Psychosom Med 47: 274-284

Epstein S (1979) The stability of behavior: I. On predicting most of the people much of the time. Pers Soc Psychol 37: 1097-1126

Epstein S (1980) The stability of behavior: II. implications for psychological research. Am Psychol 35: 790-806

Foerster F, Schneider HJ, Walschburger P (1983) Psychologische Reaktionsmuster. Minerva, München

Heberden W (1802) Commentaries on the history and cure of diseases. Payne, London, pp 362-369

Horowitz M, Schaefer BA, Hiroto D, Wilner N, Levin B (1977) Life event questionnaires for measuring presumptive stress. Psychosom Med 39: 413-431

Jenkins CD, Zyzanski SJ, Rosenman RH (1978) Coronary-prone behavior: one pattern or several? Psychosom Med 40: 25-43

Krantz DS, Glass DC, Schaeffer MA, Davia JE (1982) Behavior patterns and coronary disease: a critical evaluation In: Cacioppo JT, Petty RE (eds) Perspectives in cardiovascular physiology. Guilford, New York, pp 315-346

MacDougall JM, Dembroski TM, Musante L (1979) The structured interview and questionnaire methods of assessing coronary-prone behavior in male and female college students. J Behav Med 2: 71-83

Matthews KA, Krantz DS, Dembroski TM, Macdougall JM (1982) The unique and common variance in the structured interview and Jenkins Activity Survey estimates of Type A behavior. J Pers Soc Psychol 42: 303-313

Mischel W, Peake PK (1982) Beyond deja vu in the search for cross-situational consistency. Psychol Rev 89: 730-755

Shekelle RB, Gale M, Ostfeld AM, Paul O (1983) Hostility, risk of coronary heart disease, and mortality. Psychosom Med 45: 109-114

Williams RB Jr, Haney TL, Lee KL, Kong Y-H, Blumenthal JA, Whalen RE (1980) Type A behavior, hostility, and coronary atherosclerosis. Psychosom Med 42: 539-549

Type A as a Coping Career – Toward a Conceptual and Methodological Redefinition

H. MATSCHINGER, J. SIEGRIST, K. SIEGRIST, and K. H. DITTMANN[1]

The conceptualization and measurement of human behavior, which takes into account its variability as well as its interaction with powerful social settings, is an extremely difficult scientific enterprise. In the light of these obstacles, research on Type A behavior pattern (TABP) in its relation to premature manifestation of ischemic heart disease (IHD) must be judged as successful. This holds true despite the fact that new prospective epidemiological studies fail to replicate adequately earlier findings (Shekelle et al. 1983; Ruberman et al. 1984), and despite the fact that the pathophysiology of TABP is still controversial (Dembroski et al. 1983). The focus of shared knowledge created by research on TABP is impressive, and it is evident that certain components or elements in the TABP must be of critical importance for a premature cardiovascular vulnerability to exist. One may argue that the strength of the original concept was in its operational simplicity, as expressed in direct behavioral assessment. On the other hand, theoretical clarification of what is considered "stressful" in TABP has so far been insufficient. At this point, virtually all analyses refer to "enhanced adrenergic activity" or "increased sympathetic arousal" without specifying the different cognitive and emotional concomitants which modulate their neural and neurohumoral consequences. It seems appropriate to re-open the conceptual and methodological discussion on the stressful aspects of TABP. In this framework, we would like to present a condensed version of our work in this field, which has been accumulated over the last 5 years. The first part presents the main arguments for a theoretical reformulation of TABP in terms of an individual coping career, based on a strong personal "need for control." The second part develops the rationale for measuring "need for control" as a two-dimensional concept and describes major test-statistical properties of the instrument developed by our group. In the third part, we shall present and discuss a series of some very recent results from a prospective study on cardiovascular risk in a blue-collar population. Here, dimensions of "need for control" are considered as exogenous variables in linear structural equation models explaining parameters of cardiovascular risk, such as high blood pressure or high LDL cholesterol.

Conceptual Approach

In one of his most recent definitions, Rosenman describes TABP as a set of "behavioral dispositions such as ambitiousness, aggressiveness, competitiveness, and impatience, including specific behaviors such as muscle tenseness, alertness, rapid and

1 Department of Medical Sociology, Faculty of Medicine, University of Marburg, 3550 Marburg, Federal Republic of Germany

Biological and Psychological Factors
in Cardiovascular Disease
Ed. by T. H. Schmidt, T. M. Dembroski, and G. Blümchen

emphatic voice style and the pace of most activities, and emotional responses such as irritability and increased potential for hostility and anger" (Rosenman 1983). He concludes: "TABP is associated with hyperadrenergic responsiveness in the daily milieu, due to perception of environmental stressors and events as challenges and threats to control. ... Type A individuals perceive too many things as a threat to their control over the environment and as making demands that are incongruent with their preferred rate of activity" (loc. cit). It is important to note, that this definition no longer analyses TABP in the framework of a single personality trait but favors the notion of a "characteristic style of coping response to environmental stressors" (loc. cit.). Moreover, motivational, as well as cognitive processes, are admitted as playing a decisive role. However, these processes have never been formally investigated and neither the structured interview (SI) nor the Jenkins Activity Survey (JAS) or related techniques seem to offer appropriate tools for assessing such attributes.

Starting from impressive work reported by Glass (1977), we have suggested an approach which concentrates on a strong need for control over the immediate social environment as an important motivational basis of TABP (Siegrist et al. 1980). This need for control can be genetically determined ("high reactor syndrome"), but evidence shows that primary socialization plays an important part in two ways: Strong need for control is either the outcome of model-learning or it acts as a compensation for experience of low self-esteem or marginal socioemotional status during childhood and early adolescence. While these developmental issues have to be further established in longitudinal studies, our main argument focuses on the cognitive, perceptual consequences of enhanced need for control in adult life: Individuals experiencing high need for control tend towards unrealistic appraisal of demanding, challenging situations and of their related internal coping potential. Fear of losing control is thought to stimulate overcommitment, either in the form of underestimation of demands and associated overestimation of coping potential, or in the form of overestimation of demands and underestimation of resources. The first case is likely to occur early in adulthood where good health, professional training and achievement motivation facilitate overcommitment in terms of increased responsibility, enhanced job-involvement and extension of work-related duties to private life. Experience of rewarding feedback coming from significant others reinforces this pattern. Due to this excessive need for control, both patterns, that is the under- and overestimation of challenges, are at first experienced as successful strategies by the individual. Yet, under conditions of increased demands and obligations, continuous overcommitment may precipitate distressing experiences. Increased demands associated with limited coping abilities are likely to occur durring middle adulthood, especially so in distinct occupational groups such as low-status blue-collar workers (see below). In order to focus on duration and intensity of distressing experiences of this type, we suggest analysis of the working man during middle adulthood in terms of a "coping career": Increased demands associated with limited coping abilities precipitate further stages of such a career, leading to manifestation of premature exhaustion and "burn out", whereas moderate challenges or even increased demands which can be successfully met delay onset of these signs. In which way does need for control precipitate a coping career?

We assume that distressing experiences are not perceived in an adequate way in individuals with a strong sense of control. Cognitive patterns, established in early adulthood under more successful circumstances, persist even if increased efforts to meet demands are necessary and even if successful coping is unlikely. We expect deleterious effects on the cardiovascular system in those individuals who maintain their vigorous efforts under long-lasting, control-limiting conditions such as poor job security, forced downward mobility, and increased financial pressure. These threats to social status do exist, not only under clear-cut conditions such as job loss, but also under conditions of low control over the working environment, as expressed in situations of ambiguous or zero feedback from supervisors as well as uncertainty about pay-off of invested efforts. On the other hand, in a benign working environment even individuals with enhanced need for control may be protected against intense distress as they experience more adequate reward. Thus, harmful stages of their coping career may be experienced later in their life cycle.

A further step in the coping career of individuals with enhanced need for control can be characterized as follows: As the potential of distressing experiences increases and as signs of fatigue become more apparent, such as vividly described in the "syndrome of vital exhaustion and depression" (Appels 1983), a more realistic awareness of the "coping me" can be expected. Feelings of "immersion" are admitted, and signs of coping failure, for example, severe disturbances of the sleep-wake cycle (Siegrist et al. 1985) become evident. This is the case in the highly vulnerable period of imminent disease manifestation. In many individuals, however, realistic awareness of coping failure is established only after onset of disease such as acute myocardial infarction (AMI).

To summarize, we propose to specify "enhanced adrenergic activity" in terms of a coping career. Successful efforts, commonly experienced during early adulthood, as well as in privileged living conditions are thought to be harmless to the cardiovascular system. It is only when efforts are followed by poor pay-off or by loss of control that they develop their critical impact. In accordance with other investigators (Karasek et al. 1982; Frankenhaeuser 1983; Henry 1983), we have labeled this type of experience "active distress" (Siegrist et al. 1982). Active distress synergistically stimulates the sympathoadrenomedullary and the pituitary-adrenocortical system and by doing so promotes neurohormonal disbalance, which has been shown to impair the cardiovascular system (Schneiderman 1983).

Active distress is likely to occur under two conditions: first in social contexts that threaten acquired social status and that impose demands under conditions of low predictability; secondly in individuals who exhibit rigid cognitive strategies of formerly successful coping under these control-limiting circumstances. Individuals with high need for control are at high risk using such strategies. We therefore differentiate (1) quality of experience associated with coping (active distress), (2) social conditions or contexts which elicit or reinforce these experiences, and (3) stages of a coping career in individuals with enhanced need for control.

This approach enables us to test hypotheses, which, until now, have never been investigated in research on TABP. For example, we postulate that an enhanced need for control, in terms of vigorous effort, influences parameters of cardiovascular risk only in those middle-aged individuals who live and work under distinct control-limiting circumstances. Furthermore, we postulate that awareness of "immersion" (coping failure) in individuals with TABP discriminates persons at cardiovascular risk only in the later stages of the coping career, i. e., immediately before and after disease onset.

In the long run, differentiations of this kind can be of practical importance as they may help to clarify in which way and at which stages individuals who exhibit TABP are "coronary-prone". Before reporting results bearing on these hypotheses, we have to delineate our measurement approach in some detail.

Methodological Approach

A psychological test permits measurement of cognitions and emotions associated with enhanced need for control only in a limited, indirect way. In a trait-oriented measurement approach such as the one adopted by us, it is assumed that relevant samples of verbal stimuli act as indicators of latent dimensions, which are thought to characterize, to some extent, the principles underlying overt coping behavior. The validity of indicators of such latent dimensions is given in so far as they explain the criteria under study (indicators of cardiovascular risk) in the predicted way. We present basic information about development and test-statistical description of a scale which measures the need for control at the work site. This scale consists of a questionnaire with 44 dichotomous items measuring six aspects of cognitions and emotions associated with overt coping (see below). Each of these aspects has been considered as a latent dimension whose unidimensionality was established by means of a dichotomous logistic test model (Rasch 1960; Fischer 1974). The raw scores of each dimension provide a sufficient statistic for the location of an individual on each of the six scales.

In a second step, these six dimensions are analyzed in terms of an underlying factorial structure. Such a structure has been postulated not only as a consequence of specific operationalization (items with positive emotional connotations differ from items with negative connotations) but also as a consequence of the concept of a coping career. As mentioned earlier, we distinguish between cognitions and emotions associated with perceived successful coping and those associated with feelings of loss of control, disappointment, and fatigue. In our measurement approach, we have dealt with these two aspects in terms of two factors underlying the latent dimensions of coping behavior. The first factor is labeled "vigor", the second one "immersion". By means of a confirmatory factor analysis (Jöreskog 1973 a), we have analyzed and established the two-factorial structure of our scale "need for control". As will be shown, this structure remains fairly stable when comparing different populations, and even when comparing panel data of one population. Having checked for such an invariant latent structure of the scale, we then postulate distinct effects of "vigor" and of "immersion" on the cardiovascular risks at different stages of the coping career. This hypothesis will be tested in terms of linear structural equation models (Jöreskog and Sörbom 1979).

Development of the Scale

In order to construct an economical, well-replicable scale focusing on work-related attitudes and emotions under conditions of enhanced need for control, we started by categorizing about 600 items. (Although a few were already available, the majority were developed by us, based on a broad spectrum of answers from former interviews with coronary patients; Siegrist et al. 1980.) These items were systematized according to a number of dimensions describing active coping in the work field. Independent rating of the item pool according to those aspects by four independent raters enabled us to calculate degree of interrater concordance. A sample of 100 items with highest concordance was administered as a paper-and-pencil test in 80 coronary patients and matched controls. Classic item analysis resulted in separating out 44 items representing the following six dimensions of coping behavior:

1. Need for approval, coping with success and failure
2. Competitiveness, independence and latent hostility
3. Work commitment, hard driving
4. Perfectionism, need for making plans
5. Time urgency, impatience and irritability
6. Inability to withdraw from (work) obligations.

The probability of a specific answer to the items representing the six dimensions can be expressed as a function of two parameters: (1) the difficulty of an item, and (2) the location of an individual on the latent dimension. This function is called "item characteristic". The dichotomous logistic test model developed by Rasch (Rasch 1960) assumes equal item characteristic for all items, as well as for a defined class of situations. This allows an objective scaling of individuals on latent dimensions, i.e., a scaling independent of the item sample. As the main assumption of the Rasch model is its homogeneity with regard to different items and different individuals, estimation of model parameters is considered as independent of a specific sample under study (Fischer 1974). Testing our data with the Rasch model revealed unidimensionality for the six latent dimensions mentioned above. Further testing for unidimensionality in additional samples, as well as under repeated measurement has been undertaken and will be referred to in the next section before we finally test for the two-dimensional latent structure of the scales by means of a congeneric measurement model (Jöreskog 1971).

Test Statistics of the Scale

On the basis of a newly explored sample of 113 men (age 30-55) with established myocardial infarction and of 368 men (age 25-55) free from hard coronary events as established by ECG (for a closer description of this sample see below), we have assessed the test-statistical description as published in the German sources (Dittmann et al. 1982, 1985).

In a first step we tested uni-dimensionality of the six latent dimensions in these two samples by means of an Andersen test (Andersen 1973). Chi-square values for the original sample (113 patients with AMI) are indicated in Table 1.

Table 1. Test for groups with extreme raw scores[a]

Approval	There was no possibility to split the groups in at least two subgroups
Competitiveness	Cutting point = 2 $df = 5$ $X^2 = 7.4719$ (2 groups, 6 items)
Commitment	Cutting points = 4 and 6 $df = 14$ $X^2 = 13.576$ (3 groups, 8 items)
Perfectionism	There was no possibility to split the groups
Time urgency	Cutting points = 3 and 5 $df = 14$ $X^2 = 15.348$ (3 groups, 8 items)
Inability to withdraw	Cutting point = 5 $df = 8$ $X^2 = 16.548$ (2 groups, 9 items)

[a] AMI-patients, $n = 113$

Table 2. Stability test for the six subscales (t_1 on t_2)

Approval		$n = 259$	Perfectionism		$n = 254$
$df = 258$	Z	$= 187.60$	$df = 258$	Z	$= 157.54$
$p \leqslant 5\%$	if	$Z \geqslant 296.18$	$p \leqslant 5\%$	if	$Z \geqslant 296.18$
Competitiveness		$n = 254$	*Time urgency*		$n = 319$
$df = 253$	Z	136.17	$df = 318$	Z	$= 243.09$
$p \leqslant 5\%$	if	$Z \geqslant 290.82$	$p \leqslant 5\%$	if	$Z \geqslant 360.31$
Commitment		$n = 292$	*Inability to withdraw*		$n = 288$
$df = 291$	Z	$= 198.66$	$df = 287$	Z	$= 290.75$
$p \leqslant 5\%$	if	$Z \geqslant 331.5$	$p \leqslant 5\%$	if	$Z \geqslant 327.23$

Next, we analyzed the effect of repeated measurement on unidimensionality and homogeneity of the scales by assuming absence of interaction between item parameter and person parameter (Rost 1977) and absence of inter-individual difference in change over time. Under given restrictions, a splitting of the item sample into two parts representing two repeated applications allows the calculation of likelihood of the data for each latent dimension. These calculations have been done for the larger sample of middle-aged men without clinical coronary heart disease. Within 1 year, two measurements of the scale "need for control" have been taken. Results of the analysis of likelihood are presented in Table 2.

These results show that the measurement of each latent dimension is consistent and homogeneous for two measurement points and that no inter-individual difference in change has taken place. This result can be interpreted as expression of considerable stability of measurement where the raw score of respective dimensions prove to be a sufficient statistic for the same person parameter, at least for two points in time in the observed population.

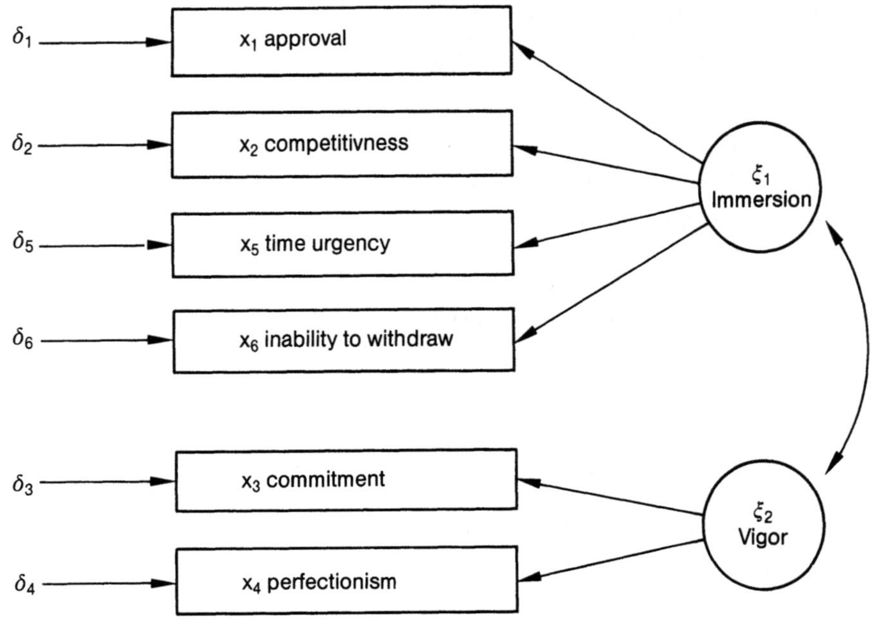

$$x = \Lambda_x \xi + \delta$$

$$\begin{bmatrix} x_1 \\ x_2 \\ x_3 \\ x_4 \\ x_5 \\ x_6 \end{bmatrix} = \begin{bmatrix} \lambda_{11} & 0 \\ \lambda_{21} & 0 \\ & \lambda_{32} \\ & \lambda_{42} \\ \lambda_{51} & 0 \\ \lambda_{61} & 0 \end{bmatrix} \begin{bmatrix} \xi_1 \\ \xi_2 \end{bmatrix} + \begin{bmatrix} \delta_1 \\ \delta_2 \\ \delta_3 \\ \delta_4 \\ \delta_5 \\ \delta_6 \end{bmatrix}$$

Fig. 1 a. The two-dimensional congeneric measurement model

To check whether or not the effect of time on individual scoring can safely be neglected we applied a three-factorial probabilistic test model including time as a third factor (Scheiblechner 1971). No significant distinction in parameters between first and second measurement was found.

The most important last step in the characterization of the scale measuring "need for control" is the demonstration of its basic latent structure in terms of two theoretically meaningful factors, "vigor" and "immersion". Such a demonstration includes stability of the basic latent structure in different samples as well as in panel data of one sample. If repeated confirmation of such a structure can be found, it becomes unlikely that we deal with an artifact. High stability of the two-factorial latent structure is a prerequisite for its inclusion into a longitudinal design studying effects of a coping career on cardiovascular risk. This enables us to test the hypothe-

AMI-patients

Factor loadings I	Factor loadings V	Error variance
x_1 1.826	0	x_1 3.012
x_2 0.854	0	x_2 2.803
x_3 0	5.83	x_3 0.244
x_4 0	0.978	x_4 17.384
x_5 1.71	0	x_5 4.423
x_6 2.45	0	x_6 5.942

Factor correlation

0.258

df = 8

χ^2 = 17.68

Blue-collar t_1

Factor loadings I	Factor loadings V	Error variance
x_1 0.956	0	x_1 1.521
x_2 0.597	0	x_2 1.182
x_3 0	1.562	x_3 0.766
x_4 0	0.828	x_4 1.839
x_5 1.072	0	x_5 1.795
x_6 1.573	0	x_6 2.105

Factor correlation

0.540

df = 8

χ^2 = 26.59

Blue-collar t_2

Factor loadings I	Factor loadings V	Error variance
x_1 1.274	0	x_1 1.136
x_2 0.675	0	x_2 1.107
x_3 0	1.546	x_3 0.996
x_4 0	0.91	x_4 1.669
x_5 1.171	0	x_5 1.72
x_6 1.249	0	x_6 2.447

Factor correlation

0.625

df = 8

χ^2 = 44.99

Fig. 1 b. Numerical results of the confirmatory factor analysis

sis that the location of an individual on the two factors changes over time, and that this change is a valid indicator of a change in an individual's coping career. By means of a confirmatory factor analysis, a stable basic latent structure in terms of the two factors "vigor" and "immersion" has been found in at least six different samples that have been tested with the scale (two samples of patients with myocardial infarction, $n = 111$ and 34; four samples of healthy subjects, $n = 416$, 163, 75

Table 3. Test of reliability for the six subscales and the two factors ("vigor" and "immersion")

Reliability			
Immersion	=0.7274	Vigor	=0.6904
Approval	=0.375	Commitment	=0.761
Competitiveness	=0.232	Perfectionism	=0.272
Time urgency	=0.390		
Inability to withdraw	=0.541		

and 41; for two samples repeated measurement after several months is available). It should be noted that the latent structure is repeatedly found in middle-aged male samples; results are less clear for older groups as well as for women. The underlying congeneric measurement model (Jöreskog 1971) is represented in Fig. 1 a and b.

As can be seen, the latent dimensions 1, 2, 5, and 6 load on the factor labeled "immersion" and the latent dimensions 3 and 4 load on the factor "vigor". Although consistently confirmed in their structure, the two factors are moderately correlated indicating their overall fit into the conceptual unit "need for control". The particular structure has a conceptual as well as an operationalizational aspect: As mentioned earlier, indicators of dimensions loading on the factor "immersion" are merely characterized by negative emotional connotations, as opposed to positive connotations associated with indicators of dimensions 3 and 4. In fact, a clear-cut separation of conceptual and methodological aspects of this two-factorial structure is not possible.

A further analysis has been set up to test the reliability of the subscales (dimensions) with respect to the maintained congeneric measurement model (Wheaton et al. 1977). Table 3 shows that subscale 6 and subscale 3 are the best representatives of the factors "immersion" and vigor respectively. This result further supports analysis of "need for control" in terms of the two-factorial concept outlined above.

Sample and Methods

In 1982, a prospective study on cardiovascular risk factors in a middle-aged (25–55 years, mean 40.8 ± 9,6) blue-collar population was launched. Men ($n = 416$) from three factories of a large enterprise in the metal industry who were initially free from hard coronary events (as established by ECG) were included in the study. The rationale for this study was based on a nation-wide investigation of occupational morbidity data in myocardial infarction where we attempted to show that metal workers are among those with highest risk for premature myocardial infarction (Bolm-Audorff and Siegrist 1983). We therefore concentrated our analysis on a intense rather than an extensive study of metal workers where follow-up of a still healthy group of workers at cardiovascular risk was of special interest. In 1983, a second screening took place where 86% of the original sample participated in medical examinations [blood pressure readings, body weight, height, serum cholesterol, high-density-lipoprotein cholesterol (HDLC), low-density lipoprotein cholesterol

(LDLC), very low-density lipoprotein cholesterol (VLDLC), triglycerides]. In addition, an extensive interview on occupational biography, workload, family life, chronic difficulties and lack of support as well as a brief inventory of recent negative life events were administered, as in 1982. The interview also included the Rose questionnaire on angina pectoris as well as extensive information about smoking, physical exercise, family history of cardiovascular diseases, medication, and sleep disturbances. Following the interview procedure the scale measuring "need for control", as described in the last section, was administered. A detailed analysis of descriptive data has already been presented in German (Siegrist et al. 1984). In this context, it should be noticed that traditional cardiovascular risk factors were present to a considerable degree in our sample. For example, the proportion of subjects with primary hypertension was 31%, with an additional 16.5% borderline hypertensives (WHO criteria). In a large male population sample including all socioeconomic groups of an urban area in West Germany, prevalence of primary hypertension was only 18%, with 21.4% borderline cases (Stieber et al. 1982). The existence of higher cardiovascular risk in lower socioeconomic groups has been well established in several industrial countries (Marmot et al. 1978; Holme et al. 1982; Ruberman et al. 1984) and has been found to hold true in our study group: 27% of the workers under study exhibited hyperlipidemia, and the mean low-density lipoprotein/high-density lipoprotein (LDL/HDL) ratio, which has been shown to be a fair marker of risk of coronary atherosclerosis, is 3.4 for the total sample (normal ratio for this sex and age group is about 2.0); 47% of the workers were slightly or markedly overweight; and 26% were heavy smokers.

In terms of socioemotional distress, these workers also exhibited rather high scores. Thus, for example, during the first interview, 29% had experienced three or more stressful negative life events during the preceding 2 years, and in every fifth worker, socioemotional support was considered very weak; 50% indicated that they suffered from repeated time pressure at their work place; and 25% experienced marked threats to their actual occupational status.

We therefore concluded that interactions between somatic risk factors and indicators of socioemotional distress might be helpful in explaining premature cardiovascular damage as expressed in excess morbidity and mortality within this sample. Very small figures already exist on incidence of new coronary events during the first year under study. The incidence of lethal and nonlethal AMI in our blue-collar population has been 3.6 times higher than that expected from calculations based on the Heidelberg WHO register on myocardial infarctions. The next section develops the specific hypotheses to be tested by linear structural models in this framework.

Hypotheses

As stated earlier, we expect deleterious effects of the factor "vigor" of need for control on the cardiovascular system in those healthy individuals who work and live under threatening social conditions such as poor job security, low occupational status, increased financial pressure, and the like. Two assumptions are made here: First, it is assumed that a still healthy middle-aged working population as a whole can be located at stages of a coping career where need for control seems to reflect a potential for misperception of challenging demands. Secondly, it is assumed that high scores on the latent factor "vigor" become critical as a cognitive concomitant of actual coping only under long-lasting conditions of restricted control. Active distress is likely to occur under circumstances where increased efforts to meet demands are followed by poor pay-off. High scores on "vigor" under these conditions reflect nonadaptive rigid cognitive strategies which are assumed to increase cardiovascular risk as evidenced by elevated blood pressure or elevated blood lipids via sustained neurohormonal activation. On the other hand, high scores on the latent factor "immersion" during the early stages of a coping career might prove to be protective. They prevent overestimation of one's own coping potential and related experiences of active distress, at least in social contexts under consideration.

The first two hypotheses to be tested are as follows:

1. The latent factor "vigor" of need for control has significant positive effects on parameters of cardiovascular risk in those sections of the blue-collar population which live and work under control-limiting circumstances such as poor job security, increased financial pressure, and low occupational status. This effect holds true after controlling for traditional risk factors such as age, weight, and cigarette smoking.
2. The latent factor "immersion" of need for control has significant negative effects on parameters of cardiovascular risk in those sections of the blue-collar population which live and work under the same control-limiting circumstances. This effect holds true after controlling for traditional risk factors, as mentioned above.

A further indirect validation of the concept of "coping career" can be found by comparing the relation between "vigor" and "immersion" in the healthy population and in the population which recently experienced AMI. If suffering from a premature AMI reflects a later stage of a coping career and a higher probability of adequate realistic assessment of the "coping me", we postulate higher mean scores on latent dimensions reflecting "immersion" in this population as compared with healthy blue-collar workers. We also expect a significantly higher "true score" on the factor "immersion" in the coronary patients as compared to healthy workers:

3. Mean scores on latent dimensions of the factor "immersion" as well as "true scores" on this factor are significantly higher in a population which recently experienced AMI than in a healthy blue-collar population.

The three hypotheses presented above are tested by linear structural equation models, which represent a highly informative combination of factor analysis and path analysis (Jöreskog 1973a, 1973b). This model allows a test of the assumption of a confirmatory factor analysis in one or more populations and a simultaneous analysis of the relations between such factors. Furthermore, one can test the model fit under certain restrictions for model parameters such as the restriction of invariance of parameters between different groups of observations. For the path model two matrices describe the relations between the latent variables (factors): The beta-matrix contains the path-coefficients between the endogenous latent variables, whereas the gamma-matrix expresses those of the exogenous latent variables. Finally, the psi-matrix contains the variance of the error in structural equations (so-called residual variance), and the phi-matrix contains the estimated correlation between exogenous factors. All other matrices contain factor loadings for endogenous and exogenous manifest variables as defined by the model and the variances of the measurement errors.

Results

Hypotheses 1 and 2 were tested by two structural equation models, with systolic blood pressure being the most endogenous variable. Its variance is thought to be explained by indicators of recurrent socioemotional activation such as "quantitative work load", "social support at work" and "sustained anger/helplessness", as well as by the two factors of "need for control" as exogenous latent variables where "vigor" has a positive and "immersion" has a negative effect on the systolic blood pressure. Additional exogenous variables are established somatic risk factors such as age, overweight (Quetelet-index), and cigarette smoking. This model has been employed first for the following groups: Workers who are members of the unskilled low-status group and who face monotonous work and relatively low job security are compared with skilled workers who do a relatively qualified job and who experience a certain degree of autonomy and job security. It is assumed that significant effects of "vigor" and "immersion" on blood pressure are expressed under the control-limiting circumstances of the unskilled group only.

A second test of the model includes a criterion measuring considerable economic pressure under difficult working conditions: A subgroup of workers who, as a consequence of low wages, is forced to do piecework is compared with a subgroup without such economic pressure. Again it is assumed that effects of "vigor" and "immersion" on blood pressure are expressed under the aggravated condition of economic pressure only. Even though the subgroups for the two group-comparison tests are overlapping to some extent, their composition is far from being identical. Similar empirical results thus add to the credibility of the approach outlined above. In either model the causal order of the dependent variables is specified as fully recursive, and no restrictions are imposed on the lower half of the coefficient-matrix B (matrix of regression-coefficients between endogenous latent constructs). As a consequence of such group-comparisons there are no restrictions on the matrix representing effects of exogenous variables on the endogenous variables mentioned above (gamma-matrix).

If the maintained factorial structure for each construct is invariant for the subgroups with respect to factor loadings and measurement errors, and if such a constraint does not greatly violate the model fit, we can then interpret estimated parameters analogous to ordinary regression coefficients, and hence can compare these parameters between the subgroups under study. Figure 2 demonstrates the structural and measurement model which underlies the following analyses. Figure 3 and Table 4 show the results of the model for different status groups. As predicted, there is a highly significant positive effect of "vigor" on the systolic blood pressure and a minor, nonsignificant negative effect of "immersion" on blood pressure in the low-status group.

"Quantitative workload" and "social support" provide significant, although smaller effects on the criterion. No direct effect is produced by the variable "sus-

Description of endogenous latent variables

η_1 = social support
measured by two five-point scaled variables

η_2 = work load
measured by two five-point scaled variables

η_3 = sustained anger/helplessness
measured by two five-point scaled variables

η_4 = systolic blood pressure

Description of exogenous latent variables

ξ_1 = immersion

ξ_2 = vigor

ξ_3 = age

ξ_4 = Quetelet index

ξ_5 = amount of cigarettes per day

$$B\eta = \Gamma\xi + \zeta$$

$$\begin{bmatrix} 1 & 0 & 0 & 0 \\ -\beta_{21} & 1 & 0 & 0 \\ -\beta_{31} & -\beta_{32} & 1 & 0 \\ -\beta_{41} & -\beta_{42} & -\beta_{43} & 1 \end{bmatrix} \begin{bmatrix} \eta_1 \\ \eta_2 \\ \eta_3 \\ \eta_4 \end{bmatrix} = \begin{bmatrix} \gamma_{11} & \gamma_{12} & \gamma_{13} & \gamma_{14} & \gamma_{15} \\ \gamma_{21} & \gamma_{22} & \gamma_{23} & \gamma_{24} & \gamma_{25} \\ \gamma_{31} & \gamma_{32} & \gamma_{33} & \gamma_{34} & \gamma_{35} \\ \gamma_{41} & \gamma_{42} & \gamma_{43} & \gamma_{44} & \gamma_{45} \end{bmatrix} \begin{bmatrix} \xi_1 \\ \xi_2 \\ \xi_3 \\ \xi_4 \\ \xi_5 \end{bmatrix} + \begin{bmatrix} \zeta_1 \\ \zeta_2 \\ \zeta_3 \\ \zeta_4 \end{bmatrix}$$

$$x = \Lambda_x \xi + \delta$$

$$\begin{bmatrix} x_1 \\ x_2 \\ x_3 \\ x_4 \\ x_5 \\ x_6 \\ x_7 \\ x_8 \\ x_9 \end{bmatrix} = \begin{bmatrix} \lambda_{11} & 0 & 0 & 0 & 0 \\ \lambda_{21} & 0 & 0 & 0 & 0 \\ 0 & \lambda_{32} & 0 & 0 & 0 \\ 0 & \lambda_{42} & 0 & 0 & 0 \\ \lambda_{51} & 0 & 0 & 0 & 0 \\ \lambda_{61} & 0 & 0 & 0 & 0 \\ 0 & 0 & \lambda_{73} & 0 & 0 \\ 0 & 0 & 0 & \lambda_{84} & 0 \\ 0 & 0 & 0 & 0 & \lambda_{95} \end{bmatrix} \cdot \begin{bmatrix} \xi_1 \\ \xi_2 \\ \xi_3 \\ \xi_4 \\ \xi_5 \end{bmatrix} + \begin{bmatrix} \delta_1 \\ \delta_2 \\ \delta_3 \\ \delta_4 \\ \delta_5 \\ \delta_6 \\ \delta_7 \\ \delta_8 \\ \delta_9 \end{bmatrix}$$

Fig. 2. The equations of the LISREL-Model which has been employed to explain the variance of SBP

$$y = \Lambda_y \eta + \varepsilon$$

$$\begin{bmatrix} y_1 \\ y_2 \\ y_3 \\ y_4 \\ y_5 \\ y_6 \\ y_7 \end{bmatrix} = \begin{bmatrix} 1 & 0 & 0 & 0 \\ \lambda_{21} & 0 & 0 & 0 \\ 0 & 1 & 0 & 0 \\ 0 & \lambda_{42} & 0 & 0 \\ 0 & 0 & 1 & 0 \\ 0 & 0 & \lambda_{63} & 0 \\ 0 & 0 & 0 & 1 \end{bmatrix} \cdot \begin{bmatrix} \eta_1 \\ \eta_2 \\ \eta_3 \\ \eta_4 \end{bmatrix} + \begin{bmatrix} \varepsilon_1 \\ \varepsilon_2 \\ \varepsilon_3 \\ \varepsilon_4 \\ \varepsilon_5 \\ \varepsilon_6 \\ \varepsilon_7 \end{bmatrix}$$

Fig. 2. Continue

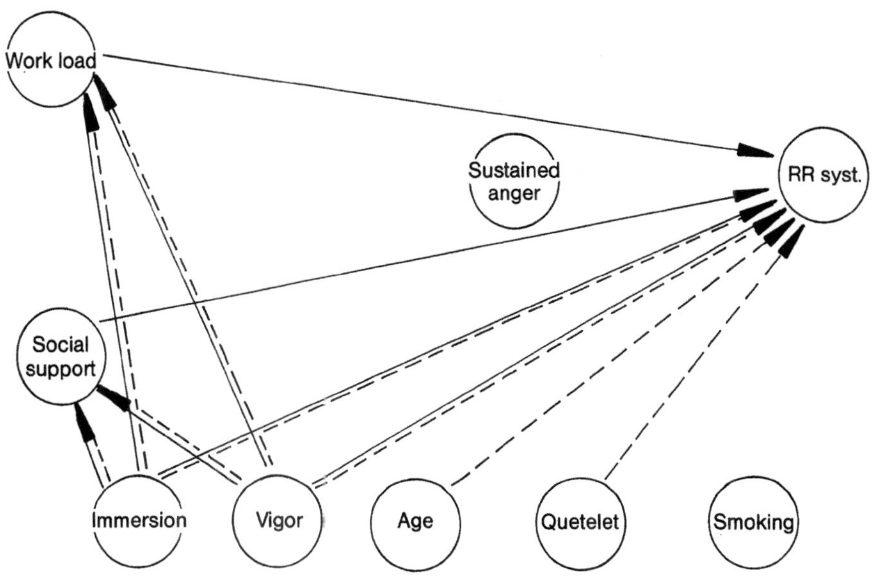

Fig. 3. LISREL-model for the subgroups: - - -, (1) higher-status group (skilled workers); —, (2) lower-status group (unskilled workers). Numerical results are shown in Table 4

tained anger/helplessness". The remaining marked positive effect of "vigor" and blood pressure under threatening socioeconomic conditions is interpreted in the framework of recurrent experience of active distress due to the disparity between personal need for control and social opportunity structure where experience of active distress is triggered by misperception of internal coping potential and of external demands. In contrast, the group working at relatively higher status under more favorable conditions shows minor effects of either factor of "need for control" on the indicator of cardiovascular risk. Moreover, the effect of "need for control" on blood pressure proved to be opposite in sign indicating a certain protective pattern,

Table 4. Numerical results for the model presented in Fig. 3[a]

Higher status (skilled workers) $n=147$

Beta = regression coefficients from endogenous on endogenous η_1 to η_4

η_1	η_2	η_3	η_4
0.000			
-0.005	0.000		
-0.002	-0.122	0.000	
0.847	7.606	-2.907	0.000

Gamma = regression coefficients from exogenous on endogenous ξ_1 to ξ_5 on η_1 to η_4

ξ_1	ξ_2	ξ_3	ξ_4	ξ_5
-0.271*	0.367*	-0.115	-0.087	-0.144
0.456*	-0.326*	0.100	-0.065	-0.029
0.389	-0.245	-0.075	0.099	0.057
7.845*	-7.324*	5.610*	3.932*	1.300

Psi = variances of structural disturbances

Eq. 1	Eq. 2	Eq. 3	Eq. 4
0.871	0.252	0.211	204.673

Lower status (unskilled workers) $n=75$

Beta = regression coefficients from endogenous on endogenous η_1 to η_4

η_1	η_2	η_3	η_4
0.000			
-0.024	0.000		
-0.099	-0.082	0.000	
-5.770*	10.623*	-0.562	0.000

Gamma = regression coefficients from exogenous on endogenous ξ_1 to ξ_5 on η_1 to η_4

ξ_1	ξ_2	ξ_3	ξ_4	ξ_5
-0.414*	0.818*	-0.353	-0.352	-0.250
0.685*	-0.592*	-0.125	0.330	0.111
0.083	-0.190	-0.025	0.114	0.079
-14.193*	18.152*	0.735	-0.741	-1.806

Psi = variances of structural disturbances

Eq. 1	Eq. 2	Eq. 3	Eq. 4
0.905	0.470	0.315	128.079

* $P \leqslant 0.05$
$Chi^2 = 185.23$; $df = 169$; $P = 0.134$

as suggested earlier. The other psychosocial variables show mainly nonsignificant effects.

The powerful influence of detrimental social contexts on blood pressure as mediated by the recurrent vigorous efforts under condition of low pay-off can be clearly demonstrated by three basic findings:

1. In the low-status group the effect of "vigor" on blood pressure is about 2.5 times larger than in the higher status group.
2. In the low-status group, total variance of blood pressure explained by the psychosocial variables under study amounts to 54%, whereas in the skilled worker-group it remains at 27%.

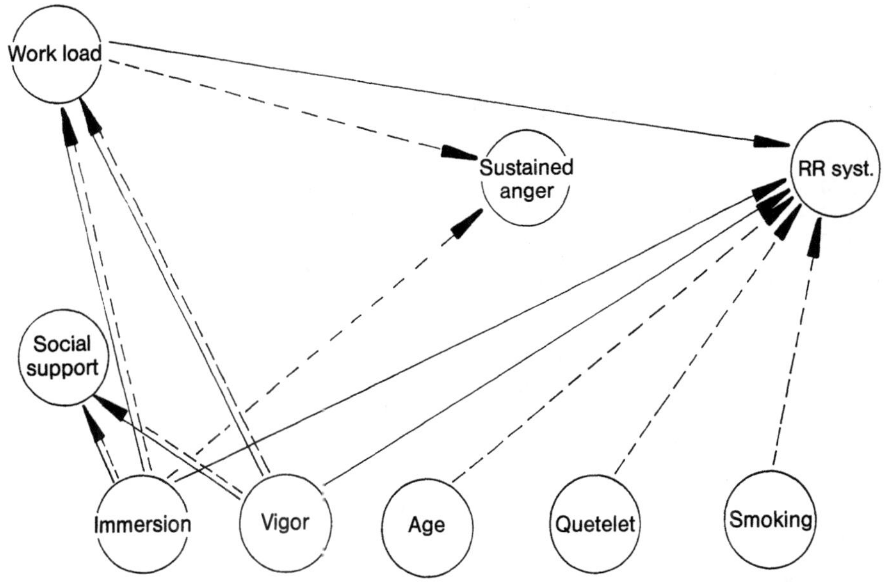

Fig. 4. LISREL-model for the subgroups: ----, (1) no piecework; —, (2) forced piecework. χ^2 $\lambda = 218.29$; $df = 175$; $P = 0.015$. Numerical results are shown in Table 5

3. Effects of latent factors of need for control in the low-status group are much more pronounced than effects produced by established somatic risk factors such as age, smoking, and overweight. In the higher status group, effects of psychosocial and of somatic risk factors are similar in magnitude (effects of gamma-matrix can be compared directly, since the variances of all exogenous latent constructs are standardized to 1). A further test of hypotheses 1 and 2 is provided by the next model where economic pressure for piecework has been chosen as a criterion to split the blue-collar population. Figure 4 and Table 5 demonstrate respective results.

Since results are very similar to those described in Table 4, only a short comment is required. Again, there is a positive effect of "vigor" on blood pressure and a negative one of "immersion" under conditions of increased economic pressure, whereas these effects are absent under more favorable social conditions. "Quantitative work load" also influences blood pressure, as well as "social support". Again, the amount of explained variance is much higher in the group under economic pressure (44%) as compared to the remaining group (14%). Effects of latent factors of "need for control" on blood pressure are once again more pronounced as compared with effects of somatic risk factors, if long-lasting critical socioeconomic circumstances prevail.

Taken together, these results give some evidence on the possibly detrimental effects of a vigorous active coping style on the cardiovascular system. What may have started as an adaptive cognitive and behavioral response in individuals under need for control in early adulthood no longer remains adequate under aggravating socioeconomic conditions of middle-adulthood, i.e., in later stages of a coping career.

Table 5. Numerical results for the model presented ~Fig. 4

Forced piecework n = 89

Beta = regression coefficients from endogenous on endogenous η_1 to η_4

η_1	η_2	η_3	η_4
0.000			
0.124	0.000		
0.073	-0.002	0.000	
-6.032	12.494*	-0.717	0.000

Gamma = regression coefficients from exogenous on endogenous ξ_1 to ξ_5 on η_1 to η_4

ξ_1	ξ_2	ξ_3	ξ_4	ξ_5
-0.347*	0.887*	-0.494	-0.331	-0.231
0.738*	-0.828*	-0.032	0.359	0.155
0.291	-0.338	0.135	0.043	0.000
-13.157*	18.956*	-0.044	0.541	-1.429

Psi = variances of structural disturbances

Eq. 1	Eq. 2	Eq. 3	Eq. 4
1.068	0.374	0.947	162.862

No piecework n = 199

Beta = regression coefficients from endogenous on endogenous η_1 to η_4

η_1	η_2	η_3	η_4
0.000			
-0.121	0.000		
0.010	0.339	0.000	
-0.104	-2.181*	-0.761	0.000

Gamma = regression coefficients from exogenous on endogenous ξ_1 to ξ_5 on η_1 to η_4

ξ_1	ξ_2	ξ_3	ξ_4	ξ_5
-0.287*	0.335*	-0.091	-0.060	-0.150
0.361*	-0.130*	0.085	-0.005	0.021
0.334*	-0.099	-0.086	0.029	0.100
0.540	0.292	4.422*	1.850*	1.754*

Psi = variances of structural disturbances

Eq. 1	Eq. 2	Eq. 3	Eq. 4
1.399	0.410	0.439	250.620

* $P \leqslant 0.05$
$Chi^2 = 218.29$; $df = 175$; $P = 0.015$

Rigid cognitive styles may prevent adequate monitoring of a misfit between invested efforts and pay-off and may even prevent adequate recognition of signs of fatique, irritation, and emotional distress. Given the important role of early development of hypertension on cardiovascular disease, it is certainly important to specify the conditions under which this development is likely to take place.

Finally, the third hypothesis was tested by comparing central tendency of the factors of "need for control" between a population which recently experienced AMI ($n = 97$) and the blue-collar population ($n = 368$). In terms of sex, age, and occupation both groups are comparable. We have stated that mean scores on latent dimensions of the factor "immersion" are significantly higher in AMI-patients than in healthy controls, thus reflecting a later stage of the coping career. We also stated

Table 6. Mean differences between AMI-patients and blue-collar workers on the six subscales of "need for control"

	Blue-collar population $n = 368$	AMI-population $n = 97$
Approval	3.606 ±0.327	4.299 ±0.3585
Competitiveness	1.731 ±0.1665	2.2371±0.3752
Commitment	5.052 ±0.2404	5.2062±0.5284
Perfectionism	4.8587±0.2134	4.9175±0.4755
Time urgency	3.1413±0.2304	4.4227±0.4936**
Inability to withdraw	3.5109±0.2573	4.4433±0.5050**

** $P \leqslant 0.01$

Table 7. Mean differences of "vigor" and "immersion". AMI-population fixed to zero

	Γ-estimates (mean differences)	t-values
Immersion	-0.725	-5.432***
Vigor	-0.153	-0.68

*** $P \leqslant 0.001$

that true scores of "immersion" are significantly higher in the group of AMI-patients. Table 6 shows mean scores for the six subscales in either group.

All four values of dimensions loading on the factor "immersion" (approval, competitiveness, time urgency, and inability to withdraw from work obligations) are markedly increased in AMI-patients as compared with healthy controls. Due to large confidence intervals, a highly significant difference in mean ($p < 0.01$) is given in dimensions 5 and 6 only, but the overall difference is much higher than in dimensions 3 and 4 (representing the factor "vigor"). A modified linear model has been employed to estimate the differences in factor means for the two subgroups (Sörbom 1974, 1982). For sake of identification of the model, factor means of the AMI-group have been fixed to zero. The estimate shows a highly significant lower "mean" of the factor "immersion" for the blue collar population, whereas the mean of "vigor" is not different between healthy controls and coronary patients (Table 7).

To summarize, there is at least indirect evidence for a decisive influence of "immersion" on cardiovascular risk in later stages of a coping career, especially under conditions of already established chronic disease.

Discussion

Our conceptual and empirical approach to the study of TABP has shown that focus on motivational and cognitive bases (over- and underestimation of demands/coping ability) as well as on their emotional concomitants (awareness of "coping me" in terms of "vigor" or "immersion") is justified in terms of its explanatory power for cardiovascular risk such as high blood pressure. This holds true if account is taken of control-limiting social contexts which trigger a career of cumulative experiences of active distress. It is clear that on both sides of the equation more evidence has to be accumulated. We therefore present additional information concerning the following questions:

1. Can we observe similar relationships of latent factors of need for control on other criteria of cardiovascular risk such as LDL or HDL?
2. Is there further evidence for a "turning point" in the coping career immediately before and/or after disease onset, as reported in results on the third hypothesis above?
3. Is additional support available from true longitudinal studies strengthening the concept of Type A as a coping career?

In recent years it has become clear that the impact of higher nervous activity (in terms of neural and neurohormonal implications of active distress, as suggested by us) on cardiovascular disease is not restricted to circumstances precipitating acute episodes - by means of cardiac arrhythmias, of acute thrombotic developments, etc. (Lown et al. 1977) - but in addition plays a role in earlier stages of the disease process, at least if some structural damage is present. Synergistic effects of somatic risk factors and psychosocial variables have been documented in animal research on atherosclerosis (Kaplan et al. 1982) and in epidemiology of IHD (Haynes et al. 1983).

Moreover, some of the traditional somatic risk factors are triggered by higher nervous activity by means of hormonal impact on processes of cell-receptor regulation. There is considerable evidence for the role of these processes in primary essential hypertension (e.g., Ganten et al. 1983). In addition to well-documented genetic influences, there might also be hormonal regulation at the level of LDL-receptors in the liver and elsewhere (Goldstein et al. 1983). In order to see whether this latter idea makes sense in terms of aggregate data analysis, as provided by the epidemiological approach, we have employed several structural models, with LDL and HDL being the most endogenous variables. It should be stated, however, that the amount of explained variance by this application of linear models is smaller than in models explaining systolic blood pressure (perhaps due to nonlinear relationships). Yet, we could find marked and consistent direct positive effects of "vigor" on LDL-level in a blue-collar group, which was already at a certain cardiovascular risk; i.e., in a group with mild hypercholesterolemia ($\geq$250 mg/%). Adding to the notion of synergism between somatic anc psychosocial influences, our data show effects of "vigor" on LDL ten times larger in the hypercholesterolemic group as compared with the group with normal cholesterol [path coefficients (pc) are 9.4 as compared with 0.91]. Our results also show that the numeric effect of "vigor" on LDL is larger than any of the effects of risk factors like age (=5.2), overweight (pc=4.4) and cigarette smoking (pc=7.6). Whereas "vigor" exerts positive effects on LDL, "immersion" exhibits negative effects. Thus the same structure of effects becomes apparent as in models explaining the variance of blood pressure.

Further substantiation is given by linear models entering HDL as the most endogenous variable. For the whole structure, symmetrical effects with opposite signs can be shown. Thus, the critical LDL/HDL-ratio is increased in a group exhibiting high scores on "vigor", at least under conditions of already established mild hypercholesterolemia.

Preliminary findings also indicate that vulnerable social contexts critically aggravate this situation. In an analysis of variance controlling for effects of age, overweight, and cigarette smoking, fear of job-loss exerts a main effect on the magnitude of LDL/HDL ratio (mean LDL/HDL in the group with fear of job-loss is 3.62 as compared to the group without this fear; mean = 3.38; $f = 2.17$; $p = \leqslant 0.10$). In addition, the mean LDL is significantly higher in the group of unskilled blue-collar workers as compared to the higher status groups after controlling for age, overweight and cigarette smoking. In explaining these preliminary findings, we should be well aware of possible intervening variables such as diet (which could not be adequately assessed). However, there is little evidence of marked differences in diet between subgroups of the blue-collar population under study. Critically increased HDL-levels, which might indicate chronic alcohol abuse, have been excluded from the sample. Nevertheless, further exploration has to be done in order to establish unequivocal relationships between indicators of sustained active distress and lipid metabolism.

Turning to the second question, we present another set of preliminary findings. Several recent prospective studies have established a relationship between the onset of severe sleep disturbances and imminent manifestation of IHD (Partinen et al. 1982). On the basis of very small numbers, we could show such an association in our blue-collar population as well in explaining 1-year incidence of new coronary events (Siegrist 1984). We wish to propose the possibility that recurrent unexplained sleep disruption can be understood in terms of coping failure, since we simultaneously found indications of high socioemotional distress associated with these disturbances. On the basis of the total blue-collar sample, we could demonstrate consistent relationships between intensity of sleep disturbances and scores on dimensions indicating high "immersion" (Siegrist et al. 1986). If this association indicates a critical stage within the coping career, we might then expect increasing explanatory power of the latent factor "immersion" on indicators of cardiovascular risk even before disease onset. We are currently analyzing cardiovascular parameters documented by ambulant polysomnographic recordings and Holter-ECG in a subgroup of blue-collar workers with reported recurrent sleep disturbances. Although definitive results are still not established, we can at least show that research designs are available for a more systematic exploration of the "turning point" of a coping career where self-awareness under the burden of fatigue and emotional distress becomes more realistic in individuals who exhibit strong need for control.

Finally, it is evident that in our blue-collar population, true longitudinal data which would allow us to establish individual coping careers are not available at present. However, we have presented data from an earlier longitudinal follow-up study which supports the concept of a coping career in coronary-prone individuals.

Of a sample of 380 male patients who survived their first myocardial infarction (for details see Siegrist et al. 1980) 75% have been followed-up for 18 months. Although presenting a less sophisticated first version of the scale measuring "need for control" (where items representing "immersion" prevailed), we found a significant increase in mean scores of need for control 18 months after the first survey, which took place in a cardiac rehabilitation center some weeks after disease onset. A closer analysis of variables associated with this increase revealed that subjects who, after their rehabilitation, experienced high actual strain in the working field had significantly higher scores of need for control after 18 months. Control-limiting social circumstances thus might precipitate later stages of a coping career where suffering from active distress is admitted and vulnerability of the cardiovascular system is increased. Unfortunately, we were not able to integrate appropriate medical information on cardiovascular parameters into this data set. Our finding of a significant relationship between indicators of a distressing coping career after the first myocardial infarction and the severity of subjectively perceived cardiac symptoms was substantiated by a most impressive recent study on the impact of psychosocial stress on mortality after myocardial infarction (Ruberman et al. 1984).

Conclusions

This paper argues for a conceptual and methodological re-definition of TABP for at least three reasons:

1. As inconsistency of reported results and lack of specificity become more evident in Type A research, explorations in the very "coronary-prone" components of this pattern are needed. At a psychophysiological level, such explorations might concentrate on a certain type of experiences of enhanced adrenergic activity, i.e., on active distress. At a cognitive level, processes linking motivation with overt coping might be considered where unrealistic appraisal of external challenges and of internal coping resources is thought to play a crucial role.
2. Although stated again and again, Type A behavior has rarely been conceptualized in terms of a systematic interaction between individual behavior and its social setting. By introducing the concept of coping career, we have linked the motivational and cognitive potential of individuals exhibiting enhanced need for control with the dynamics of control-limiting social circumstances in middle-adulthood where stressful aspects of the work environment are of special importance.
3. If cognitive processes play a role in initiating and sustaining experiences of active distress, they must be represented in the methodological approach as well. Measurement of Type A by means of direct behavioral assessment has neglected this dimension. The development of a scale measuring six aspects of need for control at the work site in terms of two basic latent factors, i.e., "vigor" and "immersion", enables us to deal with the different impact of these factors on parameters of cardiovascular risk at different stages of a coping career. Recent advances of statistical techniques, such as structural linear equation models with latent variables and confirmatory factor analysis, are available now to accomplish these tasks.

The validity of this conceptual and methodological approach, as evidenced by empirical data of a prospective study on cardiovascular risk in a male blue-collar population, is still limited. However, we have shown consistent effects of "vigor" and "immersion" on the level of systolic blood pressure under control-limiting social circumstances, which are of similar magnitude as those exerted by traditional risk factors such as smoking, overweight, and age. In addition, we have discussed preliminary findings that demonstrate comparable effects on low-density lipoprotein. The critical influence of "immersion" on cardiovascular risk at later stages of a coping career is illustrated by links that do exist between scores on its dimensions and severity of unexplained recent sleep disturbances, which might be understood as an indicator of coping failure in the presence of continuous or enhanced active distress. Longitudinal studies are needed in order to explore more fully the relationships between stages of a coping career and cardiovascular breakdown. It is clear that a more accurate and more dynamic characterization of groups at high cardiovascular risk would have wide implications for preventive and therapeutic strategies in the field of cardiovascular disease.

Acknowledgements. We are indebted to Dr. Ingbert Weber, Ruth Grünewald and Daniela Klein from our department for their cooperation in the research reported in this contribution. We are also indebted to the German Research Foundation for continuous support of this research (Si 236/4-5).

References

Andersen EB (1973) Goodness of fit test for the Rasch model. Psychometrika 38: 123-140

Appels A (1983) The year before myocardial infarction. In: Dembroski T et al. (eds) Biobehavioral bases of coronary heart disease. Karger, Basel, pp 18-38

Bolm-Audorff U, Siegrist J (1983) Occupational morbidity data in myocardial infarction. J Occup Med 25: 367-371

Dembroski T, Schmidt T, Blümchen G (eds) (1983) Biobehavioral bases of coronary heart disease. Karger, Basel

Dittmann K, Matschinger H (1982) Soziale Belastungen, Bewertungsmuster und Streß: Untersuchungen zur Bedeutung psychosozialer Risiken bei der Entstehung von Herzinfarkt. Research report to the German Research Foundation, Marburg

Dittmann K, Matschinger H, Siegrist J (1985) Fragebogen zur Messung von Kontrollambitionen (2nd ed). In: Allmendinger J et al. (eds) ZUMA-Handbuch sozialwissenschaftlicher Skalen. ZUMA, Bonn

Fischer G (1974) Einführung in die Theorie psychologischer Tests. Huber, Berlin

Frankenhaeuser M (1983) The sympathetic-adrenal and pituitary-adrenal response to challenge: a comparison between the sexes. In: Dembroski T et al. (eds) Biobehavioral bases of coronary heart disease. Karger, Basel, pp 91-105

Ganten D, Hermann K, Bayer C, Unger T, Lang RE (1983) Angiotensin synthesis in the brain and increased turnover in hypertensive rats. Science 221: 869-871

Glass DC (1977) Behavior pattern, stress and coronary disease. Erlbaum, Hillsdale

Goldstein JL, Kita T, Brown MS (1983) Defective lipoprotein receptors and atherosclerosis. N Engl J Med 309: 288-296

Haynes SG, Feinleib M, Eaker ED (1983) Type-A behavior and the 10 year incidence of coronary heart disease in the Framingham study. In: Rosenman RH (ed) Psychosomatic risk factors and coronary heart disease. Huber, Bern, pp 80-92

Henry JP (1983) Coronary heart disease and arousal of the adrenal cortical axis. In: Dembroski T et al. (eds) Biobehavioral bases of coronary heart disease. Karger, Basel, pp 365-381

Holme I, Helgeland A, Hermann I, Leren P (1982) Socio-economic status as a coronary risk factor: the Oslo study. Acta Med Scand 660: 147-151

Jöreskog KG (1971) Statistical analysis of sets of congeneric tests. Psychometrika 36: 109-133

Jöreskog KG (1973a) A general method for estimating a linear structural equation system. In: Goldberger AS, Duncan OD (eds) Structural equation models in the social sciences. Seminar, New York, pp 85-112

Jöreskog KG (1973b) Analysis of covariance structures. In: Krishnaia P (ed) Multivariate analysis III. Academic, New York, pp 263-285

Jöreskog KG, Sörbom D (1979) Advances in factor analysis and structural equation models. Abt Books, Cambridge, Mass
Kaplan JR, Manuck SB, Clarkson TB, Lusso FM, Taub D (1982) Social status, environment and atherosclerosis in Cynomolgus monkeys. Arteriosclerosis 2: 359-368
Karasek R, Russell S, Theorell T (1982) Physiology of stress and regeneration in job related cardiovascular illness. J Hum Stress 8: 29-42
Lown B, Verrier RL, Rabinowitz SH (1977) Neural and psychological mechanisms and the problem of sudden cardiac death. Am J Cardiol 39: 890-902
Marmot MG, Rose G, Shipley M, Hamilton PJS (1978) Employment grade and coronary heart disease in British civil servants. J Epidemiol Community Health 32: 244-249
Partinen M, Putkonen PTS, Kaprio J, Koskenvuo M, Hilakivi I (1982) Sleep disorders in relation to coronary heart disease. Acta Med Scand 660: 69-83
Rasch G (1960) Probabilistic models for some intelligence and attainment tests. Nielsen and Lydiche, Copenhagen
Rosenman RH (ed) (1983) Psychosomatic risk factors and coronary heart disease. Huber, Bern
Rost J (1977) Diagnostik des Lernzuwachses - ein Beitrag zur Theorie und Methodik von Lerntests. IPN-Arbeitsbericht 26, Kiel
Ruberman W, Weinblatt E, Goldberg JD, Chandhary BS (1984) Psychosocial influences on mortality after myocardial infarction. N Engl J Med 311: 552-559
Scheiblechner H (1971) CML-Parameter estimation in a generalized multifactorial version of Rasch's probabilistic measurement model with two categories of answers. Research Bulletin 4, Vienna
Schneiderman N (1983) Behavior, automatic function and animal models of cardiovascular pathology. In: Dembroski T et al. (eds) Biobehavioral bases of coronary heart disease. Karger, Basel, pp 304-364
Shekelle R, Hully S, Neaton J (1983) Type-A behavior and risk of coronary death in MRFIT. Unpublished conference report, San Diego
Siegrist J (1984) Threat to social status and cardiovascular risk. Psychother Psychosom 42: 90-96
Siegrist J, Dittmann KH, Rittner K, Weber I (1980) Soziale Belastungen und Herzinfarkt. Enke, Stuttgart
Siegrist J, Dittmann KH, Rittner K, Weber I (1982) The social context of active distress in patients with early myocardial infarction. Soc Sci Med 16: 443-454
Siegrist J, Matschinger H, Grünewald M (1986) Distress-Karriere und kardiovaskuläres Risiko. In: Klapp B (ed) Psychokardiologie. Springer, Berlin Heidelberg New York (in press)
Siegrist J, Matschinger H, Weber I, Siegrist K, Dittmann KH, Brockmeier R, Klein D (1984b) Der Einfluß sozialer Belastungen und ihrer Verarbeitung auf die Entwicklung kardiovaskulärer Risiken. (unpublished research report to the German Research Foundation, Marburg)
Sörbom D (1974) A general method for studying differences in factor means and factor structures between groups. Br J Math Stat Psychol 27: 229-239
Sörbom D (1982) Structural equation models with structured means. In: Jöreskog KG, Wold H (eds) Systems under indirect observation, vol I. North-Holland, Amsterdam, pp 183-196
Stieber J, Döring A, Keil U (1982) Häufigkeit, Bekanntheits- und Behandlungsgrad der Hypertonie in einer Großstadtbevölkerung. MMW 124: 747-752
Wheaton B, Muthen F, Alwin D, Summers G (1977) Assessing reliability and stability in panel models. In: Heise DR (ed) Sociological methodology. Jossey-Bass, San Francisco, pp 84-136

The Importance of the Type A Subcomponent Hostility for Myocardial Infarction at Young Age

W. LANGOSCH, G. BRODNER, and H. BORCHERDING[1]

Introduction

Results of recent studies suggest that hostility may be of importance in the pathogenesis of coronary heart disease (CHD). In a study by Kantor and Robertson (1977), repressed hostility as measured by the MMPI scales for "repression anxiety" and "manifest hostility", increased systematically as the level of physiological risk of developing CHD increased. This relationship persisted across social class levels and different study samples (Evans County and Buffalo, New Jersey). Siltanen et al. (1975) compared a group of 41 subjects without any symptoms or signs of CHD who had a low risk of CHD, with a group of 40 subjects with ECG signs of CHD, but without symptoms of CHD, and a group of 40 subjects with ECG signs of CHD and symptoms of CHD. In comparison with the apparently healthy men, the members of the two other groups scored significantly higher on aggression as measured by a sentence completion test. Using a factor-analytically derived aggressiveness/hostility scale of the Rating of Statements List, van Dijl (1982) was able to show, in three different studies, that myocardial infarction patients score higher on this scale.

Results of a component analysis of the interview variables used to assess the Type A behavior pattern revealed that only those items which reflected vigorous voice stylistics, hostility, and irritation were predictive for subsequent development of CHD (Matthews et al. 1977). In a prospective study by Barefoot et al. (1983), the association between the incidence of CHD events over a 25-year follow-up period and scores on a MMPI-derived hostility scale was examined. The sample consisted of 255 subjects. CHD had been cited as a factor in 15 subjects. The CHD incidence was nearly five times higher among those with higher hostility scores, and this relationship was found to be independent of smoking status, age, family history of CHD, and the presence of hypertension. These findings are similar to the results of Shekelle et al. (1983), who also assessed level of hostility using a subscale of the MMPI. Their sample consisted of 1877 employed men aged 40–45 years who were free of CHD at the intake examination. Ten-year incidence of CHD was significantly associated with the hostility scores. However, after adjustments for age, blood pressure, serum cholesterol level, cigarette smoking, and intake of alcohol were taken into accounts, the association proved no longer significant. Nevertheless, the adjusted relative odds of CHD was over 0.68 for men with hostility score $\leqslant 10$ in comparison to men with higher scores. The hostility scores were also predictive for CHD incidence over a 20-year period. This prospective relationship persisted even after adjustment for the major CHD risk factors. In the Framingham Study,

1 Benedikt Kreutz Rehabilitationszentrum, Südring 15, 7812 Bad Krozingen, Federal Republic of Germany

Biological and Psychological Factors in Cardiovascular Disease
Ed. by T. H. Schmidt, T. M. Dembroski, and G. Blümchen

men who denied showing anger to others were at increased risk of CHD, and not showing or discussing anger when provoked was found to predict CHD incidence in women (Haynes et al. 1980).

Williams et al. (1980) found that hostility level, as assessed by a subscale of the MMPI, was associated with prevalence of coronary atherosclerosis in 424 patients who had been referred to the medical center for diagnostic coronary angiography. The relationship between hostility scores and coronary atherosclerosis was nonlinear, with 48% of patients scoring $\leqslant 10$ on the hostility scale and 70% of patients with scores >10 exhibiting at least one coronary artery showing a stenosis of 75% decrease in luminal diameter. Kahn et al. (1982) used the thallium stress test for measuring severity of coronary artery disease. They observed a significant correlation between a rating of the aggressive content of patients' anwers to the Type A structured interview and severity of coronary artery disease in 37 subjects without prior history of myocardial infarction. However, this relationship was not found in 16 patients with reported prior myocardial infarction.

Psychophysiological studies have demonstrated that hostile subjects respond to laboratory challenges with exaggerated cardiovascular responses. In a study of 50 male college students, the Type A subcomponent of hostility was positively correlated with an increase in systolic blood pressure and heart rate and with heart rate variability (Dembroski et al. 1978). In another study with 84 college students, high hostility subjects responded to both high and low challenge with the same level of systolic and diastolic blood pressure increases seen in the full Type A sample only under high challenge conditions (Dembroski et al. 1979 a). A positive relationship between level of hostility and systolic blood pressure increase during a quiz was observed in a study with 64 adult male subjects who had either a history of myocardial infarction or were undergoing treatment for a disease other than CHD (Dembroski et al. 1979 b).

Although very different methods of assessment were used in all these studies, these results suggest that hostility is associated with coronary risk factors, exaggerated challenge-induced cardiovascular arousal, clinically manifest coronary artery disease, and prevalence of significant coronary atherosclerosis. In the present study, the semistructured Type A interview (Rosenman 1978) was used to assess hostility. The Type A pattern is considered to be a set of behaviors that is elicited from individuals with certain personality and behavior dispositions by an appropriately challenging environment (Rosenman and Chesney 1980). Thus, it is also necessary to look for some psychological correlates of this measure to gain a better understanding of its psychological meaning and to specify subjects' job stressors and perceived job challenges. The year before myocardial infarction is often characterized by feelings of vital exhaustion and depression (Appels 1980, 1983), and these emotional changes are found to be correlated positively with the Type A/B score of the Jenkins Activity Survey (Appels 1981). Therefore, symptoms of distress and depressed mood may also be associated with the hostility component of the Type A behavior pattern.

The present study was designed to assess whether the Type A subcomponent of hostility is related to presence and severity of stressors at the workplace and perceived challenges of the working day, as well as to achievement behavior, need for affiliation, complaints, hypochondria and depressed mood, and to indicators of exaggerated autonomic activity in response to standardized laboratory challenges. Furthermore, the relationship between hostility and coronary risk factors, as well as prevalence and severity of coronary atherosclerosis, was assessed.

Method

All 79 male subjects (mean age: 35,8 years) included in this study had suffered from a documented transmural myocardial infarction before the age of 40. They had been referred to the Benedikt Kreutz Rehabilitationszentrum Bad Krozingen, West Germany, for cardiological rehabilitation 9.5 months on average after their myocardial infarction and were subsequently entered in the study.

Measures

All patients were given the German version of Roseman's structured interview (Langosch et al. 1985). The interviews were tape-recorded, and the level of hostility was independently assessed by W. Langosch and G. Brodner. In cases of disagreement, a consensus rating was assigned using a formula adopted by MacDougall et al. (1979). The interrater reliability for the hostility rating scale was $r_{1,2} = 0.85$.

Patients completed three questionnaires:

1. The various scales of the Psychological Screening Questionnaire for Myocardial Infarction Patients (PSM; Langosch et al. 1980), which measure heart complaints, pain, emotional reactivity, bodily concern, depressed mood, speed/impatience, job concern, job competition, job responsibility, and social desirability. Additionally, patients were asked, if they regarded their former life style as healthy and if they thought that they need to change their life habits after discharge.
2. The scales of the *Freiburger Persönlichkeitsinventar* (FPI-A; Fahrenberg et al. 1978) which measure nervousness, aggressivity, depressivity, excitability, calmness, sociability, dominance, inhibition, and openness.
3. An achievement questionnaire which consists of 22 items (Modick 1977).

A total of 72 patients filled out the PSM, 60 subjects completed the FPI-A, and 73 patients completed the achievement questionnaire. A semistructured interview was used to assess the presence of the following occupational stresses: interruptions, time-pressure, deadlines, personnel shortage, need for flexibility, job conflict, vigilance, strict shift work, second part-time-job, limited self-control over vocational success, and responsibility. The severity of each stressor which had been present in the patient's job was rated on a four-point Likert-type rating scale while taking into account their frequency and intensity. The patient himself rated the stress he had perceived from each of those stressors, which had been present in his job, on a five-point Likert scale. This vocational analysis was administered to 73 patients.

A total of 78 patients took part in a psychophysiological examination after medication had been discontinued for at least 12 h. They were asked to respond rapidly and accurately while performing five stressful tasks:

1. Counting backwards by 7 beginning with 500, while a loud noise (approx. 80 dB) was heard through a headphone
2. A self-paced reaction time task which consisted of the exposition of five variously colored dots and two different tones
3. An extraneously paced reaction time task with reduction in exposure duration per stimulus of 20% in comparison to the self-paced task
4. Cognitively preparing responses to three aversive but important topics
5. Verbally presenting the answers to these three questions.

Except for the fourth task period, which was limited to 30 s, all tasks lasted 2 min. Each task was preceded and, with the exception of the fourth task, followed, by a 2-min rest period. Blood pressure was recorded immediately after each period, except after the stressor phase "cognitively preparing responses". Additionally, a blood pressure recording was taken immediately prior to the first rest period and immediately after the patient had been informed that he had to answer three questions within a time limit of 2 min, i.e., prior to the stressor phase "cognitively preparing answers". Thus, a total of 12 blood pressure recordings were taken. ECG and respiration were recorded continuously.

Relying on the results of earlier studies (Langosch et al. 1983; Brodner 1983; Langosch and Brodner 1985), the following parameters were calculated for each subject for each of the 11 phases:

Mean heart rate
Standard deviation of heart rate
Mean of relative respiration irregularity
Systolic blood pressure.

Heart rate was counted from the ECG during 10-s periods. Thus, the mean heart rate for each of 10 experimental phases was the average of 12 single values, while for the stressor phase "cognitively preparing the answers", the mean heart rate was based on 3 single values. Heart rate variability during each phase was quantified by calculating the standard deviation of these 12 or 3 single values, respectively. A change score was defined as the difference score between the corresponding values of a stressor phase and the preceding rest period. Thus, mean and standard deviation of the heart rate changes were based on 12 single difference scores for each of the 4 stressor phases and on 3 single difference scores for the stressor phase "cognitively preparing answers". Respiration irregularity during a 10-s period was calculated as the percentage of the total power spectrum that was not explained by the individual respiration rate, i.e. that part of the power spectrum that was beyond the individual respiration rate by plus or minus 1 Hz. The mean respiration irregularity of each phase was the average of the values based on the 10-s periods of the corresponding phase. Furthermore, a mean change score of respiration irregularity was calculated for each stressor period. Changes in systolic blood pressure during a stressor phase were obtained by taking the difference score between the systolic blood pressure measured immediately after a stressor phase and the recording taken immediately after the preceding rest period. In the statistical analysis, only the five change scores of each of the four parameters calculated on phase level were used, i.e., mean of heart rate changes, standard deviation of heart rate changes, mean of changes of respiration irregularity, and change of systolic blood pressure.

Additionally, total examination mean heart rate, mean standard deviation of heart rate, and mean systolic blood pressure were calculated for each subject. Thus, altogether 23 physiological parameters were calculated for each subject, i. e., 20 change scores and 3 trait scores.

Risk factors were defined as follows:
1. Nicotine: > 10 cigarettes/day
2. Hypercholesterolemia: > 260 mg%
3. Hypertriglyceridemia: > 150 mg%
4. Hyperuricemia: ⩾ 7 mg%
5. Obesity: Broca index > 10%
6. Arterial hypertension: systolic blood pressure ⩾ 160 mmHg and diastolic blood pressure ⩾ 90 mmHg
7. Diabetes mellitus: clinically manifest

Coronary angiography was performed using the Sones or Judkins technique. The only selection criterion for coronary angiography was the presence of a documented transmural myocardial infarction. Of the patients referred, 84% ($n = 66$) gave informed consent and underwent angiography. Several measures of severity of coronary atherosclerosis were employed: the number of > 50% occluded vessels (0–3); the Kaltenbach score and the Friesinger score, which take into account the hemodynamic importance in respect to perfusion type; the number of the involved segments; and the degree of narrowing. Furthermore, the type of the coronary disease was taken into account, namely, whether the patient had free coronary arteries, or a unilocular disease (i. e., only one stenosis or occlusion in one vessel and the other vessels totally normal), or a multilocular disease. Since it has been suggested that for patients with a multilocular disease the most significant process underlying a myocardial infarction at a young age is coronary arteriosclerosis (Roskamm et al. 1983), the association between degree of hostility and the severity of coronary arteriosclerosis was tested first for the total sample and secondly only for patients with a multilocular disease.

Data Analysis

When indicated, the variables were correlated with the hostility ratings. Any obtained correlation coefficient was considered to be significant if it reached the 0.05 level of significance. Next, the total sample was divided into a group of low hostility patients ($n = 32$), i. e., subjects with a rating score ⩽ 2, and high hostility patients ($n = 12$), i. e. subjects with a rating score ⩾ 4 on a five-point scale. The association between this split of the total sample and those variables which were badly skewed or which could be expressed only in ranks was tested by use of the chi-square test or, when the number of subjects was to small, by use of Fisher's Exact Test.

The significance of the difference between the means of the two groups was tested by means of the t-test, using a pooled or a separate variance estimate depending on the results of the preceding F-test, which gives the probability that the variances of the two groups differ significantly. Results were considered to be significant when the 0.05 level of significance was reached.

Results

The hostility ratings were associated with several psychological scales (see Table 1). The hostile patients were more concerned about their job, felt that they were under greater time pressure, complied less with all social rules, were less inclined to confess any weakness, reported more nervous symptoms, and described themselves as being more excitable and sociable. They also evaluated their former life-style as unhealthy and thought that they needed to change their life-style.

Furthermore, the correlational analysis indicated that it appears important to hostile subjects to achieve more than others; they strive harder for career advancement, like more to make plans, take the view that persons of the same age should drive harder, prefer to solve complicated problems, believe that friends regard them as hard-driving, regard competition as necessary, are busy most of the time, struggle to obtain self-defined goals and regard stamina as a very important personality trait (Table 2).

When the two extreme groups were compared (see Table 3), the high hostility patients proved to be more impatient, more excitable, more sociable, and more inclined to confess any weakness. In contrast to low hostility patients, high hostility

Table 1. Correlations (Pearson *r*) between hostility ratings and psychological scales

Psychological scale	Correlation coefficient	*P*
Job concern (PSM-9)	0.24	0.03
Speed and impatience (PSM-10)	0.25	0.02
Social desirability (PSM-14)	−0.21	0.04
Nervousness (FPI (A)-4)	0.28	0.02
Sociability (FPI (A)-5)	0.33	0.01
Openness (FPI (A)-9)	0.27	0.02
Former life style was healthy	−0.23	0.02
Have to change my life habits	0.21	0.04

Table 2. Correlations (Pearson *r*) between hostility ratings and aspects of achievement orientation

Achievement item	Correlation coefficient	*P*
I think it is important to achieve more than others	0.29	0.01
I strive for career advancement	0.20	0.05
I like to make plans	0.20	0.04
I think persons of same age should drive harder	0.29	0.01
I prefer solving complicated problems	0.24	0.02
I believe my friends regard me as hard driving	0.21	0.04
I am busy most of the time	0.25	0.02
I think competition is necessary	0.26	0.01
I struggle to obtain self-defined goals	0.21	0.04
I think stamina is a very important trait	0.21	0.04

Table 3. Mean differences between low hostility subjects and high hostility subjects on psychological measures

Psychological measure	Low hostility group		High hostility group		*df*	*t*	*P*
	$\bar{x}$	*s*	$\bar{x}$	*s*			
Speed and impatience (PSM -10)	15.30	4.32	19.11	3.66	37	−2.40	0.02
Excitability (FPI (A)-4)	2.71	1.90	4.64	2.06	33	−2.72	0.01
Sociability (FBI (A)-5)	7.08	3.43	10.09	2.51	33	−2.60	0.01
Openness (FPI (A)-9)	7.92	2.67	10.27	3.26	33	−2.26	0.03
I think it is important to achieve more than others	3.00	1.35	4.22	0.97	37	−2.58	0.01
I think persons of the same age should drive harder	2.00	1.11	3.22	1.56	37	−2.62	0.01
I prefer solving complicated problems	3.47	1.14	4.44	0.88	37	−2.37	0.02
I struggle to obtain self-defined goals	4.00	1.29	5.11	1.36	37	−2.24	0.03
I think stamina is a very important trait	4.27	1.02	5.11	1.17	37	−2.12	0.04

Table 4. Correlations (Pearson *r*) between hostility ratings and severity and perceived challenge of stressors at the workplace

Severity of job stressors	*Correlation coefficient*	*P*
Job conflict	0.23	0.05
Limited self-control over vocational success	0.32	0.01
Perceived challenge of job stressors		
Interruptions	0.26	0.02
Time pressure	−0.34	0.03
Strict shift work	0.40	0.05

subjects were more convinced that it is important to achieve more than others, that persons of the same age should drive harder, that they like to solve complicated problems, that they struggle more to obtain self-defined goals, and that stamina is a very important personality trait.

The presence of the 11 stressors in the workplace was not different for patients rated as high or low hostile. Concentrating on those stressors which were present in the job, it was found that the more hostile subjects were confronted with a higher degree of job conflict and more limited self-control over occupational success (see Table 4). Patients' ratings of the challenge they had perceived when they were confronted with a stressor in the workplace were correlated with the hostility ratings for the following stressors: interruptions, time pressure, and strict shift work (see Table 4). On the other hand, when the two extreme groups were compared, no significant differences could be found between low and high hostility subjects on the

Table 5. Mean differences between low hostility subjects and high hostility subjects on psychophysiological measures

Physiological parameters[a]	Low hostility group		High hostility group		df	t	P
	$\bar{x}$	s	$\bar{x}$	s			
Change in heart rate variability (bpm.): standard deviation of the difference scores between the stressor phase "continuous concentration" and the preceding rest period	2.58	2.39	5.11	4.31	42	−2.48	0.02
Change in relative respiration irregularity (%): mean difference score between the stressor phase "self-paced reaction time task" and the preceding rest period	24.30	10.11	31.22	70.86	38	−2.15	0.04
Change in systolic blood pressure (mmHg): difference score between the stressor phase "verbally presenting the answers" and the preceding rest period	12.52	8.82	19.92	7.22	41	−2.59	0.01
Heart rate (bpm): mean score across all stressor phases and all rest periods	83.19	15.13	75.51	8.49	35.19[b]	2.10	0.04
Systolic blood pressure (mmHg): mean score across all stressor phases and all rest periods	119.60	13.19	129.89	16.50	41	−2.14	0.04

[a] The definition of each parameter refers to the quantification for the single subject.
[b] t-test with separate variance estimate since the variances of the two groups are significantly different: $f=3.18$; $P=0.05$.

severity and on the perceived challenge of any job stressor which was present in the workplace.

When the psychophysiological data were correlated with the hostility ratings only two significant associations were found: The hostility ratings were positively correlated with heart rate variability when counting backwards while listening to disturbing noise ($r=0.28$, $p \leq 0.01$), and also with systolic blood pressure averaged across all experimental phases ($r=0.29$, $p \leq 0.01$). Contrasting the two extreme groups (see Table 5), it was found that the change scores for heart rate when counting backwards while listening to disturbing noise varied more in the high hostility group than in the low hostility group. High hostility patients increased their relative respiration variability more than low hostility subjects when they were confronted with a self-paced reaction time task, and high hostility patients had a more pronounced increase in systolic blood pressure immediately after emotional challenge. During the whole psychophysiological examination, the high hostility group had a lower heart rate but a higher systolic blood pressure than the low hostility group.

The prevalence of the seven standard risk factors was similar in low and high hostility subjects. Neither the coronary scoring system of Kaltenbach ($t=-0.32$, $df=37$, $p=0.19$), nor that of Friesinger ($t=-0.27$, $df=37$, $p\leqslant 0.79$) revealed any significant differences in the degree of the coronary artery obstruction between patients rated as low or high hostility. The groups did not differ in type of coronary artery disease, i.e., the presence of free coronary arteries, unilocular disease or multilocular disease ($\chi^2=0.28$, $df=2$, $p\leqslant 0.87$), or number of significantly narrowed coronary vessels, i.e., the occurence of zero-vessel disease, one-vessel disease, or multivessel disease ($\chi^2=0.00$, $df=1$, $p=1.00$). When the analyses were restricted to patients with multilocular disease, the number of significantly narrowed vessels was again not associated with low or high hostility ($\chi^2=0.00$, $df=1$, $p=1.00$).

Discussion

The young postinfarction patient rated as hostile can be characterized as a persistent, competitive striver for achievement, who has a sense that time is passing rapidly and who has a need for affiliation, although he does not comply with all social rules. Thus, hostility as assessed by the structured interview technique might be construed as instrumental, goal-directed activity (Diamond 1982).

The vocational findings do not support the hypothesis that hostile patients are confronted more frequently with stressors in the workplace; furthermore, for most stressors which are present in the job, the extent of their severity was not clearly related to the degree of hostility. Thus, in general, it cannot be concluded that hostile subjects prefer jobs with frequent stressors or jobs with few, but very severe, stressors. On the other hand, it becomes evident that hostile subjects have a conflicting attitude regarding time limits. Although they describe themselves as impatient, confronted with a high degree of job conflict and challenged by interruptions, they report that they feel less challenged by time pressure. Several explanations might be offered for this finding: hostile patients like to be under time pressure, they dislike admitting that they are under time pressure, or their perception of time pressure is affected. Whatever the true reason may be, hostile subjects seem less able to cope effectively with time pressure.

The psychophysiological data suggest that hostile subjects are prone to respond with a higher increase in systolic blood pressure and heart rate variability to environmental challenges. Considering this finding and the subjects' rather inefficient way of coping with time pressure, the hypothesis can be put forward that their complaints of nervousness and excitability may be indicative of exhaustion of their psychophysiological resources. Additionally, their coping abilities may have been impaired by a low level of social support, which is often associated with hostility (Berkman and Syme 1979).

Level of hostility is obviously not related to the prevalence of conventional risk factors for a myocardial infarction. This may, in part, be due to the fact that some risk factors are present in nearly all subjects (e.g., 96% were smokers), while other risk factors were nearly absent in this highly selected sample of postinfarction patients (e.g., only 3% had an arterial hypertension). Nevertheless, the findings of this study make it clear that in young male subjects the effect of hostility on the level of other coronary risk factors is, at best, very small.

Of the 66 patients who underwent angiography, 9% ($n=6$) had free coronary arteries, 21% ($n=14$) had unilocular disease, and 70% ($n=46$) had multilocular disease. A total of 15% ($n=10$) of the patients were classified as having zero-vessel disease, 55% ($n=36$) had single-vessel disease, 18% ($n=12$) had two-vessel disease, and 12% ($n=8$) had three-vessel disease. Thus, 70% of the patients had zero- or single-vessel disease, a finding which is in marked contrast to older patients after a myocardial infarction, in whom multivessel disease predominates (Samek et al. 1975). Similar angiographic findings have been reported by Gohlke et al. (1981), who performed angiography with 679 young postinfarction patients. It has been argued by Gohlke et al. (1981) that unilocular disease is more likely to have a thrombotic origin than an atherosclerotic origin, whereas in multivessel disease coronary arteriosclerosis is the most significant underlying process (Roskamm et al. 1983). Since high hostility and low hostility subjects do not differ in type of disease, it might be inferred that the prevalence of a significant coronary artery sclerosis is not related to hostility in young male patients. An additional finding shows that in the subgroup of patients with significant coronary atherosclerosis, i.e., patients with multilocular disease ($n=26$), the distribution of zero- or one-vessel disease ($n=13$), and multivessel disease ($n=13$) was equally common for both high hostility and low hostility patients. It may be concluded from this result, that in young postinfarction patients, the severity of coronary atherosclerosis is not associated with hostility.

It must be emphasized that in this study the only requirement for performing angiography was a documented transmural myocardial infarction. This selection criterion for coronary angiography is quite different from that which Williams et al. (1980) used in their study. Thus, it is not possible to compare the results of both studies because of differences in measurement of hostility, criteria for angiography, presence of myocardial infarction, and age of subjects.

In summary, the findings of this study make it clear that hostility as assessed by the semistructured interview technique, may be related to instrumental, goal-directed activity. Hostile subjects have, above all, difficulties in coping successfully with time pressure and they are prone to respond with exaggerated cardiovascular arousal to environmental challenge. Symptoms of distress might be indicative of exhaustion of psychophysiological resources. Hostility does not effect the level of the traditional coronary risk factors, nor is it associated with either the prevalence or the severity of significant coronary artery disease. It has been argued that at a young age thrombosis, coronary spasm, or a combination of the two, may play an important role in the development of coronary stenosis (Gohlke et al. 1981). Thus, stress-related psychophysiological mechanisms may contribute directly, indirectly, or as a triggering mechanism for the formation of significant coronary stenosis (Buell and Eliot 1980, 1983), although at the moment the exact pathways are not fully understood.

The results of this study are based, in part, on retrospective data and on a small sample. Thus, further research is clearly needed to confirm that the Type A hostility component is of importance in causing myocardial infarction at a young age.

Acknowledgment. This research was supported by a grant from the *Bundesministerium für Arbeit und Sozialordnung* (VI b A-58622).

References

Appels A (1980) Vitale Erschöpfung und Depression als Vorboten des Herzinfarkts. In: Langosch W (ed) Psychosoziale Probleme und psychotherapeutische Interventionsmöglichkeiten bei Herzinfarktpatienten. Minerva, München

Appels A (1981) The syndrome of vital exhaustion and depression and its relationship to coronary heart disease. In: Siegrist J, Halhuber MJ (eds) Myocardial infarction and psychosocial risks. Springer, Berlin Heidelberg New York

Appels A (1983) The year before myocardial infarction. In: Dembroski TM, Schmidt TH, Blümchen G (eds) Biobehavioral bases of coronary heart disease. Karger, Basel

Barefoot JC, Dahlstrom WG, Williams RB (1983) Hostility, CHD incidence, and total mortality: a 25-year follow-up study of 255 physicians. Psychosom Med 45: 59-63

Berkman LF, Syme SL (1979) Social networks, host resistance, and mortality: a nine-year follow-up study of Alameda County residents. Am J Epidemiol 109: 186-204

Brodner G (1983) Beiträge zur Prognose des Rehabilitationserfolges bei "jugendlichen Herzinfarktpatienten". Multivariate Analyse psychophysiologischer Befunde. Minerva, München

Buell JC, Eliot RS (1980) Psychosocial and behavioral influences in the pathogenesis of acquired cardiovascular disease. Am Heart J 100: 723-740

Buell JC, Eliot RS (1983) Behavior and the pathophysiology of coronary heart disease in humans. In: Dembroski TM, Schmidt TH, Blümchen G (eds) Biobehavioral bases of coronary heart disease. Karger, Basel

Dembroski TM, MacDougall JM, Shields JL, Petitto J, Lushene R (1978) Components of the Type A coronary-prone behavior pattern and cardiovascular responses to psychomotor performance challenge. J Behav Med 1: 159-176

Dembroski TM, MacDougall JM, Herd JA, Shields JL (1979a) Effects of level of challenge on pressor and heart rate responses in Type A and B subjects. J Appl Soc Psychol 9: 209-228

Dembroski TM, MacDougall JM, Lushene R (1979b) Interpersonal interaction and cardiovascular response in Type A subjects and coronary patients. J Human Stress 5: 28-36

Diamond EL (1982) The role of anger and hostility in essential hypertension and coronary heart disease. Psychol Bull 92: 410-433

Fahrenberg J, Selg H, Hampel R (1978) Das Freiburger Persönlichkeitsinventar FPI. Hogrefe, Göttingen

Gohlke H, Stürzenhofecker P, Thilo A, Droste C, Görnandt L, Roskam H (1981) Coronary angiographic findings and risk factors in postinfarction patients under the age of 40. In: Roskam H (ed) Myocardial infarction at young age. Springer, Berlin Heidelberg New York

Haynes SG, Feinleib M, Kannel WB (1980) The relationship of psychosocial factors to coronary heart disease in the Framingham Study III. Eight-year incidence of coronary heart disease. Am J Epidemiol 111: 37-58

Kahn JP, Kornfeld DS, Blood DK, Lynn RB, Heller SS, Frank KA (1982) Type A behavior and the thallium stress test. Psychosom Med 44: 431-436

Kantor S, Robertson AJ (1977) Repressed hostility and coronary heart disease: reappraisal of a relationship in terms of a meaning-focussed approach to psychological measurement. Soc Sci Med 11: 625-634

Langosch W, Brodner G (1985) Psychophysiological reactivity of Type A and Type B postinfarction patients under the age of forty. In: Orlebeke JF, Mulder G, van Doornen LJP (eds) Cardiovascular psychophysiology. Theory and methods. Plenum, New York

Langosch W, Prokoph JH, Brodner G (1980) Der psychologische Screeningbogen für Patienten mit Myokardinfarkt (PSM) bei verschiedenen kardiologischen Diagnosegruppen. In: Fassbender CF, Mahler E (eds) Der Herzinfarkt als psychosomatische Erkrankung in der Rehabilitation. Boehringer, Mannheim

Langosch W, Brodner G, Foerster F (1983) Psychophysiological testing of postinfarction patients. A study determining the cardiological importance of psychophysiological variables. In: Dembroski TM, Schmidt TH, Blümchen G (eds) Biobehavioral bases of coronary heart disease. Karger, Basel

Langosch W, Schmidt TH, Rüddel H (1985) Die deutsche Form des strukturierten Interviews zur Diagnostik des Verhaltenstyp-A-Musters. In: Langosch W (ed) Psychische Bewältigung der chronischen Herzerkrankung. Springer, Berlin Heidelberg New York

MacDougall JM, Dembroski TM, Musante L (1979) The structured interview and questionnaire methods of assessing coronary-prone behavior in male and female college students. J Behav Med 2: 71-83

Matthews KA (1982) Psychological perspectives on the Type A behavior pattern. Psychol Bull 91: 293-323

Matthews KA, Glass DC, Rosenman RH, Bortner RW (1977) Competitive drive, pattern A, and coronary heart disease: a further analysis of some data from the Western Collaborative Group Study. J Chron Dis 30: 489-498

Modick HE (1977) Ein dreiskaliger Fragebogen zur Erfassung des Leistungsmotivs - Bericht über eine deutschsprachige Weiterentwicklung des Prestatie Motivatie Test. Diagnostica 23: 298-321

Rosenman RH (1978) The interview method of assessment of the coronary prone behavior. In: Dembroski TM, Weiss SM, Shields JL, Haynes SG, Feinleib M (eds) Coronary-prone behavior. Springer, Berlin Heidelberg New York

Rosenman RH, Chesney MA (1980) The relationship of Type A behavior pattern to coronary heart disease. Act Nerv Super (Praha) 22: 1-45

Roskamm H, Gohlke H, Stürzenhofecker P, Droste C, Thomas H, Schnellbacher K, Betz P (1983) Der Herzinfarkt im jugendlichen Alter (unter 40 Jahren): Koronarmorphologie, Risikofaktoren, Langzeitprognose der Erkrankung und Progression der Koronargefäßsklerose. Z Kardiol 72: 1-11

Samek L, Roskamm H, Rentrop P, Kaiser P, Stürzenhofecker P, Schober B, Görnandt L, Velden R (1975) Belastungsprüfungen und Koronarangiogramm im chronischen Infarktstadium. Z Kardiol 64: 809-814

Shekelle R, Gale M, Ostfeld AM, Oglesby P (1983) Hostility, risk of coronary heart disease, and mortality. Psychosom Med 45: 109-114

Siltanen P, Lauroma M, Nirkko O, Punsar S, Pyorala K, Tuominen H, Vanhala K (1975) Psychological characteristics related to coronary heart disease. J Psychosom Res 19: 183-195

van Dijl H (1982) Myocardial infarction patients and heightened aggressiveness/hostility. J Psychosom Res 26: 203-208

Williams RB, Haney TL, Lee KL, Kong Y, Blumenthal JA, Whalen RE (1980) Type A behavior, hostility, and coronary atherosclerosis. Psychosom Med 42: 539-549

Hostility and Conflict as Antecedents of Arousal and Disease

S. STREUFERT and R. M. POGASH[1]

Definitions

A differential definition of "anger", "hostility", and "aggression" has escaped many a theorist or researcher - in part, probably, for good reason. The processes are often (but not always) interrelated and can be difficult to tease apart. One can, of course, argue that hostility would sensitize persons to certain kinds of information or would be likely to distort the meaning of incoming information. Anger would then be the outcome of a resulting perception, and aggression would be the obvious sequel to anger. However, even *if* these processes would function in this or some other simple fashion, they need hardly be sequential in a single direction. For that matter, hostility *can* result in anger, but anger, in turn, may produce or cue (reinforce, maintain, etc.) hostility. Anger may result in aggression, yet aggression, particularly when faced with counter-aggression from the target, may generate additional hostility and anger, and so forth. However, despite the difficulty of disentangling hostility, anger, and aggression, and despite the absence of a fixed sequence, we should try to achieve better and separate definitions of these concepts. Our understanding of the cognitive, emotional and behavioral processes that are involved can only be advanced if we communicate clearly which component we are considering - even when the resulting categorization may seem (or be) somewhat artificial. In this paper, the three concepts are considered and defined differentially - in part, because a specific focus on "hostility" (where possible) will be essential for present purposes.

To achieve a definition that will guide subsequent discussions, the views of Williams et al. (1984) will be adapted and slightly modified. These authors viewed *hostility* as an attitudinal set or personality trait. Hostility is said to originate from lack of trust in the "goodness" of other persons, i. e., from the expectation that others will behave in a mean, selfish, or undependable fashion. Williams et al. believe that hostility is probably learned. The present authors would agree that learning probably played a major role in the development of hostility, but would classify that personality characteristic not so much as a reflection of attitudinal "content," but rather as a reflection of a structural *"style"* of thinking. General (rather than specifically focused) hostility may not be reflective of "what a person thinks" (attitudinal content) but rather of "how a person thinks, how he/she deals with others, and how he/she perceives others."[2] Possibly Williams et al. (1984) had a stylistic concept in mind when they wrote about hostility as a potential "personality trait." (For more information on cognitive styles, their definitions and their cognitive/affective/behavior-

1 Pennsylvania State University College of Medicine, Hershey, PA 17033, USA

2 The finding that hostility scores are quite stable across time would add additional credence to a view of hostility as a stylistic rather than a content variable (cf., for example, Shekelle et al. 1983).

Biological and Psychological Factors
in Cardiovascular Disease
Ed. by T. H. Schmidt, T. M. Dembroski, and G. Blümchen

al outcomes, the interested reader is referred to Streufert and Streufert 1978; Streufert and Swezey 1986).

A view of general or pervasive hostility as a cognitive style is somewhat different from previous conceptions of hostility (e.g., Rosenman 1984; Spielberger et al. 1984). It differs even more widely from those views which fail to make careful distinctions between hostility, anger, and related concepts (Buss 1961; Berkowitz 1962).

In contrast to hostility, *anger* will be viewed as an *emotional* state. It reflects feelings that may range from mild irritation to rage. While hostility is located within cognition, anger is considered as an affective response. Clearly, as also suggested by Williams et al. (1984), one would expect hostility and anger to be correlated. Some authors (e.g., Schwartz et al. 1981; Frankenhaeuser 1982) view anger as an active coping response. Such a conceptualization would fit within the present definition as long as the response is primarily affective in its expression. When anger, however, is considered to be a "cognitive response associated with personal appraisal and interpretation" (Buss 1961; cf. also Diamond 1982), the distinctions between characteristics of hostility and anger become unclear. Such a view of anger does not match the definitions advanced in this paper.

Aggression may be defined as a *behavior* that is intended to be injurious or destructive (or, in some cases at least, threateningly communicative). It is frequently directed toward a target with whom conflict already exists. Generally, aggression is directly related to hostility and/or anger. However, not all hostility or anger will result in aggression (cf. the "anger-in" concept as researched by Dembroski et al. 1985). On the other hand, aggression may occur in the complete absence of anger or hostility, for example as an action which reflects a goal-oriented competitive strategy. In the latter case, no hostility may exist and the ensuing action may contain little or no (especially negative) affect.

Stylistic Hostility: a Short Review of Research Data

The primary concern of this paper, as already suggested, will be hostility, i.e., a cognitive style which may express itself in (result in) anger and aggression (as observed responses and behaviors) on the one hand, and in arousal and potential physiological damage to the hostile individual on the other. In this section, a short (and rather limited) review of relevant research will be presented. Obviously, restricted space allows only a consideration of *some* representative theoretical views and data.

The quality and appropriateness of any review of hostility and its effects depends, of course, in good part on the meaningfulness of definitions and of measures. The definition of hostility has already been discussed. The quality of measurement is quite another problem. As Spielberger et al. (1984) have pointed out, the diversity of measurement operations has probably resulted in questionable validity of findings. Recently, hostility measurement has often been considered in terms of the Ho subscale of the MMPI (Cook and Medley 1954). A cause for the repeated selection of that instrument by several researchers may be the availability of "old" MMPI scores which can be employed in longitudinal (semiprospective) data analysis procedures. There is only limited assurance that the MMPI-based Ho Subscale is as excellent a measure of hostility as might be desired. As a matter of fact, the view that this MMPI subscale actually does measure hostility, or that it measures it precisely, has been doubted. For example, Ho appears to be closely related to "cynicism" and some forms of neurotic conflict experience (e.g., suspiciousness) (cf., for example, Ostfeld et al. 1964; Costa et al. 1985; Johnson et al. 1984; Williams et al. 1984).

Whatever the Ho subscale of the MMPI does measure, there is impressive evidence showing its relationship to cardiovascular disease[3] and mortality (e.g., Barefoot et al. 1983). It correlates favorably (although not very highly) with other measures of hostility such as the Trait-Anger scale of Spielberger and associates (Spielberger et al. 1983), with behaviorally assessed "potential for hostility" (Dembroski et al. 1985) and with global structured interview-defined Type A (Rosenman 1978). It is positively associated with age, smoking, and alcohol consumption (e.g., Shekelle et al. 1983). It is especially interesting that the Ho subscale predicts not only an increased risk of coronary heart disease (CHD) but also malignant neoplasms, and overall mortality from other causes (with CHD, neoplasms, and renal diseases controlled). The predictive validity of Ho scores for overall mortality is maintained even after adjustment for smoking, alcohol consumption, systolic blood pressure, and serum cholesterol (Barefoot et al. 1983; Shekelle et al. 1983; Williams et al. 1984).

Other measurement techniques which are designed to assess hostility in particular, or the hostility/anger complex in general, corroborate these findings. Some research, however, suggests that the predictive capacity of Type A and hostility scores for coronary heart disease is generated by its "anger-in" component (Dembroski et al. 1985). Nonetheless, the behaviorally rated "potential for hostility" has been shown to be the strongest predictor of CHD in the Western Collaborative Group Study (cf. Matthews et al. 1977). Even self-reported feelings of hostility are predictive of arousal or disease such as hypertension, especially where the hostility is ineffectively managed (e.g. Weiner 1977; Baer et al. 1979; Harburg et al. 1979; Diamond 1982). In other words, the relationship between hostility experience, arousal, and hypertensive and/or cardiovascular disease has some empirical support.

There is somewhat less certainty about the cognitive and physiological mechanisms that translate hostility into disease. It goes without question that hostility is predictive of physiological arousal - yet arousal is not always a necessary predictor of disease. How, then, is hostility translated into cardiovascular damage or into other forms of disease? It is frequently assumed that vascular damage in the myocardium occurs via the initial action of catecholamines. Indeed, research shows that the myocardial infarction (MI) patients with severe disease are, in about 90% of the cases, Type A individuals (e.g., Blumenthal et al. 1978), a group for whom higher levels of epinephrine and/or norepinephrine response have been repeatedly demonstrated. Furthermore, elevated norepinephrine responsivity has been directly as-

---

3 Cynicism may increase testosterone secretion (cf. Williams et al. 1982). Testosterone has been shown to be artherogenic in animals (Uzunova et al. 1978). Estradiol, and end-product of testosterone-norepinephrine interaction, has been found at higher levels in heart attack victims (Klaiber et al. 1982; Luria et al. 1982; Castelli et al. 1983).

sociated with hostility itself, for example, in a comparison of hostile versus anxious subjects (Friedman et al. 1960). In addition, a 24-year longitudinal research effort (Harlan et al. 1967) has established a relationship between aggressive personality scores (on the Guilford-Zimmerman Temperament Survey) and higher blood lipid levels.

Assuming that the catecholamine-to-disease relationship is accepted, the data presented above (and similar data reported by other investigators) would serve to confirm that a direct physiological link between hostility and disease probably exists. However, how does hostility as a "style" function to create an "excessive" or extended arousal associated with a sufficiently damaging level of catecholamine secretion to become predictive of heart disease? It has been shown that *unexpressed* hostility (as evident in "anger-in") exacerbates and extends cardiovascular and catecholamine responses to other (potentially even unrelated) stressful stimuli (Baer et al. 1979; Goldstein 1981). Such overreactions to stimuli (cf. Nixon and Bethel 1974; Nixon 1976), whether potentially productive of hypertension or of cardiovascular disease, may not have occurred if the resulting anger had been vented (cf. Hokanson et al. 1963), or if effective counter-aggression against the target had occurred (cf. Diamond 1982). In other words, as Dembroski and associates (1985) have demonstrated, hostility *per se* is not enough. It probably takes the *maintenance* of hostility and its anger effects over time (e.g., "anger-in") to generate sufficient physiological responsivity of a kind and degree that can damage the myocardium. In other words, disease may result when social conflicts with the targets of hostility and anger are frequently maintained, at least until the hostile person forgets the situation over a period of time or until he or she has a chance to "get even". Incidentally, that "revenge" may be less than obvious. In short, *conflict maintenance* across time may well be a decisive factor in the hostility/disease relationship. We shall return to that point later.

Beyond Hostility and Anger

Can all arousal, all hypertension, and all damage to the myocardium - to the degree to which it is caused by or related to behavioral characteristics - be explained by the hostility/anger syndrome or by its "anger-in" component? It is not likely. There is a great deal of evidence which also points to other, quite unrelated antecedents. For example, Williams et al. (1984) report that covariation of Ho scores with Type A diminishes the measured damaging effects of Type A but does not eliminate them entirely. Such a finding should be expected when hostility and, to some extent, the "anger-in" dimension are measured as part of the Type A profile. Several earlier writers (cf. the discussions of Manuck and Polefrone 1985) have postulated or observed a number of "intrapsychic conflicts" that may be related to hypertension and/or to cardiovascular disease. Such conflicts include the effects of suppressed hostility, ineffective social interaction and assertion, defensive interaction stylistics, and lack of social support. More recently, observations and research have combined to identify interpersonal conflict (McKegney and Williams 1967), anticipation of aversive stimulation (Shapiro et al. 1963), demanding cognitive tasks (Shapiro et al. 1963; Nestel 1969; Lorimer et al. 1971; Baumann et al. 1973), situational demands for active coping and requirements for vigilance (Obrist 1976, 1981), task-relevant incentives (Elliott 1969), attentional demands (Williams 1975), stimulus novelty (Light and Obrist 1980), and anxiety (Thailer et al. 1982) as situations in which excessive cardiovascular and/or catecholamine responsivity may be obtained. Some of the research suggests that persons with identified vascular or cardiac problems tend to show especially elevated responsivity to stressors or demands of these kinds.

It would be difficult to argue that all of the obtained/observed responsivity or hyperreactivity in these various stressor task or demand settings was generated by hostility and/or anger. For that matter, there now is evidence that some non-hostility-producing settings may generate excess cardiovascular responsivity that far exceeds responses generated in settings which foster hostility. For example, Streufert et al. (1984) had their subjects participate in a potentially hostility-producing Type A structured interview, in a very gentle and apparently clinical "complexity interview", and in a challenging video game. Considerable increases in systolic blood pressure (SBP) and diastolic blood pressure (DBP) over resting baseline were observed for all tasks[4]. Yet by far the greatest delta values for both blood pressure and heart rate were obtained in the gentle complexity interview, not in the hostility-producing structured (Type A) interview. Moreover, while Type A persons with previously identified heart disease responded with excess delta blood pressure values to both the Type A interview and the complexity interview, Type B disease victims responded with excess delta values *only* to the gentle complexity interview. Anger or "anger-in" appeared not to be involved in the hyperresponsivity. Their reactivity was probably generated by purely cognitive phenomena. In other words, cognitively experienced conflict probably elevated their autonomic and associated neuroendocrine responses.

Is it possible to find a "common denominator" for the various antecedents of excess physiological responses? Moreover, can we find a denominator which would include hostility, and especially its "anger-in" correlate, and place them in a sufficiently prominent - but not necessarily dominant - position? It appears that such a feat should be possible. Let us, for the moment, explore the various theoretical suggestions that have been advanced by previous writers. The "components" of Type A (e.g., Rosenman 1978) are well known and the reader need hardly be reminded of them. Glass (1977) and Glass and Contrada (1982) have favored an emphasis on control as the explanation for Type A behavior and its physiological effects, i.e., behaviorally initiated physiological hyperresponsivity. Rosenman (1984) would modify that view toward an emphasis on "competitiveness". Achievement orientation has been implicated as well (Rosenman et al. 1964; Frankenhaeuser 1980; Ray and Bozek 1980; Rosenman and Chesney 1982). Gutmann and Benson (1971), at least with hypertension as an outcome, view the requirement for continuous behavioral adjustments to changes in the environment as a causal antecedent. Streufert et al. (1979) have reported a relationship between cognitive complexity and arousal, a re-

4 While SBP, DBP, and HR increases paralleled each other for the interview setting and another "resting" condition in the presence of another person, pressor responses became disparate for the video game. For most subjects, increases in DBP considerably exceeded increases in SBP, with some persons producing the inverse relationship.

lationship that has been extended to myocardial infarctions in more recent cross-sectional research (cf. Streufert 1984).

In view of the apparent diversity of behavioral factors that have been theoretically postulated or have received research support, one might be tempted to conclude that there may be many independent behavioral antecedents to physiological hyperreactivity and to potential disease. Yet, as scientists, we are often uncomfortable about postulating a multitude of causal factors. At the cognitive antecedent level, do these factors have anything in common - at least those that have received some research support? A careful analysis of the cognitive underpinnings of these factors suggests that physiological cardiovascular and neuroendocrine hyperreactivity may be caused or, at least, cognitively initiated by the *frequency, degree,* and *length* of experienced *cognitive* conflict. Certainly, hostility experience would generate such conflict. When hostility is maintained via "anger-in", that conflict would extend over considerable time. But let us go beyond hostility and consider whether some of the other proposed or validated predictors of arousal and disease fit into the "conflict" theory. Trying to cope in the presence of adversity (but not giving up) would probably maintain severe conflict as attempts to cope continue. Problems with assertiveness, demanding tasks, stimulus novelty, desired incentives, and, in some cases, anxiety (when there is some attempt to deal with it) would also be likely to generate cognitive conflict. In other words, conflict need not arise from "interpersonal" settings. It may clearly relate to concerns with "control." It may be an outcome of frustrations that are experienced in the attempt to reach blocked goals, as long as the person involved has not given up. It may be a reflection of cognitive competition among dimensional judgments with alternate implications, i.e., in cognitively complex (multidimensional) persons. Cognitive conflict in complex persons may also arise from an anticipation of alternate potential outcomes created by actions that are currently being considered, that is, anticipations that may require a high level of "vigilance."[5] Among all of these potential sources of cognitively generated conflict (all of which have been discussed by previous writers as potential or demonstrated antecedents of serious arousal or disease), unexpressed hostility ("anger-in") could certainly play a major part. In some cases, non-hostility-produced conflicts may even be displaced and could be experienced as anger or expressed as aggression. The next section will deal with the causation of such "interpretive" effects.

Stylistic Conflict: Perceptions, Interpretations, and Responses

This paper has already defined "hostility" as, in part, a stylistic phenomenon. That style would determine, or influence, whether some stimulus is perceived as threatening, challenging, etc. The responsive hostility and anger, or its level and endurance over time, would be a function of this style. Such a "style" argument can be ex-

5 An alternative explanation for "cynical" and "vigilant" responses in some persons may be based on complexity theory. For example, to a more multidimensional (cognitively complex) person, a friend can be *both* a good and loving companion and a useful means toward an end (cf. the various interpretations of the MMPI Ho scale discussed above).

tended to the conflict notion. A person's cognitive style would determine whether social or nonsocial cognitive conflict is maintained, accelerated, and translated into physiological responses. Certainly, there are many situations where nearly anyone would view his or her environment as laden with conflict. Good examples might be such events as: "Should I buy this car or that one?" or "Why did he hit me, I didn't do anything to him?" Under such conditions, emerging cognitive conflict is practically inevitable. On the other hand, many conflicts are the result of an interaction between person and environment, or a result of cognitive mismatches within the person's thought processes. Here, the characteristics of a person's own interpretive processes are of considerable importance. Yet not everyone experiences cognitive conflicts and dilemmas with frequency; some of us almost always know (or think we know) what "the right thing to do" is - and act accordingly. Some of us do not respond to challenge or do not find it interesting. Some of us ignore the other person who is trying to compete or pick a fight, and some of us do not even generate anger toward that person, an anger which we would have had to hide. Some of us do not become time urgent. And, some of us perceive our world along single fixed dimensions that negate the possibility of self-generated cognitive conflict. If we do belong to such a group, behavioral factors in our make-up are probably less likely to be responsible for cardiovascular disease.[6]

For many of us, however, stylistically generated conflict experience is frequent and may be enduring and severe. What *kind* of conflict perceptions we experience, however, what kind of affective/physiological response to that conflict we would generate, and what resultant action may be typical for us may vary greatly from person to person. For many who live in the competitive western world, stylistic perceptions and cognitions may reflect hostility, leading to anger and aggression. For those of us who are cognitively complex, frequent, often severe, and at times enduring conflicts among perceptions, among decision options and their interrelationships may emerge (especially where the environment contains multiple uncertainty). For those of us with a considerable need for novelty (and, possibly, variety) (cf. the GIAL theory of Streufert and Streufert 1978), cognitive conflict and its sequelae may be generated by the varied, unfamiliar, and sometimes threatening input (or its sequelae) which we seek or manage to provide for ourselves. For those of us who have been described as "cynical" or "suspicious," cognitive conflict experience may be due to either perceptual multidimensionality or due to perceptual distortion. Of course, multiple stylistic antecedents of potential cognitive conflict experience might join to form an overall style that exposes us to diverse levels, diverse frequencies, and diverse durations of more or less severe conflict. The resulting emotional and physiological arousal responses would covary with the cognitive antecedents, and may, over the long run, produce potential disease states.

A low or moderate degree of conflict experience, if the GIAL theory is correct, may arouse the "interest" of the experiencing person, leading to information search and motivated attention. However, once the perceived cognitive conflict exceeds an "adaptation level," cognitive and physiological responses may turn more toward a

6 Unless, of course, we must live in an ever-changing environment that tends to overload us with the unexpected, that requires continual readjustment, or imposes frequent and lasting *external* conflict experience.

"fight or flight" orientation (cf. the predictions and physiological findings of Williams et al. 1984, 1982, for various task settings).

Physiological responses to experienced levels and durations of conflict would, if they are strong enough, be directly experienced, and would likely be recognized as a physiological change by the person involved. That perceptual experience may become part of a feedback loop (Schachter and Singer 1962): the person may interpret his or her physiological arousal in the light of previous experience, beliefs, etc. In other words, he or she would likely generate some "cognitive" interpretation of those physical experiences.[7] Krantz and associates (Durel and Krantz 1984) have clarified the processes involved in such feedback loop systems. From the present point of view, past experience and previous learning, possibly in association with some genetic factors, could help the person identify (1) whether a perceived physiological feeling is or is not a reflection of a cognitive conflict; (2) what that conflict is all about (for example, a suspicious, hostile person who is experiencing a physiological arousal response might seek and find a nonexistent external foe); (3) how serious this conflict is; and (4) whether it requires a response, which kind of response is needed, and when that response should occur. These interpretations of a physiological feedback loop would interact with already existing cognitions (e.g., interpretations of an external situation or internal conflict) to maintain, amplify, diminish, or change affective/physiological and subsequent behavioral outcomes. In turn, feedback loop effects would be continued, increased, or diminished (for more detail, the interested reader is referred to the excellent discussion of such a feedback system by Krantz and his associates). In other words, a person's stylistic cognitions about conflict, as they are created or influenced by perceptual and interpretive thought processes, would be augmented by additional interpretive processes that are based on perceptions of physiological changes. This allows those styles to do "double work" in generating a particular person's more-or-less typical and presumably quite stable cognitive, affective/physiological, and behavioral responses. The frequency, degree, and length of such conflict experience is likely to translate into physiological reactivity, and possibly into subsequent disease. Of course, the kind of physiological response, its level, frequency and duration would probably be of considerable importance. How, when, and at what levels cognitive conflict responses translate into physiological characteristics still need to be explored.

Preliminary Data on Conflict and Disease

Research has demonstrated that "hostility" and/or "anger" (if that is what the Ho subscale does measure) can result in excessive arousal and in potential subsequent cardiovascular damage. Similar data have been provided for "potential for hostility" scores based on structured interviews. If hostility experience, especially in the "anger-in" format, is considered as part of an overall "cognitive conflict" concept, then these findings could be used to support a conflict-disease theory. However, be-

7 Of course, that process of perception, cognitive interpretation of the perceived physiological change, and subsequent response may (e.g., via reinforcement) have long ago become "automated" as a part of an individual's overall cognitive style with its behavioral sequelae.

fore a "conflict" view can replace a "hostility" view, it must be demonstrated that conflicts which are not related to anger and hostility can and do predict arousal and can lead to cardiovascular damage. Some data - however preliminary - are now available from our research lab and will be reported here. We will first consider data on cognition and arousal, and conclude with preliminary findings on cognition and coronary artery disease.

Arousal

Predicting either arousal or disease from cognition necessitates having some reasonable way of assessing cognition; in the present case, a reasonable way to assess a cognitive style (or styles) related to conflict experience. Our measurement grew out of an interest in styles such as complexity and incongruity adaptation (Streufert and Streufert 1978). Initially we used a subjective measure of multidimensional differentiation and integration to assess cognitive complexity. This technique, known as Sentence (Paragraph) Completion Test (Schroder and Streufert 1963; Schroder et al. 1967) has been widely validated. It obtains information on a person's perception and resolution of multidimensional cognitive conflict. While persons found to be generally "unidimensional" are less likely to experience conflicts among cognitions, persons who are scored as differentiators and integrators do experience at least choice conflict and often consequential conflict problems (Streufert and Streufert 1978; Streufert and Swezey 1986).

Measurement via subjective tests, such as the Sentence Completion technique, which require training of scorers is far from ideal. Objective measures, where available, are certainly preferable *if* they can measure the appropriate phenomenon adequately. However, measurement of *styles* via objective tests is quite difficult. The problems of measurement of coronary-prone behavior via the structured interview (SI) of Rosenman and Friedman, versus its measurement via objective techniques (Jenkins et al. 1971; Jenkins 1978) come to mind. As Durel and Krantz (1984) have pointed out, the Jenkins Activity Scale is a measure of *content*, while the SI is primarily a measure of *style*. Indeed, it is very difficult to measure style in objective tests. People know and may be willing to tell you *what* they think, i.e., they understand the contents of their own thoughts. However, it is unlikely that they know, and probably have never even considered, *how* they think. Consequently they cannot tell the researcher about their own stylistic characteristics. As a result, the researcher has to tease the stylistic structure out of content responses. This necessity, aggravated by the effects of social desirability in items that are designed to elicit structural consequences, make the task of developing tests for style very cumbersome and quite slow. Our research group, for example, has been working on the development of objective measures for two styles for quite some time. We have been interested in measuring both "cognitive complexity" and "incongruity adaptation". While our objective tests are certainly not yet in their final form, they have progressed considerably and are useful for some purposes. For example, they should be able to predict the degree of conflict experience which are "typical" for certain persons - at least where conflict is based on multidimensional cognition and on incongruity adaptation. In turn, if the proposed theoretical view of cognitive conflict is correct, items from these stylistic tests should be able to predict (where they are conflict relevant) arousal and potential disease.

Our initial analysis of conflict items and their prediction of arousal employed noninvasive techniques (SBP, DBP, HR). We chose to work only with noninvasive technology because (1) we wanted to compare potentially diverse arousal responses to a relatively rapid succession of different tasks, and (2) we wanted to avoid secondary stressor experiences that might confound our findings. Our data analysis employed regression techniques to identify questionnaire items that would significantly predict systolic versus diastolic (or both) arousal responses. We found that arousal was predicted by quite diverse items which, in most cases, appeared unrelated to hostility and anger. For example, systolic arousal (in the absence of considerable increases in diastolic arousal) for social stress settings was predicted by items such as "There is no quick answer to life's problems," "I have changed my view of others frequently during the last few years," and "When there are several decisions I could make and all of them seem to have some - but different - advantages, I usually think through all the possibilities again, but still find it hard to make up my mind." In general, these and similar items seem to reflect intentionally generated or maintained conflict. Diastolic arousal for social task settings (in the absence of considerable increases in systolic arousal) was predicted by items such as "When people argue because they have different opinions, I try to show them that they are probably both right; it depends on how one looks at the situation," "When I have to make a decision in an unclear or confusing situation, I do what best fits my current strategy, but I may change my approach if the outcome is not quite what I expected," and "When someone points out to me that I have just said something which is inconsistent with some previous remark I made, I feel quite pleased because consistency is the hobgoblin of little minds." Again, an openness to conflict appears present. Clearly all of these items (and, of course, others which similarly predicted excess systolic or diastolic arousal) were conflict oriented but *generally not hostility oriented*. Items predicting low systolic arousal in social tasks were associated with taking a long time in decision settings, e.g., "When I have to make a decision in an unclear or confusing situation, I tend to take a very long time to decide - I prefer to be right rather than quick," or with the experience of anxiety rather than excitement in response to novelty. Low diastolic arousal in social task settings was predicted by items that would avoid conflict or would maintain consistency, e.g., "I have changed my views of others only when those people have changed a lot" or "I set goals for myself that I can achieve."

Excessive or high levels of systolic arousal in a nonsocial challenging task was predicted by items which reflect flexibility and the use of alternate strategies in handling complex situations, e.g., "Different ideas and opinions come from different assumptions. Despite their differences they may all be justified," "When there are several decisions I could make and all of them have some - but different - advantages, I try to imagine what the various long-term outcomes of my possible decisions would be and how they relate to the goals I have," and "If I must make a decision in an unclear or confusing situation I try to think of which parts of the available alternatives can be combined to achieve the purposes I have in mind for the moment." Excessive or high diastolic arousal for nonsocial challenging tasks, in contrast, was predicted by items like "When someone disagrees with me, it usually means that one of us is wrong," "It would be best for everyone if all of us had the same correct ideas and opinions," and "If I must make a decision in an unclear and confusing situation, I focus only on the most important component of the situation." Apparently, intentional self-exposure to conflict settings predicts systolic elevation for nonsocial tasks, and the attempt to rid oneself of conflict appears to predict greater diastolic elevations. Not surprisingly, the same items which predicted high systolic deltas for nonsocial tasks often predicted low diastolic deltas, and vice versa. For example, while persons who responded with high systolic arousal responded favorably to the item "If I get information that disagrees with a strong opinion of mine, I think about or try to find out whether still other opinions exist. Maybe one of them would be best, but it is difficult to decide which one that might be," persons with high diastolic arousal to nonsocial task settings rejected that item.

In sum, conflict as a predictor of arousal appeared to be a component of all statistically significant items. Apparently, the kind of conflict, its origin, the setting in which it occurs, and the kind of arousal it produces can vary. Nonetheless, conflict appears to be ever-present and pervasive. Furthermore, our data suggest that hostility as an item component was not required for the prediction of arousal. Yet, as previously discussed, there was some evidence for "interest" as a component of systolic arousal and for "vigilance" as a component of at least diastolic arousal that occurred in nonsocial task settings.

Coronary Artery Disease

As stated earlier, not all arousal - not even all excessive arousal - is necessarily related to subsequent coronary artery disease (CAD). It is of importance to determine, (1) what kind of arousal, if any, in response to diverse tasks (settings, challenges, requirements, etc.); (2) what level and frequency of arousal experience; and (3) what combination of factors that may include arousal can be identified as antecedents of CAD. To begin to explore these and related questions, we assembled items from our previous research that had been predictive of arousal. We added 21 items from three of Siegel's (1985) factors [General Anger (nine items), Hostile Outlook (six items), and Anger-in (six items)] representing hostility/anger responses. Siegel's items were selected since they represented a spectrum of items utilized by other researchers and since they appeared to be more clearly related to hostility and anger in a "pure" sense; i.e., it was thought that they might be less confounded with other characteristics such as cognitive complexity, suspiciousness, etc. The total inventory of arousal plus anger statements consisted of 100 items. It was administered to patients who had either undergone cardiac catherization during the last 3 years at the Hershey Medical Center, or who had been hospitalized for other noncardiovascular reasons. The patients were classified into three groups: those with serious CAD as established by catheterization procedures, using the classification system employed by researchers such as Williams and associates (1984), and Dembroski and associates (1985) (two or more occluded arteries at 75% or higher occlusion). Occlusion of one artery at 75% or above was considered moderate disease. Occlusion of less than 75% in all arteries or absence of disease was considered mild/absent CAD. Patients hospitalized for other (noncardiac or vascular problems) were classified together with patients of the disease mild/absent group.[8]

A regression procedure for disease incidence and for a coronary index score produced nearly equivalent data. Of the 100 inventory items, 17 were significantly predictive of CAD. Only two of the hostility items reached significance: "I tend to get angry more frequently than most people" ($P<0.02$), and "It irritates me a lot when people get in my way" ($P<0.05$). An additional hostility-related item, "I am secretly quite critical of others," reached a P level of 0.15. The remaining 15 significant predictor items suggested little or no affinity to hostility or anger. Their significance level was in some cases as high as $P<0.005$, e.g., "When someone disagrees with me in a discussion, I usually find it extremely interesting" (CAD disease victims agreed with the item) and "When people say that a problem has several solutions, I must agree; solutions must depend on the situation" (CAD victims disagreed). It is quite interesting to note that most of the items which were significantly related to CAD in our regression analysis had in our previous research been predictive of *systolic* arousal in *social* settings.

To begin to validate the obtained 17 significant inventory items, to again test the hostility factors of Siegel (1985), and to attempt to replicate our previous finding that had identified heart disease patients as more cognitively complex, we continued to administer our 100-item inventory of hostility/arousal items and the Sentence (Paragraph) Completion Test of Schroder and Streufert (1963) to patients with CAD and to control patients. At the time of writing this paper, the responses of 25 patients with CAD and 19 control patients had been observed. Their responses to the 17 predictive inventory items were summed to a single score. Comparisons between the CAD and control groups were made for that combined score, for factor-based scores on General Anger, Hostile Outlook and Anger-In (cf. Siegel 1985) and for cognitive complexity.[9]

The data were analyzed with one-way ANOVA techniques. The single factor in each analysis was disease incidence (CAD present versus absent, as previously defined). In addition, correlations among the various dependent measures were calculated. In one case, a covariance analysis was introduced. The purpose of data analysis was to gain a preliminary validity estimate for the previously discussed findings. Even though this second sample was small, it appeared useful to estimate whether the significant prediction of CAD from the 17 previously discussed inventory items and from cognitive complexity could be substantiated.

The results indicated that the summed 17 predictor items successfully predicted disease incidence in the second sample ($f=4.216$; 1/37 *df*; $P=0.044$). It should be noted that this result was obtained from responses on six-point scales with evenly weighted scale points. Future analysis will carefully study the distribution of CAD victims and controls on these six-point scales, to provide potentially useful weights or cut-off values for each scale.

---

8 It is, of course, recognized that some of the patients who did not undergo catheterization may have CAD. If so, this condition would weaken rather than strengthen our data.

9 The results below should be considered preliminary since they are based on only those subjects that had responded at the time of writing and since CAD patients and control patients have not yet been matched on some of the relevant variables. Matching will be done, once more responses to the tests have been obtained.

The results for predictive validity of cognitive complexity were strikingly strong ($f=9.583$; 1/31 *df*; $P=0.004$). (The smaller value for degrees of freedom is due to the fact that some Sentence Completion tests were not appropriately filled out and could not be scored.) Sentence Completion scores and the summed scores for the 17 predictor items were correlated ($r=0.333$), suggesting more than 10% common variance of the two measures. Consequently, an analysis of covariance with CAD as the independent variable, cognitive complexity as the dependent variable, and the summed 17 predictor items as the covariate was run. In this analysis, an *f* value of 3.66 (1/30 *df*) was obtained, reducing the *P* value for cognitive complexity to 0.06. Similarly, employing complexity as a covariate reduced the summed 17 predictor item effect to a nonsignificant *f* ratio. In other words, some of the predictor variance of the cognitive complexity scores was also reflected in the 17 inventory items and vice versa. Such a finding fits well with theoretical assumptions about cognitive conflict as an antecedent of heart disease. We suggested above that cognitive complexity should be one, but not the only, conflict-producing style with relevance to CAD. A more general stylistic measure would probably contain some of the same predictive characteristics that could be contained in cognitive complexity scores. As long as a general test does not capture all conflict effects, one would also expect some remnant predictive capacity of complexity scores.

None of the anger/hostility factors of Siegel (1985) included in this analysis predicted CAD. The *f* values for the General Anger score, the Hostile Outlook score, and for Anger-In remained below 1.0. With relatively small variance values obtained for these analyses, the absence of any meaningful effect was clearly due to near identical mean values.[10]

We may then conclude that preliminary data analysis of CAD patients and controls (drawn primarily from central Pennsylvania) does provide initial support for a conflict theory. Two findings, however, are especially striking: (1) the replication of a (previously equally strong) finding relating cognitive complexity to CAD and/or MI, and (2) the finding that hostility and anger, as obtained via Siegel's (1985) factor-based items, appear unrelated to CAD. Certainly, our data collection is not complete, and some changes in our data may yet be obtained with more extensive matching of patients and controls and with the more balanced data that are due to a greater number of subjects. However, the complete absence of hostility/anger effects and the very strong complexity results will probably not change drastically. One may wonder whether the status of hostility and anger, especially "anger-in" as an antecedent to cardiovascular disease should not be re-examined. Are we indeed dealing with the same kind of hostility/anger when we employ Siegel's scales and when we base our data on the MMPI Ho subscale? Is Potential for Hostility, as measured in the SI, pure hostility? It might be that the MMPI subscore and the Potential for Hostility measure are in some part concerned with a phenomenon that is something more than a hostile outlook. Both measures may, in part, focus on a response tendency that is closely associated with a conflict experience that may only in part be due to a hostile style or a hostile attitude.

10 It should be noted, however, that one Anger-In item produced an extreme bimodal response only from CAD victims.

References

Baer PE, Collins FH, Bourenoff GC, Ketchel MF (1979) Assessing personality factors in essential hypertension with a brief self-report instrument. Psychosom Med 16: 321-330
Barefoot JC, Dahlstrom WG, Williams RB (1983) Hostility, CHD incidence and total mortality: I. 25-year follow-up study of 255 physicians. Psychosom Med 45: 59-63
Baumann R, Ziprian H, Godicke W, Hartrodt W, Nauman E, Lauter J (1973) The influence of acute psychic stress situations on biochemical and vegetative parameters of essential hypertensives at the early state of the disease. Psychother Psychosom 22: 131-140
Berkowitz L (1962) Aggression: a social psychological analysis. McGraw-Hill, New York
Blumenthal JA, Williams RB, Kong Y, Schanberg SM, Thompson LW (1978) Type A behavior pattern and coronary atherosclerosis. Circulation 58: 634-639
Buss AJ (1961) The psychology of aggression. Wiley, New York
Cook WW, Medley DM (1954) Proposed hostility and pharisaic-virtue scales for the MMPI. J Appl Psychol 38: 414-418
Costa PT, Zonderman AB, McCrae RR, Williams RB (1985) Content and comprehensiveness in the MMPI: an item factor analysis in a normal adult sample. J Pers Soc Psychol 48: 925-933
Dembroski TM, MacDougall JM, Williams RB, Haney TL, Blumenthal JA (1985) Components of Type A, hostility, and anger-in: relationship to angiographic findings. Psychosom Med (to be published)
Diamond EL (1982) The role of anger and hostility in essential hypertension and coronary heart disease. Psychol Bull 92: 410-433
Durel LA, Krantz DS (1984) The possible effects of beta-adrenergic blocking drugs on behavioral and psychological concomitants of anger. In: Chesney MA, Goldston SE, Rosenman RH (eds) Anger and hostility in behavioral medicine. Hemisphere/McGraw-Hill, New York
Elliott R (1969) Tonic heart rate: Experiments on the effects of collative variables lead to hypothesis about its motivational significance. J Pers Soc Psychol 12: 211-228
Frankenhaeuser M (1980) Psychobiological aspects of life stress. Coping and health. Plenum, New York
Frankenhaeuser M (1982) The sympathetic-adrenal and pituitary-adrenal response to challenge: comparison between the sexes. In: Dembroski TM, Schmidt TH, Blumchen G (eds) Biobehavioral bases of coronary heart disease. Karger, Basel
Friedman M, St George S, Byers SO, Rosenman RH (1960) Excretion of catecholamines, 17-ketosteroids, 17-hydroxy-corticoids, and 5-hydroxyindole in men exhibiting a particular behavior pattern (A) associated with high incidence of clinical coronary artery disease. J Clin Invest 39: 758-764
Glass DC (1977) Behavior patterns, stress, and coronary disease. Erlbaum, Hillsdale
Glass DC, Contrada RJ (1982) Type A behavior and catecholamines: A critical review. In: Lake CR, Ziegler M (eds) Norepinephrine: clinical aspects. Williams and Wilkins, Baltimore
Goldstein IB (1981) Assessment of hypertension. In: Prokop CK, Bradley LA (eds) Medical psychology: contributions to behavioral medicine. Academic, New York
Gutmann MC, Benson H (1971) Interaction of environmental factors and systemic arterial blood pressure: a review. Medicine 50: 543-553
Harburg E, Blakelock EH, Roeper PJ (1979) Resentful and reflective coping with arbitrary authority and blood pressure: Detroit. Psychosom Med 41: 189-202
Harlan WR, Oberman A, Mitchell RE, Graybiel A (1967) Constitutional and environmental factors related to serum-lipid and lipoprotein levels. Ann Intern Med 66: 540-555
Harrell JP (1980) Psychological factors and hypertension: a status report. Psychol Bull 87: 482-501
Hokanson JE, Burgess M, Cohen MF (1963) Effects of displaced aggression on systolic blood pressure. J Abnorm Soc Psychol 67: 214-218
Jenkins CD (1978) A comparative review of the interview and questionnaire methods in the assessment of the coronary-prone behavior pattern. In: Dembroski TM, Weiss SM, Shields JL, Haynes SG, Feinleib M (eds) Coronary-prone behavior. Springer, Berlin Heidelberg New York
Jenkins CD, Zyzanski SJ, Rosenman RH (1971) Progress toward validation of a computer scored test for the Type A coronary prone behavior pattern. Psychosom Med 33: 193-202
Johnson JH, Butcher JN, Null C, Johnson KN (1984) A replicated item level factor analysis of the MMPI. J Pers Social Psychol 47: 105-114

Klaiber EL, Broverman DM, Haffajee CI, Hochman JS, Sacks GM, Dalen JE (1982) Serum-estrogen levels in men with acute myocardial infarction. Am J Med 73: 872-881
Light KC, Obrist PA (1980) Cardiovascular response to stress: Effects of opportunity to avoid, shock experience and performance feedback. Psychophysiology 17: 243-252
Lorimer AR, MacFarlane PW, Provan G, Duffy T, Lawrie TDV (1971) Blood pressure and catecholamine response to 'stress' in normotensive and hypertensive subjects. Cardiovasc Res 5: 169-173
Luria MH, Johnson MW, Pego R, Seuc CA, Manubens SJ, Wieland MR, Wieland RG (1982) Relationship between sex hormones, myocardial infarction, and occlusive coronary disease. Arch Intern Med 142: 42-44
Manuck SB, Polefrone JM (1984) Behavioral factors in hypertension: cardiovascular responsivity, anger, and social competence. In: Chesney MA, Goldston SE, Rosenman RH (eds) Anger and hostility in behavioral and cardiovascular disorders. Hemisphere/McGraw-Hill, New York
Matthews KA, Glass DC, Rosenman RH, Bortner RW (1977) Competitive drive, pattern A, and coronary heart disease: a further analysis of some data from the Western Collaborative Group Study. J Chronic Dis 30: 489-498
McKegney FP, Williams RB (1967) Psychological aspects of hypertension II: The differential influence of interview variables on blood pressure. Am J Psychiatry 123: 1539-1545
Nestel PJ (1969) Blood pressure and catecholamine excretion after mental stress in labile hypertension. Lancet 1: 692-694
Nixon PGF (1976) The human function curve. Practitioner 217: 765-771, 935-944
Nixon PBB, Bethel JN (1974) Preinfarction ill health. Am J Cardiol 33: 446-449
Obrist PA (1976) The cardiovascular-behavioral interaction - as it appears today. Psychophysiology 13: 95-107
Obrist PA (1981) Cardiovascular psychophysiology: a perspective. Plenum, New York
Ostfeld AM, Lebovits BZ, Shekelle RB, Paul O (1964) A prospective study of the relationship between personality and coronary heart disease. J Chronic Dis 17: 265-276
Ray JJ, Bozek R (1980) Dissecting the A-B personality type. Br J Med Psychol 53: 181-186
Rosenman RH (1978) The interview method of assessment of the coronary-prone behavior pattern. In: Dembroski TM, Weiss SM, Shields JL (eds) Coronary prone behavior. Springer, Berlin Heidelberg New York
Rosenman RH (1984) Health consequences of anger and implications for treatment. In: Chesney MA, Goldston SE, Rosenman RH (eds) Anger and hostility in behavioral and cardiovascular disorders. Hemisphere/McGraw-Hill, New York
Rosenman RH, Chesney MA (1982) Stress, Type A behavior and coronary disease. In: Goldberger L, Breznitz S (eds) The handbook of stress: theoretical and clinical aspects. MacMillan, New York
Rosenman RH, Friedman M, Straus R, Wurm M, Kositchek R, Hahn W, Werthessen NT (1964) A predictive study of coronary heart disease: the Western Collaborative Group Study. JAMA 189: 15-22
Schachter S, Singer JE (1962) Cognitive, social, and physiological determinants of emotional state. Psychol Rev 69: 379-399
Schroder HM, Streufert S (1963) The measurement of four systems of personality structure varying in level of abstractness: sentence completion method. ONR Technical Report 11, Princeton University
Schroder HM, Driver JM, Streufert S (1967) Human information processing. Holt, Rinehart and Winston, New York
Schwartz GE, Weinberger DA, Singer JA (1981) Cardiovascular differentiation of happiness, sadness, anger and fear following imagery and exercise. Psychosom Med 43: 343-364
Shapiro AP, Moutsos SE, Krifcher E (1963) Patterns of pressor responses to noxious stimuli in normal, hypertensive and diabetic subjects. J Clin Invest 42: 1890-1898
Shekelle RB, Gayle M, Ostfeld AM, Paul O (1983) Hostility, risk of coronary heart disease, and mortality. Psychosom Med 45: 109-114
Siegel JM (1984) The measurement of anger as a multidimensional construct. In: Chesney MA, Goldston SE, Rosenmann RH (eds) Anger and hostility in behavioral and cardiovascular disorders. Hemisphere/McGraw-Hill, New York
Spielberger CD, Jacobs G, Russel S, Crane R (1983) Assessment of anger: The state-trait anger

scale. In: Butcher JN, Spielberger CD (eds) Advances in Personality Assessment, vol 2. Hemisphere/McGraw-Hill, New York

Spielberger CD, Johnson EH, Russell SF, Crane RJ, Jacobs GA, Worden TJ (1984) The experience and expression of anger. In: Chesney MA, Goldston SE, Rosenman RH (eds) Anger and hostility in behavioral medicine. Hemisphere/McGraw-Hill, New York

Streufert S (1984) The dilemma of excellence: how strategic decision-making can kill you. Int Management 39: 36-40

Streufert S, Streufert SC (1978) Behavior in the complex environment. Winston, Washington DC (Wiley, New York)

Streufert S, Swezey R (1986) Complexity, Managers and Organizations. Academic, New York

Streufert S, Streufert SC, Dembroski TM, MacDougall JM (1979) Complexity, coronary prone behavior and physiological response. In: Osborne DJ, Gruneberg MM, Eiser JR (eds) Research in psychology and medicine, vol 1. Academic, London, pp 206-218

Streufert S, Streufert SC, Denson AL, Lewis J, Henderson R, Shields JL (1984) Differential effects of work related stressors on cardiovascular responsivity. Stress Anxiety 9: 191-203

Thailer SA, Friedman R, Harshfield GA, Kleinert HD, Pickering TG (1982) Analysis of behavioral interactions in blood pressure variability. Presented at meeting of the Association for Advancement of Behavior Therapy, Los Angeles, 19-21 November, 1982

Uzunova AD, Ramey ER, Ramwell PW (1978) Gonadal hormones and pathogenesis of occlusive arterial thrombosis. Am J Physiol 234: 454-459

Weiner H (1977) Psychobiology and human disease. Elsevier North Holland, New York

Williams RB (1975) Physiological mechanisms underlying the association between psychological factors and coronary disease. In: Gentry WD, Williams RB (eds) Psychological aspects of myocardial infarction and coronary care. Mosby, St Louis

Williams RB, Lane JD, Kuhn CM, Melosh W, White AD, Schanberg SM (1982) Type A behavior and elevated physiological and neuroendocrine responses to cognitive tasks. Science 218: 483-485

Williams RB, Barefoot JC, Shekelle RB (1984) The health consequences of hostility. In: Chesney MA, Goldston SE, Rosenman RH (eds) Anger, hostility and behavioral medicine. Hemisphere/McGraw-Hill, New York

Psychological Stress and Sudden Cardiac Death

R. A. De Silva[1]

The three clinically identifiable endpoints of coronary artery disease (CAD) are angina pectoris, myocardial infarction, and sudden cardiac death (SCD). Angina pectoris and myocardial infarction may both result in SCD; indeed, in over two-thirds of cases of CAD, this is the ultimate mode of death (American Heart Association 1984). In fully 25% of persons with CAD, the initial and only presentation of coronary disease is that of sudden death and 450000 deaths annually are attributed to this cause alone in the United States. It is not suprising that, until recently, attention had been focused almost exclusively on angina and myocardial infarction, since the swift onset of death and the brevity of the terminal event made medical interception for SCD difficult and largely futile. Sudden death was seen as the inexorable culmination of advanced coronary heart disease. In the last decade or so, however, advances in cardiopulmonary resuscitation, electrical defibrillation, pacemaker technology, and drug therapy have made it possible not only to reverse, but also to study in detail, a process which in centuries past had been uniformly fatal (Lown 1979; DeSilva et al. 1981; Cobb et al. 1975; Graboys et al. 1982). The observation that the victim of cardiac arrest can often be resuscitated suggests that the acute process is potentially reversible and that death is due to an "electrical accident" (Lown 1979; DeSilva et al. 1978). This realization has spurred new research into both the precipitating factors for SCD and its prevention.

Among the many risk factors studied, both acute and chronic forms of psychological stress have been proposed as precipitants of SCD. Acute emotional perturbations have long been associated with sudden death in the folklore of many cultures and in anecdotal observations in the medical literature. Based on clinical considerations, it is extremely unlikely that acute psychological stress is *solely* and *directly* responsible for sudden death in the absence of preexisting heart disease and other permissive factors. Clinical and experimental studies indicate that neural signalling between the brain and the heart plays a powerful role in modifying cardiac electrical properties, so that cardiac arrhythmias which predispose to sudden death occur. These studies support the view that acute psychological stress may be a putative risk factor for SCD. Since acute emotional perturbations do not occur in isolation, but rather in a life setting, the relevant clinical and epidemiologic backgrounds need to be explored for an understanding of the process whereby death occurs following exposure to acute psychological stress. The relevant clinical and psychosocial studies which reveal a connection between sudden death and presumed sources of psychological stress are reviewed here. For the purpose of this discussion, acute

1 Assistant Clinical Professor of Medicine, Harvard Medical School, Boston, Massachusetts 02115, USA; Section of Cardiology, Department of Medicine, New England Deaconess Hospital, Boston, Massachusetts 02215, USA

Biological and Psychological Factors
in Cardiovascular Disease
Ed. by T. H. Schmidt, T. M. Dembroski, and G. Blümchen

psychological stress is defined as a situation which results in an acute emotional perturbation and which may be associated with measurable cardiovascular changes.

Risk Factors for Sudden Cardiac Death

The established risk factors for angina and myocardial infarction include hypertension, hyperlipidemia, smoking, diabetes, and a number of other subsidiary factors. These risk factors do not differentiate between the victims of angina and myocardial infarction on the one hand and victims of SCD on the other. The lack of precision in differentiating between these subsets is not suprising, since the usual common substrate for angina, myocardial infarction, and SCD is CAD, and standard risk factors, when present, point to the development of this disease.

Several epidemiologic and clinical studies point to an additional risk factor which serves to distinguish a subset of patients with CAD who are at higher risk for SCD than others. This group of patients exhibits certain ventricular arrhythmias which are linked to the subsequent occurrence of SCD (Lown 1979). Ventricular arrhythmias, or ventricular premature beats (VPB), are virtually ubiquitous in an elderly population. In the concomitant presence of CAD, some characteristics of these arrhythmias reflect the presence of underlying *electrical instability* of the heart (Lown 1979; Cobb et al. 1975). Electrical instability of the ventricular myocardium is considered a prerequisite for the development of *ventricular fibrillation* (VF), which is the primary electrophysiologic derangement responsible for SCD. In two-thirds of cases, acute myocardial injury is absent (Cobb et al. 1975). VF is a chaotic, disorganized, and ineffectual contraction of the heart, which rapidly results in cardiovascular collapse and death if the heart is not promptly defibrillated. Clinical studies indicate that the arrhythmia usually responsible for SCD is VF, while sudden and complete cessation of heart action (asystole) is only a subsidiary mechanism. In epidemiologic studies on sudden death, it is implicitly assumed that death is due to a cardiac cause, since in the vast majority of victims, autopsy shows the presence of coronary heart disease. In this discussion, therefore, the terms *sudden death* and *sudden cardiac death* are used interchangeably; the primary arrhythmia, unless otherwise defined, is assumed to be VF. Sudden death is defined as unexpected, naturally occurring death occurring in a person with or without known heart disease within 24 h of developing symptoms. In cases where death is instantaneous, prodromal symptoms are absent. By clinical convention, sudden death is said to have occurred even when the victim is resuscitated and survives.

Psychosocial Risk Factors for Sudden Death

Acute psychological stress does not occur in isolation from other aspects of a person's life. Rather, such stress occurs in a psychosocial setting which is ongoing at the time of death. It is thus relevant to examine psychosocial factors which may have a bearing on SCD. A variety of epidemiologic studies attest to the correlation between sudden death and certain indices of presumed psychosocial distress. Of the many factors which may play a role, the contribution of educational level, social class, bereavement, life event changes, and certain behavioral factors will be examined in relation to SCD.

Educational Level and Social Class

Educational level and social class may be used as markers of the level of psychosocial distress, because they constitute an index of social and economic status and because they reflect success and accomplishment in contemporary society. Comstock (1971) showed that, among deaths in 189 men aged 45-64 years in Washington County, Maryland, those with 8 years or fewer of education had a greater than expected death rate from degenerative and atherosclerotic heart disease than men with more education. A history of smoking and lack of church attendance also correlated with mortality. Among 1829 Army veterans, Hrubec and Zukel (1971) found that physicians had the best long-term prognosis over an 18-year period following "first attacks of coronary heart disease." If physicians were excluded, professional men with college education had a better survival than other occupational or educational groups. A British study comparing 100 sudden deaths with 100 cases of nonfatal myocardial infarction found an association of the fatal events with a „lower social class", which may be assumed to have a lower level of education (Myers and Dewar 1975). A continously rising incidence of coronary heart disease as an inverse function of educational attainment was also demonstrated in the Framingham study (Dawber et al. 1959). In studying 122 men in Seattle who died suddenly, Bainton and Peterson (1963) found that fewer than expected deaths occurred in men with professional-managerial occupations than in men engaged in service trades. They concluded that lower education and lower median incomes were consistent with differences in occupational categories. In a prospective 5-year study, Hinkle et al. (1968) followed 270000 men in the Bell System throughout the continental U.S. They found that the number of new coronary events, including cardiac deaths, higher in men with no college education. Men who attained the highest level of management did not exhibit this higher risk, despite transfers to new companies or frequent promotions to new jobs. Hinkle et al. did not implicate education itself in explaining these differences in mortality between the groups of higher and lower levels of education. Rather, they related the onset of cardiac events to differences in social, economic, and possibly biological backgrounds which were, in part, linked to educational level.

The large demographic studies of Kitagawa and Hauser (1973) found a consistent inverse relationship in adults between cardiovascular mortality and educational attainment. The apparent effect of educational level on cardiovascular mortality was most evident in the age group 25-64 years and was greater in women than men. For example, among white men in this age group, mortality ratios scaled by educational level decreased from a high of 1.15 for men with less than 5 years of schooling to a low of 0.70 for men with 4 or more years of college, a differential of 64%. Similarly, comparable ratios for women were 1.60 vs. 0.78, a 105% differential. These workers demonstrated that education and income have distinctive and inverse associations with cardiovascular mortality.

The classic studies of Kitagawa and Hauser assume a special importance in view of the findings of the Health Insurance Plan of New York study (Weinblatt et al. 1971). The HIP study showed that blue collar workers had a higher cardiovascular mortality than white collar workers during a 6–47-month period after a clinically documented myocardial infarction. In 1978, the same group of investigators reported an association between educational level and the presence of complex forms of ventricular arrhythmia. Among 1739 men who survived myocardial infarction and were monitored electrocardiographically for 1 h, men with 8 or fewer years of schooling exhibited over three times the risk of SCD if complex ventricular arrhythmias were present (Weinblatt et al. 1971). In contrast, men who were better educated with the same grade of arrhythmias had a significantly lower risk for death. The cumulative mortality rates were 33% and 9% respectively for the two groups. This observed difference in mortality rates was not accounted for by either standard risk factors or a variety of clinical characteristics studied. This landmark study established for the first time a relationship between an epidemiologic variable, ventricular arrhythmia, and SCD.

Obviously, educational level is not the causal factor in the onset of premature death from coronary heart disease. Rather, education constitutes an index of success in society, as it is considered one of the most highly valued of social attainments. Lack of education may be handicapping and socially entrapping and constitute a source of stress in later life. A low educational level is associated with lower median imcome and differences in occupational category and contributes to job boredom (Bainton and Peterson 1963). Differences in biologic, social, and economic backgrounds may also influence the educational level a person may attain, so that the early development of cardiac disease and premature death may in fact relate to these factors.

Bereavement

The death of a close person, especially that of a spouse, ruptures a longstanding bond of great personal significance. Bereavement has been noted in several epidemiologic studies to have a powerful effect on subsequent mortality of the bereaved. Young et al. (1963) noted in a cohort of 4486 widowers 55 years or older that mortality rates were significantly higher than among nonwidowers. The increment in mortality for widowers was 40% over that for nonwidowers in the 6-month period following bereavement. Focusing on a semirural Welsh community of 5184 persons, Rees and Lutkins (1967) also arrived at a similar conclusion. They found that in the 1st year of bereavement, seven times as many bereaved relatives died as control subjects. Ten times as many recently widowed people died during the 1st year as in the control population. This finding was especially true among widowers, who had a mortality rate of 12.2% compared with 1.2% for a control group. Moreover, persons who died following bereavement were younger than the relatives who predeceased them, and they died at a younger age than was usual for their community. While these studies show a powerful effect of bereavement on mortality of the bereaved, neither of these studies shed light on the causes of death. Besides confirming the above findings in a study of 4486 widowers, Parkes et al. (1969) additionally examined causes of death. They found that deaths due to cardiovascular disease accounted for the only significant increase in mortality, and they suggested that the psychological impact of bereavement may have accounted for these cardiac deaths. In a careful case control study of 81 sudden death victims, Cottington et al. (1980) showed that, among the numerous life changes examined, the death of a close person was the only significant factor affecting mortality from CAD. These victims were six times as likely to have experienced the death of a close person within the preceding 6 months as controls. Other significant life events, such as financial, legal, family, or work-related problems, did not have the same impact on mortality.

Life Event Changes

Studies utilizing the method of weighting of life events described by Rahe et al. (1973; 1974) have demonstrated that the accumulation of various types of psychological stresses, such as marriage, separation, sexual difficulties, divorce, job loss, financial problems, violations of law, imprisonment, and bereavement, has an increased association with sudden death. A Schedule of Recent Events (SRE) containing 42 such events is used retrospectively to assess the magnitude of life changes by assigning an arbitrary but proportionally scaled numeric weight to each important event. The patient, or the spouse in cases of a deceased patient, provides the necessary information. A summation of such scores, expressed as Life Change Units (LCU), yields a total score which provides an estimate of the magnitude and the extent of important life changes in a defined period of time. Using the SRE, Rahe et al. (1973) studied 279 survivors of documented myocardial infarction and 226 cases of abrupt coronary death in Helsinki. Marked elevations in LCU were seen in the 6 months immediately prior to both myocardial infarction and sudden death. This elevation was particularly evident in sudden death victims, and women and men showed similar increases in LCU. Changes in LCU have been correlated with acute increases in urinary catecholamine excretion in subjects with coronary heart disease by Theorell and coworkers (1972). It is a tenable argument that heightened sympathetic adrenergic activity during stressful life changes may contribute to the onset of both myocardial infarction and SCD in susceptible individuals.

This approach to assessing important life changes, though innovative and conceptually important, suffers from some unavoidable deficiencies. In cases of SCD, the victim is unavailable to provide the crucial information, which has to be obtained from the spouse. Furthermore, antecedent, psychologically important events may be subconsciously weighted more heavily by both subjects and spouses if they appear to be linked to occurrences such as myocardial infarction or sudden death. Other intervening illnesses, which may be an independent source of stress, introduce a confounding variable. Furthermore, comparison of life events from chronologically different epochs separated by a year introduces error through problems of recall. These considerations may introduce a bias in favor of the impact of life changes on SCD. These objections are answered in part by two other studies which controlled for errors between reports by victims and spouses and for chronologic separation between the two 6-month periods during which LCU were measured. In comparing scores obtained from 20 men and their respective spouses, Theorell (1970) could find no significant differences in total LCU scores between the groups. Ulf (1975) studied monozygotic twins who were death discordant; i.e., one twin died during the study period. In comparing mean LCU scores, pairs of monozygotic twins showed significant differences between deceased and surviving partners, the former showing higher scores. This careful study also accounts for genetic differences that may alter predisposition to the development of CHD and SCD.

Retirement

Retirement is an important aspect of aging and represents an important life change. Though retirement may be viewed positively by some, it is likely that, for many people, it represents a loss of status, reduction in income, and decreased social usefulness. Such an important life change may have an important effect on longevity. Casscells et al. (1980) examined this hypothesis indirectly among men living in Florida in a study carefully matched for age, occupation, and several coronary risk factors. Among 568 men so matched, 76 of the test group had retired, while the corresponding controls had not; in contrast, in the case of 26 members of the control group who had retired, the corresponding member of the test group had not. The crude matched pair relative-risk ratio for retirement and fatal CHD was 2.9 (95% confidence limits; range, 1.9-4.9). After adjustment for age and history of previous hospitalization for myocardial infarction, the relative risk was 1.8 (95% confidence limits; range, 1.0-3.3). These data suggest that retirement increases the risk for coronary mortality by 80%.

Behavioral Factors

Certain behavioral and psychological factors have been associated with the onset of premature death and disease states. In a broad approach to this problem, Thomas (1976), who prospectively evaluated healthy medical students at Johns Hopkins University, found certain features, such as nervous tension, anxiety, anger under stress, insomnia, smoking, and alcohol intake to be associated with higher rates of premature death and onset of disease. These precursors were assessed with regard to the later occurrence of suicide, cancer, hypertension, myocardial infarction, and mental illness; no specific mention is made of sudden death as a separate end point. While such a comprehensive evaluation has not been made with regard to sudden death, other investigators have attempted to study the impact of certain specific emotional or behavioral factors in this connection.

Depression has been noted as a precedent to sudden death. Greene (1972) reported a high prevalence of depression and agitation prior to death when the next of kin of sudden death victims were interviewed. This study was small, rather empirical, and indirect, since direct assessment of psychological and behavioral characteristics was not possible, given the design of the study. A prospective study by Bruhn et al. (1974) of patients with myocardial infarction indicated that elevated depression scores, a pattern of "joyless striving at work", and type A behavior characteristics correlated with the occurrence of SCD. Bruhn et al. used a semistructured interview for identifying what they termed the "Sisyphus pattern," a structured interview for characterizing type A behavior and the Welsh pure depression subscale of the MMPI. A total of 35 of 67 patients and two of 67 controls died during the 10-year period of the study. The depression scale alone was not a powerful predictor of sudden death, but it appeared to add to the predictive strength of the interview data. It was the authors' conclusion that "joyless struggle" - which they labelled the "Sisyphus pattern" - and type A behavior were predictive of sudden death. (Sisyphus, a king of Corinth, was banished to Hades after being accused of a certain levity with regard to the gods. He was doomed to push a massive stone up the side of a mountain, whence the stone would roll back of its own weight. He had to toil ceaselessly without success as his punishment - hence the term "Sisyphean toil".)

Studies designed to characterize patients psychologically and behaviorally in order to predict victims of a particular disease process are conceptually attractive. However, as noted by Aiken (1972), such studies are extremely difficult to conduct and validate because of current methodological deficiencies in psychosomatic research, such as the accurate measurement of psychological variables, problems with controlling observations, fallacies in the deduction of causality, proper case identification, and sampling error.

Sudden Death During Acute Psychological Stress

The notion that death may occur during acute psychological stress is one which is found in both primitive and contemporary societies. It is an observation which spans centuries and finds expression in Greek and other mythologies, in Apocryphal stories, the Bible, and anecdotes in the lay literature. The foregoing discussion provides a background for discussing the occurrence of sudden death in psychologically stressful situations. In the studies cited, however, there is no clear indication whether death occurred under conditions of acute or ongoing psychological stresses and whether other concomitant factors played a provocative role. A number of observers have examined the roles of psychological stress and other relevant variables in contributing toward sudden death.

In an anecdotal, but now classic descriptive paper, Engel (1971) chronicled the circumstances of death in 170 individuals culled from press reports. Deaths where suicide was suspected were excluded, and in 16 instances, additional information was obtained from witnesses, attending physicians, and the medical examiner. Based on these reports, Engel created eight categories, listed below, which may be associated with sudden death:

1. Death or collapse of a close person
2. Acute grief
3. Threat of loss of a close person
4. Loss of status or self-esteem
5. Mourning or an anniversary
6. Personal danger or threat of injury
7. After a period of danger
8. Triumph or extreme joy

The 170 deaths usually occurred within 1 h after emotional arousal, when the victims were considered still to be reacting to the precipitating event. Engel speculated on the possible pathophysiologic processes which may be in play in such deaths. He suggested that either sympathetic or parasympathetic excitation may be responsible; the contribution of each will be discussed later.

Autopsy Studies

In a review of 100 men dying suddenly from coronary heart disease, Myers and Dewar (1975) found that 23 had experienced intense stress in the 30 min preceding death and that 40 had experienced such stresses within the preceding 24 h. These stresses varied from visits to a surgical clinic, an attack by dogs, fights over games, involvement in traffic accidents, notification of divorce, and so forth. Moderate physical activity, recent meals, especially with alcohol, and time of day or week were significantly related to mortality. Chronic psychological stress, strenous exercise, season of the year, and environmental temperature were unrelated to sudden death. Rissanen et al. (1978) interviewed the next of kin in evaluating the circumstances surrounding the sudden death of 118 victims. The prevalence of acute and chronic stresses, heaviness of the arms, dyspnea, fatigue, sweating, and nervousness was evaluated. "Acute" stress was noted in 19% of patients, "chronic" stress occurred in 25%, and unusual fatigue in 32% of cases. An important observation was that in 32 victims experiencing "acute" stress, death was rapid, resulting within 2 h; myocardial infarction was unusual in this group. Of the 32 victims, 14 died instantaneously. These observations suggest that acute psychological stress may have provoked rapid perturbations in electrical activity of the heart resulting in ventricular fibrillation (and sudden death) rather than the slower evolution of myocardial infarction. In contrast, victims with long-standing stresses had a longer duration of symptoms, and the evolution of acute myocardial infarction was more common than in the previous group.

Cebelin and Hirsch (1980) reviewed 497 deaths due to homicidal assault in Cuyahoga County, Ohio, and found 15 victims without unequivocal evidence for trauma as the cause of death. In all these cases, the victims had been assaulted by relatives, spouses, strangers, or others. Though there were some external injuries, there was no internal damage or blood loss to account for death. In ten cases, arguments or fights had preceded death, and in several cases the victim, sometimes a child, had been tied down or forcibly restrained. In 11 of the 15 deaths, microscopic studies showed myofibrillar degeneration of the heart, usually in the subendocardium. Such changes were absent from the heart of 15 victims of motor vehicle accidents used as controls. The authors concluded that the acute stress of the homicidal attack with threats and forcible restraint produced an acute stress-related cardiomyopathy with the subsequent development of VF and sudden death.

Clinical Studies

The studies cited above deal with the circumstances of death in deceased victims of sudden death. Clinical studies on the role of acute psychological stress in SCD are sparse. A number of investigators report the relationship of psychological stress and ventricular arrhythmias (Sigler 1961; Taggart et al. 1969; Orth-Gomer et al. 1980). The assumption here is that ventricular arrhythmias are a risk factor for developing SCD, but in none of these studies is long-term follow-up provided to indicate which of the subjects in fact suffered SCD. Other investigators have reported the occurrence of SCD in the midst of acute psychological stress while under observation (Jarvinen 1955; Lown et al. 1976). Lown et al. (1976) reported the detailed clinical, psychiatric, and psychological analysis of a man with normal coronary arteries who suffered repeated episodes of cardiac arrest in the setting of life crises presumed to relate to his personality, profession, and sexuality.

We utilized another approach in appraising the prevalence of acute psychological stresses prior to the onset of sudden death (Reich et al. 1981). Patients who were admitted to the clinical service at our hospital in Boston for treatment of serious ventricular arrhythmias were studied retrospectively for the occurrence of acute psychological stress prior to the provocation of their major arrhythmias. The 117 patients had had either VF or ventricular tachycardia (VT) that was not temporally related to acute myocardial infarction. Of these, 62 patients (53%) had been resuscitated by electrical defibrillation from VF following cardiac arrest, 13 (11%) had experienced VT with syncope, and 42 (36%) had suffered VT that was considered serious enough to require pharmacologic treatment for prevention of SCD. Clinical evaluation included Holter monitoring, echocardiography, exercise stress testing, and, where appropriate, coronary angiography, to establish the nature of underlying heart disease. The majority (65%) of patients had coronary heart disease (CHD), while the remainder had other types of heart disease or no demonstrable structural heart disease. Each patient was interviewed separately by a cardiologist and a psychiatrist. The interviews focused on the recent clinical history, life situations, and the sequence of events and psychological experiences of the 24 h preceding the life-threatening arrhythmia. Detailed information, where available, was also obtained from the spouse or others to corroborate or complete the sequence of events. In some instances, the major arrhythmic event occurred in hospital, while the patient was under electrocardiographic monitoring, and information was immediately available from the attending medical personnel. Only those disturbances identified by the patient and recognized by both of the interviewers as unusual and notable psychological experiences involving strong affective states were catalogued for analysis. In all cases, the actual arrhythmia, either VF or VT, was recorded and confirmed at the time of occurrence. Psychological tests were administered to each patient to detect abnormal personality traits or emotional states and for evidence of brain damage. These tests included the Minnesota Multiphasic Personality Inventory (MMPI), the Multiple Affect Adjective Check List (MAACL) and the Bender-Gestalt Visual Motor Retention Test.

Using the above methods, 25 (21%) of the 117 patients were identified who had experienced acute psychological experiences within the 24 h preceding their arrhythmic episode. In ten of these patients, episodes occurred in the hospital where the timing and details of the psychological disturbances could be readily documented. In the remaining 15, the details of the antecedent psychological experiences were reconstructed from historical material. Of the 25 patients, 18 had two or more arrhythmic episodes which were preceded by psychological perturbations; in several, the recurrence of the arrhythmia was associated with the recurrence of specific and meaningful situations in the patient's life. The other seven patients had single episodes of arrhythmia, six of which were cardiac arrest due to VF. The specific situations associated with the major arrhythmia and the accompanying affective states are summarized in Table 1.

Table 1. Major situations and affective states associated with VF or VT in 25 patients with psychological antecedents to arrhythmia

Situation	Affective state
Public humiliation	Anger
Threat of or actual marital separation	Acute anxiety, Fear
Bereavement	Acute depression
Business failure	Acute depression
Nightmares	Fear

VF, ventricular fibrillation; VT, ventricular tachycardia

Table 2. Prevalence of acute psychological stress preceding sudden death (Reprinted with permission from DeSilva 1982)

Investigators	Population sample	Time frame	Total cases (*n*)	Cases with APS (*n*)	Prevalence (%)
Myers and Dewar (1975)	postmortem	30 min-24 h	100	23 40	23 40
Rissanen et al. (1978)	postmortem	2 h	118	23	19
Reich et al. (1981)	clinical	24 h	117	25	21

APS, acute psychological stress

The predominant affective state associated with the psychological disturbances was anger; other leading states included acute anxiety, fear, and anticipatory excitement. In 15 (60%) of the 25 cases, the onset of VF or VT was less than 1 h from the onset of the psychological disturbance. In seven cases, the time lag was between 1 and 6 h duration and in the remaining three, the time lag between the onset of the disturbances and the arrhythmia was 12-24 h. Psychological testing failed to differentiate between patients with putative psychological triggers for arrhythmias when they were compared with matched controls who had similarly serious arrhythmias but no such triggers. Trends which were not statistically significant toward elevations in the hypochondriasis, hysteria, and depression scales of the MMPI and in the anxiety and depression scales of the MAACL were seen in the group of 25 patients with presumed psychophysiologically triggered arrhythmias when compared with the controls.

In this group of 117 patients, all of whom were alive at the time of study, 21% experienced acute states of emotional arousal prior to the precipitation of a life-threatening arrhythmia. This estimate lies within the range reported by Myers and Dewar (1975) and Rissanen et al. (1978). Myers and Dewar found that as many as 40% of sudden deaths occurred within 24 h after the occurrence of acute psychological stress. The estimate of Rissanen et al. is lower, with 19% of deaths occurring in the same time frame (Table 2).

It should be recognized that in none of the studies is causality proven; in each study, the proximity of the psychologically stressful event to sudden death was con-

Table 3. Biobehavioral models used for the study of SCD (Reprinted with permission from DeSilva 1982)

Investigators	Year	Biological model	Proposed mechanism of death
Cannon	1957	"voodoo death"	sympathoadrenal activation
Richter	1957	swimming rats	vagally mediated asystole
Raab	1966	stress in rats	catecholamine release and myofibrillar damage
Wolf	1967	"dive reflex" in man	vagally induced asystole
Lown et al.	1973	stress in dogs	transient risk factors for VF
Haft	1979	stress in rats	platelet microthrombi and myocardial necrosis
Corley et al.	1975	stress in monkeys	asystole from myocardial degeneration
Johansson et al.	1974	stress in pigs	myocardial necrosis and ventricular arrhythmias
Skinner et al.	1975	stress in pigs	sympathetic activation and VF
Lown and DeSilva	1978	potential or resuscitated SCD victims	sympathetic arousal and ventricular arrhythmias
Cebelin and Hirsch	1980	autopsy cases	stress-induced myocardial necrosis
Reich et al.	1981	potential or resuscitated SCD victims	sympathetic arousal and ventricular arrhythmias

sidered to be the principal contributory factor to the occurrence of death. Additionally, in the study of Reich et al. (1981), recurrence of serious ventricular arrhythmias within the same or similar emotional settings suggested that a linkage existed between the psychological state of the individual and the cardiac event. The psychophysiologic basis for this linkage will be discussed later.

Biobehavioral Models for Sudden Cardiac Death

Animal and Human Models

The unexpectedness of death in an individual who is usually presumed to be healthy, the brevity of the terminal event, and the almost certain outcome do not easily allow the systematic study of the problem of sudden death. The study of the contribution of biobehavioral factors to the genesis of SCD is even more difficult. Nonetheless, certain animal and clinical models have been developed to probe the association between psychological factors and SCD. These studies are summarized in Table 3.

Cannon, who did not actually study the victims, used "voodoo death" as a prototype for a theoretical discussion of the role of psychological factors in the provocation of sudden death (Cannon 1957). He postulated that the casting of a curse, tribal castigation, and superstitious beliefs and fears relating to the occult resulted in a sympathoadrenal response in susceptible individuals. In turn, this response presumably sets off fluid shifts and osmotic changes in the body, producing a shock-like state eventually leading to death. While he noted that such persons manifested a rapid, thready pulse terminally, he did not implicate a cardiac cause directly. It would be a theoretical assumption to state that such persons may have had a cardiac arrhythmia, such as VT, preceding death.

Other investigators have used a variety of animal and human models to study the manner in which psychological stress affects the electrical integrity of the heart (Richter 1957; Raab 1966; Wolf 1967; Johansson et al. 1974; Corley et al. 1975; Skinner et al. 1975; Lown and DeSilva 1978; Haft 1979; Lown et al. 1973). These models employ rats, dogs, pigs, and man to determine biochemical changes, structural effects on heart muscle, and rhythmic alterations leading to ventricular arrhythmias and sudden death during the induction of acute psychological stress. Several of these studies have been described above. Those studies which shed light on the mechanisms of SCD during psychological stress are discussed below.

Pathophysiologic Mechanisms for SCD

Vagal Mechanisms

In the studies cited above, two cardiac arrhythmic mechanisms are implicated in the onset of death, viz., *asystole* (complete cessation of all electrical and mechanical activity of the heart) and *VF* (disorganized electrical and mechanical activity of the heart). Though both pathophysiologic mechanisms result in the ineffective ejection of blood from the heart and eventual death if left uncorrected, it is important to discuss the relative importance of each of these mechanisms in relation to acute psychological stress.

Much of the psychological literature has concentrated on asystole as the mechanism of SCD. In large part, this perception is due to studies conducted in animals where vagal responses are relatively easily evoked by acute, psychologically stressful situations (Hughes and Lynch 1978). Albutt, in 1915, proposed that cardiac death in man was due to reflex vagal inhibition of the heart. Richter's experimental investigations in rats greatly influenced thinking in that direction. Those rats made to swim in water tanks died from bradycardia and asystole, rather than from drowning (Richter 1957). Removal of whiskers accelerated the onset of death, presumably due to loss of normal orientation. Richter equated the experience of drowning in this situation to the human experience of "helplessness." In Richter's view, "voodoo" death in primitive societies possibly results from severe, vagally mediated cardiac slowing. This hypothesis was further promoted by Wolf (1967), who suggested that vagal slowing of the heart is part of a complex pattern of reactions related to the "dive reflex" found in seals, whales, and raptorial birds. In man, this is an atavistic reflex recalling an ancient phylogeny and is elicited by facial exposure to a cold stimulus. In Wolf's view, certain emotional responses are capable of evoking this response, thereby causing vagally mediated cardiac slowing and cessation of heart action or permitting the emergence of ventribular arrhythmias. Though short periods of asystole, heart block, and ventricular arrhythmias may occur during diving or upon facial exposure to a cold stimulus, a review of the literature on this subject fails to disclose deaths attributable to this reflex. Our own investigations of the "dive reflex" conducted on patients with malignant arrhythmias or resuscitated from SCD have not supported this hypothesis (Lown and DeSilva 1978). Further, in these same patients, evocation of other vagal reflexes such as carotid sinus pressure and Valsalva's maneuver caused slowing of heart rate, but did not evoke significant arrhythmias.

Clinical experience indicates that vagally induced cessation of cardiac action is not a major mechanism of SCD in man (Lown 1979; DeSilva et al. 1978). MacWilliam (1923) had already noted half a century ago that, when normal sinus node activity is suppressed, escape pacemakers invariably take over to reestablish normal cardiac activity. It is true that anxiety may momentarily cause bradycardia or second- and third-degree heart block, but death from such events has not been documented with certainty. Rarely, vagal stimulation by direct pressure on the carotid bulb may induce cardiac standstill and death, but in this situation, death is due to cardiac conduction system disease and an inability of subsidiary pacemakers to sustain cardiac rhythm. Anxiety and psychological mechanisms do not play a role here. Following acute myocardial infarction, especially of the inferior wall, severe bradycardia and heart block may occasionally cause death with or without intervening ventricular arrhythmia. Massive anterior wall myocardial infarction may result in extensive damage to heart muscle and the cardiac conduction system, and death from asystole may result. Again, in these situations, the arrhythmia induced does not derive from psychological factors, but rather from reflex vagal activation and from myocardial damage.

Sympathetic Neural Mechanisms

The heart is richly innervated by both divisions of the autonomic nervous system. The linkage between the brain and the heart is perhaps most strikingly demonstrated by the series of abnormalities collectively referred to as the "long QT syndrome" (LQTS) (Jervell and Lange-Nielsen 1957; Romano et al. 1963; Schwartz 1976; Wellens et al. 1972). The QT interval of the electrocardiogram represents repolarization of the heart, and abnormalities during this phase are associated with increased electrical instability of the heart and an increased propensity for VF. The syndrome may be either congenital or acquired. In the congenital variety of LQTS, the heart is frequently normal structurally, with no evidence of either coronary artery disease or ventricular dysfunction. There is a marked proclivity for the emergence of VT or VF during emotional or physical stress. The mechanism of action is thought to be direct neural stimulation of the heart by cardiac sympathetic pathways via the stellate ganglia. Schwartz (1976) have postulated an imbalance in sympathetic neural input between the right and the left stellate ganglia which innervate different regions of the heart. Such an imbalance leads to a differential repolarization sequence in the heart, leading to an ongoing state of electrical instability. Sensory inputs such as loud noises may evoke life-threatening arrhythmias and lead to cardiac arrest. In one case report by Wellens et al. (1972), VF was initially provoked by a thunderclap. Subsequently, recurrent episodes could be provoked by an alarm clock, loud rock and roll music, and the noise of a falling bedpan, even during sleep. Cardiac catheterization failed to reveal any significant abnormalities and electrophysiologic studies showed normal results, with failure to provoke arhythmia. Treatment with propranolol prevented provocation of further episodes of VF by auditory stimuli. Since VF is frequently not sustained, spontaneous recovery following loss of consciousness often occurs in these patients. However, early demise is the rule if the patient is left untreated. Beta-adrenergic blockade, phenytoin, and bretylium have been used successfully to prolong life.

Coumel and coworkers (1978) described another syndrome in four children without organic heart disease in whom VT and syncope could be triggered by effort or emotion in the absence of LQTS. Electrical stimulation of the heart could not reproduce the arrhythmia, but infusion with the sympathetic agonist isoproteronol did so consistently. Treatment with beta-adrenergic antagonists alone or in combination with other drugs was successful in suppressing ventricular arrhythmia.

Studies in animals, reviewed extensively elsewhere, show that direct stimulation of the central nervous system using drugs and other chemical substances or electrical probes evokes a variety of ventricular arrhythmias, including VF (Levy 1913; Korteweg et al. 1957; DeSilva 1982). Stimulation or ablation of neural structures demonstrates that the efferent pathway arises in the midbrain and quadrigeminal bodies, traverses the reticular formation, and is finally channelled to the heart via the stellate ganglia and the cardiac sympathetic nerves. With a normal heart, it is difficult to provoke VF, even with potent nonphysiologic stimuli. In contrast, stimulation of the midbrain in dogs after the induction of myocardial ischemia results in a tenfold increase in the incidence of VF as compared with the control setting when ischemia alone is induced (Satinsky et al. 1971). This experiment demonstrates the powerful co-action between the CNS and the heart when the latter has been rendered electrophysiologically unstable by coronary occlusion.

Induction of heat, cold, and noise stress in rats (Haft 1979), psychological stress in monkeys (Corley et al. 1975), and electric shock in pigs (Johansson et al. 1974) leads to myocardial degeneration and sudden death. The cardiac arrhythmias leading to death have been defined in some studies. Corley et al. (1975), studying yoked monkeys, showed that electric shock led to the development of bradyarrhythmias and death through asystole. This arrhythmis probably resulted from cardiac muscle damage occurring during psychological stress. As originally shown by Raab (1966) prolonged psychological stress may result in myocardial damage and cardiac arrhythmias, presumably as a result of catecholamine release. The myocardial lesions consist of necrosis and subepicardial hemorrhage. These lesions resemble those seen in patients receiving prolonged infusions of catecholamines or in patients dying from pheochromocytoma, a catecholamine-secreting adrenal tumor. Haft (1979) noted intravascular aggregations of platelets in the coronary circulation with subepicardial areas of hemorrhage in rats subjected to noise and thermal stress. These effects may have been due to release of catecholamines engendered by the experimental condition. In conscious dogs, Liang et al. (1979) correlated marked increases in plasma epinephrine and norepinephrine in association with changes in ventricular electrical stability induced by acute psychological stress. Besides surges in catecholamines, it is likely that psychological stress releases substances such as thrombin, thromboxane, and adenosine diphosphate, which enhance platelet aggregation, alter the rheologic properties of blood, and change both coronary blood flow and the electrical properties of the heart.

A series of investigators have shown that coronary occlusion performed in animals placed in surroundings that are unfamiliar to them or otherwise stressful yields a high incidence of VF. For example, Skinner et al. (1975) showed that experimental coronary occlusion in pigs produced a marked increase in the occurrence of VF when the animals were placed in an environment that was unfamiliar to them, compared with an environment to which they had previously become acclimatized. In subsequent experiments utilizing cryoablation techniques, Skinner and Reed (1981) demonstrated that frontothalamic-brain stem tracts were involved in the response to psychological stress leading to the development of VF. Verrier and Lown (1984) who performed coronary occlusion in conscious dogs in a psychologically stressful setting, showed a severalfold increase in the incidence of VF as compared with a nonstressful environment. They further demonstrated that both increased sympathetic neural tone and withdrawal of vagal tone were important neural mechanisms in the process leading to the occurrence of VF.

That adrenergic mechanisms play a role in destabilizing the heart is also demonstrated indirectly by the observation that ventricular electrical stability is affected by treatment with beta-adrenergic agents such as propranolol and tolamolol (Matta et al. 1974; Rosenfeld et al. 1978). These agents are assumed to act by attachment to beta-adrenergic receptors, thus interdicting the effect of epinephrine and norepinephrine on these receptors. For example, Matta et al. (1974) showed that, during acute psychological stress in conscious dogs provoked by the Sidman shock avoidance procedure, tolamolol could ablate the changes in threshold for repetitive firing in the heart, thereby stabilizing the heart electrically. Rosenfeld et al. (1978) also demonstrated a beneficial result on ventricular arrhythmias in conscious dogs undergoing coronary occlusion when tolamolol was used. In humans, the beneficial results of beta-adrenergic blockers during psychological stress was shown by Taggart and coworkers (1969), who demonstrated that ventricular arrhythmias provoked by psychological stress during public speaking may be reduced or prevented by a dose of oxyprenolol prior to reexposure to such stress. When this protective effect of beta-adrenergic agents extends to the prevention of VF in man remains to be determined.

Although these studies indicate an important role for adrenergic mechanisms in the emergence of VT and VF, it should not be assumed that these are the exclusive conduits for the destabilizing effects of the CNS on the heart. Additional neural and humoral interactions may exist which have yet to be elucidated. Neural mechanisms, in particular in the provocation of VF, have been inadequately studied in man. We examined the possible role of sympathetic stimulation in a small group of patients with ventricular arrhythmias, some of whom were resuscitated from SCD. We were able to increase both heart rate and VPB frequency by psychological stress testing. In this same group of patients, evocation of autonomic vagal and sympathetic reflexes was also performed. High grades of arrhythmia could not be provoked by sympathetic activation such as head-up tilt, hyperventilation, breath holding, or the overshoot phase of Valsalva's maneuver. Evocation of the "dive reflex," which is a combined sympathetic and vagal reflex, did not avoke arrhythmia, save in one patient who also became agitated during application of the cold stimulus to the face. From these observations, it appears that passive evocation of autonomic reflexes alone is not a sufficient trigger for the occurrence of life-threatening ventricular arrhythmias.

Electrophysiologic Mechanisms

As mentioned previously, the major mechanism of SCD is VF, with asystole accounting for a minority of cases. The hypothesis that psychological stress is a potent risk factor for sudden death from VF is best supported by animal investigations. Since these studies have been extensively reviewed elsewhere, only a summary will be provided (DeSilva 1982; DeSilva and Lown 1978; Verrier and Lown 1984).

Whether important changes in ventricular electrophysiologic changes occur in response to acute psychological stress is a relevant question. In the conscious animal, induction of VF would result in serious psychological and autonomic nervous system disruptions, rendering serial observations invalid as the animal would have to be resuscitated repeatedly. We devised an alternative to inducing VF in the conscious dog by utilizing a precursor to VF, designated the *repetitive extrasystole* (RE) threshold (Matta et al. 1976; DeSilva et al. 1979). Experimentally, electrical stability of the heart is measured by using a graded electrical impulse to induce VF via a cardiac pacing catheter. This electrophysiologic event is not sensed by the animal. As the RE threshold reliably tracks the VF threshold, rapid estimates of the latter can be obtained when the dog is studied in control and stressful environments. Rapid, sequential measurements of the propensity for fibrillation can be gauged in response to exposure to acute psychological stress induced by electrical shock conditioning. These studies were conducted by instrumenting the dogs with intracardiac pacing and intra-arterial pressure catheters. The animals were then conditioned for 3 successive days with electrical shocks while under restraint in a Pavlovian sling. Following these sessions, the animals were allowed to recover in a large, well-ventilated cage which functioned as the control environment. Various experimental interventions may be performed and the effect of such interventions measured by assessing the VF threshold. Following shock conditioning in a sling, mere exposure and restraint in this environment resulted in increases of up to 50% in vulnerability to VF as measured by the RE threshold method. When VF was electrically induced in the sling environment, the threshold was also markedly reduced, again indicating that acute psychological stress produces prodigious increases in susceptibility to this fatal arrhythmia (DeSilva et al. 1978a). There were also marked increases in heart rate, blood pressure, and surges in plasma catecholamine levels (Liang et al. 1979).

The above experiments were conducted in the nonischemic heart in the absence of myocardial disease. In the clinical setting, the heart is often afflicted by CAD even when the subject is asymptomatic. Such hearts may already be electrically unstable, and the addition of acute psychological stress may lead to the precipitous development of VF. It is not known why VF can be provoked in some hearts which appear to be grossly normal on clinical study or pathologic examination. One of the most potent factors in the provocation of VF is the onset of myocardial ischemia or infarction. Not only is the threshold for VF reduced, but there is an accompanying increase in sympathetic neural tone which further lowers the threshold for VF. A third factor is the degree of pain and distress the person feels at the inception of an ischemic event. When myocardial ischemia or infarction is present, a relatively small increase in vulnerability for VF is sufficient to allow the heart to reach the threshold for this fatal arrhythmia. Though acute myocardial infarction is absent in the majority of instances of SCD, the presence of transient ischemia in such cases cannot be discounted. Thus, in the diseased heart, the above factors may act in concert to precipitate the fatal event.

These experiments provide several insights into the psychophysiologic and electrophysiologic mechanisms which are engaged when a subject is exposed to acute psychological stress. Based on these considerations, DeSilva and Lown (1978) and Lown et al. (1980) have proposed the existence of *transient risk factors* which originate in the CNS and impinge on electrically unstable myocardium and provoke VF. Such transient risk factors include the phasic activity of the sympathetic nervous system, as discussed. The following conclusions may thus be drawn:

1. Electrical instability of the heart is a prerequisite for the provocation of VF.
2. Acute psychological stress produces marked increases in vulnerability of VF in normal and ischemic myocardium.
3. In the ischemic heart (or in the heart otherwise predisposed to VF by disease), such stress may actually precipitate this fatal arrhythmia and cause sudden death.
4. In the normal heart, without evidence for preexisting myocardial instability, acute psychological stress does not ordinarily provoke VF and sudden death.

Clinical Presentations

The sudden collapse of a person following exposure to acute psychological stress is both dramatic and frightening. Though death may occur in the predisposed individual, it cannot always be assumed that sudden collapse presages a fatal condition. Palpitations, faintness, dizziness, and even syncope are not uncommonly associated with emotional or stressful situations. It is useful to segregate the types of cardiovascular reactions which may occur with acute psychological stress. In many cases, the person may become dizzy or actually faint and then recover completely. It is important to determine whether there is an underlying cardiac cause for this presentation in order to stratify the victim for treatment according to risk.

Cardiovascular Responses to Acute Psychological Stress

The cardiovascular system may display a repertoire of responses to acute psychological stress (DeSilva 1984). There are essentially three groups of responses which may be associated with acute psychological stress, and these are summarized in Table 4. The usual cardiovascular response (Type I response) is sinus tachycardia with a sensation of palpitations, flushing, tremor, and sweating. There is generally no change or an elevation in blood pressure, but the subject may feel "faint" or light-headed. The clinical outcome is not serious, and complete recovery is the rule. Constant or continuing exposure to stressful situations may however produce a sustained state of sinus tachycardia and produce labile or sustained hypertension. This type of cardiovascular response does not result in loss of consciousness, and specific treatment is not necessary unless hypertension is present.

In other subjects, acute psychological stress causes a set of more unusual responses (Type II response). Though these cardiovascular responses are also self-limiting and rarely cause death, far more distinctive clinical and electrocardio-

Table 4. Cardiovascular responses to acute psychological stress (Reprinted with permission from DeSilva 1984)

Type of response	EKG rhythm	Somatic correlates	Clinical outcome
Type I (usual response)	sinus tachycardia (hypertension)	flushing, anxiety, tremor, sweating, rapid pulse	self-limited with recovery
Type II (unusual response)	(A) bradycardia (hypertension)	pallor, sweating, faintness, syncope	spontaneous recovery, may need medical intervention
	(B) atrial arrhythmias	palpitations, dizziness, fatigue, chest pain, syncope	spontaneous recovery, may need medical intervention
	(C) isolated VPB	palpitations, chest discomfort, syncope	self-limited or may require medical treatment
Type III (extreme response)	arrhythmias of sudden death (VF, asystole, electromechanical dissociation)	cardiac arrest	death if untreated

graphic states can be identified, and the subject may require treatment. Three subsets may be identified in this category. The first response is one of bradycardia, hypotension, and even asystole. This response is manifest by many subhuman mammals and similar to that described by Richter (1957) and Engel (1978). The physiologic mechanism is referred to as *vasovagal syncope* if the subject actually faints. Fainting is often due to slowing of heart rate and a sudden decrease in blood pressure. Recovery is often spontaneous. The second subset Type II responses consists of the occurrence of atrial arrhythmias, including atrial premature beats, atrial fibrillation, atrial flutter, and supraventricular tachycardia. These arrhythmias are accompanied by palpitations, dizziness, chest pain, fatigue, and syncope, either singly or severally. As with the previous subset, medical treatment is not often required. In troublesome cases, drug treatment, counselling, and instruction in relaxation methods are of value. Reassurance that this condition will not cause sudden death is useful in preventing progression to a state of cardiac neurosis which may easily become established. The third subset of Type II responses is the occurrence of ventricular premature beats in association with acute psychological stress. The clinical behavior of this arrhythmia (if it is uncomplicated by VT or VF) is almost exactly the same as in the preceding subset. Again, treatment is often not necessary, and reassurance is adequate. In some cases, symptomatic palpitations may require treatment with antiarrhythmic drugs. However, careful clinical screening is necessary to exclude the possibility that the arrhythmia is not a progenitor of SCD.

The most serious or extreme outcome in association with acute psychological stress is a type III response. The arrhythmias which occur are those associated with SCD. These arrhythmias include VT, VF, asystole, and electromechanical dissociation. Current evidence, reviewed above, would indicate that VT and VF are the rhythm disturbances most often associated with acute psychological stress. Sustained asystole and electromechanical dissociation (where electrical activity of the heart is maintained, but there is no mechanical activity) are not commonly associated with acute psychological stress, but rather with organic heart conditions. These rhythm disturbances are serious and life-threatening and cause sudden death if untreated. Treatment consists of administering antiarrhythmic or cardiotonic drugs, defibrillation, or pacemaker insertion, as appropriate.

If the person dies following the acute episode, clearly, clinical studies other than an autopsy cannot be performed. Opportunities for repeated examination and laboratory evaluation do not exist in such cases. If a person survives the acute state, whether spontaneously or following cardiopulmonary resuscitation, certain clinical and psychological studies can be performed to assess risk for a fatal arrhythmia and whether a psychological trigger exists.

Cardiac Assessment of Risk for Sudden Death

Changes in cardiovascular functioning accompany emotional behavior. A complete analysis of cardiovascular responses to both physical and emotional stress is therefore necessary to profile the individual's proclivity for sudden death. A complex array of cardiovascular studies is available for assessing heart disease and its correlates. Application of these methods requires a judicious, selective, and systematic approach. The clinical methods for analyzing the subject with rhythm alterations in relation to acute psychological stress has been discussed in detail elsewhere, and a summary will be provided (DeSilva 1984). Since acute psychological stress may evoke various cardiovascular responses ranging from faintness, dizziness, syncope, to cardiac arrest, it is necessary to distinguish between these clinical presentations. For example, an acute response to a psychologically stressful situation may present as syncope. Such an episode of syncope may merely be due to sinus bradycardia accompanied by hypotension (vasodepressor syncope), or it may be a more serious and life-threatening presentation such as ventricular tachycardia or nonsustained VF. The treatment for each of these presentations is different. The clinical studies performed on a patient undergoing an event such as dizziness, syncope, or cardiac arrest should answer the following questions:

1. Was the episode due to a cardiovascular or a central nervous system cause?
2. What was the type of arrhythmia?
3. Was the arrhythmia provoked by psychological stress?

Noninvasive Testing

The objective of cardiac testing is to uncover rhythm alterations which will disclose the arrhythmia causing cardiovascular collapse. When a person collapses, the nature of the rhythm disturbance may be uncovered at the time of revival if electrocardiographic monitoring is undertaken immediately. Such monitoring will determine whether the diagnosis is sinus bradycardia, asystole, ventricular tachycardia, or VF.

If, however, the person has already recovered spontaneously, it becomes necessary to establish by further testing the cardiac rhythm responsible for recurrent episodes of dizziness, faintness, or syncope. Though recurrent episodes of fainting are not very likely to be due to ventricular tachycardia or VF the very first episode must be taken seriously, as the symptoms may well presage a future episode of VF in some cases. Thus, further cardiac testing needs to be performed to disclose the rhythm disturbance which occurs in conjunction with episodes of loss of consciousness.

The standard methods for assessing the patient who has suffered loss of consciousness include ambulatory electrocardiographic (Holter) monitoring and exercise stress testing. These methods will disclose the arrhythmia allegedly causing the symptoms associated with acute psychological stress. Holter monitoring is accomplished with a compact cassette tape recorder equipped with a timing track. The monitor is attached to the chest via electrodes and the subject keeps a time log of important events. During playback of the tape, correlations can be made between recorded arrhythmias and physically and emotionally stressful events. Dimsdale and Moss (1980) have added the sampling of blood by a timed withdrawal method for the assay of catecholamines in order to correlate observed arrhythmias with elevations in epinephrine and norepinephrine. They have demonstrated that the stress of events like public speaking produces marked increases in these vasoactive amines.

Exercise stress testing provides a further method of assessing the other circumstances under which the arrhythmia may occur. The exercise stress test itself is a somewhat fearful and psychologically stressful event for many subjects. In some cases, serious and life-threatening ventricular arrhythmias may be uncovered by exercise stress testing when they are not evident by Holter monitoring (Graboys et al. 1978).

Echocardiography will help determine the presence or absence of structural heart disease. This easily administered ultrasonic examination provides a simple noninvasive method of assessing the heart for the presence of previous scarring from a myocardial infarction, cardiac muscle disease, or valvular heart disease. All of these conditions may be associated with both atrial and ventricular arrhythmias. Radionuclide assessment of cardiac function has gained favor for the assessment of the pumping function of the heart. This method has applications in biobehavioral research, since the pumping action of the heart is modified by the level of prevailing sympathetic tone.

Invasive Testing

Invasive evaluation of patients with unexplained syncopal episodes or cardiac arrest include cardiac catheterization, coronary angiography, and electrophysiologic testing of the heart. Cardiac catheterization and coronary angiography serve to identify the presence or absence of structural heart disease such as coronary artery disease, mitral valve prolapse, and cardiomyopathy, all of which may be associated with serious ventricular arrhytmias. Electrophysiologic studies are performed by placing a catheter in either the atrial or the ventricular chambers and stimulating the heart electrically in an attempt to reproduce the arrhythmia. Such a study serves to establish whether a specific arrhythmia is the cause of the episode of syncope. If the patient has a known ventricular arrhythmia, proclivity for cardiac arrest from VF can also be determined. Electrophysiologic studies are becoming increasingly important in the assessment of survivors of cardiac arrest and in gauging the efficacy of drug treatment. Experimentally, this method is used in both anesthesized and conscious dogs to study the effects of neural stimulation, ablation of neural structures, drugs, and psychological stress on the electrical properties of the heart. Frequently, however, invasive studies are not necessary to establish the nature of heart disease or the type of arrhythmia, as these can be determined by a careful history, a thorough physical examination and noninvasive studies.

By establishing the nature of the cardiovascular mechanism responsible for the clinical presentation and by correlating the event with an psychologically stressful event, it is possible to determine whether there is a link between the emotional state of the subject and the cardiac event. It is also possible, by performing the above testing, to establish a more complete picture of the underlying state of health of the heart. A therapeutic approach including both behavioral and medical components can thus be fashioned.

Psychological Stress Testing

It would seem logical that, if an arrhythmia occurs during psychological stress, attempts should be made to reproduce the rhythm disturbance in the laboratory by psychological stress testing. Although there is frequent documentation of spontaneously occurring arrhythmia during psychological stress, attempts to reproduce arrhythmia during induced stress has met with variable success. Schiffer et al. (1976) used a quiz under time pressure in men with coronary heart disease to determine the cardiac effects. Continuous electrocardiographic monitoring was performed. Though heart rate and ST segment changes were noted, provocation of arrhythmia was not reported. Taylor et al. (1982) performed a similar quiz during exercise stress testing in postmyocardial infarction patients in an attempt to disclose abnormalities not evident with physical stress alone. No significant differences in maximal heart rate, systolic blood pressure, or in the prevalence of ST segment change were noted for patients or for controls. Evidently, no significant arrhythmia was provoked in these patients. Donlon et al. (1979) tested the effect on heart rhythm and blood pressure of an hour-long interview by a psychiatrist and a cardiologist. The interview was filmed, and the subject's global reaction (expressive movements, content, and emotional response) was scored separately by the two observers. The frequency of VPB was also scored and a correlation made between relaxed, stressful, and very stressful periods, as judged by the ratings. Significant differences between frequency of arrhythmia and periods of relaxation and stress were found. The test was conducted on only one patient who had indicated, several weeks after an acute myocardial infarction, that emotional factors had been involved in the genesis of his heart attack.

In an initial attempt to determine whether psychological stress played a role in provocation of arrhythmia, we used a three-part test to screen 19 patients with known arrhythmias documented by Holter monitoring and exercise stress testing (Lown and DeSilva 1978). The test consisted of mental arithmetic and reading from Stroop color cards for 5 min each and a 10-min discussion of important life situations such as illness, finances, and marriage. A control period of electrocardiographic monitoring was recorded with the patient reading quietly. Electrocardiographic monitoring was continued during the stress test, and the control and test periods were scored for heart rate and ventricular arrhythmia frequency and grade. Statisti-

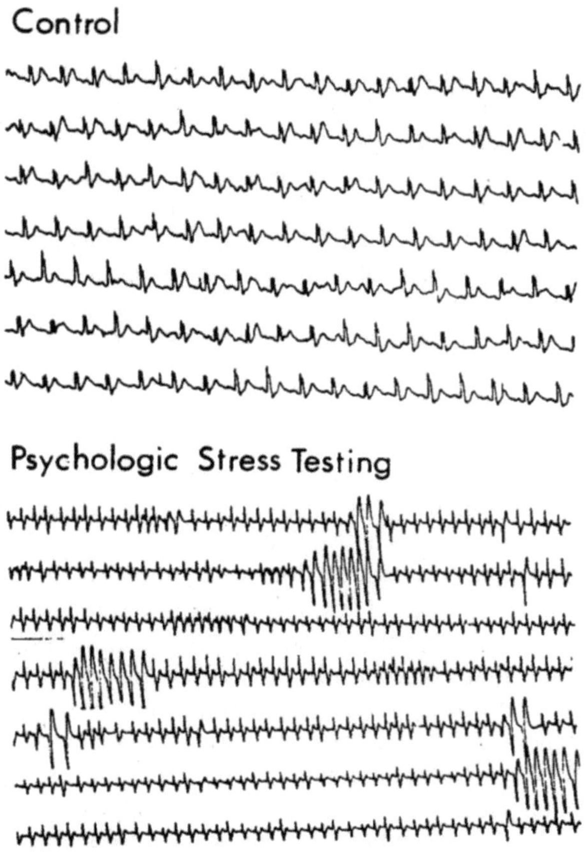

Fig. 1. Psychological stress testing in a man with previous myocardial infarction and recurrent cardiac arrest. The control tracing *(upper panel)* shows normal sinus rhythm at 65 beats per min. During a discussion of his illness and possible death, he wept, and recurrent runs of supraventricular and ventricular tachycardia were recorded *(lower panel)*; heart rate is 92 beats per min. (Reproduced with permission from Lown and DeSilva 1978)

cally significant increases in both heart rate and arrhythmia frequency were noted. In one patient, serious runs of VT, which on previous occasions had degenerated to VF, were recorded (Fig. 1). Though group means for VPB frequency were significantly affected, no arrhythmia was provoked in several of the patients who had presented with cardiac arrest due to VF and who had collapsed while in the throes of acute psychological stress. The probable reason for this result is that the situation of the stress test does not realistically simulate the actual environmental and psychological circumstances under which cardiac arrest took place. Particular situations which are both uniquely meaningful to the individual and powerful enough to provoke a major cardiovascular event can hardly be reproduced effectively in the laboratory. Psychological stress testing, therefore, has certain difficult limitations and has thus not seen wider application.

Management of the Patient

Management of a patient who has succumbed to cardiac arrest and who has been successfully resuscitated is a complex problem which requires the attentive involvement of the cardiologist as well as other professionals, including the psychiatrist and the social worker (DeSilva and Dimsdale 1982). Treatment of such patients will, of course, follow clearly established lines and include antiarrhythmic drug prophylaxis against the recurrence of VF. In the foregoing discussion, two groups of patients with cardiac arrest were recognized, i.e., those with a psychophysiologic trigger and those without such a basis for cardiac arrest. Though this discussion focuses on resuscitated patients for whom there was a strong probability that the arrest was linked to a psychological event, clinical management of these two groups of patients is not very different. This is because any resuscitated person will have a residual fear of the recurrence of cardiac arrest. Furthermore, even if a specific psychophysiologic trigger cannot be identified preceding cardiac arrest, already existing or newly occurring stressful situations may act as a trigger for another episode of cardiac arrest. Psychosocial issues therefore become relevant in both groups of patients. Hence, attention to behavioral, psychological, and social issues must constitute part of the overall treatment plan.

A detailed clinical analysis of the events which ostensibly precipitated cardiac arrest should be made in order to provide insights into management of the problem. The intention of obtaining such a history is twofold: to be able to attend to the psychological situations in the patient's life which may need redress, and to avoid as far as possible recurrence of similar situations. In several of our patients who suffered serious and life-threatening arrhythmias, there was a pattern of recurrent situations such marital or job-related conflicts (Reich et al. 1981). Recognition of these situations is crucial to the management of these patients and to the prevention of life-threatening arrhythmias. It must be realized that these patients are not psychiatrically ill, but are enmeshed in common life situations which have evolved into a state of affairs causing extreme psychological distress. In these situations, counseling for the patient and the family should be included as part of the treatment plan. In only some cases have we found it necessary to recommend long-term therapy if the occurrence of arrhythmia is related to uncontrollable anger or rage reactions on the part of the patient or if there is a seemingly self-destructive behavioral pattern conductive to the emergence of arrhythmia. Although there are insufficient data to state decisively the nature of these behavioral patterns, our preliminary observations suggest that some high-energy individuals who engage in prolonged periods of excessive physical and emotional activity coupled with travel, sleep deprivation, hunger, and fatigue may succumb to VT or VF at the end of such activity. While the physiologic basis for this occurrence is unclear, some individuals may undergo a recurrence of arrhythmia if this scenario is repeated. Recognition of this pattern and directive counseling may be useful in preventing the next episode.

In patients who are at high risk for sudden cardiac death (i.e., who have had a myocardial infarction or who have serious ventricular arrhythmias in conjunction with heart disease), but who have not yet suffered cardiac arrest, it would seem a reasonable precaution to evaluate any major life event change., since such changes may be associated with the future occurrence of premature cardiac death. Thus, fol-

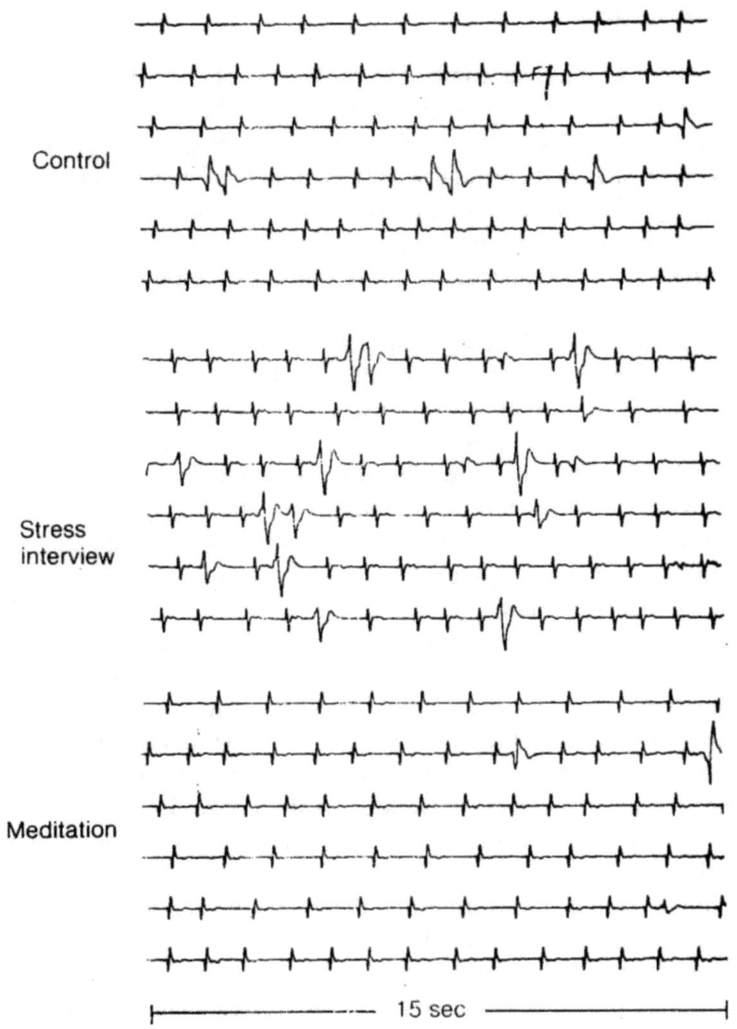

Fig. 2. Effect of stress interview and meditation on a man with recurrent cardiac arrest. During the control period *(upper panel)*, unifocal ventricular premature beats (VPB) and one couplet are seen. When he discussed domestic and job-related problems, the frequency of VPB and couplets increased *(middle panel)*. During a quiet period of meditation, a marked reduction in VPB and couplet frequency is seen *(lower panel)*. (Reproduced with permission from DeSilva and Lown 1978)

lowing marital disruption, bereavement, sudden loss of a job or retirement, attention needs to be paid to the psychological and physical impact of these events on such patients. Though precise tools for the objective measurement of the impact of such events on cardiovascular health are still lacking, our practice is to evaluate the patient clinically soon after the occurrence of a major psychological event with exercise stress testing and Holter monitoring to uncover the emergence of serious arrhythmias which may presage the occurrence of SCD. Such arrhythmia may require specific antiarrhythmic drug treatment as a prophylactic measure against SCD. Angina may also be exacerbated following serious psychological disruptions, and treatment with beta-adrenergic blocking and other agents may be necessary to protect the patient from both myocardial infarction and sudden death.

Anxiety is a frequent component of cardiac disease. Since acute psychological stress is associated with an increase in ventricular arrhythmia frequency, it is our practice to teach patients with such arrhythmias a relaxation procedure. This noncultic form of meditation consists of three phases: muscular relaxation, breathing, and repetition of a word such as "one" or "breathe." Benson et al. (1975) used this method to evaluate the effect on ventricular arrhythmia. Patients were instructed to perform the relaxation method for 20 min daily, and after 6 weeks, Holter monitoring was performed. When compared with the control period of monitoring, a reduction in ventricular arrhythmia frequency was noted. Since much of the reduction in arrhythmia was observed during sleep, it is likely that the observation was related to the suppression of arrhythmia during sleep. Voukidis and Forwand (1977) found that the results were very variable using a similar technique. In some patients, arrhythmia frequency during meditation was reduced, while in others it was unaffected or increased. Our preliminary observations suggested that in about one-half of patients studied, a noticeable reduction in VPB frequency occurred (R. A. DeSilva and B. Lown, Effect of a noncultic form of meditation on ventricular premature beat frequency, unpublished work). In three patients, bursts of VT were terminated. Taken as an aggregate group, however, a statistically significant reduction in VPB frequency did not occur. These observations suggest that spontaneous variability of arrhythmia may be affecting the results, so that it may be difficult to assess the effect of meditation on VPB frequency. In some patients, however, a consistent reduction in arrhythmia frequency is noted. In such cases, the method is recommended if the effect can be documented (Fig. 2). In most subjects, a subjective sensation of great relaxation is achieved, and this effect is useful as a coping mechanism during periods of acute emotional stress.

The precise mechanism whereby relaxation or meditation may affect heart rate, blood pressure, and arrhythmia frequency is unknown. Davidson et al. (1979) found that heart rate decreases were directly correlated with decreases in plasma norepinephrine levels during relaxation therapy. Whether the same mechanism obtains when a reduction in ventricular arrhythmia is observed requires investigation. Weiss and Engel (1971) and Pickering and Miller (1977) have shown that ventricular arrhythmias can be decreased with biofeedback techniques. The mechanism is probably related to overdrive suppression of the arrhythmia through an increase in heart rate. Because the procedure and instrumentation for teaching biofeedback is more complex than for a simple relaxation procedure, the latter is preferred.

Future Directions

In the above discussion, it is assumed that drug therapy is the primary approach to the management of patients deemed at high risk for sudden death or resuscitated from sudden death. Some new approaches focusing on interventions in the CNS have been proposed based on animal experimentation. These studies have focused on the role of adrenergic and serotonergic receptors in the brain and periphery. Increasing central stores of cathecholamines or serotonin by using their amino acid precursors, tyrosine and tryptophan, has been found to limit sympathetic outflow to the heart and peripheral vasculature. This effect results in increased electrical stability of the heart and protects against vulnerability to VF in the intact dog (Rabinowitz and Lown 1978; Scott et al. 1981). The dopamine agonist, bromocriptine, also has a similar protective effect (Falk et al. 1981). Other chemical substances which have a more complex effect on both the sympathetic and parasympathetic nervous systems, such as morphine, protect the heart electrically in anesthesized dogs and in animals undergoing psychological stress (DeSilva et al. 1978a, 1978b). Part of the protective effect of morphine on electrical stability is mediated by an increase on vagal tone, and hence, a withdrawal of sympathetic neural tone on the heart. Since morphine also affects the endorphin system in the brain, a more complex interaction may be involved with this drug. These experiments not only underscore the effects of neural and biochemical systems on electrical stability of the heart, but also suggest alternative approaches for therapy in the future. If a central neural trigger exists for provoking VF, therapy may be targeted towards intercepting the adverse effects of sympathetic discharge arising from the brain and impinging on the heart. The development of such centrally acting drugs for clinical use awaits further research.

Despite the lack of conclusive proof for causality, we cannot afford to ignore the evidence indicating that neural and psychological factors play a role in the provocation of sudden death. Each year, about 450000 people in the United States succumb to SCD, which alone constitutes the single most important cause of mortality. SCD is also the leading cause of mortality in Europe and the Soviet Union. Current estimates indicate that such deaths are preceded by acute psychological disturbances in 20%-40% of cases. Thus, analysis of risk factors for SCD must perforce include not only characterization of the nature and extent of heart disease, but also behavioral, psychophysiologic, and psychosocial attributes of the potential victim. Identification of the intermediary neurochemical mechanisms involved in precipitating sudden death may permit the introduction of innovative treatments aimed at interdicting neural traffic to the heart. Closer attention to the behavioral and psychological factors which may affect recurrence of cardiac arrest will provide a more comprehensive basis for the management of the resuscitated patient.

References

Aikin RCB (1972) Methodology of research in psychosomatic medicine. Br Med J 4: 285

Albutt C (1915) Diseases of the heart, including angina pectoris, vol 2. MacMillan, London

American Heart Association (1984) Heart facts. Dallas, Texas, p 2

Bainton CR, Peterson DR (1963) Deaths from coronary heart disease in persons fifty years and younger. N Engl J Med 268: 569

Benson H, Alexander S, Feldman CL (1975) Decreased ventricular premature beat contractions through the use of the relaxation response in patients with stable ischaemic heart disease. Lancet 2: 380

Bruhn JG, Paredes A, Adsett CA, Wolf S (1974) Psychological predictors of sudden death in myocardial infarction. J Psychosom Res 18: 187

Cannon WB (1957) "Voodoo" death. Psychosom Med 19: 182

Casscells SW, Hennekens CH, Evans D, Rosner B, DeSilva RA, Lown B, Davies JE, Jesse MJ (1980) Retirement and coronary mortality. Lancet 2: 1288
Cebelin MS, Hirsch CS (1980) Human stress cardiomyopathy. Hum Pathol 11: 123
Cobb LA, Baum RS, Alvarez HA III, Schaffer WA (1975) Resuscitation from out-of-hospital ventricular fibrillation: 4 years' follow-up. Circulation 51-52 [Suppl 3]: 223-228
Comstock GW (1971) Fatal arteriosclerotic heart disease, water hardness at home, and socioeconomic characteristics. Am J Epidemiol 94: 1
Corley KC, Mauck HP, Shiel FOM (1975) Cardiac responses associated with "yoked-chair" shock avoidance. Psychophysiology 12: 439
Cottington EM, Matthews KA, Talbott A, Kuller LH (1980) Environmental events preceding sudden death in women. Psychosom Med 42: 567
Coumel P, Fidelle J, Lucet V, Attuel P, Bouvrain Y (1978) Catecholamine induced severe ventricular arrhythmias with Adams-Stokes syndrome in children: report of four cases. Br Heart J 40 [Suppl]: 28
Davidson DM, Winchester MA, Taylor CB et al. (1979) Effects of relaxation therapy on cardiac performance and sympathetic activity in patients with organic heart disease. Psychosom Med 41: 303
Dawber TR, Kannel WB, Penkoskie N, Stokes J III, Kagan A, Gordon T (1959) Some factors associated with the development of coronary heart disease: six years' follow-up experience in the Framingham Study. Am J Publ Health 49: 1349
DeFaire U (1975) Life change patterns prior to death in ischemic heart disease: a study of death in discordant twins. J Psychosom Res 19: 273
DeSilva RA (1982) Central nervous system risk factors for sudden cardiac death. In: Greenberg HM, Dwyer EM (eds) Sudden coronary death. New York Academy of Sciences, New York, pp 143-160
DeSilva RA (1984) Electrocardiographic responses to behavioral stimuli. In: Herd JA, Gotto AM, Weiss SM (eds) Cardiovascular instrumentation: proceedings of the working conference on applicability of new technology to biobehavioral research. U.S. Dept. of Health and Human Services, National Institutes of Health Publication No. 84-1654, p 121
DeSilva RA, Dimsdale JE (1982) Biobehavioral issues in the assessment, continuing care and rehabilitation of patients at risk for life-threatening arrhythmias. In: Biobehavioral factors in sudden cardiac death. National Academy of Sciences Press, Washington, D.C., pp 97-107 (Institute of medicine interim report, no 3)
DeSilva RA, Lown B (1978) Ventricular premature beats, stress and sudden death. Psychosomatics 19: 649
DeSilva RA, Verrier RL, Lown B (1978a) Effects of psychological stress and vagal stimulation with morphone on vulnerability to ventricular fibrillation (VF) in the conscious dog. Am Heart J 34: 692
DeSilva RA, Verrier RL, Lown B (1978b) Protective effect of the vagotonic effect of morphine sulphate on vulnerability to ventricular fibrillation. Cardiovasc Res 12: 161
DeSilva RA, Verrier RL, Lown B (1979) Repetitive extrasystole threshold as an index of vulnerability to ventricular fibrillation during psychological stress. Clin Res 27: 562A
DeSilva RA, Hennekens CH, Lown B, Casscells SW (1981) Lignocaine prophylaxis in acute myocardial infarction: an evaluation of randomized trials. Lancet 2: 855
DeSilva RA, Graboys TB, Podrid PJ, Lown B (1980) Cardioversion and defibrillation. Am Heart J 100: 881
Dimsdale JE, Moss J (1980) Plasma catecholamines in stress and exercise. JAMA 243: 340
Donlon PT, Meadow A, Amsterdam EA (1979) Emotional stress as a factor in ventricular arrhythmias. Psychosomatics 20: 233
Engel GL (1971) Sudden and rapid death during psychological stress: folklore or folk wisdom? Ann Intern Med 74: 771
Engel GL (1978) Psychologic stress, Vasodepressor (vasovagal) syncope and sudden death. Ann Intern Med 89: 403
Falk RH, DeSilva RA, Lown B (1981) Reduction to vulnerability to ventricular fibrillation by bromocriptine, a dopamine agonist. Cardiovasc Res 15: 175
Graboys TB, DeSilva RA, Lown B (1978) Ambulatory monitoring and exercise stress testing in the management of patients with malignant arrhythmias. Am J Cardiol 41: 400

Graboys TB, Podrid PJ, Lown B, DeSilva RA (1982) Long-term survival of patients treated with antiarrhythmic drugs. Am J Cardiol 50: 437
Greene WA, Goldstein S, Moss AJ (1972) Psychosocial aspects of sudden death. Arch Intern Med 1129: 725
Haft JI (1979) Role of platelets in coronary artery disease. Am J Cardiol 43: 1197
Hinkle LE Jr, Whitney LH, Lehman EW, Dunn J, Benjamin B, King R, Plakun A (1968) Occupation, education and coronary heart disease. Science 161: 238
Hrubec Z, Zukel WJ (1971) Socioeconomic differentials in prognosis following episodes of coronary heart disease. J Chronic Dis 23: 881
Hughes CW, Lynch JJ (1978) A reconsideration of psychological precursors of sudden death in infrahuman animals. Am Psychol 33: 419
Jarvinen KAJ (1955) Can ward rounds be a danger to patients with acute myocardial infarction? Br Med J 1: 318
Jervell A, Lange-Nielsen F (1957) Congenital deaf-mutism, functional heart disease, with prolongation of the Q-T interval and sudden death. Am Heart J 54: 59
Johansson G, Johnsson N, Lannek N, Blomgren L, Lindberg P, Poupa O (1974) Severe stress cardiopathy in pigs. Am Heart J 87: 451
Kitagawa FM, Hauser PM (1973) Differential mortality in the United States: a study in socioeconomic epidemiology. Harvard University Press, Cambridge, pp 11-13, 78-79
Korteweg GCJ, Boeles JTF, Tencate J (1957) Influences of stimulation of some subcortical areas on the electrocardiogram. J Neurophysiol 20: 100
Levy AG (1913) The exciting causes of ventricular fibrillation in animals under chloroform anesthesia. Heart 4: 319
Liang B, Verrier RL, Lown B (1979) Correlation between circulating catecholamine levels and ventricular vulnerability during psychological stress in conscious dogs. Proc Soc Exp Med Biol 161: 166
Lown B (1979) Sudden cardiac death: The major challenge facing contemporary cardiology. Am J Cardiol 41: 313-328
Lown B, DeSilva RA (1978) Roles of psychologic stress and autonomic nervous system changes in provocation of ventribular premature complexes. Am J Cardiol 41: 979
Lown B, Temte JV, Reich P, Gaughan C, Regestein Q, Hai H (1976) Basis for recurring ventricular fibrillation in the absence of coronary artery disease and its management. N Engl J Med 294: 623
Lown B, DeSilva RA, Reich P, Murawski BJ (1980) Psychophysiologic factors in sudden cardiac death. Am J Psychiatry 137: 1325
Lown B, Corbalan R, Verrier RL (1973) Psychologic stress and threshold for repetitive ventricular response. Science 182: 834
Matta RJ, Lawler JE, Lown B (1974) Ventricular electrical stability in the conscious dog: effects of psychologic stress and beta-adrenergic blockade. Am J Cardiol 34: 692
Matta RJ, Verrier RL, Lown B (1976) The repetitive extrasystole threshold as an index of vulnerability to ventricular fibrillation. Am J Physiol 230: 1469
MacWilliam JA (1923) Ventricular fibrillation and sudden death. Br Med J 2: 215
Myers A, Dewar HA (1975) Circumstances attending 100 sudden deaths from coronary artery disease with coroners' necropsies. Br Heart J 37: 1133
Orth-Gomer K, Edwards ME, Erhardt L, Sjogren A, Theorell T (1980) Relation between ventricular arrhythmias and psychologic profile. Acta Med Scand 207: 31
Parkes CM, Benjamin B, Fitzgerald R (1969) Broken heart: statistical study of increased mortality among widowers. Br Med J 1: 740
Pickering TG, Miller NE (1977) Learned voluntary control of heart rate and rhythm in two subjects with premature ventricular contractions. Br Heart J 39: 152
Raab W (1966) Emotional and sensory factors in myocardial pathology. Am Heart J 72: 538
Rabinowitz SH, Lown B (1978) Central neurochemical factors related to serotonin metabolism and cardiac ventricular vulnerability for repetitive electrical activity. Am J Cardiol 41: 516
Rahe RH, Bennett L, Romo M, Siltanen P, Arthur RJ (1973) Subjects' recent life changes and coronary heart disease in Finland. Am J Psychiatry 130: 1222
Rahe RH, Romo M, Bennett L, Siltanen P (1974) Recent life changes, myocardial infarction and abrupt coronary death. Arch Intern Med 133: 221

Rees WD, Lutkins SG (1967) Mortality of bereavement. Br Med J 4: 13
Reich P, DeSilva RA, Lown B, Murawski BJ (1981) Acute psychological disturbances preceding life-threatening ventricular arrhythmias. JAMA 246: 233
Richter CP (1957) On the phenomenon of sudden death in animals and man. Psychosom Med 19: 91
Rissanen V, Romo M, Siltanen P (1978) Premonitory symptoms and stress factors preceding sudden death from ischemic heart disease. Acta Med Scand 204: 389
Romano G, Gemme G, Pongilione R (1963) Aritmie cardiache rare dell'età pediatrica: II. accesi sincopali per fibrillazione ventriculare parosistica (presentazione del primo caso della letterature pediatrica italiana). Clin Pediatr (Bologna) 45: 656
Rosenfeld J, Rosen MR, Hoffman BF (1978) Pharmacologic and behavioral effects of arrhythmias that immediately follow abrupt coronary occlusion: a canine model of sudden coronary death. Am J Cardiol 41: 1075
Satinsky J, Kosowsky B, Lown B (1971) Ventricular fibrillation induced by hypothalamic stimulation during coronary occlusion (abstract) Circulation [Suppl 2]: 60
Schiffer F, Hartley HH, Schulman CL, Abelmann WH (1976) The quiz electrocardiogram: a new diagnostic and research technique for evaluating the relation between emotional stress and ischemic heart disease. Am J Cardiol 37: 41
Schwartz PJ (1976) Cardiac sympathetic innervation and the sudden infant death syndrome. Am J Med 60: 167
Scott NA, DeSilva RA, Lown B, Wurtman RJ (1981) Tyrosine administration decreases vulnerability to ventricular fibrillation in the normal canine heart. Science 211: 727
Sigler LH (1961) Abnormalities in the electrocardiogram induced by emotional strain. Am J Cardiol 8: 807
Skinner JE, Lie JT, Entman ML (1975) Modification of ventricular fibrillation latency following coronary artery occlusion in the conscious pig: the effects of psychological stress and beta-adrenergic blockade. Circulation 51: 656
Skinner JE, Reed JC (1981) Blockade of frontocortical-brainstem pathway prevents ventricular fibrillation of ischemic heart. Am J Physiol 240: H156
Taggart P, Carruthurs M, Somerville WW (1969) Electrocardiogram, plasma catecholamines and lipids and their modification by oxprenolol when speaking before an audience. Lancet 2: 341
Taylor CB, Davidson DM, Houston N, Agras WS, DeBusk RF (1982) The effect of a standardized psychological stressor on the cardiovascular response to physical effort soon after myocardial infarction. J Psychosom Res 26: 263
Theorell T (1970) Psychosocial factors in relation to the onset of myocardial infarction and to some metabolic variables: a pilot study. Academic Thesis, Karolinska Institute, Sweden
Theorell T, Lind E, Froberg J, Karlsson C-G, Levi L (1972) A longitudinal study of 21 subjects with coronary heart disease: life changes, catecholamine excretion and related biochemical reactions. Psychosom Med 34: 505
Thomas CB (1976) Precursors of premature death and disease. Ann Intern Med 85: 653
Verrier RL, Lown B (1984) Behavioral stress and cardiac arrhythmias. Annu Rev Physiol 46: 155
Voukidis P, Forwand S (1977) The effect of elicitation of the relaxation response in patients with intractable ventricular arrhythmias. Circulation 55-56 [Suppl 3]: 157
Weinblatt E, Shapiro S, Frank CW (1971) Changes in personal characteristics of men over five years, following first diagnosis of coronary heart disease. Am J Public Health 61: 831
Weinblatt E, Ruberman W, Goldberg JD, Frank CW, Shapiro S, Chaudhury BS (1978) Relation of education to sudden death after myocardial infarction. N Engl J Med 299: 60
Weiss T, Engel BT (1971) Operant conditioning of the heart in patients with premature ventricular contractions. Psychosom Med 33: 301
Wellens HJJ, Vermuelen A, Durrer D (1972) Ventricular fibrillation occurring on arousal from sleep by auditory stimuli. Circulation 46: 661
Wolf S (1967) The bradycardia of the dive reflex: a possible mechanism of sudden death. Cond Reflex 2: 89
Young M, Benjamin B, Wallis C (1963) The mortality of widowers. Lancet 2: 454

II. Cardiovascular Psychophysiology

Behavioral Correlates of Cardiovascular Reactivity in School Children*

T. H. SCHMIDT[1,2], H. THIERSE[3], and J. ESCHWEILER[2]

Introduction

Biological and behavioral factors have been isolated in animal and human research that are associated with both enhanced cardiovascular reactivity and elevated cardiovascular risk. Evidence related to this subject has been compiled in several chapters of this book supporting the hypothesis that pronounced and repeated transient rises of blood pressure and heart rate might accelerate the development of arteriosclerosis (see Anderson et al., Manuck et al., Koolhaas et al., von Holst, Stöhr, Dembroski and MacDougall, Herd, Matthews and Rakaczky, and Obrist et al., this volume). Such cardiovascular reactions may lead to intimal lesions (Hirsch et al. 1984) that increase the permeability of the arterial wall, allowing the passage of low-density lipoprotein (LDL) and very low-density lipoprotein (VLDL) cholesterol into the subendothelial region, where it induces the proliferation of smooth muscle cells (Ross and Glomset 1976). These changes are thought to be the beginning of the atherosclerotic process, which may start early in life (Enos et al. 1955; Paffenbarger and Wing 1967; McNamara et al. 1971; Newman et al. 1986). Investigations of children which include the testing of their cardiovascular reactivity therefore appear to be of special interest. A number of psychophysiologic studies in adults indicate an association between behavioral characteristics which are typical of the type A behavior pattern (TABP) and enhanced cardiovascular responses during challenging circumstances that are relevant to type A characteristics, although there are notable exceptions (Matthews 1982, 1983; Myrtek 1983; Myrtek and Greenlee 1984, Krantz and Manuck 1984).

In children, it has been shown that the TABP can be observed reliably and that it is related to the same behavioral correlates seen in adult studies: When threatened with the possibility of failure, both type A children and type A adults try to exert active control (Glass 1977; Matthews 1979); while performing a strenuous task, both ignore fatigue (Carver et al. 1976; Matthews and Volkin 1981) and have high performance standards (Matthews and Siegel 1983; Suls et al. 1981). With regard to psychophysiologic aspects, only a few studies have investigated cardiovascular reactiv-

* We should like to thank the *Deutsche Forschungsgemeinschaft* for supporting this study.

1 Abteilung Epidemiologie und Sozialmedizin, Arbeitsgruppe Verhaltensmedizin, Medizinische Hochschule Hannover, Konstanty-Gutschow-Straße, 3000 Hannover 61, Federal Republic of Germany (Correspondence and requests should be addressed to the first author)

2 This work was done while authors were with the Psychosomatische Abteilung, Universitätskliniken, 5000 Köln 41, Federal Republic of Germany

3 Psychologisches Institut I, Lehrstuhl 2, Universität zu Köln, Meister-Ekkehart-Straße 9, 5000 Köln 41, Federal Republic of Germany

Biological and Psychological Factors
in Cardiovascular Disease
Ed. by T. H. Schmidt, T. M. Dembroski, and G. Blümchen

ity in type A and B children or adolescents. Although differing somewhat in results, these studies support the hypothesis that type A children exhibit enhanced cardiovascular responses during challenging circumstances (Lawler et al. 1981; Lundberg 1983; Matthews and Jennings 1984; Siegel et al. 1983).

In previous investigations, we have shown that pronounced type A behavior (type A1) is related to enhanced cardiovascular responses during the structured interview in a sample of 212 German policemen, supporting the intercultural validity of the hyperreactivity concept in type A adults to some extent (Schmidt 1983; Schmidt et al. 1985a, b). The study described in this chapter was designed to substantiate this hypothesis further with respect to German elementary school children. Our aim was to find answers to the following questions:

1. Can German teachers recognize components of TABP such as impatience, competitiveness, aggressiveness, and dominance with sufficient accuracy in children they know well?
2. Do children who are prone to such behavior also exhibit elevated cardiovascular reactions in competitive tasks?
3. Can persons who do not know the children but only observe them during these tasks also perceive similar differences in their behavior, and are components of type A behavior assessed in such a way also related to indices of increased cardiovascular reactivity during these tasks?
4. Is TABP related to better psychomotor performance?
5. Is psychomotor performance related to cardiovascular reactivity?

Methods

As there are no German instruments for assessing TABP in children, we translated the Matthews Youth Test for Health (MYTH) into German (see Appendix, Eschweiler 1986; Schmidt et al. 1985a). The MYTH is a 17-item questionnaire developed by Karen Matthews to assess TABP in children (Matthews and Angulo 1980); it measures elements of type A behavior such as competitive achievement-striving and impatience-aggression. The questionnaire is completed by teachers and others who know the children well. The teachers rate how characteristic each item or statement is of the child on a scale of 1 (extremely uncharacteristic) to 5 (extremely characteristic). Items 5, 11, and 13 are reverse coded, and all items are summed to yield an overall type A score. Possible total MYTH scores range from 17 (extreme type B) to 85 (extreme type A).

After a pretest, we revised the first German translation, added another item asking on a five-point scale for certainty of judgment, and distributed this German version of the MYTH to several schools and one kindergarten in the Cologne area. The teachers completed the questionnaire for every child in their respective classes. From 27 teachers (24 female and 3 male), we received 583 completed questionnaires concerning children aged 4–16 years. To determine the test-retest reliability, 395 children were evaluated according to the MYTH in two elementary schools a second time by the same teacher after an interval of 6 weeks–6 months. To determine inter-rater reliability, the behavioral characteristics of 126 children in six classes of these elementary schools were assessed by six pairs of teachers.

In order to investigate the relationship between MYTH scores and cardiovascular reactivity, we tested 94 children of both sexes aged 6–11 years in a psychophysiologic experiment conducted in both these elementary schools. These were selected from 459 children (244 girls and 215 boys) in 21 elementary school classes, grades 1–4, by means of their scores on the German version of the MYTH. In each class, we chose the two to four boys and girls with either the highest (type A) or the lowest score values (type B). These children were asked to participate in the psychophysiologic study; their parents were acquainted with the purpose of the study in a letter and signed an informed consent in which they agreed to allow their children to participate. About 95% of the parents agreed, and only one child did not want to participate. A total of 43 girls (22 type A and 21 type B) and 51 boys (25 type A and 26 type B) were then invited to play competitive video games (VG) and to test their eye-hand coordination in a multiple choice reaction time task (RTT).

The children were guided through the experiment by two investigators; these were: (a) a female experimenter (J. E.) taking part in all experiments, and (b) either the second (H. T.) or the principal investigator (T. S.); J. E. and one of the two male investigators were continually present in the room with the children when the experiment took place. The female experimenter collected each child from her/his classroom. After the child's weight, height, and the circumference of the upper nondominant arm had been measured, the male investigator explained the VG, the multiple choice RTT, and the whole procedure of the experiment. When the child had understood the details of the tasks and tried them out, a blood pressure (BP) cuff was applied to the nondominant arm, and some test measurements were carried out so that the child would understand the function of the BP apparatus. A cuff of either size 8 or 12 cm in width was chosen; the bigger size was used when the circumference of the upper arm was 20 cm or more. At rest periods, as well as during the tasks, BP and heart rate (HR) were determined at 1-min intervals with an automatic electronic BP device (Bosomat II-D, suitable for ergometric exercise), which was operated by the female experimenter.

At three rest periods (before the tasks, between the first and second task, and after the second task), each child was told that we then wanted to test how well she/he could relax. During the first rest period before the tasks, cardiovascular parameters were measured at minute intervals until BP values stopped declining (about 7–10 min). The last 5 min were used as a baseline. In the first task, the children were asked to play competitive VG to the best of their abilities against standards preset by a computer; for 6 min they played about 8–9 games (8.68 ± 1.49) of Interton Electronic, VC 4000, cassette 3, no. 47. The children were to return a video ball with a video racket via a joy stick placed in front of them, knocking out bars in a square field. Each knockout raised the score shown on the screen; in each game, they were allowed six balls. After each game, the children were praised by the male investigator for the score they achieved; they were also encouraged to aim for a higher score in the next game. The score values of each game were recorded. As some children from grade 1 school classes could not count up to more than 20, we used for all grade 1 children another VG (no. 41) with the same characteristics and rules, but during which only a lower score could be reached; all children could thus follow their scores. After the VG, the children were again asked to relax for a rest period of 5 min.

For the multiple choice RTT, which was performed during the following 6 min, the *Wiener Determinationsgerät* (manufactured by Schuhfried, Vienna, Austria) was used. The children were told that we wanted to test how fast and accurately they could react to optical and accoustic stimuli. The test started at a low speed during the 1st min. As soon as a colored light (red, blue, green, yellow, and white) lit up, the children had to press a button of the same color. The presentation rate of the stimuli was raised during the first 3 min from 20 to 30 and from 30 to 40 per minute; at the 4th min, an additional accoustic stimulus (high or low tone) was added. In the 5th min, the speed was increased again to 50 stimuli per minute; this rate was retained during the 6th and final minute. Correct, wrong, delayed, and omitted reactions were recorded. The RTT was followed by the third rest period of 5 min duration, after which we thanked the children for their participation and took them back to their classrooms.

Both the male and female experimenter observed the children's behavior during the experiment, and they scored independently the following behavioral variables on five-point rating scales:

1. *During rest periods:* physical rest, inner relaxation, exploratory behavior, contact seeking, speech activity[4]
2. *During the tasks:* tension, engagement, impatience, mimicry, speech activity, excessive demand, enjoyment, resignation
3. *At the end concerning the whole experiment:* quickness of comprehension, motoric restlessness, emotional excitement, ambition, cooperation, unfriendly-friendly, extraversion-introversion, TABP, contact to observer,[5] and global certainty of judgment for each child

From pretests, these variables seemed to us particularly striking and sufficiently easy to observe and score and to include important TABP components; in pretests, the observers practiced coding the behavior. The rate of agreement was determined by testing inter-rater reliability.

During rest periods and during both task situations, mean values for systolic (SBP) and diastolic blood pressure (DBP) and HR were calculated, together with maximal values during the VG and RTT. Mean and maximal reactions of these parameters during the tasks were determined by substracting the mean values of rest period 1 from the values during the task.

Statistical analyses were carried out in the computer center of the University of Cologne on a Control Data Cyber76 using the program systems SPSS and BMDP.

4 Although children were asked to relax and not to speak during rest periods or tasks, pretests showed that the children did not comply to this; therefore, we included this variable.

5 This variable was not introduced at the beginning of the psychophysiologic study, but was included later when it appeared to the observers to be an important behavioral characteristic of the children.

Results

The German Version of the MYTH

As shown by factor-analytic procedures (principal component analysis) the German version of the MYTH is composed of three factors (eigenvalues over 1) which account for 67.5% of the variance. Factor 1 comprises 70.4% of the explained variance, factor 2, 18.4%, and factor 3, 11.3%. According to the factor loadings (see Appendix), factor 1 is mainly composed of questions 3, 5, 6, 8, 11, 13, and 17, which ask about impatience, anger, and quarrelling; factor 2 mainly comprises questions 1, 2, 4, 9, 12, 14, and 16, which deal with an inclination toward competition and speeding things up; factor 3 is mainly composed of questions 7, 10, and 15, which investigate leadership qualities. Three subscales were formed by the sum of the questions corresponding to each of the three factors and designated according to the leading behavioral quality, i.e., impatience (factor 1), competitiveness (factor 2), and dominance (factor 3). All three subscales correlate highly with the total MYTH score and are not independent of each other, as can be seen in Table 1. This indicates that the subscales are influenced by one common factor. The internal consistency (Cronbach's alpha coefficient) of the MYTH score and the three subscales is considerably high.

Table 2a shows the test-retest reliability for an interval of 6 weeks-3 months for 211 children and for an interval of 3-6 months for 184 children, as well as for the entire group of 395 children for the whole interval of 6 weeks-6 months. The correlation coefficients indicate good stability for these scales, although the coefficients are usually somewhat higher for the shorter period of time.

During the first scoring, the teachers were significantly more certain about their assessments of the children's behavior than during the second (Table 2b); this was

Table 1. Intercorrelations of three subscales and MYTH score and internal consistency of these scales ($n=583$)

	Impatience	Competitiveness	Dominance	MYTH score
Impatience		0.58***	0.43***	0.86***
Competitiveness			0.61***	0.87***
Dominance				0.72***
Internal consistency (Cronbach's α coefficient)	0.91	0.88	0.85	0.93

Table 2a. Test-retest correlation coefficients of MYTH score and three subscales for different time intervals

	6 weeks-3 months	3-6 months	All
n	211	184	395
MYTH score	0.86***	0.78***	0.83***
Impatience	0.85***	0.77***	0.81***
Competitiveness	0.82***	0.74***	0.78***
Dominance	0.76***	0.79***	0.77***

Table 2b. Teachers' certainty of judgment in the MYTH during first and second test after 6 weeks–3 months or 3–6 months

	Mean rank				
	First test	Second test	*z*	*p*	*n*
6 weeks–3 months	46.83	43.05	-4.88	<0.001	211
3–6 months	41.25	31.40	-6.19	<0.001	184

Table 2c. Inter-rater reliability of the total MYTH score and the three subscales in six pairs of teachers

Pair of teachers	MYTH score	Impatience	Competitiveness	Dominance	*n*
1	0.86***	0.81***	0.70***	0.74***	23
2	0.79***	0.78***	0.73***	0.82***	20
3	0.67***	0.69***	0.46*	0.54**	20
4	0.66**	0.72***	0.78***	0.71***	18
5	0.63***	0.74***	0.45**	0.59***	29
6	0.45*	0.62**	0.41	0.69**	16
Pooled	0.62***	0.66***	0.44***	0.70***	126

*** $p<0.001$; ** $p<0.01$; * $p<0.05$

Table 3. Mean German MYTH scores (± standard deviation) for different age groups of boys and girls*

Age (years)	MYTH score		
	Boys *(n)*	Girls *(n)*	*p*
6–7	51.6 ± 11.6 (29)	47.8 ± 11.9 (56)	ns
8–9	52.3 ± 13.2 (119)	45.3 ± 11.6 (127)	0.001
10–11	53.9 ± 12.0 (86)	45.7 ± 12.3 (88)	0.001
>11	51.1 ± 11.6 (27)	43.8 ± 10.3 (25)	0.021
Total	52.6 ± 12.4 (261)	45.7 ± 11.7 (296)	0.001

* Children under the age of 6 years were not taken into account because of the small-sized group ($n=18$); another eight children could not be considered because of missing age data.

independent of whether the second scoring was carried out within a period of 3 or 6 months. This might have to do with the fact that the first scoring took place shortly before the end of the school year; the second scoring was thus made after the long summer vacation, so that the teachers had not seen their pupils for some time. Furthermore, some teachers had also taken over new classes.

The inter-rater reliability, both individually and pooled, of six different pairs of teachers in six school classes is shown in Table 2c. For the total MYTH score, the correlation coefficients range from $r=0.86$ to 0.45, and for the three subscales, from $r=0.82$ to 0.41. These differences in inter-rater agreement are due to the fact that some teachers knew the children better than others. Each class had only one teacher responsible for the children for at least 1 year, whereas some of the teachers who did the second ratings only taught the children for 1 or only a few hours per week. Therefore, these teachers were also significantly less certain in their scoring of the children's behavior ($z = -4.07$; $p < 0.001$). These results indicate that, although most teachers show good agreement, inter-rater reliability might depend on how well the teachers know the children. Pooled correlation coefficients between both ratings determined for the total number of 126 children in the six school classes range from $r = 0.70$ (dominance subscale) to 0.44 (competitiveness subscale).

As can be seen in Table 3, boys were scored significantly higher by their teachers on the MYTH than girls; this was also true for each separate age group with the exception of the youngest group of 6- to 7-year old children. For all questions except for questions 2 and 14, teachers assessed boys as being significantly more type A than girls (Eschweiler 1986). These results are in overall accordance with those described by Matthews (1980), but in her studies some other questions (5, 12, 16) did not differentiate between boys and girls. Older children showed more dominant behavior according to their teachers' ratings [dominance subscale (age): $F(3{,}556) = 2.62$; $p = 0.05$]; the other scales were not age dependent.

To summarize: The German version of the MYTH appears to be a reliable, stable, and internally consistent measure of type A behavior in children. In our study of German elementary school children, boys are regarded as being more impatient, aggressive, competitive, dominant, and more ambitious than girls, the children becoming more dominant with increasing age.

The Psychophysiologic Study

In Table 4a, mean values and standard deviations of the MYTH type A score, as well as of the subscales for impatience, competitiveness, and dominance, are shown for each subgroup of the 94 children selected for the psychophysiologic study. As expected, compared with type B children in the analysis of variance (ANOVA), type A children have significantly higher MYTH scores [$F(1{,}90) = 306.3$; $p < 0.001$], as well as higher values for the subscales impatience [$F(1{,}90) = 255.2$; $p < 0.001$], competitiveness [$F(1{,}90) = 182.2$; $p < 0.001$], and dominance [$F(1{,}90) = 72.9$; $p < 0.001$]. Moreover, compared with girls, boys had higher MYTH scores [$F(1{,}90) = 10.4$; $p = 0.0017$] and higher scores on the impatience subscale [$F(1{,}90) = 19.78$; $p < 0.001$]. No significant sex differences were seen for the subscales for competitiveness and dominance. Furthermore, there were no significant interactions between type A/B status and sex for any of these scales.

Physical Variables

The ANOVA results did not reveal any significant differences between sexes or behavior types for age, height, weight, circumference of the upper nondominant arm, or right- or left-handedness. The mean age for the whole group was 8.9 ± 1.1 years. When two age groups were formed (6–8 and 9–11 years), as expected, the older group showed higher measurements for height, weight, and circumference of the upper arm. There was also a weak interaction between sex and age concerning height [$F(1{,}86) = 3.4$; $p < 0.07$] and weight [$F(1{,}86) = 4.0$; $p < 0.05$], indicating that girls aged 9–11 are somewhat taller and heavier than boys in the same age group.

Table 4a. Mean values (±standard deviation) of MYTH score and of subscales impatience, competitiveness, and dominance for 25 type A boys, 22 type A girls, 26 type B boys, and 21 type B girls

Age	Type	Boys	Girls
MYTH score	A	67.88±7.91	62.09±7.13
	B	37.89±8.83	32.71±8.71
Subscale	A	28.72±3.85	24.05±4.25
Impatience	B	14.77±4.01	12.29±3.33
Subscale	A	28.04±4.47	26.96±3.39
Competitiveness	B	16.15±5.19	14.33±4.10
Subscale	A	11.12±2.30	11.09±2.31
Dominance	B	6.96±3.09	6.10±2.51

Table 4b. Mean (±standard deviation) height and weight for type A and B boys and girls in two age groups

		Height (cm)	
Age	Type	Boys *(n)*	Girls *(n)*
6–8 years	A	133.9±7.2 (10)	128.4± 3.4 (9)
	B	131.2±4.8 (6)	131.5± 5.1 (8)
9–11 years	A	140.1±5.8 (15)	142.4±10.0 (13)
	B	140.3±8.7 (20)	144.8± 8.9 (13)
		Weight (kg)	
6–8 years	A	29.6±3.6 (10)	26.6± 3.6 (9)
	B	28.3±1.9 (6)	27.8± 3.2 (8)
9–11 years	A	34.1±5.6 (15)	35.8± 8.5 (13)
	B	33.6±5.1 (20)	38.5± 8.1 (13)

Table 4b shows mean height and weight for type A and B boys and girls in both age groups.

Cardiovascular Parameters at Rest

During rest period 1 before the tasks, ANOVA shows no significant differences in SBP, DBP, and HR between behavior types and no significant differences in DBP and HR between the sexes. However, as can be seen in Table 5, compared with girls, boys exhibited higher SBP levels [$F\,(1{,}89)=5.03$; $p=0.027$]. Essentially the same results were found for rest periods 2 and 3, although SBP was slightly lower for these two rest periods. This effect was more enhanced with type B as compared with type A children [rest 2 – rest 1: $F\,(1{,}89)=8.29$; $p=0.005$; rest 3 – rest 1: $F\,(1{,}89)=3.67$; $p=0.059$], as well as with girls as compared with boys [rest 2 – rest 1: $F\,(1{,}89)=3.80$; $p=0.054$; rest 3 – rest 1: $F\,(1{,}89)=3.13$; $p=0.08$]. This indicates that after the tasks, both type A children and boys needed longer to calm down to comparable SBP values. Therefore, we used rest period 1 as a reference value to calcu-

Table 5. Mean values (±standard deviation) of SBP, DBP, and HR during the 5-min rest period 1 before the tasks for 25 type A boys and 22 type A girls, as well as for 26 type B boys and 21 type B girls, and mean differences *(Δ)* between rest periods 2 and 1 and between rest periods 3 and 1

Rest period 1	Type	Boys	Girls
SBP (mmHg)	A	102.2±11.7	94.9±10.4
	B	100.9±11.7	98.2±10.4
DBP (mmHg)	A	64.4± 8.8	66.7± 9.5
	B	66.7± 7.0	68.4± 7.3
HR (bpm)	A	89.1±13.7	90.6±12.2
	B	87.2±13.0	85.5±12.6
Rest 2 – rest 1			
Δ SBP (mmHg)	A	-0.3± 6.8	-2.0± 4.7
	B	-3.1± 6.5	-6.4± 5.4
Δ DBP (mmHg)	A	0.0± 5.1	0.3± 3.6
	B	-0.4± 3.6	0.3± 5.4
Δ HR (bpm)	A	-1.6± 5.1	-1.5± 5.2
	B	0.3± 5.0	-0.5± 6.9
Rest 3 – rest 1			
Δ SBP (mmHg)	A	-2.4± 6.0	-3.0± 5.1
	B	-3.2± 6.4	-7.1± 6.6
Δ DBP (mmHg)	A	-1.7± 5.3	-0.3± 4.7
	B	0.0± 5.5	-1.5± 4.0
Δ HR (mmHg)	A	-0.3± 5.9	-1.5± 6.4
	B	1.1± 6.7	1.0± 7.5

late cardiovascular reactions during both tasks. No such differences were seen between behavior types or between boys and girls for DBP or HR.

In order to determine the influence of factors such as age (years), sex (boys = 1; girls = 2), height (cm), weight (kg), weight index,[6] and type A/B status (type B = 1; type A = 2) as well as the subscales for impatience, competitiveness, and dominance, on cardiovascular parameters at rest, stepwise multiple regression analyses[7] were carried out (Table 6). For SBP at rest, weight and sex were main predictors, both together explaining about 28% of the variance; for DBP, weight alone explained more than 25% of the variance, but none of the above factors predicted HR at rest.

6 Log_{10} (weight/height^3); this index appeared to be an important factor for children's SBP in the Bogalusa Heart Study (Voors et al. 1976).

7 The lowest *F* value for a variable to enter multiple regression analyses was limited to 3.8, as this is the lower limit for significant *F* values with 1 *df* in the numerator. By this procedure, only those factors are considered which contribute essentially to the prediction of the dependent variable.

Table 6. Results of stepwise multiple regression analyses for SBP and DBP at rest before the tasks

Factor	Regression coefficient	Multiple *R*	R^2	*F*	*df*	*p*
SBP at rest						
Weight	0.79	0.459	0.210	24.49	1,91	<0.001
Sex	-5.82	0.526	0.277	8.42	2,90	0.005
Constant	81.79					
DBP at rest						
Weight	0.62	0.512	0.263	32.75	1,91	<0.001
Constant	46.33					

Table 7. Mean and maximal SBP, DBP, and HR responses (±standard deviation) during the video game (VG) and during the multiple choice reaction time task (RTT)

		VG	RTT
ΔSBP	(mmHg)	9.7±7.6	7.5±7.4
ΔSBP_{max}	(mmHg)	15.8±8.9	13.0±7.8
ΔDBP	(mmHg)	11.5±5.7	12.2±5.7
ΔDBP_{max}	(mmHg)	17.7±6.9	17.3±6.4
ΔHR	(bpm)	10.0±7.7	10.3±7.1
ΔHR_{max}	(bpm)	17.9±9.8	17.0±8.9

Cardiovascular Reactions During the Tasks

In Table 7, mean and maximal responses of SBP, DBP, and HR during both the VG and the multiple choice RTT are shown. Differences between sexes and behavior types with respect to mean and maximal cardiovascular reactions during these tasks were tested by two-way ANOVA.

During the VG. Compared with girls, boys exhibited significantly higher mean and maximal SBP reactions during the VG as can be seen in Fig. 1a [Δ SBP: $F(1,89)=6.38$, $p=0.0133$; ΔSBP_{max}: $F(1,89)=6.3$, $p=0.0139$]. The main effect of behavior types was marginally significant, indicating slightly higher reactions in type A children [Δ SBP: $F(1,89)=3.69$, $p=0.078$; ΔSBP_{max}: $F(1,89)=2.66$, $p=0.107$]. There were no significant interactions between type A/B status and sex for SBP reactions, although there were for DBP reactions (Fig. 1b), indicating higher mean and maximal DBP rises in type A boys, but not in type A girls during this task [Δ DBP: $F(1,89)=7.19$, $p=0.0087$; ΔDBP_{max}: $F(1,89)=12.62$, $p=0.0006$]. The main effects for mean DBP reactions are only marginally significant [type A/B status: $F(1,89)=3.46$, $p=0.066$; sex: $F(1,89)=2.9$, $p=0.0921$]. For maximal DBP reactions, there is a significant effect of behavior types [DBP_{max}: $F(1,89)=6.59$, $p=0.0119$] and a marginal sex effect [DBP_{max}: $F(1,89)=3.49$, $p=0.065$]. There were no significant effects at all for HR.

In order to determine the relative influence of different factors on mean and

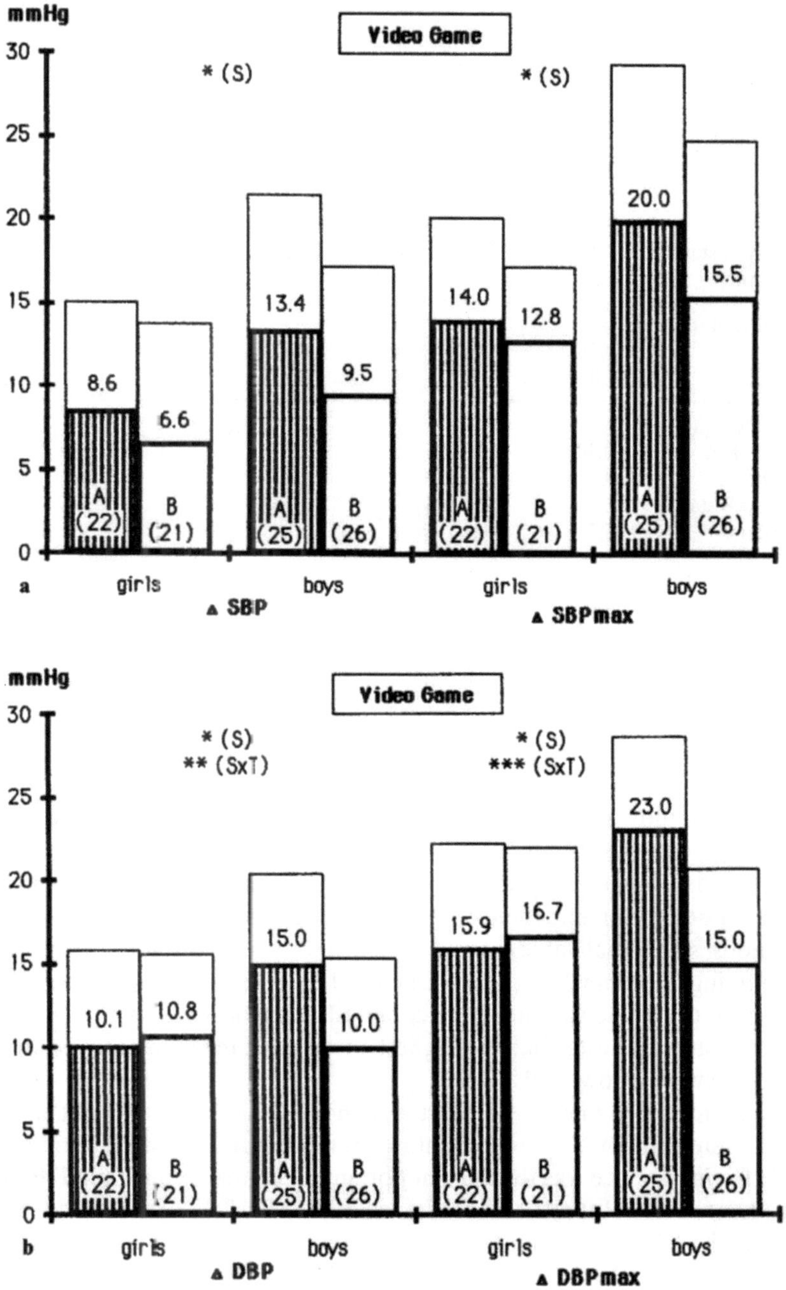

Fig. 1 a, b. Mean and maximal systolic (**a**) and diastolic (**b**) BP reactions during the VG in 22 type A and 21 type B girls, as well as in 25 type A and 26 type B boys [*thin lines* indicate +1 SD; *(S)* indicates a significant sex difference and *(S × T)* a significant interaction between sex and behavior types; *$p<0.05$; **$p<0.01$; ***$p<0.001$]

Table 8a. Results of stepwise multiple regression analyses of mean and maximal SBP and DBP reactions during the video game (VG)

Factor	Regression coefficient	Multiple *R*	R^2	*F*	*df*	*p*
ΔSBP during VG						
Sex	-5.08	0.250	0.063	6.07	1,91	0.016
SBP at rest	-0.21	0.324	0.105	4.26	2,90	0.042
Height	0.23	0.400	0.160	5.80	3,89	0.018
Type A/B status	3.37	0.457	0.209	5.46	4,88	0.022
Constant	3.59					
ΔSBP_{max} during VG						
Sex	-4.35	0.246	0.060	6.01	1,91	0.018
Constant	22.07					
ΔDBP during VG						
DBP at rest	-0.30	0.285	0.081	8.04	1,91	0.006
Height	0.26	0.459	0.211	14.82	2,90	<0.001
Type A/B status	2.40	0.505	0.255	5.29	3,89	0.024
Constant	-5.71					
ΔDBP_{max} during VG						
Subscale impatience	0.24	0.297	0.088	8.81	1,91	0.004
DBP at rest	-0.34	0.394	0.155	7.10	2,90	0.009
Height	0.25	0.490	0.240	9.93	3,89	0.002
Constant	0.77					

maximal cardiovascular reactions during the VG, stepwise multiple regression analyses were carried out, including the following factors: age, sex, height, weight, weight index, initial values at rest before the task, and type A/B status, as well as the three subscales for impatience, competitiveness, and dominance. For mean SBP reactions, sex, initial values at rest, height, and type A/B status are main predictors accounting for about 21% of the variance of these reactions, whereas sex accounted for about 6% of the variance of maximal SBP responses during the VG (Table 8a). These results indicate that the highest mean SBP reactions can be found in tall type A boys with low SBP at rest.

With regard to mean DBP reactions, initial values at rest, height, and type A/B status were main predictors accounting for more than 25% of the variance. The subscale for impatience was the most important predictor for maximal DBP responses, together with DBP at rest and height accounting for 24% of the variance (Table 8a). During the VG task, tall and especially impatient type A children with low DBP at rest show the most marked DBP reactions. None of the factors investigated predicted HR reactions during the VG task.

During the Multiple Choice RTT. None of the cardiovascular reactions investigated during the multiple choice RTT showed a significant interaction between sex and behavior type. SBP (Fig. 2a) showed a marginally significant main effect for sex [ΔSBP_{max}: $F(1,89)=3.06$, $p=0.084$], as well as for type A/B status [ΔSBP_{max}: $F(1,89)=3.43$, $p=0.067$], indicating somewhat higher maximal SBP reactions in boys

Table 8 b. Stepwise multiple regression analyses for mean and maximal reactions of SBP, DBP, and HR during the multiple choice reaction time task (RTT)

Factor	Regression coefficient	Multiple *R*	R^2	*F*	*df*	*p*
ΔSBP_{max} during RTT						
Subscale competitiveness	0.27	0.259	0.067	6.53	1,91	0.012
Constant	7.11					
ΔDBP during RTT						
Age	1.50	0.311	0.097	9.76	1,91	0.002
DBP at rest	-0.30	0.435	0.189	10.20	2,90	0.002
Weight	0.25	0.491	0.241	6.17	3,89	0.015
Constant	10.79					
ΔDBP_{max} during RTT						
Age	1.93	0.323	0.104	10.59	1,91	0.002
DBP at rest	-0.38	0.477	0.228	14.38	2,90	<0.001
Weight	0.26	0.520	0.270	5.16	3,89	0.026
Constant	16.66					
ΔHR During RTT						
HR at rest	-0.25	0.448	0.201	22.90	1,91	<0.001
Constant	32.06					
ΔHR_{max} during RTT						
HR at rest	-0.26	0.376	0.142	15.01	1,91	<0.001
Constant	39.96					

and in type A children. Stepwise multiple regression analysis, showed the subscale for competitiveness to be the only predictor, accounting for about 7% of the variance of maximal SBP reactions during the RTT (Table 8 b). None of the other factors investigated (age, sex, height, weight, weight index, initial values at rest period 1, type A/B status, or the other subscales) predicted mean or maximal SBP reactions.

Significantly different mean or maximal DBP responses were seen neither between boys and girls nor between type A and B children during the multiple choice RTT (Fig. 2 b). In stepwise multiple regression analysis, age, initial values at rest period 1, and weight were predictors accounting for 24% and 27% respectively of the variance of mean and maximal DBP reactions during this task (Table 8 b). Sex, height, weight index, type A/B status, and the three subscales failed to predict DBP reactions.

DBP responses exceed those of SBP, which can be seen in Fig. 3 a, where BP responses during each of the 6 min of the RTT are shown separately. SBP reactions show a continuous rise for both behavior types, with type A children reaching the maximum in the 4th min and type B children in the 5th min. This might be a reflection of the minute-by-minute increasing difficulty of the task up to the 5th min. A significant type A/B effect of these SBP reactions was found during the 2nd [Δ SBP: $F(1,87)=4.63$, $p=0.034$] and 3rd min [Δ SBP: $F(1,87)=4.53$, $p=0.036$]; a marginally significant type A/B effect was also found during the last minute of this

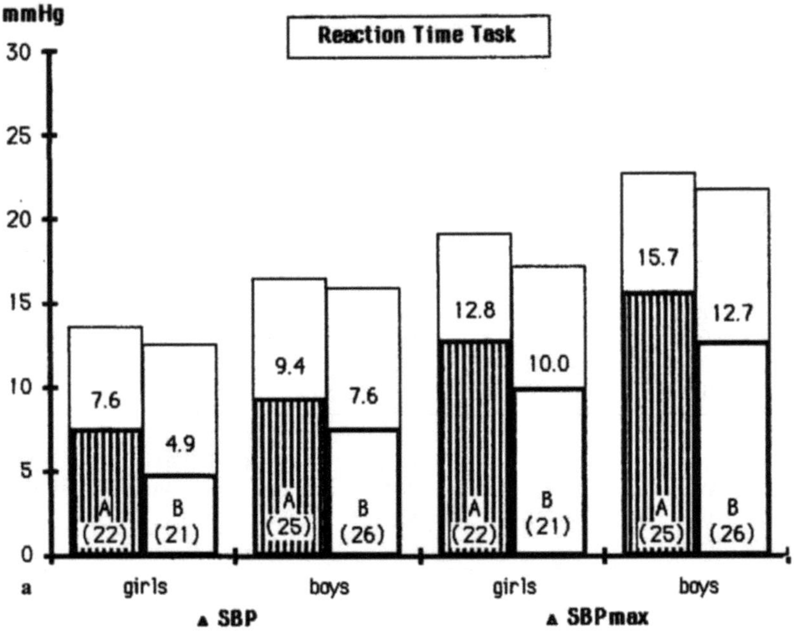

a

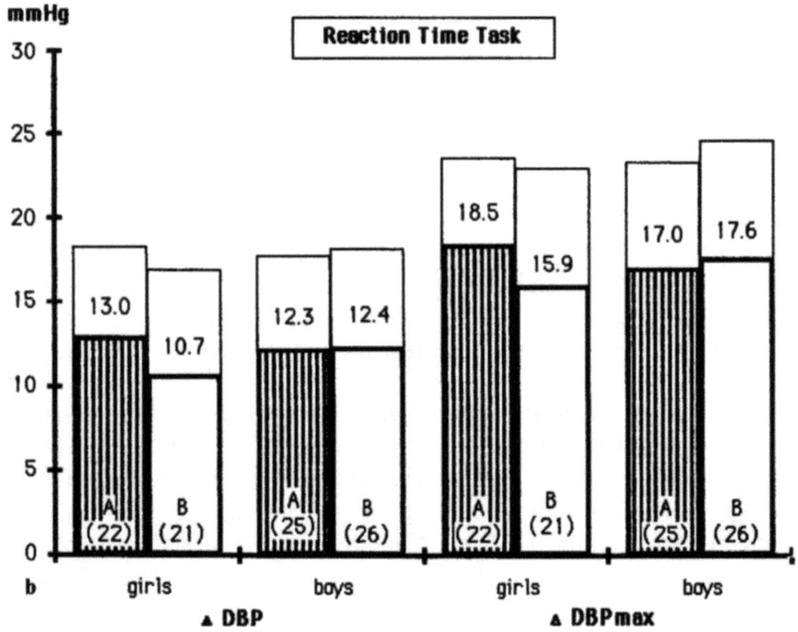

b

Fig. 2 a, b. Mean and maximal systolic **(a)** and diastolic **(b)** BP reactions during the multiple choice RTT in 22 type A and 21 type B girls, as well as in 25 type A and 26 type B boys (*thin lines* indicate +1 SD)

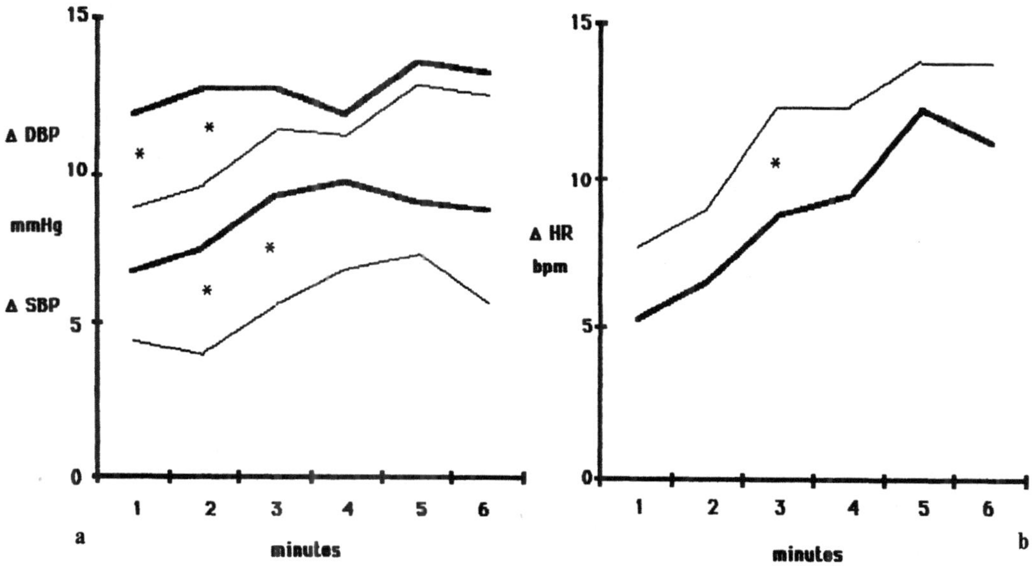

Fig. 3 a, b. Minute-by-minute diastolic *(two upper curves)* and systolic BP reactions *(two lower curves)* **(a)** and HR responses **(b)** during the multiple choice RTT in type A *(thick lines)* and type B children *(thin lines)* (*$p < 0.05$)

task [Δ SBP: $F\,(1,87) = 3.26$, $p = 0.074$]. This indicates higher SBP responses in type A children with a medium degree of task difficulty. The marginally significant effect during the 6th min might be due to the decline of SBP responses in type B children when the degree of task difficulty was not further increased; type A children did not exhibit such a marked decline.

A continuous rise in DBP responses up to the 5th min can also be seen in type B children, whereas from the beginning of this task, type A children exhibited rather high DBP reactions, which became only slightly more pronounced with increasing task difficulty. Type A children show significantly more marked DBP responses during the 1st [Δ DBP: $F\,(1,87) = 5.05$, $p = 0.027$] and 2nd min [Δ DBP: $F\,(1,87) = 4.60$, $p = 0.035$]. In SBP and DBP responses, neither significant differences between sexes nor significant interactions between sex and type A/B status were found when each of the 6 min of this task were analyzed separately.

There were no significant interactions between sex and type A/B status in HR reactions during the RTT and no significant sex differences. Contrary to the type A hyperreactivity hypothesis, however, mean HR reactions were significantly higher in type B children: [Δ HR: 8.8 vs 11.9 bpm; $F\,(1,89) = 4.25$, $p = 0.042$]; when each minute was analyzed separately, a continuous rise in HR responses could again be seen up to the 5th min. The unexpected difference between type A and type B children was significant only during the 3rd min [$F\,(1,87) = 5.17$, $p = 0.026$] (Fig. 3 b). During multiple regression analysis, only initial values at rest period 1 predicted mean and maximal HR reactions, accounting for about 20% and 14% of the variance respectively. Neither type A/B status nor any other factor predicted HR reactions (Table 8 b).

Higher HRs at rest period 1 are related to less pronounced HR reactions during the RTT. The higher HR responses in type B children seen in the ANOVA results might be due to an insignificantly higher HR in type A children during rest period 1, which is most pronounced in type A girls: ($HR_{at\ rest\ 1}$: 90.6 vs 85.5 bpm). When HR reactions during the RTT are determined by taking the mean value of rest period 2 (just before this task) as a reference value, ANOVA results do not show any significant differences between behavior types. These results indicate that type A behavior does not play a role here in HR reactions and that the unexpected ANOVA effect is instead an artifact caused by differing initial values during rest period 1.

Performance Parameters

During the VG the average score per game was analyzed as a measure of psychomotor performance for the 78 children who played game no. 47. The children from the first grade ($n=16$) were not included, as they played a different video game (no. 42) in which they could only reach a lower score (see above). Of the first grade children, 25% had experience with VG, compared with 53% of the older group; with increasing age, children had significantly more VG experience ($Chi^2=11.38$, $p=0.001$). In the ANOVA, the effects of sex, type A/B status, and VG experience were investigated, but none of these factors had a significant influence on performance. When age was included as a factor, there was a significant interaction only between age and VG experience, indicating that older experienced children could play better, i.e., had higher averaged scores [$F(1,77)=4.15$, $p=0.046$]. These results show that this performance parameter is not able to differentiate between type A and B children with these VG.

When the average score during the VG was correlated to BP and HR and BP and HR reactions in this task, significant results were found in mean [$r=0.21$, $p=0.033$] and maximal HR reactions [$r=0.20$, $p=0.037$]; this points to somewhat higher HR reactions in children who perform better during the VG.

In the multiple choice RTT, indices of psychomotor performance were assessed in 84 children by recording correct, delayed, omitted, and wrong responses during the 6 min of the task; the first ten of the 94 children taking part in the experiment had to be excluded from further analyses, as these performance parameters could not be recorded because of a technical defect. Age was expected to have an influence on psychomotor performance in this test; therefore, two-way analysis of covariance was carried out for the factors sex and behavior type using age as covariate. The results show that older children performed significantly better as measured by correct ($r=0.61$***), delayed ($r=-0.46$***), and omitted responses ($r=-0.59$***), but the child's age did not influence the number of wrong responses in this task. There were no significant sex differences or significant interactions between sex and type A/B status, but as can be seen in Fig. 4, type A children had significantly more correct responses: [$F(1,79)=5.28$, $p=0.024$] and omitted fewer responses: [$F(1,79)=7.3$, $p=0.008$]; this indicates better psychomotor performance for type A children.

When the indices of psychomotor performance were related to cardiovascular parameters, significant correlations were found between mean and maximal SBP and DBP during the RTT and correct and omitted responses (Table 9); the same was true when correlating the responses of SBP and DBP to these two performance

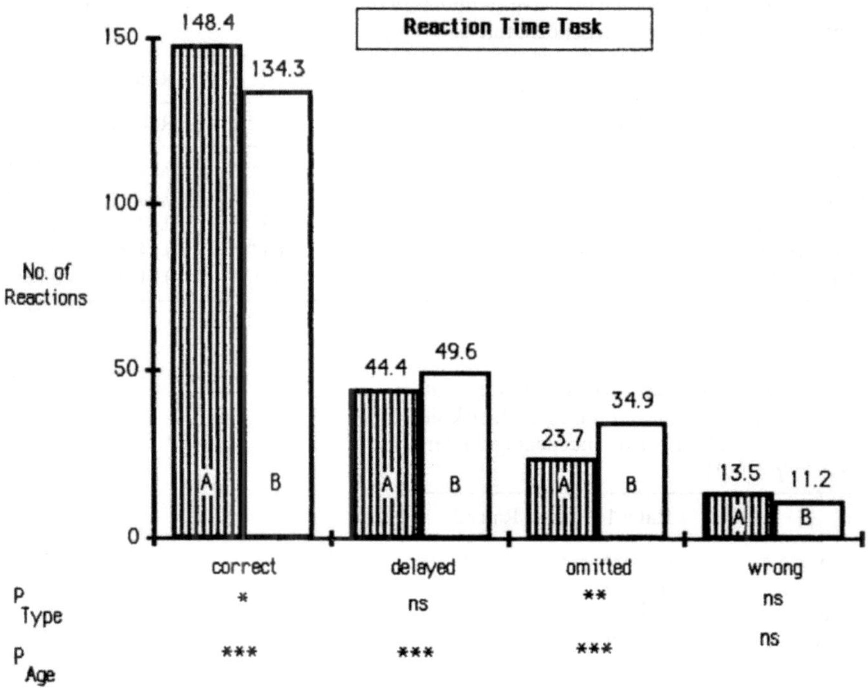

Fig. 4. Psychomotor performance parameters during the multiple choice RTT for 42 type A and 42 type B children with age as covariate (***$p<0.001$; **$p<0.01$; *$p<0.05$; *ns*, non significant)

Table 9. Pearson correlation coefficients between mean and maximal SBP and DBP and their reactions during the multiple choice reaction time task (RTT) and indices of psychomotor performance during this test ($n=84$)

	Indices of psychomotor performance during RTT (no. of reactions)			
	Correct	Delayed	Omitted	Wrong
SBP	0.24*		-0.24*	
SBP_{max}	0.28**		-0.28**	
DBP	0.29**		-0.32**	
DBP_{max}	0.29**		-0.32**	
ΔSBP				
ΔSBP_{max}	0.19*		-0.21*	
ΔDBP	0.21*		-0.30**	
ΔDBP_{max}	0.20*		-0.28**	

* $p<0.05$ ** $p<0.01$

Table 10a. Correlation coefficients between ratings of the children's behavior during different rest periods as observed by two independent raters ($n=94$)

	Rest 1/rest 2		Rest 1/rest 3		Rest 2/rest 3	
	Rater 1	Rater 2	Rater 1	Rater 2	Rater 1	Rater 2
Physical rest	0.70***	0.72***	0.57***	0.58***	0.79***	0.73***
Relaxation	0.51***	0.43***	0.40***	0.36***	0.60***	0.47***
Exploratory behavior	0.53***	0.64***	0.38***	0.45***	0.49***	0.64***
Contact seeking	0.59***	0.61***	0.53***	0.64***	0.64***	0.74***
Speech activity	0.57***	0.60***	0.46***	0.49***	0.81***	0.76***

Table 10b. Correlation coefficients between ratings of the children's behavior during both task situations as observed by two independent raters ($n=94$; ***$p<.001$)

	Rater 1	Rater 2
Tension	0.50***	0.52***
Engagement	0.60***	0.63***
Impatience	0.56***	0.62***
Mimicry	0.47***	0.58***
Speech activity	0.53***	0.60***
Excessive demand	0.41***	0.47***
Enjoyment	0.42***	0.54***
Resignation	0.26***	0.51***

*** $p<0.001$

parameters. The results indicate that better psychomotor performance, i.e., more correct as well as fewer omitted responses, is accompanied by higher SBP and DBP, as well as higher SBP and DBP increases during this task.

Behavioral Ratings

The behavioral ratings made by two independent observers of the children during the experiment were analyzed with regard to stability in the different situations, inter-rater reliability, correlations with MYTH-assessed TABP, differences between type A and B children, and correlations with cardiovascular parameters. Results were considered to be reliable only when they were significant for both observers.

As can be seen in Tables 10a and 10b, physical rest, speech activity, and contact seeking were scored by both observers as the most stable behavioral variables during rest periods, whereas during the tasks, engagement, impatience, and speech activity were seen by both observers as somewhat stable during the tasks.

As can be seen in Table 11, inter-rater reliability is quite different for the various behavioral variables. This might depend on how easy or difficult it is to observe certain types of behavior. For instance, during rest periods, speech activity, contact seeking, and physical rest show good inter-rater reliability, whereas inter-rater reliability for relaxation is rather low. The latter variable was contrasted to physical rest

Table 11. Inter-rater reliability of behavioral ratings during different phases of the experiment and correlation coefficients between behavioral ratings and MYTH-assessed TABP for both observers. Differing *n* are due to missing data

	Inter-rater reliability *(n)*	MYTH-assessed TABP	
		Rater 1	Rater 2
Rest 1			
Physical rest	0.62*** (93)		
Relaxation	0.31*** (93)	−0.30**	
Exploratory behavior	0.49*** (87)		
Contact seeking	0.66*** (93)		0.19*
Speech activity	0.89*** (94)	0.19*	0.24**
Video Game			
Tension	0.41*** (94)	0.23*	0.20*
Engagement	0.60*** (94)	0.30**	0.23*
Impatience	0.65*** (94)	0.36**	0.23*
Mimicry	0.50*** (94)	0.17*	0.30**
Speech activity	0.77*** (94)	0.27**	0.32***
Excessive demand	0.48*** (93)	0.22*	
Enjoyment	0.51*** (94)		0.34***
Resignation	0.50*** (87)	0.29**	
Rest 2			
Physical rest	0.64*** (93)		
Relaxation	0.39*** (93)	−0.51***	
Exploratory behavior	0.61*** (87)		
Contact seeking	0.74*** (93)	0.28**	
Speech activity	0.93*** (94)		
Reaction Time Task			
Tension	0.35*** (94)	0.28**	
Engagement	0.53*** (93)	0.20*	0.30**
Impatience	0.61*** (94)	0.23*	0.18*
Mimicry	0.34*** (93)		
Speech activity	0.69*** (94)		
Excessive demand	0.57*** (93)		
Enjoyment	0.49*** (93)		0.29**
Resignation	0.58*** (86)		
Rest 3			
Physical rest	0.81*** (93)		
Relaxation	0.24* (93)	−0.26**	
Exploratory behavior	0.56*** (87)		
Contact seeking	0.66*** (93)		0.23*
Speech activity	0.86*** (94)		
For the whole experiment			
Quickness of comprehension	0.70*** (87)		0.25*
Motoric restlessness	0.65*** (94)	0.23*	
Emotional excitement	0.51*** (94)	0.22*	
Ambition	0.63*** (94)	0.49***	0.33***
Cooperation	0.60*** (87)		
Unfriendly/friendly	0.45*** (87)		0.30**
Extraversion/introversion	0.80*** (87)	−0.53***	−0.42**
TABP	0.70*** (94)	0.65***	0.38***
Contact to observers	0.75*** (54)		0.36**
Certainty of judgment	0.32** (87)		

* $p<0.05$ ** $p<0.01$ *** $p<0.001$

as inner relaxation, but results indicate that the inner state is more difficult to observe than externally exhibited behavior. During the tasks, both raters show most agreement in scoring speech activity and impatience. In the scales of global behavioral assessment at the end of the experiment, inter-rater reliability is best for extraversion-introversion, contact to rater, TABP, quickness of comprehension, motoric restlessness, and ambition, whereas it is rather low for certainty of judgment, indicating that both observers often experienced different degrees of certainty in assessing a child's behavior.

As can also be seen in Table 11, MYTH-assessed TABP is related by both observers to more speech activity during rest period 1; to more tension, engagement, impatience, mimicry, and speech activity during the VG; and to more engagement and impatience during the RTT. Both observers also attribute more ambition, more extraversion, and more type A behavior to children who had been assessed as type A by their teachers. The correlation coefficients between TABP assessed on the one hand in the experiment and on the other in the MYTH are, however, too low for the short-term behavioral observation during the experiment to be able to replace the teachers' type A assessment in the MYTH.

In order to investigate behavioral differences between type A and B children and between boys and girls, Mann-Whitney *U* tests were also performed independently for each observer. Again, both observers attributed significantly more speech activity during rest period 1; more tension, engagement, impatience, mimicry, and speech activity during the VG; and more engagement and impatience during the RTT to type A children. Moreover, MYTH-assessed type A children were seen by both observers to be more ambitious, extraverted, and type A (Table 12).

During the VG, both observers considered the boys to be more engaged, impatient, and talkative, and during the RTT, to be more tense, engaged, and impatient. Boys were also rated as being more ambitious, extraverted, and type A; both observers showed more certainty in assessing behavioral characteristics of boys (Table 13).

When cardiovascular parameters were correlated to behavioral variables, a striking difference could be seen between boys and girls (Table 14): Boys exhibited considerably more significant and higher correlations than girls, which was true for rest periods, tasks, and the behavioral scales encompassing the whole experiment. This was also true for both the female and male observers; the latter had no knowledge of the children's BP or HR. Only those correlation coefficients are reported which are significant for both observers.

During rest periods, boys but not girls who showed more signs of physical rest had a lower HR; the more activity they developed during this phase, such as exploratory behavior and contact seeking, the higher their HR was. During the VG, tension, engagement, impatience, mimicry, ambition, emotional excitement, and TABP correlated significantly and positively with BP and/or its reactions in boys, whereas during the RTT, only impatience was related to higher HR and SBP responses. Motoric restlessness was connected with slighter responses of HR during the VG and of SBP and DBP_{max} during the RTT.

To summarize: In boys, tension, engagement, impatience, emotional excitement, ambition, and TABP are mainly related to elevated BP responses.

Table 12. Mann-Whitney *U* tests of MYTH-assessed types A/B differences in behavioral ratings of both observers

	Rater	Mean rank		*U*	*p*
		Type A	Type B		
Rest 1					
Physical rest	1				
	2				
Relaxation	1	39.53	54.63	730	0.004
	2				
Exploratory behavior	1				
	2				
Contact seeking	1				
	2	52.21	42.79	883	0.073
Speech activity*	1	51.45	43.55	919	0.062
	2	52.66	42.34	862	0.020
Video Game					
Tension*	1	53.48	41.52	824	0.025
	2	52.37	42.63	876	0.059
Engagement*	1	54.86	40.14	759	0.004
	2	53.39	41.61	828	0.026
Impatience**	1	56.97	38.03	660	0.001
	2	55.15	39.85	745	0.005
Mimicry*	1	51.77	43.23	904	0.096
	2	55.26	39.74	740	0.003
Speech activity**	1	54.07	40.93	796	0.010
	2	55.65	39.35	722	0.002
Excessive demand	1	51.69	42.21	861	0.036
	2				
Enjoyment	1				
	2	56.31	38.69	691	0.001
Resignation	1	50.09	38.05	684	0.008
	2				
Rest 2					
Physical rest	1				
	2				
Relaxation	1	34.24	60.03	482	<0.001
	2				
Exploratory behavior	1				
	2				
Contact seeking	1				
	2	54.62	40.38	770	0.007
Speech activity	1				
	2				
Reaction Time Task					
Tension	1	54.65	40.35	769	0.007
	2				
Engagement**	1	52.07	41.82	843	0.050
	2	54.43	39.41	732	0.004
Impatience*	1	53.34	41.66	830	0.029
	2	52.17	42.83	885	0.084
Mimicry	1				
	2				
Speech activity	1				
	2				

Table 12 (Continue)

	Rater	Mean rank		U	p
		Type A	Type B		
Excessive demand	1				
	2				
Enjoyment	1				
	2	54.21	39.63	742	0.006
Resignation	1				
	2				
Rest 3					
Physical rest	1				
	2				
Relaxation	1	40.35	53.79	769	0.011
	2				
Exploratory behavior	1				
	2				
Contact seeking	1				
	2	53.28	41.72	833	0.025
Speech activity	1				
	2				
During the whole experiment					
Quickness of comprehension	1				
	2	49.87	38.26	694	0.022
Motoric restlessness	1	53.61	41.39	818	0.025
	2				
Emotional excitement	1	52.94	42.06	849	0.037
	2				
Ambition**	1	60.13	34.87	511	<0.001
	2	56.17	38.83	697	0.001
Cooperation	1				
	2				
Unfriendly/friendly	1				
	2	51.06	37.10	643	0.005
Extraversion/introversion**	1	30.86	56.84	381	<0.001
	2	33.70	54.07	503	<0.001
TABP**	1	30.38	64.62	638	<0.001
	2	37.57	57.43	638	<0.001
Contact to observer	1				
	2	32.59	22.02	222	0.008
Certainty of judgment	1				
	2				

* Significant for one rater and marginally significant for the other rater
** Significant for both raters

Table 13. Mann-Whitney *U* tests of sex differences in behavioral ratings of both observers

	Rater	Mean rank		*U*	*p*
		Boys	Girls		
Rest 1					
Physical rest	1				
	2				
Relaxation	1				
	2				
Exploratory behavior	1				
	2				
Contact seeking	1				
	2				
Speech activity	1				
	2				
Video Game					
Tension	1	54.17	39.59	757	0.007
	2				
Engagement**	1	53.34	40.57	799	0.013
	2	56.14	37.26	656	<0.001
Impatience**	1	52.92	41.07	820	0.029
	2	54.39	39.33	745	0.006
Mimicry	1				
	2				
Speech activity**	1	53.80	40.02	775	0.007
	2	53.93	39.88	769	0.009
Excessive demand	1				
	2				
Enjoyment	1				
	2				
Resignation	1				
	2				
Rest 2					
Physical rest	1				
	2				
Relaxation	1				
	2				
Exploratory behavior	1				
	2				
Contact seeking	1				
	2				
Speech activity	1				
	2				
Reaction time task					
Tension*	1	55.18	38.40	705	0.002
	2	51.75	42.47	880	0.078
Engagement**	1	55.10	37.58	670	0.001
	2	53.82	39.07	734	0.005
Impatience**	1	52.83	41.17	825	0.029
	2	52.74	41.29	830	0.035
Mimicry	1				
	2				
Speech activity	1				
	2				

Table 13 (Continue)

	Rater	Mean rank		*U*	*p*
		Boys	Girls		
Excessive demand	1				
	2				
Enjoyment	1				
	2				
Resignation	1				
	2				
Rest 3					
Physical rest	1				
	2	42.83	51.85	867	0.094
Relaxation	1				
	2				
Exploratory behavior	1				
	2				
Contact seeking	1				
	2				
Speech activity	1				
	2				
During the whole experiment					
Quickness of comprehension	1				
	2	49.29	37.79	692	0.024
Motoric restlessness	1	52.30	41.80	852	0.055
	2				
Emotional excitement	1	51.67	42.56	884	0.082
	2				
Ambition**	1	53.92	39.88	769	0.010
	2	57.61	35.51	581	0.001
Cooperation	1				
	2	48.43	38.80	732	0.050
Unfriendly/friendly	1				
	2				
Extraversion/introversion*	1	39.41	49.39	725	0.060
	2	38.22	50.79	669	0.017
TABP	1				
	2	40.24	56.12	726	0.003
Contact to observer	1	31.45	22.92	248	0.035
	2				
Certainty of judgment*	1	49.64	37.38	675	0.010
	2	47.85	39.48	759	0.081

* Significant for one rater and marginally significant for the other rater
** Significant for both raters

Table 14. Spearman correlation coefficients between behavioral ratings and cardiovascular parameters for boys and girls according to both observers

		Boys		Girls	
		Rater 1	Rater 2	Rater 1	Rater 2
Rest 1					
Physical rest	HR	-0.32*	-0.38**		
Exploratory behavior	HR	0.39**	0.48**		
Contact seeking	HR	0.42***	0.46***		
Speech activity	HR	0.32*	0.29*		
Video Game					
Tension	DBD	0.25*	0.28*		
	DBD_{max}	0.32*	0.33*		
	ΔSBP	0.33**	0.27*		
	ΔSBP_{max}	0.33**	0.26*		
	ΔDBP	0.45***	0.28*		
	ΔDBP_{max}	0.49***	0.30*		
Engagement	SBP	0.28*	0.26*		
	DBP	0.29*	0.36**		
	DBP_{max}	0.33**	0.41**		
	ΔSBP	0.34**	0.37**		
	ΔSBP_{max}	0.36**	0.33**		
	ΔDBP	0.47***	0.45***		
	ΔDBP_{max}	0.49***	0.42**		
Impatience	DBP	0.33**	0.29*		
	DBP_{max}	0.39**	0.33**		
	ΔSBP	0.36**	0.41**		
	ΔSBP_{max}	0.35**	0.35**		
	ΔDBP	0.49***	0.42**		
	ΔDBP_{max}	0.52***	0.43***		
	ΔHR_{max}			-0.51***	-0.28*
Mimicry	DBP	0.27*	0.37**		
	DBP_{max}	0.30*	0.45**		
Speech activity	DBP			-0.28*	-0.32*
	DBP_{max}			-0.26*	-0.27*
Enjoyment	SBP_{max}	-0.42**	-0.25*		
	ΔSBP			0.29*	0.27*
	ΔSBP_{max}			0.33*	0.32*
	ΔHR_{max}	-0.33**	-0.27*		
Rest 2					
Physical rest	HR	-0.41**	-0.40**		
Relaxation	DBP	-0.33**	-0.34**		
Exploratory behavior	HR	0.34**	0.29*		
Speech activity	SBP	-0.27*	-0.27*		
Reaction time task					
Tension	HR_{max}			0.40**	0.27*
Impatience	HR_{max}	0.26*	0.26*		
	ΔSBP	0.26*	0.26*		
	ΔSBP_{max}	0.37**	0.43***		
Resignation	SBP	-0.37**	-0.34**		
	SBP_{max}	-0.32*	-0.25*		

Table 14 (Continue)

		Boys		Girls	
		Rater 1	Rater 2	Rater 1	Rater 2
Rest 3					
Physical rest	HR	-0.48***	-0.40**		
Relaxation	HR	-0.27*	-0.40**		
Exploratory behavior	HR	0.41**	0.47***		
Contact seeking	HR	0.38**	0.48***		
During the whole experiment					
Motoric restlessness					
During VG:	ΔHR	-0.25*	-0.27*		
	ΔHR_{max}	-0.30*	-0.33**		
During RTT:	ΔSBP	-0.24*	-0.24*		
	ΔDBP_{max}	-0.24*	-0.29*		
Emotional excitement					
During VG:	DBP	0.28*	0.35**		
	DBP_{max}	0.29*	0.38**		
	ΔDBP	0.28*	0.32*	-0.27*	-0.29*
	ΔDBP_{max}	0.24*	0.29*	-0.26*	-0.29*
Ambition					
During VG:	DBP	0.33**	0.39**		
	DBP_{max}	0.39**	0.45***		
	ΔSBP	0.34**	0.31*		
	ΔSBP_{max}	0.30*	0.32*		
	ΔDBP	0.50***	0.37**		
	ΔDBP_{max}	0.50***	0.38**		
During RTT:	ΔSBP	0.32*	0.29*		
TABP					
During VG:	DBP	0.42***	0.35**		
	DBP_{max}	0.51***	0.40**		
	ΔSBP_{max}	0.34**	0.24*		
	ΔDBP	0.49***	0.34**		
	ΔDBP_{max}	0.52***	0.35**		

* $p<0.05$ ** $p<0.01$ *** $p<0.001$

In MYTH-assessed type A children, tension, engagement, and impatience are related to elevated BP and/or more pronounced BP reactions during the VG (Table 15); SBP, DBP, and maximal DBP responses are elevated in the more impatient type B children during this task. During the RTT, speech activity is related to slighter SBP reactions in type A children, and tension to a higher HR and elevated maximal SBP and SBP reactions only in type B children. Further, ambition is related to a higher BP during both tasks only in type B children. When MYTH-assessed type B children were rated as type A by the observers, SBP was higher during both tasks; when MYTH-assessed type A children were rated as type A by both observers, DBP reactions were higher during the VG. Motoric restlessness was related to lower BP and BP reactions during both tasks in type B children. For further details, see Table 15.

In short, the correlations between the various behavioral ratings and cardiovascular parameters in type A and B children are not uniform. This might be due to be-

Table 15. Spearman correlation coefficients between behavioral ratings and cardiovascular parameters for type A and B children according to both observers

		Type A		Type B	
		Rater 1	Rater 2	Rater 1	Rater 2
Rest 1					
Exploratory behavior	HR	0.28*	0.30*		
Speech activity	HR			0.25*	0.26*
Video game					
Tension	ΔSBP	0.31*	0.31*		
	ΔSBP_{max}	0.34**	0.33*		
	ΔDBP	0.37**	0.39**		
	ΔDBP_{max}	0.40**	0.40**		
Engagement	SBP_{max}	0.30*	0.27*		
	DBP_{max}	0.29*	0.24*		
	ΔSBP	0.27*	0.32*		
	ΔSBP_{max}	0.31*	0.36**		
	ΔDBP_{max}	0.26*	0.42**		
Impatience	SBP			0.41**	0.26*
	DBP			0.35**	0.24*
	DBP_{max}			0.36**	0.25*
	ΔDBP	0.28*	0.32*		
	ΔDBP_{max}	0.28*	0.33*		
Mimicry	DBP_{max}			0.30*	0.34**
Rest 2					
Physical rest	HR	-0.37**	-0.28*		
Contact seeking	SBP			-0.36**	-0.30*
Reaction time task					
Tension	SBP_{max}			0.31*	0.25*
	HR			0.43**	0.25*
	HR_{max}			0.42**	0.35**
	ΔSBP_{max}			0.40**	0.25*
Impatience	SBP_{max}			0.29*	0.27*
	ΔSBP_{max}				
Speech activity	ΔSBP	-0.30*	-0.46***		
	ΔSBP_{max}	-0.26*	-0.37**		
Resignation	HR	0.28*	0.39**		
Rest 3					
Relaxation	HR			-0.25*	-0.27*
Speech activity	SBP			-0.33*	-0.32*
	HR			0.33*	0.39**
During the whole experiment					
Motoric restlessness					
During VG:	SBP_{max}			-0.33*	-0.39*
	ΔSBP_{max}			-0.29*	-0.30*
	ΔHR			-0.29*	-0.32*
	ΔHR_{max}			-0.28*	-0.40**
During RTT:	SBP			-0.28*	-0.32*
	SBP_{max}			-0.29*	-0.30*
	ΔDBP			-0.31*	-0.34*
	ΔDBP_{max}			-0.27*	-0.29*
Ambition					
During VG:	SBP			0.35**	0.36**
	SBP_{max}			0.33**	0.34**

Table 15 (Continue)

		Type A		Type B	
		Rater 1	Rater 2	Rater 1	Rater 2
During RTT:	SBP			0.32*	0.32*
	SBP_{max}			0.32*	0.36**
	DBP_{max}			0.27*	0.25*
TABP					
During VG:	SBP			0.40**	0.31*
	SBP_{max}			0.35**	0.26*
	ΔDBP	0.32*	0.29*		
	ΔDBP_{max}	0.35**	0.33*		
During RTT:	SBP			0.35**	0.25*
	SBP_{max}			0.39**	0.29*
	HR			0.36**	0.27*
	HR_{max}			0.37**	0.28*

* $p<0.05$ ** $p<0.01$ *** $p<0.001$

Table 16a. Results of stepwise multiple regression analyses of mean and maximal SBP, DBP, and HR reactions, including parameters of behavioral observation during the video game (VG) for 85 children

Factor	Regression coefficient	Multiple *R*	R^2	*F*	*df*	*p*
ΔSBP during VG						
Tension	1.39	0.297	0.088	8.04	1,83	0.006
Unfriendly/friendly	-2.20	0.398	0.158	6.81	2,82	0.011
Extraversion/intro-version	-0.87	0.455	0.207	4.97	3,81	0.029
Constant	19.51					
ΔSBP_{max} during VG						
Tension	2.18	0.284	0.080	7.25	1,83	0.009
Unfriendly/friendly	-1.72	0.389	0.151	6.85	2,82	0.011
Constant	11.15					
ΔDBP during VG						
Impatience	1.08	0.333	0.111	10.34	1,83	0.002
DBP at rest	-0.31	0.417	0.174	6.28	2,82	0.014
Height	0.28	0.577	0.333	19.36	3,81	<0.001
Unfriendly/friendly	-0.29	0.610	0.372	4.85	4,80	0.030
Constant	-4.43					
ΔDBP_{max} during VG						
Impatience	1.19	0.370	0.137	13.13	1,83	<0.001
DBP at rest	-0.32	0.443	0.197	6.13	2,82	0.015
Height	0.25	0.535	0.286	10.13	3,81	0.002
Unfriendly/friendly	-1.21	0.575	0.330	5.27	4,80	0.024
Type A/B status	2.88	0.606	0.368	4.68	5,79	0.034
Constant	6.35					
ΔHR_{max} during VG						
Enjoyment	-2.55	0.278	0.078	6.98	1,83	0.010
Cooperation	2.91	0.451	0.203	10.45	2,82	0.001
HR at rest	-0.16	0.500	0.250	8.98	3,81	0.001
Constant	4.65					

Table 16b. Results of stepwise multiple regression analyses of mean and maximal SBP, DBP, and HR reactions, including parameters of behavioral observation during the multiple choice reaction time task (RTT) for 85 children

Factor	Regression coefficient	Multiple *R*	R^2	*F*	*df*	*p*
ΔSBP during RTT						
Tension	2.10	0.299	0.089	8.19	1,83	0.005
Unfriendly/friendly	-1.33	0.394	0.155	6.38	2,82	0.013
Resignation	-0.87	0.444	0.197	4.19	3,81	0.044
Constant	3.84					
ΔSBP_{max} during RTT						
Impatience	2.12	0.397	0.157	15.49	1,83	<0.001
Unfriendly/friendly	-1.63	0.479	0.229	7.63	2,82	0.007
Subscale competitiveness	0.22	0.524	0.274	5.03	3,81	0.028
Motoric restlessness	-0.75	0.562	0.315	4.81	4,80	0.031
Constant	15.47					
ΔDBP during RTT						
Age	1.91	0.345	0.119	11.21	1,83	0.001
Unfriendly/friendly	-1.41	0.468	0.219	10.54	2,82	0.002
DBP at rest	-0.30	0.550	0.303	9.70	3,81	0.003
Weight	0.23	0.592	0.351	5.91	4,80	0.017
Subscale competitiveness	0.15	0.622	0.387	4.65	5,79	0.034
Constant	14.69					
ΔDBP_{max} during RTT						
Age	2.26	0.356	0.127	12.04	1,83	0.001
DBP at rest	-0.36	0.481	0.231	11.14	2,82	0.001
Unfriendly/friendly	-1.38	0.570	0.324	11.17	3,81	0.001
Weight	0.24	0.602	0.363	4.81	4,80	0.031
Constant	23.76					
ΔHR during RTT						
HR at rest	-0.26	0.438	0.192	19.67	1,83	<0.001
Impatience	1.26	0.499	0.249	6.23	2,82	0.014
Motoric restlessness	-0.74	0.548	0.300	5.94	3,81	0.017
Constant	31.80					
ΔHR max during RTT						
HR at rest	-0.28	0.354	0.125	11.86	1,83	<0.001
Impatience	1.86	0.433	0.188	6.31	2,82	0.014
Motoric restlessness	-0.84	0.493	0.243	5.93	3,81	0.017
Sex	3.59	0.531	0.282	4.31	4,80	0.041
Constant	33.59					

havioral differences as well as differences mainly in cardiovascular reactions between type A and B children.

In order to determine the relative importance of the behaviors exhibited by the children during the experiment for the prediction of cardiovascular reactions, we introduced the behavioral ratings of both observers into stepwise multiple regression analyses. Together with the other 10 variables tested previously (sex, age, weight, weight index, height, initial values at rest, type A/B status, and the three subscales for impatience, competitiveness, and dominance), the following behavioral variables were also included: tension, engagement, impatience, mimicry, speech activity, excessive demand, enjoyment, resignation, as well as quickness of comprehension, motoric restlessness, emotional excitement, ambition, cooperation, unfriendly-friendly, extraversion-introversion, and TABP as observed by the experimenters. For each of these variables, the behavioral ratings of both observers were added, thus forming a scale of 2-10; the resulting score could be used for further analyses of 85 children.

As can be seen in Tables 16a and 16b, the observed behavioral variables improved the prediction of cardiovascular reactions, and on the whole, they appear to be more important than the other parameters. Tension and impatience predict more pronounced responses during both tasks. A child's friendliness, however, is related to reduced BP reactions; this is also true for introversion during the VG and for resignation during the RTT. Enjoyment during the VG and motoric restlessness during the RTT predict reduced HR responses.

With respect to the VG, the scales of tension, unfriendly-friendly, and extraversion-introversion account for about 21% of the variance of mean SBP responses. Tension and unfriendly-friendly alone account for 15% of the variance of maximal SBP responses, while 37% of the variance of mean and maximal DBP responses is explained by the variables impatience, DBP at rest, height, unfriendly-friendly, and type A/B status (the latter only for $\Delta\ DBP_{max}$). Enjoyment of the VG was related to reduced maximal HR responses and the children's increased cooperation to elevated maximal HR responses; both variables, together with HR at rest, accounted for 25% of the variance. As the children were encouraged by one of the experimenters after each single game to aim for a higher VG score in the next game, a high degree of cooperation might have elevated maximal HR reactions. None of the factors investigated predicted mean HR responses. When the average VG score was corrected for the infuence of age and of the different VG which first grade schoolchildren played, and then additionally introduced into stepwise multiple regression analysis, this variable was positively related only to maximal HR responses; this accounted after the variables enjoyment and cooperation, and together with HR at rest for 29% of the variance.

During the RTT, the scales of tension, unfriendly-friendly, and resignation explained about 20% of mean SBP reactions. Impatience and unfriendly-friendly were main predictors and, together with the subscale for competitiveness and motoric restlessness, accounted for nearly 32% of the variance of maximal SBP responses. The scale unfriendly-friendly improved the prediction of mean and maximal DBP responses by about 10% and, together with the factors age, DBP at rest, weight, and the subscale for competitiveness (the latter affecting only mean DBP responses), accounted for about 39% and 36% respectively of the variance. Together with HR at rest, impatience and motoric restlessness accounted for 30% of the variance of mean HR reactions during the RTT; sex was an additional predictor for maximal HR reactions, accounting altogether for 28% of the variance, with girls exhibiting the most pronounced HR responses. When performance parameters were additionally introduced into stepwise multiple regression analyses, they did not predict cardiovascular reactions.

These results indicate that observations of children's momentary behaviors can predict their cardiovascular responses even better than teachers' type A/B classification. To further substantiate this hypothesis, a number of various tasks should be investigated with trained observers who are unaware of the test subjects' cardiovascular responses.

Discussion

The German version of the MYTH appears to be a reliable, internally consistent measure of children's type A behavior. Factor analysis of the German MYTH items revealed three components of the TABP: impatience, competitiveness, and dominance. The first two factors correspond very well with the two factors Matthews found in her original MYTH-Form O which reflect competitive achievement-striving and impatience-aggression (Matthews and Angulo 1980). As Matthews noted, these factors bear some resemblance to factors H (hard-driving competitiveness) and S (speed and impatience) in the Jenkins Activity Survey. The assessment of inter-rater reliability was impeded by the fact that each class usually has only one teacher; only in a few classes did a second teacher sometimes teach a special subject for 1 or more h per week. Although these teachers were less certain in their judgment, with few exceptions, mainly with regard to the competitiveness subscale, most of the correlation coefficients are quite good. Test-retest reliability indicates that the MYTH-assessed TABP and its three subscales are stable behavioral characteristics, at least for up to 6 months.

In this German sample, substantial gender differences in mean type A scores emerged, which is in agreement with Matthews' data: Both the American and German MYTH norms for boys and girls are very similar. In adulthood, the TABP also appears to be more prevalent among males than among females (Waldron 1978). Our results support once more the hypothesis that behavioral gender differences in adulthood have an early beginning in childhood.

Observation of the children's actual behavior during the experiment provides further evidence for behavioral differences between boys and girls, as boys were scored by both observers as being more impatient, engaged, and ambitious. However, this might also partly be due to the kind of tasks we used, as especially the VG appeared to us to be more challenging for boys than for girls. These behavioral gender differences, however, are in concordance with previous findings that boys are more competitive and aggressive than girls (Maccoby and Jacklin 1974; Matthews and Angulo 1980).

MYTH-assessed TABP correlates significantly and moderately with impatience and engagement during the tasks, as well as with ambition and extraversion, as shown during the whole experiment. Moreover, significant differences between type A and B children can be demonstrated in these observed behaviors. Although this supports our assumption that elements of type A behavior can be scored reliably during short-term behavioral observations, the teachers' judgment cannot be replaced by these ratings. As others have shown, different assessment techniques of the TABP in children and adults correlate only moderately; this can be seen when comparing the Adolescent Structured Interview and the MYTH (Matthews and Jennings 1984), as well as the Structured Interview and the Jenkins Activity Survey (Matthews 1982; Myrtek 1983). The main purpose of this study, however, was to investigate behavioral factors influencing cardiovascular parameters and responses in children, and both measures of type A behavior, MYTH and behavioral ratings during the experiment, were significantly related predominantly to BP reactions.

At rest, weight was the most important predictor of SBP and the only predictor of DBP, explaining 21% and 26% of the variance respectively. As expected, the TABP did not predict BP or HR at rest, but compared with girls, boys exhibited an elevated SBP, which was also observed during all periods of the experiment. These results are in agreement with those of several epidemiologic studies, not only of adults but also of children (Laaser and Schütt 1978; Lauer et al. 1975; Voors et al. 1976), in which body weight was found to be an important factor determining BP and in which a higher SBP was also seen in boys. It was also only in boys that we found behavioral correlates of cardiovascular parameters during rest periods: Higher scores of physical rest were related to lower HRs, whereas active behaviors such as exploratory behavior, contact seeking, and speech activity correlated positively with elevated HRs. This gender-related difference between observed behaviors and their relation to cardiovascular parameters might also partly have to do with the fact that scoring the boys' behavior seemed to be easier for both observers, male and female, although the reason for that remains obscure.

During the VG and to some extent during the RTT as well, boys exhibited elevated SBP responses. During both tasks, they were seen to be more engaged and impatient; both these behaviors correlated positively with elevated BP and pronounced SBP and DBP reactions during the first task. During the second task, only boys' impatience was related to elevated SBP reactions. These results indicate that SBP reactivity is enhanced in boys, although it has to be considered that this might be a task-specific effect. Being male is a risk factor for coronary heart disease, and perhaps such task- or stimulus-specific cardiovascular hyperreactivity in males does contribute to this elevated coronary risk they present.

MYTH-assessed TABP was related to elevated BP reactions during both tasks. Although the TABP is only marginally significant in the ANOVA, stepwise multiple regression analysis shows that the TABP, along with the factors sex, SBP at rest, and height, predicts mean SBP reactions during the VG, accounting for about 21% of the variance of SBP reactions, with each single factor explaining about 4%-6% of the variance. The most pronounced SBP reactions during the VG are seen in tall type A boys with low SBP at rest, but type A girls also show somewhat enhanced SBP reactions during this task. However, when the ratings of the behaviors observed during the experiment were introduced, only tension, unfriendliness-friendliness, and extraversion-introversion predicted SBP reactions. During the RTT, type A children also exhibited marginally significant greater maximal SBP responses, as shown by the ANOVA results, but in multiple regression analyses, only the subscale for competitiveness predicted maximal SBP responses. When behavioral ratings were included, tension, unfriendly-friendly, and resignation improved prediction and accounted for 20% of the variance of mean SBP responses, while impatience, unfriendly-friendly, the competitiveness subscale, and motoric restlessness accounted for 32% of the variance of maximal SBP responses.

The TABP also contributes in multiple regression analysis toward explaining about 26% of the variance of DBP reactions during the VG, although DBP at rest and height appear to be more important factors, explaining 8% and 13% of the variance respectively. These results indicate that not only initial values, but also height might be important factors determining the extent of BP reactions in children and should be considered in future investigations. For maximal DBP reactions, the impatience subscale is the most important predictor, which, together with DBP at rest and height, accounts for 24% of the variance. When behavioral ratings were included, impatience and unfriendly-friendly improved prediction and, together with DBP at rest, height, maximal DBP responses, and type A/B status, accounted for 37% of the variance of DBP reactions. However, multiple regression analysis masks another important result, which can clearly be seen by the significant interaction between sex and type A/B status in two-way ANOVA: During the VG, only type A boys exhibit DBP reactions of about 50% greater than those of type B boys or type A and B girls. These behavioral observations support the view that the VG might be a task stimulating DBP reactions mainly in type A boys, who are tense, engaged, impatient, ambitious, and emotionally excited.

During the RTT, there were no significant ANOVA effects seen in DBP responses. In stepwise multiple regression analyses, age, DBP at rest, and weight were predictors of mean and maximal DBP responses explaining 24% and 27% of the variance respectively. The scale unfriendly-friendly improves prediction; this variable, together with the other variables just mentioned and the competitiveness subscale (the latter only for Δ DBP_{max}), account for 39% and 36% of the variance of mean and maximal DBP responses respectively. It remains open why weight is related to DBP reactions during this task independently of DBP at rest. In both tasks, lower BP values at rest were related to more pronounced BP reactions, which is in accordance with Wilder's law of initial values (Wilder 1967); the same is true for HR, which is significant only in the second task.

Age was the most important predictor of DBP reactions during the RTT. This might have been partly due to the fact that older children were better able to cope with this task; i.e., older children presented more correct, but fewer delayed and omitted responses; wrong responses only were not significantly related to age. More correct and fewer omitted responses, however, correlate also significantly and positively with DBP responses (Table 9). Multiple regression analysis did not allow these performance parameters to enter additionally after age, because of their high correlation with this variable (multiple R for correct, delayed, omitted, and wrong responses with age $= 0.67$; $p < 0.001$); this is an example for multicollinearity in multiple regression analysis (Cohen and Cohen 1975). This association of performance and cardiovascular reactivity indicates that one has to pay for better psychomotor performance by an increased level of physiologic arousal, i.e., during the RTT with more pronounced BP responses and during the VG with elevated HR

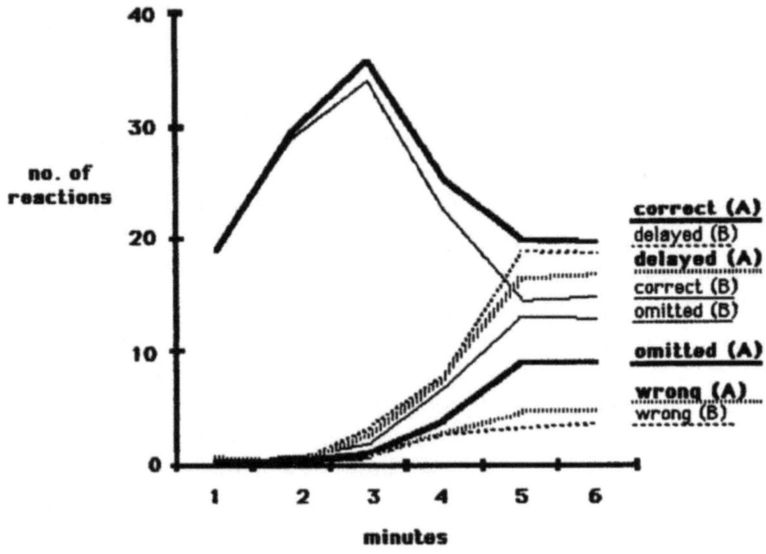

Fig. 5. Psychomotor performance during the multiple choice RTT of 42 type A and 42 type B children at minute intervals

Table 17. Total possible reactions (TPR) and correct (c) and omitted reactions (o) per minute during the multiple choice RTT for 42 type A and 42 type B children at minute intervals; for delayed and wrong reactions, there were no significant differences

Min	TPR		Type A	Type B	*F*	*df*	*p*
1	20	c:	19.05	19.07			
		o:	0.05	0.34	9.10	1,79	0.003
2	30	c:	29.45	28.74	4.95	1,79	0.029
		o:	0.10	0.53	8.07	1,79	0.006
3	40	c:	35.74	33.89			
		o:	0.94	1.93			
4	40	c:	25.40	22.56	3.53	1,79	0.064
		o:	4.00	6.96	7.01	1,79	0.010
5	50	c:	19.90	14.50	5.95	1,79	0.017
		o:	9.08	12.97	5.50	1,79	0.022
6	50	c:	19.56	14.95	3.83	1,79	0.054
		o:	8.98	12.66	6.54	1,79	0.012

reactions. Type A children also exhibit better psychomotor performance during the RTT; that is, they make more correct responses and omit fewer responses. Their BP responses were also more marked during some phases of this task (Fig. 4 a). Better performance has also been seen in some adult type A studies (Frankenhaeuser et al. 1980, 1983; Blumenthal and McKee 1980; MacDougall et al. 1981), although a greater number of studies have not found performance differences (Myrtek 1983). Future studies should identify the dimensions of suitable tasks in which these behavioral characteristics have an effect on performance.

Degree of difficulty during the RTT appears to be related to SBP reactions in a kind of dose-response relationship whereby the SBP reaction curve of type A children is above that of type B children throughout the 6 min of the task. However, only in the 2nd and 3rd min of the RTT and with a medium degree of difficulty is this A/B difference significant. This supports Dembroski's hypothesis that type A/B differences in cardiovascular reactivity might be evoked by stimuli of medium intensity, whereas too weak challenges stimulate neither type A a nor type B individuals enough, and too strong stimuli trigger maximal reactions in type A and B persons (Dembroski et al. 1979). DBP reactions also increase in a dose-response relationship, together with the degree of task difficulty, but only in type B children, while the DBP of type A children appears to be raised nearly to its maximum from the very beginning of this task; this results in significant A/B differences during the 1st and 2nd min of the task.

Up to the 3rd min, both type A and type B children could cope with the task very well, as can be seen in Fig. 5, but in the 4th min, when accoustic stimuli are added, the number of correct responses decreases dramatically to nearly half of the total possible reactions, although the speed of presentation is not increased further. When the speed is increased to 50 stimuli per minute during the last 2 min of the task, both type A and type B children make fewer than even half of the total possible responses. With the exception of the 3rd min, type A children omitted from the 1st min onward significantly fewer responses and already during the 2nd min exhibited more correct responses (Table 17); this was also true during the 5th min whereas such differences were marginally significant during the 4th and 6th min.

During the last 2 min of the RTT, type B children showed nearly as many omitted as correct responses (*upper and lower thin solid lines* in Fig. 5), whereas type A children exhibited more than twice as many correct as omitted responses *(upper and lower thick solid lines);* moreover, in type B children, delayed responses *(upper thin dotted line)* exceeded correct responses, while type A children still showed more correct than delayed responses *(upper thick dotted line).* This indicates that better psychomotor performance is most pronounced in type A children during the last 2 min but that during this time BP responses do not differ markedly. DBP reactions are very similar in type A and B children; SBP reactions are just marginally significant only in the 6th min and somewhat lower in type B children. With regard to cardiovascular responses, however, this signifies better psychomotor performance for type A children during the more difficult part of the RTT without increased physiologic costs.

This means that type A children perform better from the very beginning, when it is easy to cope with the RTT, and this improved performance is related to more pronounced SBP and DBP responses; when the task becomes very difficult to cope with, type B children perform even worse, although their BP responses increase nearly to type A levels. If this can be generalized, type A behavior might be seen as a strategy by which early enhanced physiologic activation guarantees good performance, which, compared with type B behavior, does indeed cost more in easy but not in difficult tasks. If, as we may presume, there are such and even more complex relations between various behaviors, preparatory cardiovascular reactions, and performance, the differing results in the type A literature with regard to physiologic reactivity and performance are not surprising. However, it points to the necessity of more sophisticated approaches for the investigation of these relationships. For instance, continuous noninvasive BP recording, which is available today (see Wesseling et al., this volume), would allow a closer and more accurate comparison of behavioral and performance parameters with cardiovascular responses.

Most of the present findings are, however, in agreement with other studies of children (Matthews and Jennings 1984; Lundberg 1983; Lawler et al. 1981), adolescents (Siegel et al. 1983) and adults (Matthews 1982; Krantz and Manuck 1984; Myrtek 1983, 1984) demonstrating more pronounced SBP responses in type A individuals; this appears to be the most reliable cardiovascular response reported in the type A literature. Similarly to our results, Matthews and Jennings also found greater DBP elevations in type A boys aged 9-12 years when they played a competitive VG against the computer; differences in DBP responses, however, were only seen when TABP was assessed with the Adolescent Structured Interview. Lawler and coworkers and Matthews and Jennings were also able to find enhanced HR responses in type A children, whereas in our investigation during the RTT, HR responses were elevated in type B children. This adverse A/B effect, however, was due to nonsignificant HR differences at rest, which is revealed by the results of multiple regression analysis. Unexpectedly, Matthews and Jennings also found the lowest HR during a difficult mental arithmetic task in type A children, and this finding is not without precedent in the adult literature (Diamond et al. 1984).

The study findings provide the first data from a sample of German children regarding the association between the TABP, together with other related behavioral components, and BP responses. At least among boys, the extent of their competitiveness, impatience, tension, engagement, and ambition is related to enhanced BP responses. However, those circumstances which together with these behaviors elicit enhanced cardiovascular responses still have to be specified. Competition stimulated by the experimenter might be one factor, task difficulty another. There might also be more appropriate tasks for studying individual differences of behaviorally induced cardiovascular responses in female subjects. Future research should identify the dimensions of the environment which elicit enhanced cardiovascular reactions from type A individuals, both male and female. Our results, however, also indicate that a broad spectrum of various behavioral characteristics can be specified which predict cardiovascular reactivity even better than the simple type A/B classification, and these behaviors need further investigation.

Although there are doubts about global TABP in its present form being a risk factor for the development of coronary heart disease (see Shekelle et al., Kittel, and Appels et al., this volume), some of its core elements, such as hostility, aggression, and anger, are still thought to elevate cardiovascular risk, as demonstrated in prospective (Shekelle et al. 1983; Barefoot et al. 1983; Haynes et al. 1980) and case control studies (Dembroski et al. 1985; MacDougall et al. 1985; Williams et al. 1980, 1983). The most prominent hypothesis is that enhanced neuroendocrine and cardiovascular reactions might be one of the mediators between such behaviors and future disease. Atherosclerosis seems to have its roots in childhood or adolescence. At present, it is not known to what extent behaviorally induced enhanced cardiovascular responses in children can contribute to this process. Cardiovascular reactivity, however, appears to be a stable individual difference variable already visible in childhood (Obrist 1981; Giordani et al. 1981; Glass et al., to be published; Manuck and Garland 1980). As Matthews and Jennings also conclude in their study, we can state that, to the extent that physiologic reactivity does enhance coronary risk, the present findings suggest that elements of the TABP may begin to exert their pathogenic influence early in life.

Summary

The German version of the MYTH appears to be a reliable, stable, and internally consistent measure of type A behavior in children. As in American children, type A behavior observed in German elementary school children from 6 to 11 years show substantial gender differences. Boys are seen by their teachers as being more impatient, aggressive, competitive, dominant, and ambitious. Compared with girls, SBP at rest is elevated in boys, whereas DBP and HR do not differ. Weight is the main predictor of SBP and DBP in boys and girls. During a competitive VG and during a multiple choice RTT, boys seem to be more engaged and impatient, and they exhibit somewhat enhanced SBP responses.

The TABP is not related to BP and HR at rest, but it is significantly associated with SBP and DBP responses during both tasks. During the VG, DBP reactions are most pronounced in type A boys, but there are no gender or type A/B differences seen in the average scores in the games; better performance, however, is related to elevated HR responses. During the RTT, better psychomotor performance is related to enhanced BP responses, and type A children perform better. An easy-to-medium degree of task difficulty stimulates SBP and DBP responses mainly in type A children, whereas the BP of type B children increases to type A levels during the more difficult part of the task, although the children perform less well. Components of the TABP observed during the experiment, such as tension, impatience, engagement, emotional excitement, and ambition, are also related to enhanced BP responses, but mainly in boys. The question arises of whether such behavior-related and pronounced cardiovascular responses start to contribute to the elevated coronary risk of male individuals already at this young age. A friendly child, however, whether boy or girl, may be somewhat protected from pronounced BP responses.

Acknowledgements. The authors should like to express their thanks to Dr. Karen Matthews for her stimulating help and advice which made this study possible. We should also like to thank the children participating in the study and their parents; our special thanks go to all the teachers who laid the groundwork for this study through their conscientious recording of the children's behavior and especially to

G. Kraft and W. Leßmann, the directors of the two public elementary schools where the psychophysiologic investigations were carried out (*Gemeinschaftsgrundschule* in Cologne, Freiligrathstraße, and in Quadrat-Ichendorf), for their support and assistance in this study. We should like to express our particular thanks to D. Wippermann for her skillful organizational assistance. For the statistical analysis, we should like to thank Dr. Dipl. math. H. Lüpsen of the Computer Center, University of Cologne. The preparation of this manuscript was greatly facilitated by the untiring support of Hazel Schmidt.

Appendix

Items of the German Version of the MYTH and Factor Loadings after Orthogonal Varimax Rotation

Item	Factor 1	Factor 2	Factor 3
1. Wenn dieses Kind spielt, versucht es immer zu gewinnen.	0.473	0.491	0.485
2. Dieses Kind arbeitet eher schnell und energisch als langsam und gemächlich.	−0.048	0.717	0.291
3. Dieses Kind wird ungeduldig, wenn es auf andere warten muß.	0.659	0.480	0.131
4. Dieses Kind erledigt viele Dinge in Eile.	0.332	0.681	0.188
5. Bis dieses Kind sich über seine Spielkameraden ärgert, muß schon viel passieren.	0.729	0.169	0.147
6. Dieses Kind unterbricht andere.	0.742	0.191	0.327
7. Dieses Kind ist bei vielen Tätigkeiten Anführer.	0.240	0.208	0.862
8. Dieses Kind reagiert schnell gereizt.	0.819	0.248	0.183
9. Wenn dieses Kind mit anderen im Wettbewerb steht, leistet es mehr als gewöhnlich.	0.105	0.623	0.350
10. Dieses Kind argumentiert oder debattiert gerne.	0.167	0.295	0.711
11. Dieses Kind ist geduldig, wenn es mit anderen spielt, die langsamer sind.	0.745	0.233	0.017
12. Dieses Kind versucht beim Arbeiten oder Spielen alles besser als andere Kinder zu machen.	0.304	0.716	0.321
13. Dieses Kind kann lange still sitzen.	0.768	−0.030	0.192
14. Bei Spielen oder Schularbeiten ist es für dieses Kind wichtiger, möglichst Bester zu sein, als daran Spaß zu haben.	0.224	0.766	−0.044

Item	Factor 1	Factor 2	Factor 3
15. Dieses Kind wird von anderen Kindern als Anführer angesehen.	0.135	0.202	0.869
16. Dieses Kind möchte immer Erster sein.	0.404	0.641	0.383
17. Dieses Kind gerät leicht in Streitereien.	0.835	0.184	0.089

References

Barefoot JC, Dahlstrom G, Williams RB (1983) Hostility, CHD incidence, and total mortality: A 25-year follow-up study of 255 physicians. Psychosom Med 45: 59-63

Blumenthal JA, McKee DC (1980) Task incentives, type A behavior pattern, and verbal problem solving performance. J Appl Soc Psychol 10: 101-114

Carver CS, Coleman AE, Glass DC (1976) The coronary prone behavior pattern and the suppression of fatigue on a treadmill test. J Pers Soc Psychol 33: 460-466

Cohen J, Cohen P (1975) Applied multiple regression/correlation analysis for the behavioral sciences. John Wiley, New York

Dembroski TM, MacDougall JM, Herd JA, Shields JL (1979) Effects of level of challenge on pressor and heart rate responses in type A and B subjects. J Appl Soc Psychol 9: 209-228

Dembroski TM, MacDougall JM, Williams RB, Haney TL, Blumenthal JA (1985) Components of type A, hostility and anger: Relationship to angiographic findings. Psychosom Med 47 (3): 219-233

Diamond EL, Schneiderman N, Schwartz D, Smith JC, Vorp R, Pasin RD (1984) Harrassment, hostility, and type A as determinants of cardiovascular reactivity during competition. J Beh Med 7: 171-189

Enos WF Jr, Beyer JC, Holmes RH (1955) Pathogenesis of coronary disease in American soldiers killed in Korea. JAMA 158: 912

Eschweiler J (1986) Psychophysiologische Untersuchungen zum Typ-A-Verhalten bei Kindern. MD Dissertation, University of Cologne

Frankenhaeuser M (1983) The sympathetic-adrenal and pituitary-adrenal response to challenge: Comparison between the sexes. In: Dembroski TM, Schmidt TH, Blümchen G (eds) Biobehavioral bases of coronary heart disease. Karger, Basel, pp 91-105

Frankenhaeuser M, Lundberg U, Forsman L (1980) Dissociation between sympathetic-adrenal and pituitary-adrenal responses to an achievement situation characterized by high controllability: Comparison between type A and type B males and females. Biol Psychol 10: 79-91

Giordani B, Manuck SB, Farmer JK (1981) Stability of behaviorally induced heart rate changes in children after one week. Child Dev 52: 533-537

Glass DC (1977) Behavior pattern, stress and coronary disease. Lawrence Erlbaum, Hillsdale, NJ

Glass DC, Lake CR, Contrada RJ, Kehoe K, Erlanger LR (to be published) Stability of individual differences in physiologic responses to stress. J Health Psychol

Haynes SG, Feinleib M, Kannel WB (1980) The relationship of psychosocial factors to coronary heart disease in the Framingham study. III. Eight-year incidence of coronary heart disease. Am J Epidemiol 3 (1): 37-58

Hirsch EZ, Maksem JA, Gagen D (1984) Effects of stress and propranol on the aortic intima of rats. Arteriosclerosis 4: 526

Krantz DS, Manuck SB (1984) Acute psychophysiologic reactivity and risk of cardiovascular disease: A review and methodologic critique. Psychol Bull 96: 435-464

Laaser U, Schütt A (1978) The cardiovascular risk-profile of adolescents in Cologne: A representative study including 6302 pupils. Z Kardiol 67: 837-846

Lauer R, Connor W, Leaverton P, Reiter M, Clarke W (1975) Coronary heart disease risk factors in school children: The Muscatine study. J Pediatr 86: 697-706

Lawler K, Allen M, Critcher E, Standard B (1981) The relationship of physiological responses to the coronary-prone behavior pattern in children. J Behav Med 4: 203-216
Lundberg U (1983) Note on type A behavior and cardiovascular responses to challenge in 3-6-year-old children. J Psychosom Res 27: 39-42
MacDougall JM, Dembroski TM, Krantz DS (1981) Effects of types of challenge on pressor and heart rate responses in type A and B women. Psychophysiology 18: 1-9
MacDougall JM, Dembroski TM, Dimsdale JE, Hackett TP (1985) Components of type A, hostility, and anger in further relationships to angiographic findings. Health Psychol 4 (2): 137-152
Maccoby EE, Jacklin CN (1974) The psychology of sex differences. Stanford University Press, Stanford, CA
Manuck SB, Garland FN (1980) Stability of individual differences in cardiovascular reactivity: A thirteen-month follow-up. Physiol Behav 24: 621-624
Matthews KA (1979) Efforts to control by children and adults with the type A coronary prone behavior pattern. Child Dev 50: 842-847
Matthews KA (1983) Assessment issues in coronary-prone behavior. In: Dembroski TM, Schmidt TH, Blümchen G (eds) Biobehavioral bases of coronary heart disease. Karger, Basel, pp 62-78
Matthews KA (1982) Psychological perspectives on the type A behavior pattern. Psychol Bull 91: 293-323
Matthews KA, Angulo J (1980) Measurement of the type A behavior pattern in children: Assessment of children's competitiveness, impatience-anger, and aggression. Child Dev 51: 466-475
Matthews KA, Volkin JI (1981) Efforts to excel and the type A behavior pattern in children. Child Dev 52: 1283-1289
Matthews KA, Siegel JM (1983) Type A behaviors by children, social comparison and standards for self-evaluation. Dev Psychol 19: 135-140
Matthews KA, Jennings JR (1984) Cardiovascular responses of boys exhibiting the type A behavior pattern. Psychosom Med 46: 484-497
McNamara SS, Molot MA, Stremple JF, Cutting RT (1971) Coronary artery disease in combat casualties in Vietnam. JAMA 216: 1185-1187
Myrtek M (1983) Typ-A-Verhalten: Untersuchungen und Literaturanalysen unter besonderer Berücksichtigung der psychophysiologischen Grundlagen (Research report of the research group on psychophysiology, Freiburg). Minerva, Munich
Myrtek M, Greenlee MW (1984) Psychophysiology of type A behavior pattern: A critical analysis. J Psychosom Res 28 (6): 455-466
Newman WP, Freedman DS, Voors AW, Gard PD, Frinivasan SR, Cresanta YL, Williamson GD, Webber LS, Berenson GS (1986) Relation of serum lipoprotein levels and systolic blood pressure to early atherosclerosis: The Bogalusa heart study. N Engl J Med 314: 138-144
Obrist PA (1981) Cardiovascular psychophysiology: A perspective. Plenum, New York
Paffenbarger RS, Wing AL (1967) Characteristics in youth predisposing to fatal stroke in later years. Lancet 1: 753
Ross R, Glomset JA (1976) The pathogenesis of atherosclerosis, (II). N Engl J Med 295: 420
Shekelle RB, Gayle M, Ostfeld AM, Paul O (1983) Hostility, risk or coronary heart disease, and mortality. Psychosom Med 45: 109-114
Schmidt TH (1983) Cardiovascular reactions and cardiovascular risk. In: Dembroski TM, Schmidt TH, Blümchen G (eds) Biobehavioral bases of coronary heart disease. Karger, Basel, pp 130-174
Schmidt TH, Dembroski TM, MacDougall JM, Leidig P, Eschweiler J, Thierse H, Schug S (1985 a) Various perspectives on cardiovascular reactivity and the type A behavior pattern. In: Orlebeke JF, Mulder G, van Doornen LJP (eds) Psychophysiology of Cardiovascular Control. Plenum, New York, pp 745-766
Schmidt TH, Rüddel H, Langosch W, Undeutsch K, Neus H, Hahn R, Dembroski TM, MacDougall JM (1985 b) Psychophysiologische Untersuchung zum Typ-A-Verhalten und seine Beziehung zu traditionellen kardiovaskulären Risikofaktoren bei Polizeibeamten aus dem Raum Köln. In: Langosch W (ed) Psychische Bewältigung der chronischen Herzerkrankung. Springer, Berlin Heidelberg New York Tokyo, pp 79-113
Siegel JM, Matthews KA, Leitch CJ (1983) Blood pressure variability and the type A behavior pattern in adolescence. J Psychosom Res 27: 265-272

Suls J, Becker MA, Mullen B (1981) Coronary-prone behavior, social insecurity, and stress among college-aged adults. J Human Stress 7: 27-34

Voors A, Foster T, Frerichs R, Webber L, Berenson G (1976) Studies of blood pressures in children, ages 5-14 years, in a total biracial community: The Bogalusa heart study. Circulation 54: 319-327

Waldron J (1978) Sex differences in the coronary-prone behavior pattern. In: Dembroski T, Weiss S, Shields J, Haynes S, Feinleib M (eds) Coronary-prone behavior. Springer, Berlin Heidelberg New York, pp 199-205

Wilder J (1967) Stimulus and response: The law of initial value. Bristol, Wright

Williams RB (1983) Behavioral correlates of angiographic findings. In: Dembroski TM, Schmidt TH, Blümchen G (eds) Biobehavioral bases of coronary heart disease. Karger, Basel, pp 39-54

Williams RB, Haney TL, Lee KL, Kong Y, Blumenthal JA, Whalen RE (1980) Type A behavior, hostility, and atherosclerosis. Psychosom Med 42: 539-549

Familial Aspects of the Type A Behavior Pattern and Physiologic Reactivity to Stress

K. A. Matthews and C. J. Rakaczky[1]

Introduction

It has become increasingly clear that familial factors play an important role in the etiology and course of coronary heart disease (CHD). First-degree relatives of patients with CHD are at elevated risk for a coronary event (Slack and Evans 1966). In the Western Collaborative Group Study (WCGS), men who were 39-49 years old at study onset and had a family history of CHD were at elevated risk for CHD during the 8½-year follow-up period (Rosenman et al. 1975). Although the mechanisms by which family history of CHD exerts its pathogenic influence are not entirely clear, they are likely to be due in part to basic morphological features of the coronary arteries present at birth, which provide the foundation for subsequent development of atherosclerosis (see Neufeld and Blieden 1978). They are also likely to be due to familial clustering of major risk factors for CHD and their associated pathophysiological processes. For example, blood pressure levels of biologically related parents and children correlate between 0.28 and 0.37 in various studies, whereas the blood pressure levels of parents and adopted children do not correlate significantly (Feinleib et al. 1980). Part of the familial clustering of blood pressure, at least in adulthood, appears to be due to the familial clustering of another risk factor, obesity (e.g., Carney et al. 1976). Cholesterol levels and diabetes also appear to aggregate in the family (e.g., Sing et al. 1980). Furthermore, life-style factors that influence health, such as diet preferences, exercise habits, and smoking, are clearly behaviors that result from the attitudes, role models, and social milieu to which persons are exposed in early family life.

The major purpose of this paper is to review comprehensively what is known about the contribution of familial factors to another important risk factor for CHD, the Type A coronary-prone behavior pattern. Type A behavior is characterized by extremes of aggressiveness, vigorous voice stylistics, easily aroused hostility, and a chronic sense of time urgency. It is related to approximately a twofold risk for CHD, controlling statistically for the effects of the other major risk factors (Rosenman et al. 1975). Because Type A is an independent risk factor, it is thought to exert its pathogenic influence via mechanisms other than the standard risk factors. The current major hypothesis is that Type A individuals respond to daily challenges and stresses which they confront with a heightened sympathetic activation, and this physiological pattern accounts for their elevated risk. Indeed, such reactivity does seem to characterize the Type A individual's style of interacting with the environment (see Matthews 1982 and Houston 1983, for reviews). Given the relationships

1 Department of Psychiatry, University of Pittsburgh, 3811 O'Hara Street, Pittsburgh, PA 15213, USA

Biological and Psychological Factors
in Cardiovascular Disease
Ed. by T. H. Schmidt, T. M. Dembroski, and G. Blümchen

proposed among Type A, sympathetic reactivity, and coronary risk (see Krantz and Manuck 1984, for a review), this paper also reviews what is known about familial aspects of physiological responses to stress. That is the starting point of this paper.

Physiological Reactivity to Stress

Twin Studies

A basic question in understanding the familial contributions to physiological reactivity to stress is whether or not it has an inherited base. There are solid data suggesting genetic components of individual differences in basal or resting levels of sympathetic-related processes such as blood pressure. Are there, however, genetic contributions to individual differences in responses to psychological or physical stressors? The first study addressing this question was reported in 1968 by Shapiro and his colleagues. The neuroendocrine and cardiovascular responses of 12 monozygotic (MZ) and 12 dizygotic (DZ) twin pairs were measured before and after performing the Stroop Color Naming Task and experiencing ischemic arm pain. Analyses showed a greater resemblance within MZ twin pairs than within DZ twin pairs in the pressor response after ischemic arm pain, but not in the other measures.

To our knowledge, the only other investigation of genetic contributions to physiological reactivity was conducted by Rose et al. (1982a, b).[2] They evaluated the cardiovascular responses of 239 pairs of normotensive adolescents and young adults. The sample included 111 pairs of MZ twins, 66 pairs of DZ twins, and 54 unrelated individuals; their age range was 14-33 years. Participants completed five tasks interspaced with a relaxation/recovery period. The tasks included three "psychological" stressors: serial subtraction, the Stroop Color Naming Task, and tracing a star using the star's mirror image; and two "physical" stressors: isometric hand grip, and cold pressor. Preliminary data analyses from the project have been presented at the American Heart Association meetings and show a greater resemblance in blood pressure response to the stressors within MZ twin pairs than within DZ twin pairs, who, in turn, are more similar than unrelated pairs. Such a pattern is consistent with a genetic hypothesis. An interesting observation made by Rose et al. is that the evidence for a genetic component appears stronger for pressor responses to stress than for pressor levels prior to the presentation of the stressor.

Further studies of the ambulatory blood pressure of the same and additional twin pairs have been completed and also reported at the American Heart Association meetings (Rose et al. 1983). Analyses thus far show that systolic blood pressure lability is stable over time in the twins and that measures of ambulatory systolic blood pressure lability, controlling for level, are more concordant for MZ pairs than for DZ pairs, who, in turn, are more concordant than unrelated pairs. Should this pattern of findings be supported by additional analyses, they strongly suggest a genetic component to individual differences in pressor responses to stress.

2 Several additional articles have been published or come to our attention since this paper was written in early 1984.

Familial History of Cardiovascular Disease

Another basic question to be addressed in order to understand familial factors in physiological reactivity is whether or not "reactive" parents have offspring who are reactive because of modeling, specific childrearing practices, genetic influences, or some combination thereof. Unfortunately, there are no data bearing directly on this question. However, if one assumes that hypertensives are reactive to stress, and there are strong data suggesting they are (e.g., Goldstein 1983), then studies concerning the reactivity of offspring of hypertensive parents are pertinent here.

Table 1 summarizes the results of 27 studies in the existing literature (through spring 1984) concerning the physiological responses of persons with a family history of cardiovascular diseases. The first column lists author(s) and year of publication; the complete reference can be found in the list at the end of this paper. The second column describes the subject characteristics and how family history of cardiovascular disease was defined and verified. The third and fourth columns indicate the measures of behavior and psychological states, and the tasks and performance on those tasks respectively. The last two columns list the physiological measures and the results from analyses of those measures.

A careful review of this table shows that a wide variety of participants were studied: pregnant women, office workers, elementary school-aged children, and undergraduates. Moreover, diverse stressors were used, ranging from the immersion of the hand or foot in cold water, through serial subtraction to ingestion of caffeine; and diverse physiological indicators were employed, ranging from blood pressure to catecholamines and renal blood flow, although the majority measured only blood pressure and heart rate. Twenty-four studies included only persons with a family history of hypertension, whereas three considered persons with any cardiovascular disease, most typically hypertension, CHD, and stroke. A common problem with the studies is that very few verified the family history of disease; i.e., the report of the child was taken as a sufficient indicator of disease. Nonetheless, the results of these studies are most instructive.

Of the 27 studies, 19 (70%) found clear evidence that those with a family history of cardiovascular disease showed greater levels of blood pressure, heart rate, or plasma renin activity than those without a family history of cardiovascular disease during the challenge of performing both physically and psychologically demanding tasks. In those studies in which the data are analyzed controlling for basal levels, it still appears that healthy persons with a family history of cardiovascular disease show a greater physiological response to stress than persons without a family history of cardiovascular disease.

One of the 19 studies is particularly informative because it measured catecholamines in addition to blood pressure and heart rate; it included a hypertensive comparison group; and it verified the parental history of high blood pressure through health records (Falkner et al. 1979). In addition to showing the above pattern for blood pressure in this investigation of 75 adolescents, the catecholamine results showed that normotensives with a family history of hypertension and hypertensives had greater catecholamine responses to the stress of performing mental arithmetic than did normotensives without a family history of hypertension.

Table 1. Physiologic responses to stress in persons with and without a family history of cardiovascular disease

Reference	Subjects/family history definition	Behavioral measures	Tasks/outcomes	Physiological measures	Physiological results
Dieckmann and Michel (1935)	173 women, no ages given. 70 were not pregnant; 31 were pregnant with no complications due to elevated BP; 72 were pregnant with complications of toxemia, preeclampsia, or eclampsia, but these data were not presented./ Hypertension in at least 1 parent was reported by 13 of the 31 pregnant women with no complications and in 28 of the 70 nonpregnant women	None	Cold pressor. (testing month for pregnant women not given)	BP: TYCOS aneroid sphygmomanometer	In nonpregnant women with FH: mean Δ SBP=35.5 mmHg; and mean Δ DBP=34.5 mmHg. In nonpregnant women without FH: mean Δ SBP=18.7 mmHg; and mean Δ DBP=23.3 mmHg. In pregnant women with FH: mean Δ SBP=35.4 mmHg; and mean Δ DBP=26.1 mmHg. In pregnant women without FH: mean Δ SBP=19.6 mmHg; and mean Δ DBP=19.8 mmHg. No significance tests presented
Hines and Brown (1936)	288 normotensives who show minimal pressor response, aged 4-86; 90 normotensives who show BP increases of 22 mmHg, aged 4-15; 193 hypertensives, aged 24-64. Both sexes included but not identified	None	Cold pressor	BP: method not reported	87% of hyperreactive normotensives and 14% of nonhyperreactive normotensives report a FH of hypertension. Hypertensives have a strong pressor response. No significance tests presented
Briggs and Oerting (1937)	233 pregnant women, aged 16-40; 137 multiparas and 96 primaparas. / Hypertension in 2 parents was reported by 10 *Ss*. Hypertension in 1 parent was reported by 44 *Ss*. Verified by parental BP measured in clinic when possible	None	Cold pressor administered between 4 and 9 months of gestation	BP: method not reported	No criteria given for reactivity assessment. All 10 *Ss* with FH in 2 parents were hyperreactive; of 44 *Ss* with FH in one parent, 13 were hyperreactive; of the remaining 179, 2 were hyperreactive. No significance tests presented
Chesley and Chesley (1939)	517 pregnant women during the 3rd and 4th month of gestation. / Cardiovascular disease or diabetes was reported in the parents of 208 *Ss*	None	Cold pressor administered at 4 months gestation	BP: method not reported; 4th phase DBP used	FH *Ss* did not differ in BP during baseline or task compared to those *Ss* reporting no FH
Feldt and Wenstrand (1942)	260 male and 90 female normotensive office workers; mean age=37, range 21-67. / Hypertension in at least one parent was reported by 96 *Ss*	None	Cold pressor	BP: method not reported	Hyperreactors were those 80 men and 24 women with largest BP response: mean Δ SBP=27.7 mmHg; and mean Δ DBP=24.4 mmHg; 29% had a FH. Hyporeactors were those 180 men and 66 women with smaller BP responses: mean Δ SBP=11.4 mmHg; and mean Δ DBP=11.9 mmHg; 26% had a FH. No significance tests presented

Δ, difference between baseline and task levels; ACT, general motor activity; CHD, coronary heart disease; DBP, diastolic blood pressure; FBF, forearm blood flow; FPA, finger pulse amplitude; FVR, forearm vascular resistance; FH, family history; HR, heart rate; IBI, inter beat interval; JAS, Jenkins Activity Survey; PEP, pre-ejection period; PRA, plasma renin activity; PTT, pulse transit time; *Ss*, subjects; SBP, systolic blood pressure; SCL, skin conductance level; SCR, skin conductance response; SI, structured interview; SRR, electrodermal activity.

Table 1 (continue)

Reference	Subjects/family history definition	Behavioral measures	Tasks/outcomes	Physiological measures	Physiological results
Russek (1942)	200 normotensives aged 40-69. / 53 reported having at least 1 parent with hypertension	None	Cold pressor	BP: method not reported	Hyperreactors were those 82 *Ss* with largest BP response: mean Δ SBP=32.0 mmHg; and mean Δ DBP=21.5 mmHg; 28% had a FH. Hyporeactors were those 118 *Ss* with smaller BP responses: mean Δ SBP=14.0 mmHg; and mean Δ DBP=10.4 mmHg; 25% had a FH
Brod (1960)	101 normotensives. / 39 reported having at least one parent with hypertension	None	Cold pressor	BP: method not reported	54% of the FH *Ss* had exaggerated BP responses compared to only 11% of the *Ss* without a FH
Remington et al. (1960)	50 children aged 8-18. / At least 1 parent was attending a hypertension clinic. Matched with 50 controls	None	Cold pressor; breath holding; exercise (knee bends)/None reported	BP: standard aneroid sphygmomanometer, 5th phase DBP used. Pulse rate: manually from right wrist	FH *Ss* had higher SBP and lower pulse rate, across all tasks and rest periods, than those *Ss* without a FH. No difference detected for DBP
Shapiro (1961)	50 hypertensives and 36 normotensive males and females. Of the 36 normotensives, 18 were psychiatric patients, and 18 were medical students. / 14 normotensives reported having at least 1 parent, grandparent, or sibling with hypertension	Clyde Mood Scale	Repeated venipuncture because of *Ss* supposed error; cold pressor; Stroop Color Test/ None reported	BP: Gulford Instruments Model 110 Automated BP recorder; mercury measures also taken to verify BP. Pulse rate: cardiotachometer	FH normotensives had larger Δ SBP in all three tasks compared to those normotensive *Ss* without a FH. FH normotensives had larger Δ pulse rate during the venipuncture compared to those normotensive *Ss* without a FH. FH normotensives had higher baseline SBP levels than those normotensive *Ss* without a FH
Falkner et al. (1979)	25 white male, 17 white female, 12 black male, and 21 black female adolescents aged 14-16. / Of the 75, 25 were normotensive with no FH of hypertension; 33 were normotensive with a FH of at least 1 parent having hypertension; 17 had DBP above the 95% for their age and sex and also had at least 1 parent with hypertension. Parental hypertension verified by health records	None	Mental arithmetic./None reported	HR, BP: Arteriosonde; Plasma catecholamines: assessed via technique of Von Euler and Lishajko	FH normotensives had larger Δ DBPs and Δ HRs than the group without a FH. FH normotensives had larger Δ catecholamines than the group without a FH. FH normotensives had larger DBP levels during recovery than the group without a FH. No baseline differences in BP, HR, or catecholamines detected
Light and Obrist (1980)	60 undergraduate men, aged 18-29. 29 had casual SBP> 135 mmHg. / Parents verified FH. No breakdown of FH of hypertension group given	None	Cold pressor; erotic film; shock avoidance./None reported	HR: cardiotachometer; BP: Korotkoff-detecting microphone verified by direct measures of BP	Normotensive *Ss* were divided into two groups on the basis of the median of Δ HR. The range of Δ HR for low HR responders was 2-33 bpm and the range of Δ HR for the high HR responders was 34-69 bpm. Of those *Ss* classified as high HR responders, 30% had a FH. Of those *Ss* classified as low HR responders, only 6% had a FH. Of those *Ss* having casual SBP> 135 mmHg and who were classified as high HR responders, 57% had a FH, and of those classified as low HR responders, only 9% had a FH

Table 1 (continue)

Reference	Subjects/family history definition	Behavioral measures	Tasks/outcomes	Physiological measures	Physiological results
Warren and Fischbein (1980)	166 children aged 5 and 5 attending a regularly scheduled pediatric checkup. Of the 166, 91 were boys and 13 were black. / 18 children had a hypertensive father; 21 had a hypertensive mother; and 8 had both parents hypertensive. Parents verified FH	None	Regularly scheduled DPT booster, BP assessed before and immediately after shot	BP: no method reported	*Ss* with FH in 2 parents or in father had higher SBP and DBP after shot than *Ss* without a FH. *Ss* with a FH in mother did not differ in BP from those *Ss* without a FH. Preshot levels not compared
Collins et al. (1981)	53 children aged 8-13. / 26 had hypertensive fathers	None	Reaction time to white noise stimulus./None reported	HR, PTT, FPA, and SRR: method not reported	FH *Ss* had increases in HR. *Ss* without a FH had decreases in HR. FH *Ss* had shorter PTT, than those without a FH. FH *Ss* also habituated in their PTT shortening across trials while those *Ss* without a FH did not. FH *Ss* were more reactive on SRR than those *Ss* without a FH across all trials
Hollenberg et al. (1981)	24 normotensives who were potential kidney donors aged 22-66 years and 15 hypertensive patients aged 22-65 years. / 8 of the normotensives reported having at least 1 parent with hypertension	None	Slide presentations where *Ss* had to verbally identify optical illusions; Raven's Progressive Matrices, a nonverbal IQ test./None reported	BP: arterial via Statham P23 DC transducer connected to a catheter and recorded on a Electronics in Medicine polygraph. Urography, selective renal arteriography, and renal blood flow assessed by the Xenon washout technique. PRA, plasma angiotensin II, aldosterone, and cortisol were assayed by radioimmunoassay. Plasma and urine creatine, sodium, and potassium were assessed by the autoanalytic method	Normotensive *Ss* without a FH had increases in renal blood flow during stress while normotensive *Ss* with a FH had decreases in renal blood flow. Normotensive *Ss* with a FH had increases in plasma renin activity compared to those normotensive *Ss* without a FH. BP and HR effects not significant
Jorgenson and Houston (1981)	31 female and 27 male undergraduates. / 16 females and 14 males reported hypertension in at least 1 parent. Only nondiabetic parents included in FH group	Taylor Manifest Anxiety Scale and a measure of apprehension during shock avoidance	Stroop Color Task; mental arithmetic; shock avoidance. / FH *Ss* reported more apprehension during shock avoidance; FH females had higher anxiety levels than females without a FH	BP, HR: Narco BioSystems Korotkoff microphone, recorded on Narco physiograph	FH females had higher SBP levels during trials compared to females with no FH. FH *Ss* had higher DBP and HR levels during task compared to *Ss* without a FH. FH *Ss* had less variable Δ DBP than those *Ss* without a FH. No baseline or recovery differences for FH group
Lawler and Allen (1981)	19 boys and 20 girls aged 11-13. / 15 *Ss* had at least one parent with hypertension. Parents verified FH	Bortner Type A Psychomotor Test Battery; MYTH Type A Scale	Reaction time; anagram task/No differences	BP: Arteriosonde. HR: EKG. Skin conductance: via technique described in Lawler (1978)	FH *Ss* had higher SBP levels at baseline and tasks than those *Ss* without a FH. FH *Ss* tended to have larger Δ DBP ($P<0.08$) from baseline to task than those *Ss* without a FH. A/B effects reported elsewhere

Table 1 (continue)

Reference	Subjects/family history definition	Behavioral measures	Tasks/outcomes	Physiological measures	Physiological results
Manuck et al. (1981)	69 undergraduate men aged 17-21. / 20 reported at least 1 parent with hypertension	None	Concept formation/None reported	HR: Grass PTT-6 photoelectric transducer. BP: Standard occluding cuff. All measures recorded on Grass Model 7 polygraph	FH *Ss* had higher SBP levels during task, but not DBP or HR. FH *Ss* who were assessed as high HR reactors (mean Δ HR = 18.3 bpm) had larger SBP levels during task than those *Ss* without a FH who were high HR reactors. No baseline differences for FH were detected for SBP, DBP, and HR
Hastrup et al. (1982)	104 college-aged men. / Hypertension in 2 parents was reported by 9 *Ss*, hypertension for 1 parent was reported by 16 *Ss*	JAS Type A Scale. No differences between FH groups on Type A assessment	Reaction time/ None reported	HR, BP: method not reported	FH *Ss* had higher SBP and HR levels during the task compared to those *Ss* without a FH
Manuck and Proietti (1982)	36 undergraduate men, mean age 19. / 18 reported having at least 1 parent with hypertension, which was confirmed by parent	None	Concept formation; mental arithmetic; isometric handgrip. / No differences detected	HR: Lafayette # 76624 photoelectric transducer recorded on a Datagraph recorder. BP: Dinamap 850	FH *Ss* had higher SBP levels during all tasks than those *Ss* without a FH. FH *Ss* had higher DBP levels during handgrip than those *Ss* without a FH. FH *Ss* had higher HR levels during concept formation and mental arithmetic than those *Ss* without a FH. FH *Ss* who were assessed as high HR reactors (mean Δ HR = 18.4 bpm) had higher SBP levels at baseline than those *Ss* who were high HR reactors without a FH
Newlin and Levenson (1982)	47 undergraduate men aged 18-25. / 23 reported having at least 1 parent with CHD	JAS Type A; Psychomotor Symptomatology Questionnaire (PSQ); FH *Ss* had higher scores on PSQ than *Ss* without a FH. Type A *Ss* had higher scores on PSQ than Type B *Ss*	Reaction time with shock; Stroop Color Test; isometric handgrip. / Type A *Ss* were faster in their reaction times than Type B *Ss*. No differences for FH groups	BP, IBI, PTT, PEP, FPA, SCL, SCR, and ACT: all measures recorded on a Grass Model 7 polygraph	FH *Ss* had higher FPA levels during reaction time and Stroop Color Test than those *Ss* without a FH. Type A *Ss* had larger Δ DBP during all tasks than those *Ss* without a FH. Type A *Ss* had smaller Δ SBP during hand-grip task than those *Ss* without a FH. No baseline differences reported
Williams et al. (1982)	31 undergraduate men, 11 were rated as Type A by both JAS and SI. / Of those 11 assessed as Type A, 7 reported having hypertension or MI in at least one parent. No FH breakdown for Type B *Ss*	JAS Type A; SI Type A	Mental arithmetic; reaction time./None reported	HR, BP: Arteriosonde. FBP, FVR: via venous plethysmography strain gauge. Blood samples obtained to assess catecholamines via radioenzymatic technique. Cortisol, prolactin, and testosterone	Type A *Ss* had larger decreases in FVR, and larger Δ epinephrine, Δ norepinephrine, and Δ cortisol, during mental arithmetic, as compared with Type B *Ss*. Type A *Ss* had larger Δ testosterone during reaction time compared with Type B *Ss*. Type A *Ss* who had a FH had larger Δ cortisol during reaction time than other groups
Allen et al. (1983)	64 undergraduate men aged 17-29. Four were black. / 24 reported having at least 1 parent with hypertension and confirmed by parent	JAS Type A; SI Type A	Cold pressor; isometric handgrip; digit span; reading comprehension. / Type A *Ss* reported putting forth more effort than Type B *Ss*	HR, PTT: Grass Model 7 polygraph. BP: Arteriosonde and verified by standard mercury readings	Type A FH and Type B no FH *Ss* had higher SBP and DBP during baseline and tasks, larger Δ DBP during a face to face confrontation with experimenter, and larger decreases in PTT during hand-grip than Type A no FH and Type B FH *Ss*.

Table 1 (continue)

Reference	Subjects/family history definition	Behavioral measures	Tasks/outcomes	Physiological measures	Physiological results
					FH *Ss* had higher HR during baseline, smaller Δ DBP during reading comprehension, and larger decreases in PTT during digit span than the *Ss* with no FH. Type A no FH *Ss* had smaller Δ SBP during hand-grip than all other *Ss*. Type A FH *Ss* had larger Δ HR during reading comprehension than all other groups
Greenberg (1983)	36 normotensive men, aged 18-30. / 18 reported having at least 1 parent with hypertension and FH verified by parents. All *Ss* were caffeine or coffee drinkers (2-5 cups/day)	None	Mental arithmetic; *Ss* were administered 3 levels of caffeine: 3 mg, 125 mg, or 250 mg./ None reported	SBP: beat to beat tracking method which was a Narco Korotkoff microphone. HR: EKG via a Beckman R611 Dynograph	FH *Ss* had higher post-caffeine baseline SBP levels, larger Δ SBP during the task and recovery, and higher HR levels during task and recovery than *Ss* without a FH. No HR differences for FH *Ss* during post-caffeine baseline. No pre-caffeine baseline differences detected for SBP or HR
Hohn et al. (1983)	141 children aged 10-17; 62 were black. / 76 children had at least 1 parent who had DBP > 95 mmHg at rest during three separate occasions. Parental BP verified by health records	None	Treadmill exercise	BP: baseline-standard mercury-column, phase 4 DBP used. Task: Narco programmable electrosphygmomanometer. Blood samples used to analyze sodium, potassium, creatine, hemoglobin, hematocrit, plasma renin activity, norepinephrine. Urine analyzed for sodium, potassium, creatine, immunoreactive prostaglandin, and kallikrein	White FH *Ss* had higher HR levels at recovery than black FH *Ss* and white *Ss* without a FH. Black FH *Ss* had higher SBP and DBP levels during baseline than those black *Ss* without a FH and higher DBP during maximum exercise than those black *Ss* without a FH and all white *Ss*. No BP difference within white *Ss* during baseline or exercise
Holroyd and Gorkin (1983)	35 undergraduate men aged 18-22. / 18 reported having at least 1 parent with hypertension. Verified by parents	Novaco Anger Scale; JAS Type A	Role playing anger-inducing situations. / FH *Ss* reported more anxiety during task than those *Ss* without a FH	HR: recorded on a Grass Model 7 polygraph. BP: Narco sphygmomanometer	*Ss* were classified as anger inhibitors or anger reporters via the Novaco Anger Scale. *Ss* assessed as anger inhibitors had higher HR and SBP during tasks than those *Ss* who were assessed as anger reporters. FH *Ss* had higher HR levels during baseline and task than those *Ss* without a FH. When baseline HR is covaried, the above effect for anger inhibitors and HR levels during task remains, but the FH effect does not. FH *Ss* had higher DBP levels during task than those *Ss* without a FH. *Ss* assessed as anger reporters without a FH had lower SBP levels during the task than all other *Ss*

Table 1 (continue)

Reference	Subjects/family history definition	Behavioral measures	Tasks/outcomes	Physiological measures	Physiological results
Lane et al. (1984)	29 undergraduate women. / 8 reported having at least 1 parent with hypertension	JAS Type A	Mental arithmetic./No differences	BP: Arteriosonde. HR: EKG (R-wave). FBF, Respiration: Strain gauge recorded on Beckman R611 polygraph	The fight-flight (FF) response is described as increases in HR, SBP, DBP, and FBF. FH *Ss* had larger Δ FF and Δ HR than those *Ss* without a FH. Type A FH *Ss* had larger Δ FF and Δ HR than those *Ss* classified as Type A no FH and all Type B *Ss*. Type B FH *Ss* had smaller Δ HR than Type B *Ss* without a FH
Manuck et al. (1985)	44 undergraduate men, mean age of 19. / 22 reported having at least 1 parent with hypertension. FH verified by parent	Spielberger State-Trait Anxiety Inventory (STAI); State-Trait Anger Inventory (STAgI)	Mental arithmetic. / *Ss* reporting high anxiety achieved fewer correct solutions and worked at a slower pace. No effects for FH groups or high/low anger groups	BP, HR: Omron Hem-77 electrosphygmomanometer	FH *Ss* had larger Δ HR and Δ DBP during task than those *Ss* without a FH. FH *Ss* reporting high anxiety had larger Δ HR than FH *Ss* reporting low anxiety. No Δ HR difference in low anxiety *Ss*. FH *Ss* who reported high anxiety had increases in SBP across minutes of the task. *Ss* without a FH who reported high anxiety had decreases in Δ SBP across minutes of the task. *Ss* reporting high anger had larger Δ HR during task than those *Ss* reporting low anger. FH *Ss* who reported high anger had larger Δ HR than those *Ss* without a FH who reported high anger

Of the remaining eight studies, four showed no effects for family history of cardiovascular disease, whereas four showed significant interactions between family history of cardiovascular disease and another behavioral variable, usually Type A. Of the four studies reporting null effects, three were published between 1939 and 1942 and used the cold pressor test to elicit blood pressure responses (Chesley and Chesley 1939; Feldt and Wenstrand 1942; Russek 1942). Although these were pioneering studies at the time, perhaps they were less sophisticated, even in the measurement of basic variables like blood pressure, than current studies. Also, perhaps the cold pressor test alone is not an adequate challenge to discriminate hyperreactors from nonreactors.

The "interaction" studies showed that participants who were both Type A and had a family history of cardiovascular disease had a heightened physiological response compared with those who were Type B with, and Type A without, a family history of cardiovascular disease, respectively. The pattern of results was consistent across measures of cortisol (Williams et al. 1982); fight-flight pattern of blood pressure, heart rate, and forearm blood flow (Lane et al. 1984); and blood pressure and pulse transit time (Allen et al. 1983). An anomolous result of these studies is that the physiological response of Type B participants without a family history of cardiovascular disease resembled more closely the response of Type A participants with a family history of cardiovascular disease than the other two groups. There is no ready explanation for these findings, but they do suggest that future studies should measure Type A and family history of cardiovascular disease, in an effort to understand their independent and combined relationships with physiological responsivity to stress.

The final "interaction" study to be discussed here is especially interesting (Light et al. 1983). Male undergraduates performed a competitive mental task while their blood pressure and heart rate were monitored and periodic urine samples were collected. Participants were divided into a low-risk group, i. e., normotensives without a family history of hypertension, and a high-risk group; i. e., either borderline systolic hypertensives or normotensives with a family history of hypertension. Although the data were not presented in such a way to show the independent effect of family history of hypertension on physiological function, they did show that among the high-risk group, heart rate responsivity was directly related to the decrease in sodium and fluid excretion from the kidney. This study, therefore, suggests one potential mechanism by which family history of hypertension, in interaction with cardiovascular responses to psychological stress, may confer risk in an apparently healthy population.

In summary, the studies on physiological reactivity to stress and familial history of cardiovascular disease do suggest that important familial factors contribute to individual differences in physiological reactivity. Furthermore, there is evidence that at least one index of reactivity - pressor response to stress - is, in part, under some genetic control. The relevance of these findings to understanding the familial determinants of Type A individuals' physiological responses to stress is not completely clear, however. The data on reactivity of offspring of parents with cardiovascular disease are based primarily on studies of offspring of hypertensive parents, and Type A individuals are not more likely to become hypertensive than are Type B individuals. Furthermore, Type A individuals who are physiologically reactive to stress may be those who also have hypertensive parents. Thus, what we know at present is that familial factors predict physiological reactivity, which, in turn, predicts Type A and risk for hypertension, two independent risk factors for coronary heart disease. The specific mechanisms causing the familial associations are not yet specified, and how they interact in producing the reactive individual is not yet clear. Progress depends, in part, on defining the types of reactivity and their associated mechanisms.

Other Familial Factors

Although genetic influences may be involved in accounting for the association between family history of hypertension and reactivity, and for individual differences in pressor responses to stress, other family variables deserve attention. For example, childrearing practices, modeling of parents, and specific health habits pertinent to coronary risk that are encouraged and maintained by family attitudes and practices are important.

To our knowledge, only Baer and his colleagues at the University of Houston have attempted to study the interrelationships among childrearing practices, reactivity, and family history of hypertension. In their series of four studies (Baer et al. 1980, 1983), three-member families consisting of a father, mother, and a boy or girl between the ages of 8 and 13 years were videotaped as they interacted under standard conditions calling for disagreement or conflict. The family members' blood pressures were recorded before and after the interactions. In approximately half of the families, the father was diagnosed as hypertensive and under treatment. Individuals with disabling target organ damage, secondary hypertension, other chronic illness, or psychiatric disturbance were excluded. The videotapes were later reliably coded into 14 categories and summarized by 4 dimensions: positive verbal remarks (e.g., agree); negative verbal remarks (e.g., complain); positive nonverbal behavior (e.g., nodding of the head); and negative nonverbal behavior (e.g., averting gaze from speaker).

In the first of these studies (Baer et al. 1980), families with a hypertensive father differed in their behavior from families with a normotensive father while performing a skit in which the family members were to display their unhappiness with each other. More specifically, more negative nonverbal behaviors were expressed in families with a hypertensive father. Individual comparisons showed that this effect was particularly due to more negative nonverbal behaviors being displayed by the mother and the child in the hypertensive families. Hypertensive fathers also showed more negative nonverbal behavior in the presence of a male child than did normotensive fathers. Furthermore, the greater frequency of negative nonverbal behaviors of the parents during the skit was accompanied by higher systolic blood pressure measured immediately after the skit in the child ($r = 0.52$; $P < 0.05$). No similar relationships for blood pressure were found for normotensive families, largely because of the low rate of negative nonverbal behaviors in these families.

In another task in which families were trying to resolve their disagreements about the best solutions to a series of problems, they were asked either to express or to withhold their feelings. Results showed that, relative to normotensive families, families with a hypertensive father demonstrated more negative nonverbal behavior and less positive behavior when instructed to express their feelings, but when instructed to withhold their feelings, showed less negative verbal behavior and more positive verbal behavior.

A subsequent report by Baer et al. (1983) described three separate investigations of the frequency of gaze aversion, the behavior most frequently coded as a negative nonverbal behavior, in families with hypertensive and normotensive fathers. These studies also showed a pattern of results consistent with the first report. That is, hypertensive fathers and their normotensive wives and children engaged in more negative nonverbal behavior, i.e., looked at each other less both while listening and speaking, than did members of normotensive families. This difference occurred most prominently during emotionally negative verbalizations.

Taking the results of the four Baer et al. studies together, they suggest that persons with a family history of hypertension may experience a distinctive pattern of childrearing practices when the family faces difficult decisions, attempts to resolve conflict, or engages in activities in which feelings should be expressed or withheld. That is, although persons with a family history of hypertension experience just as many negative verbal messages as persons without a family history of hypertension, they experience and express more negative nonverbal behaviors, particularly gaze aversion, when trying to express dissatisfaction and disagreement. Other research indicates that gaze aversion is not as controllable as verbal behavior and may reflect psychological processes when verbal behavior is not informative, and that, furthermore, it reflects conflict avoidance via reduction of both information and confrontation. Extrapolating from these findings, it is not unreasonable to assume that the offspring of hypertensives acquire at an early age a diminished capacity to freely express and resolve hostile feelings. This interpretation is further supported by the findings that when families are specifically instructed to express their feelings, the hypertensive families express even more negative nonverbal behavior than do normotensive families, and that negative nonverbal behaviors are positively associated with systolic blood pressure levels of the children of hypertensive fathers.

It is intriguing to speculate about whether or not childrearing practices leading to conflict avoidance in the offspring of hypertensives may lead to the subsequent development of hypertension, and may, in part, account for the risk for hypertension associated with having an immediate family member who is hypertensive. The findings from the above studies are based on cross-sectional data, and, as such, cannot offer definitive statements about causal relationships. Nonetheless, they are remarkably consistent with previous observations that hypertensives have difficulty expressing anger and hostility, tend to be sociable, but at the same time unassertive (e.g., Esler et al. 1977).

Type A Behavior

Twin Studies

There have been several studies of the heritability of Type A behavior measured by the structured interview (SI) and the Jenkins Activity Survey (JAS), the two most common measures of Type A used in epidemiological studies (Jenkins 1978; Rosenman 1978). In the most comprehensive study (Rahe et al. 1978; Rosenman et al. 1974), Rosenman and his colleagues administered both the SI and JAS to 89 MZ and 93 DZ twin pairs and also measured other coronary risk factors and behavioral variables related to Type A. Results showed no significant heritability of Type A assessed by the SI. However, some of the behavioral variables correlated with Type A did show significant heritability (e.g., Thurstone Temperament Activity Scale, although the DZ intraclass correlations for these variables did not differ significantly from zero). Furthermore, analyses of the JAS Type A scores did reveal significant heritability, although again the DZ intraclass correlations did not differ significantly from zero. This conflicting state of affairs is clarified somewhat by subsidiary heritability analyses of the JAS factor scores. The JAS factor which measures speed and impatience showed significant heritability, but speed of behavior is only one of several secondary factors contributing to the overall interview assessment of Type A. In sum, these findings do not support the heritability of overall Type A, but they do suggest that facets of Type A may have a heritable base.

Table 2. Twin analyses of clinical ratings factor and its items

Item	MZ twins			DZ twins			Probability level for significance tests:		
	AMS	WMS	r	AMS	WMS	r	Within pair estimate of genetic variance	Holzinger's H/Falconer's estimate	Harter average difference test
Clinical ratings	0.77	0.20	0.58[a]	0.61	0.25	0.41[a]	0.17	0.08	0.04
Response latency	1.27	0.57	0.38[a]	1.10	0.69	0.23[a]	0.21	0.16	0.12
Explosiveness of speech	1.61	0.59	0.46[a]	1.18	0.59	0.34[a]	0.52	0.18	0.45
Rapid, accelerated speech	1.82	0.59	0.51[a]	1.58	0.62	0.44[a]	0.43	0.29	0.50
Potential for hostility	1.54	0.64	0.41[a]	1.19	0.85	0.17[b]	0.11	0.05	0.01
Loudness of voice	1.35	0.44	0.51[a]	0.85	0.57	0.20[a]	0.01[c]	0.01	-
Competition for control of interview	1.63	0.57	0.48[a]	1.45	1.01	0.18[a]	0.01	0.02	0.01

[a] $P<0.05$.
[b] $P<0.10$.
[c] The significance level of the among component estimate of genetic variance is presented because the probability level of equal MZ and DZ total variances was <0.20.
AMS, among pair mean square; WMS, within pair mean square; *r*, intraclass correlation coefficient. $n=80$ twin pairs for both MZ and DZ samples.

To further pursue this last possibility, Rosenman, Dembroski, and I sought to identify those Type A dimensions in the SI, if any, that have a heritable base (Matthews et al. 1984). The tape-recorded Type A interviews of the 80 MZ and 80 DZ twin pairs available for auditing in the Rosenman study were coded for the extent of self-reported Type A behaviors, the major speech stylistics considered to be indicative of Pattern A, and the observable Type A behaviors, e.g., signs of hostility and extremes of competition for control of the interview. Then scores for the four major dimensions measured by the SI were calculated, and those scores for which there were sufficient data were subjected to twin analyses by the Christian et al. (1974) method.

Analyses revealed that for the clinical ratings factor, the MZ intraclass correlations were about twice the size of the comparable DZ correlations factor, and that the estimates of genetic variance approached conventional levels of significance ($P<0.05$-$P<0.08$) for the Harter average difference test, Holzinger's H, and Falconer's estimate, respectively (see Table 2). This is precisely the pattern of results expected, given an additive model of genetic variance. The clinical ratings factor constitutes the sum of six ratings of the major speech stylistics and observable Type A behaviors exhibited throughout the interview and is the factor most highly associated with overall assessment in this sample ($r=0.84$, $P<0.001$), as well as in other samples (Matthews et al. 1982). The findings for the remaining factors were not consistent with a genetic hypothesis.

Subsidiary analyses of the individual ratings loading on the clinical ratings factor are shown in Table 2. Inspection of this table reveals that all items loading on the factor show a similar pattern of results with both MZ and DZ intraclass correlations significantly or nearly significantly different from zero, suggesting some familial similarity in clinical ratings or interview behaviors. Furthermore, the MZ correlations for loudness of speech, competition for control of the interview, and potential for hostility are about twice the size of the comparable DZ correlations, and the estimates of genetic variance were, on the whole, significant for these three items.

These results are intriguing because individual differences in the clinical ratings factor, particularly in loudness of voice, competition for control of the interview, and potential for hostility, may share a common element. All may reflect a general hyperresponsivity to environmental challenge and, in the present case, to the challenge presented in the SI. Consistent with this notion are data showing that specific overt Type A behaviors exhibited during an interview, e.g., frequent interruptions of the interviewer and a loud voice, can be the result of mutual imitation between the interviewer and interviewee (Matthews 1982); that they can be used to dominate and control social interactions (Dembroski et al. 1984); and that they are reduced in intensity following beta-adrenergic blockage (Schmeider et al. 1983). The evidence reviewed above indicates that cardiovascular hyperreactivity to environmental challenge, which does characterize the Type A, may have a heritable base. Should there be a modest heritable base in individual differences in the clinical ratings factor, the available findings may indicate that underlying aspects of Pattern A is a general hyperresponsivity that has a heritable base. Stated differently, underlying Pattern A may be a general temperament to be responsive to environmental demands and stressors.

A temperament is considered to be a broad predisposition to behave in a certain style that emerges early in life, is relatively consistent over time, and has a heritable component. Building upon this predisposition are the early familial and cultural factors that shape the specific ways the individuals perceive, understand, and respond to their environment. Similarly, in the case of Type A, the early familial and cultural factors may build upon the proposed temperament substrate, and, given the twin data, these factors certainly play the greatest role in shaping the ways the individual with the Type A pattern perceives, understands, and behaves in western society. Nonetheless, according to the temperament perspective, a necessary, but insufficient condition for producing specific aspects of Type A is a general, perhaps heritable hyperresponsivity to environmental challenge.

Parental Childrearing Practices and Modeling

Even if there is a temperament substrate underlying Pattern A, parents probably have a very powerful impact on their children's Type A behaviors by modeling certain behaviors, and by using specific childrearing practices. Evidence regarding the former mechanism comes from two studies. Among a sample of male and female college undergraduate twins and their parents, JAS Type A scores of the co-twin mean were positively associated with the Type A scores of the same-sex parents (Matthews and Krantz 1976). Similarly the Bortner Type A test battery scores of adolescent boys and their fathers were significantly associated (Bortner et al. 1970). Although these two investigations are not population-based, they do concur in suggesting that children imitate the Type A behavior of the same-sex parent.

Evidence regarding the childrearing practices associated with the development of Pattern A comes from two observational studies of the childrearing practices used with Type A and Type B sons. In the first of these studies (Glass 1977), mothers interacted with their elementary-school-aged sons, who had been rated by their teachers as exhibiting Type A or Type B behavior. The boys were required to complete three tasks: stack a set of oddly shaped blocks with one hand while blindfolded, copy a pictoral representation of a geometric figure with a set of cubes, and throw bean bags into a basket. The mothers were allowed to assist their sons in any way they wished, with the exception of completing the tasks for the children. An observer present in the testing room coded the behavior of the mothers and children. After completion of the testing period, the mothers administered the Type A SI. In this way, the potential childrearing practices used by Type A and Type B mothers with their Type A and Type B boys were examined.

The results revealed that Type A boys were treated differently from Type B boys. Specifically, Type A and Type B mothers gave fewer positive evaluations of task performance to Type A boys than to Type B boys, and Type A boys were pushed to try harder than were Type B boys, particularly by Type B mothers. An example of the latter is, "You're doing fine, but next time, let's try for 5." Because of the nature of the study, it could not be concluded that the differences in childrearing practices associated with the Type A and Type B boys caused the children's behavior pattern. In fact, children have such an impressive range of effects on caregivers that the differences in maternal behavior may have been elicited by the children's characteristic behavior (Harper 1975).

To test this possibility, the study was essentially repeated with two modifications (Matthews 1977). First, the boys in this study were actual As or Bs who exhibited Type A or Type B behavior, respectively, according to a prearranged script. They did this during the performance of the bean bag tossing task while a female stranger (a mother of another same-age boy) observed. In this way, the women had an opportunity to form an initial impression of the children's behavior. The second modification was that following the bean bag performance, the children interacted with the women on the other two tasks. The boys did not follow a script during this portion of the experiment. It was expected that if the female strangers responded to Type A and Type B boys in a manner similar to the mothers in the previous study, then it is likely that the Type A children in the previous study were causing their own mothers to behave as they did. However, if the female strangers responded to the Type A and Type B boys in a manner different from the boys' own mothers, then it is likely that the maternal childrearing practices in the previous study were not caused by the children and may have contributed, in fact, to the children's Type A behavior.

Analyses of the coded interactions of the children and women revealed that, in contrast to the previous findings, Type A boys received more positive evaluations of their task performance than did Type B boys from female strangers. Similar to the previous findings, Type A boys were pushed to accelerate their efforts more often than were Type B boys. However, only the Type B women consistently showed the above pattern of results.

Taking the results of the two studies together, it seems probable that the Type A boys do not cause their own mothers to give them few positive evaluations, because they do not elicit such from female strangers. Rather, a low intrafamilial frequency of positive evaluation of task performance and a high extrafamilial frequency may play a causal role in the development of Pattern A. On the other hand, it does appear that Type A behavior by boys elicits comments designed to improve the children's performance from Type B mothers and strangers. Thus, a curious phenomenon results: Type A boys elicit precisely that behavior from Type B women that may encourage them to continue striving to achieve ever-escalating goals. Thus, this adult/Type A child interaction is likely to be a self-perpetuating dynamic which should also maintain the Type A child's continual struggle to achieve into adulthood.

Summary and Concluding Comments

This paper reviews and evaluates existing data on the familial determinants of Type A behavior pattern and its associated physiological reactivity to stress. Genetic factors contribute to individual differences in pressor responses to physical and psychological challenge, and those with a family history of cardiovascular disease, particularly hypertension, are most likely to show blood pressure and heart rate responses to stress. It is unclear how these findings relate to understanding the familial determinants of the physiological reactivity associated with Type A, because Type A is not associated with risk for hypertension, and because specification of types and levels of reactivity is lacking. Nonetheless, the available data encourage systematic investigations into the mechanisms associated with familial aspects of sympathetic reactions to stress.

Based on reanalyses of the Rosenman et al. twin study, the present chapter suggests that there might be a temperamental underpinning of aspects of the Type A behavior pattern. Should a child who is temperamentally prone to be Type A initially express some approximation of Type A characteristics, then these characteristics would be encouraged and maintained by families in which the same-sex parent exhibits Type A behaviors and by the very childrearing practices that the temperamentally prone Type A child elicits from his or her parents. Thus, the Type A behavior pattern is likely to be self-reinforcing and resistant to change.

References

Allen MT, Lawler KA, Mitchell VP (1983) The Type A behavior pattern, family history of hypertension, and cardiovascular reactivity in college-age males: results using the Jenkins Activity Survey. (Unpublished manuscript, available from MT Allen, Department of Psychiatry, University of North Carolina, Chapel Hill, NC 27514)

Baer PE, Vincent JP, Williams BJ et al. (1980) Behavioral response to induced conflict in families with a hypertensive father. Hypertension [Suppl I] 2: 70–77

Baer PE, Reed J, Bartlett PC, et al. (1983) Studies of gaze during induced conflict in families with a hypertensive father. Psychosom Med 45: 233–242

Bortner RW, Rosenman RH, Friedman M (1970) Familial similarity in pattern A behavior: fathers and sons. J Chronic Dis 23: 39–43

Briggs JF, Oerting H (1937) The prognostic value of the cold test in pregnancy. Minn Med 20: 382–384

Brod J (1960) Essential hypertension. Hemodynamic observations with a bearing on its pathogenesis. Lancet 2: 773–778

Carney E, Goodman HC, McBride M, et al. (1976) Childhood antecedents of adult obesity: do chubby infants become obese adults? N Engl J Med 295: 6–9

Chesley LC, Chesley ER (1939) The cold pressor test in pregnancy. Surg Gynecol Obstet 69: 436–440

Christian JC, Kang KW, Norton JA (1974) Choice of an estimate of genetic variance from twin data. Am J Hum Genet 26: 154-161

Collins FH, Baer PE, Bourianoff GG (1981) Orienting behavior of children with hypertensive fathers. Psychophysiology 18: 181 (abstract)

Dembroski TM, MacDougall JM, Musante L (1984) Desirability of control versus locus of control: relationship of paralinguistics in the Type A interview. Health Psychol 3: 15-26

Dieckmann WJ, Michel HL (1935) Thermal study of vasomotor lability in pregnancy. Arch Int Med 54: 420-430

Esler M, Julius S, Zweifler A, et al. (1977) Mild high-renin essential hypertension. N Engl J Med 296: 405-411

Falkner B, Onesti G, Angelakos ET (1979) Cardiovascular response to mental stress in normal adolescents with hypertensive parents. Hemodynamics and mental stress in adolescents. Hypertension 1: 23-30

Feinleib M, Garrison RJ, Havlik RJ (1980) Environmental and genetic factors affecting the distribution of blood pressure in children. In: Lauer RM, Shekelle RB (eds) Childhood prevention of atherosclerosis and hypertension. Raven, New York

Feldt RH, Wenstrand EW (1942) The cold pressor test in subjects with normal blood pressure. Am Heart J 23: 766-771

Glass DC (1977) Behavior patterns, stress, and coronary disease. Erlbaum, Hillsdale

Goldstein DS (1983) Plasma catecholamines and essential hypertension: an analytical review. Hypertension 5: 86-99

Greenberg WP (1983) The effects of caffeine and stress on blood pressure in individuals with parental history of hypertension. (Unpublished manuscript, available from Greenberg WP, Department of Psychiatry, University of California, Los Angeles, CA 90024)

Harper L (1975) The scope of offspring effects: from caregiver to culture. Psychol Bull 82: 784-801

Hastrup JL, Light KC, Obrist PA (1982) Family history of cardiovascular disorders as a predictor of individual differences in response to stress. Psychophysiology 19: 615-622

Hines EA, Brown GE (1936) The cold pressor test for measuring the reactibility of the blood pressure: data concerning 571 normal and hypertensive subjects. Am Heart J 11: 1-9

Hohn AR, Riopel DA, Keil JE, et al. (1983) Childhood familial and racial differences in physiologic and biochemical factors related to hypertension. Hypertension 5: 56-70

Hollenberg NK, Williams GH, Adams DF (1981) Essential hypertension: abnormal renal vascular and endocrine responses to a mild psychological stimulus. Hypertension 3: 11-17

Holroyd KA, Gorkin L (1983) Young adults at risk for hypertension: effects of family history and anger management in determining responses to interpersonal conflict. J Psychosom Res 27: 131-138

Houston BK (1983) Psychophysiological responsivity and the Type A behavior pattern. J Res Personal 17: 22-39

Jenkins CD (1978) A comparative review of the interview and questionnaire methods in the assessment of the coronary-prone behavior pattern. In: Dembroski TM, Weiss S, Shields J, et al. (eds) Coronary-prone behavior. Springer, Berlin Heidelberg New York

Jorgensen RS, Houston BK (1981) Family history of hypertension, gender, and cardiovascular reactivity and stereotypy during stress. J Behav Med 4: 175-189

Krantz DS, Manuck SB (1984) Acute psychophysiologic reactivity and risk of cardiovascular disease: A review and methodologic critique. Psychol Bulk 96: 435-464

Lane JD, White AD, Williams RB Jr (1984) Cardiovascular effects of mental arithmetic in Type A and Type B females. Psychophysiology 21: 39-46

Lawler KA (1980) Cardiovascular and electrodermal response patterns in heart rate reactive individuals during psychological stress. Psychophysiology 17 (5): 464-470

Lawler KA, Allen MT (1981) Risk factors for hypertension in children: their relationship to psychophysiological responses. J Psychosom Res 23: 199-204

Light KC, Obrist PA (1980) Cardiovascular reactivity to behavioral stress in young males with and without marginally elevated casual systolic pressures. Comparison of clinic, home, and laboratory measures. Hypertension 2: 802-808

Light KC, Koepke JP, Obrist PA, et al. (1983) Psychological stress induces sodium and fluid retention in men at high risk for hypertension. Science 220: 429-431

Manuck SB, Proietti JM (1982) Parental hypertension and cardiovascular response to cognitive and isometric challenge. Psychophysiology 19: 481-489

Manuck SB, Giordani B, McQuaid KJ, et al. (1981) Behaviorally-induced cardiovascular reactivity among sons of reported hypertensive and normotensive parents. J Psychosom Res 25: 261-269
Manuck SB, Proietti JM, Rader SJ, et al. (1985) Parental hypertension, affect, and cardiovascular response to cognitive challenge. Psychosom Med 41: 189-200
Matthews KA (1977) Caregiver-child interactions and the Type A coronary-prone behavior pattern. Child Dev 48: 1752-1756
Matthews KA (1982) Psychological perspectives on the Type A behavior pattern. Psychol Bull 91: 293-323
Matthews KA, Krantz DS (1976) Resemblances of twins and their parents in pattern A behavior. Psychosom Med 28: 140-144
Matthews KA, Krantz DS, Dembroski TM, et al. (1982) The unique and common variance in the structured interview and Jenkins activity survey measures of the Type A behavior pattern. J Personal Social Psychol 42: 303-313
Matthews KA, Rosenman RH, Dembroski TM, et al. (1984) Familial resemblance in components of the Type A behavior pattern: a reanalysis of the California Type A twin study. Psychosom Med 46: 484-497
Neufeld HN, Blieden LC (1978) Pediatric atherosclerosis: genetic aspects. In: Strong WB (ed) Atherosclerosis: its pediatric aspects. Grune and Stratton, New York
Newlin DB, Levenson RW (1982) Cardiovascular responses of individuals with Type A behavior pattern and parental coronary heart disease. J Psychosom Res 26: 393-402
Rahe RH, Hervig L, Rosenman RH (1978) The heritability of Type A behavior. Psychosom Med 40: 478-486
Remington RD, Lambarth B, Moser M, et al. (1960) Circulatory reactions of normotensive and hypertensive subjects and of the children of normal and hypertensive parents. Am Heart J 59: 58-70
Rose RJ, Miller JZ, Grim CE (1982a) Familial factors in blood pressure response to laboratory stress: a twin study. Psychophysiology 19: 583 (abstract)
Rose RJ, Miller JZ, Grim CE (1982b) Blood pressure response to laboratory stressors in young normotensive twins and singletons. Paper presented at the annual meeting of the American Heart Association, Council of Epidemiology, San Antonio, Texas, March, 1982
Rose RJ, Tanner CK, Christian JC (1983) Familial influences on lability of blood pressure. Data from normotensive twins. Circulation 68 [Suppl III]: 344
Rosenman RH (1978) The interview method of assessment of the coronary-prone behavior pattern. In: Dembroski TM, Weiss S, Shields J et al. (eds) Coronary-prone behavior. Springer, Berlin Heidelberg New York
Rosenman RH, Rahe RH, Borhani NO, et al. (1974) Heritability of personality and behavior pattern. Acta Genet Med Gemeloll 23 37-42
Rosenman RH, Brand RJ, Jenkins CD, et al. (1975) Coronary heart disease in the Western Collaborative Group Study: final follow-up experience of 8½ years. JAMA 233: 872-877
Russek HI (1942) The significance of vascular hyperreaction as measured by the cold pressor test. Am Heart J 42: 398-404
Schmeider R, Friedrich G, Neus H, et al. (1983) The influence of beta blockers on cardiovascular reactivity and Type A behavior pattern in hypertensives. Psychosom Med 45: 417-424
Shapiro AP (1961) An experimental study of comparative responses of blood pressure to different noxious stimuli. J Chronic Dis 13: 293-311
Shapiro AP, Nicotero J, Sapira J, et al. (1968) Analysis of the variability of blood pressure, pulse rate, and catecholamine responsivity in identical and fraternal twins. Psychosom Med 30: 506-520
Sing CF, Orr JD, Moll PP (1980) Review of factors that predict serum cholesterol in the general population. In: Lauer RM, Shekelle RB (eds) Childhood prevention of atherosclerosis and hypertension. Raven, New York
Slack J, Evans KA (1966) The increased risk of death from ischemic heart disease in first degree relatives of 121 men and 96 women with ischemic heart disease. J Med Gen 3: 239-257
Warren P, Fischbein C (1980) Identification of labile hypertension in children of hypertensive parents. Conn Med 44: 77-79
Williams RB Jr, Lane JD, Kuhn CM, et al. (1982) Type A behavior and elevated physiological neuroendocrine responses to cognitive tasks. Science 218: 483-485

Stress and Cigarette Smoking: Implications for Cardiovascular Risk

T. M. DEMBROSKI[1] and J. M. MACDOUGALL[2]

We have previously argued in the literature that coronary-prone behaviors can be usefully divided into two categories - *consumatory behaviors* which directly or indirectly insult the cardiovascular system, and *stress-inducing behaviors* or traits which act to promote inappropriate, excessive, and protracted bouts of sympathetic nervous system and neuroendocrine arousal in the person's daily interactions with the environment (Dembroski and MacDougall 1982). The former category includes smoking, immoderate alcohol consumption, excessive intake of high calorie, fat-laden diets, *failure* to maintain medication regimens, and the like. The latter includes trait characteristics such as Type A and hostility, as well as overt maladaptive behaviors, such as excessive social aggressiveness and inappropriate ways of dealing with anger.

Although it is conceptually useful to distinguish between these two categories, in many cases behaviors within and across categories act additively and, in some instances interactively, to enhance cardiovascular risk. For example, considerable research suggests that cigarette, caffeine, and alcohol consumption frequently covary in frequency (e.g., Matarazzo and Saslow 1960; Ferguson 1973). Some data suggest that concurrent consumption of caffeine and nicotine interactively increases blood pressure to pathological levels in untreated and diuretic-treated hypertensives (Freestone and Ramsay 1982) and is epidemiologically associated with unusually high levels of total cholesterol and low density lipoproteins (LDL) (Heyden et al. 1979).

Psychological "stress" increases consumption of cigarettes, particularly in certain predisposed individuals (Schachter 1978; Conway et al. 1981), and cigarette consumption has been reported to interact with various stress-related psychological traits in increasing risk for myocardial infarction (MI) (Grossarth-Maticet 1980; Friedman et al. 1983). Similar research in our laboratory has revealed that *hostility*, as assessed by component scoring of the Type A structured interview (SI), interacted with the level of cigarette consumption in predicting the number of prior MIs in patients undergoing coronary arteriography, such that increasing hostility was associated with increased MI frequency only for smokers (T. M. Dembroski, J. M. MacDougall, and R. B. Williams, unpublished data).

A plausible interpretation of these findings is that the pathophysiological effects of cigarette smoking are enhanced in some individuals as a result of existing behavioral or psychological characteristics, or particular environmental situations (e.g., high stress). These existing characteristics may operate to make the individual more

1 University of Maryland at Catonsville, MD 21228, USA
2 Stress and Cardiovascular Research Center, Eckerd College, St. Petersburg, FL 33733, USA

Biological and Psychological Factors in Cardiovascular Disease
Ed. by T. H. Schmidt, T. M. Dembroski, and G. Blümchen

susceptible to the effects of smoking or they may magnify the pathogenic effects of smoking through as yet poorly understood mechanisms.

The very few studies that have previously attempted to investigate the effects of smoking and stress on physiological response have suffered from a variety of limitations, including the use of passive stressors, lack of appropriate control groups, or use of inappropriate and incomplete measures of physiological response parameters (Nesbitt 1963; Fuller and Forest 1977; Gilbert and Hagen 1980; Golding and Mangan 1982; Hatch et al. 1983).

A recent study from our laboratory sought to circumvent these limitations (MacDougall et al. 1983). The purpose of the study was to examine how cigarette smoking and coping with situational stress combined to influence the blood pressure and heart rate of young male smokers. The rationale for this study derived from the fact that, although smoking has been implicated in the atherogenic process (Herbert 1975; Auerbach et al. 1976; Vlietstra et al. 1980; Chesebro et al. 1982), some research suggests that smoking may contribute to acute cardiac events through other dynamic pathways. These include thrombotic occlusion (McKenna et al. 1980; Zalokar et al. 1981), myocardial O_2 depletion (Aronow et al. 1974), and increased frequency of ventricular arrythmias (Bellet et al. 1972; Hennekens et al. 1980). These processes are believed to be induced by the two primary toxic constituents of tobacco smoke - carbon monoxide (CO) and nicotine - which combine to simultaneously deprive the myocardium of oxygen, increase oxygen demand through elevations in heart rate (HR) and blood pressure (BP), and destabilize myocardial electrical activity, leading to disorders of cardiac rhythm (Bekheit and Fletcher 1976; Cryer et al. 1976, 1977; Trap-Jensen et al. 1979; Koch et al. 1980). Such consequences would be catastrophic in hearts already compromised by extant coronary artery disease (CAD), and, indeed, smoking exerts its greatest risk for MI in the presence of elevated serum cholesterol and coronary atherosclerosis (Doyle 1972; Hartz et al. 1981). Another argument favoring the above pathways is the fact that the risk for acute cardiovascular events declines significantly after cessation of the smoking habit (Gordon et al. 1974).

Many of the pathogenic effects of cigarette smoking arise from the net excitatory effects of nicotine on sympathetic nervous system (SNS) control of the heart and vascular system. Moreover, many of the SNS effects of nicotine ingestion are also induced by external stressors. For example, both stress and nicotine increase HR, cardiac output, total systemic resistance, and BP, and cause systemic release of catecholamines affecting the myocardium, smooth muscle, and vascular beds. Mobilization of free fatty acids from adipose tissue and perhaps resultant increases in circulating lipids may also be involved. Similarly, release of the neuropeptides vasopressin and beta-endorphins is enhanced, as well as other neuroregulators such as acetylcholine and dopamine (Pomerleau and Pomerleau 1984). In addition, nicotine stimulates the central cholinergic pathways, including those in the reticular activating system, which results in desynchronization of cortical electrical activity and probable effects on central integrative mechanisms that influence SNS activity. In fact, nicotine in cigarette smoke penetrates the blood/brain barrier within 7 s following inhalation (Jarvik 1970). Thus, during stressful activity, nicotine could potentiate stress-induced SNS activity as well as mimic it (MacDougall et al. 1983).

In our study, young male smokers either smoked or sham smoked three moderate nicotine-CO cigarettes while either relaxing or playing a mildly stressful video game. The time sequence of the events in the experiment was as follows: After completing a consent form, subjects filled out questionnaires and read magazines in a relaxed atmosphere for a 1-h period while a research assistant ensured compliance with our request to abstain from smoking. Thereafter, subjects were escorted into the experimental room, where they were fitted with BP and HR recording leads. All subjects then relaxed for a 10-min period while baseline data were recorded. The average baseline BP and HR values for the entire group were as follows: Systolic blood pressure (SBP = 118.4 mmHg; diastolic blood pressure (DBP) = 71.6 mmHg; HR = 68.8 bpm. Afterwards, all subjects were told that their "eye-hand coordination and psychomotor skill" would be evaluated by having them play a video game (Atari "Breakout"). The purpose of this procedure was to ensure that the groups of randomly assigned subjects in all experimental conditions were statistically homogeneous both in baseline values and challenge-induced reactivity levels of BP and HR. In addition, the test game provided us with the opportunity to determine (1) whether performance levels would be affected by the subsequent experimental maneuvers and (2) whether physiological reactivity levels produced by the test game would correlate with cardiovascular response induced by smoking a cigarette. After the test game, the experimental sequence began and, depending upon group assignment, consisted of a 3.5-min period of either smoking or sham smoking an unlit 80-mm filter-tipped cigarette (Marlboro) containing 1.0 mg of nicotine and 16.0 mg of tar. At the conclusion of the smoking session, one half of the subjects in each of the two smoking conditions relaxed for 2 min, while the other half played the video game, again under instructional conditions to improve performance on "the eye-hand coordination and psychomotor skill task." This testing sequence was repeated three times. Thus, at the conclusion of the experiment each subject had smoked or sham smoked three cigarettes and played the video game or relaxed three times.

The results were clear-cut in demonstrating that smoking and stress combined in a purely additive fashion to double SBP and HR increases over those seen with either smoking or stress alone. These results can be seen in Fig. 1, panels A and C. Note here, also, that we included an additional experimental group, which was subjected to the experimental paradigm without first participating in the pretest video game (smoke/no stress, NG). This group was included to control for any possible "carry-over" effects of the pretest video game.

The data for DBP suggested that the joint effects may have been interactive and cumulative over time. As can be seen in panel B of Fig. 1, repeated episodes of the stress and smoking combination resulted in a markedly increased DBP by the third smoking/stress period. Inspection of panel D, in which the rate-pressure product index (RRPI $\times$ HR $\times 10^{-2}$) data are presented, offers additional limited support for the operation of a synergistic effect beyond the primarily additive effects observed for SBP alone and HR alone. RPPI provides a crude index of myocardial oxygen consumption and is relevant to some potential pathophysiological mechanisms engendered by the stress/smoking interaction that were discussed earlier.

Thus, stress, which tends to induce individuals to increase smoking, also operates to exaggerate its potential pathogenic effects. An additional finding of considerable interest was the observation that the magnitude of reaction to the test game

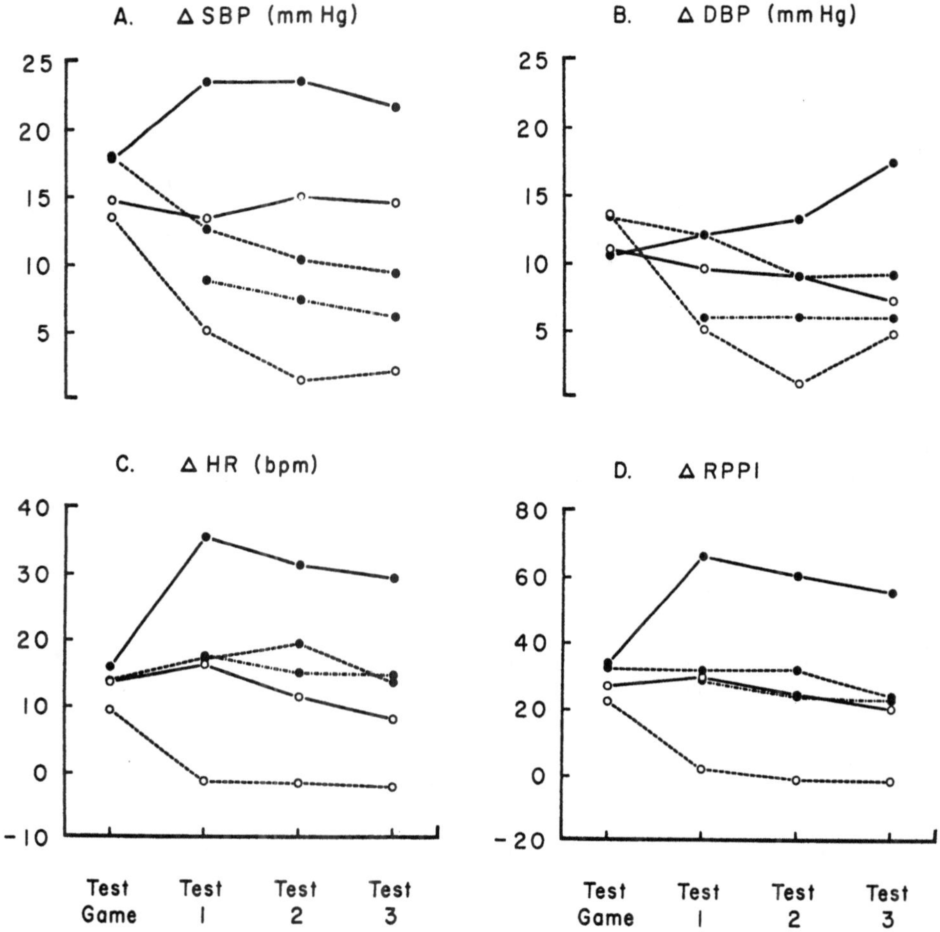

Fig. 1. Changes in BP, HR, and rate-pressure product index (RPPI) for all experimental groups across the test game and three test periods of experiment. ●——●, smoke/stress; ● – – – ●, smoke/no stress; ○——○, no smoke/stress; ○ – – – ○, no smoke/no stress; ● - · · · - ●, smoke/no stress, NG

prior to smoking predicted the magnitude of cardiovascular reaction to smoking alone, suggesting the presence of individual differences in autonomic lability which mediate the magnitude of cardiovascular reactions shown by individuals to either stress or smoking. Finally, performance may also be affected by the stress and smoking combination. Those who smoked before the video game evidenced a significant decrement in performance, whereas those who sham smoked showed performance enhancement.

As a next step in this program of research, we designed a study to investigate how the combination of stress and smoking would affect cardiovascular reactions in young women. Although smoking apparently carries a very strong risk for CHD, MI, and sudden death in women (Mann et al. 1976; Slone et al. 1978; Talbott et al. 1981; Willett et al. 1981; Chesebro et al. 1982), relatively little is known concerning how women react physiologically to cigarette smoking. The extant physiological literature on smoking appears to be largely based on male subjects, and when small numbers of females have been included (e.g., Trap-Jensen et al. 1979; Freestone and Ramsay 1982), separate analyses have not been reported. It is known, however, that women frequently evidence lower neuroendocrine and cardiovascular reactions to external stress than do men, both in the laboratory and in natural settings (e.g., Frankenhaeuser et al. 1976; Frankenhaeuser et al. 1978; MacDougall et al. 1981; Frankenhaeuser 1983). In this connection, recent preliminary research has suggested that nicotine affects the body weight and eating behavior differently in female rats relative to male rats (N. E. Grunberg 1984, personal communication). Taken together, the data suggest that nicotine may interact with hormones such as estrogen and progesterone, and perhaps with other hormones that differ between the sexes.

The study design was similar to that described above, which was used to evaluate the effects of stress and smoking on cardiovascular responses of young males, except for the following three differences:

1. In an earlier study, the findings suggested that males may take the challenge of the video game more seriously than women (MacDougall et al. 1981). We therefore included a monetary incentive to heighten the involvement of women subjects in the task.
2. Because most biomedical research typically evaluates the effects of only one or two cigarettes on physiological response, and because several males complained of discomfort following the smoking of three cigarettes, we reduced the number of cigarettes from three to one consumed just prior to the video game task.
3. Since nicotine effects on physiological responses generally begin to diminish after 10 or 15 min, we extended the time of exposure to the video game to determine whether the stress and smoking combination would potentiate cardiovascular reactions over the entire time frame of the task.

In addition, for reasons which are described below, we also included the Type A structured interview (SI) as a second task. As with the video game, subjects either smoked or sham smoked one cigarette immediately prior to the SI.

Following a 1-h period of questionnaire administration, during which smoking was not permitted, subjects were escorted into the experimental room and fitted with HR and BP recording leads. Thereafter, all communications were delivered through tape-recorded messages, beginning with baseline instructions. At the end of the 10-min baseline period, subjects played an initial video game ("Breakout"), which the recorded message described as a test of their "psychomotor skill." The latter was followed by a 3-min recovery period, which preceded the actual experimental sequence. Subjects were randomly assigned to either a 4.5-min smoke or sham smoke condition, followed by a 12-min period of either stress (video game) or relaxation. The same brand of cigarette (Marlboro) used for males was also used for the women subjects. The game was described as a continuation test of their "eye-hand coordination and psychomotor skill" and subjects were told that they would earn a penny a point for their highest score, giving them the chance to earn an additional $ 10.00 for their participation. Subjects in the relaxation condition were instructed to "relax and take it easy for the next several minutes." BP and HR were recorded during smoking activity and during the test phase which followed.

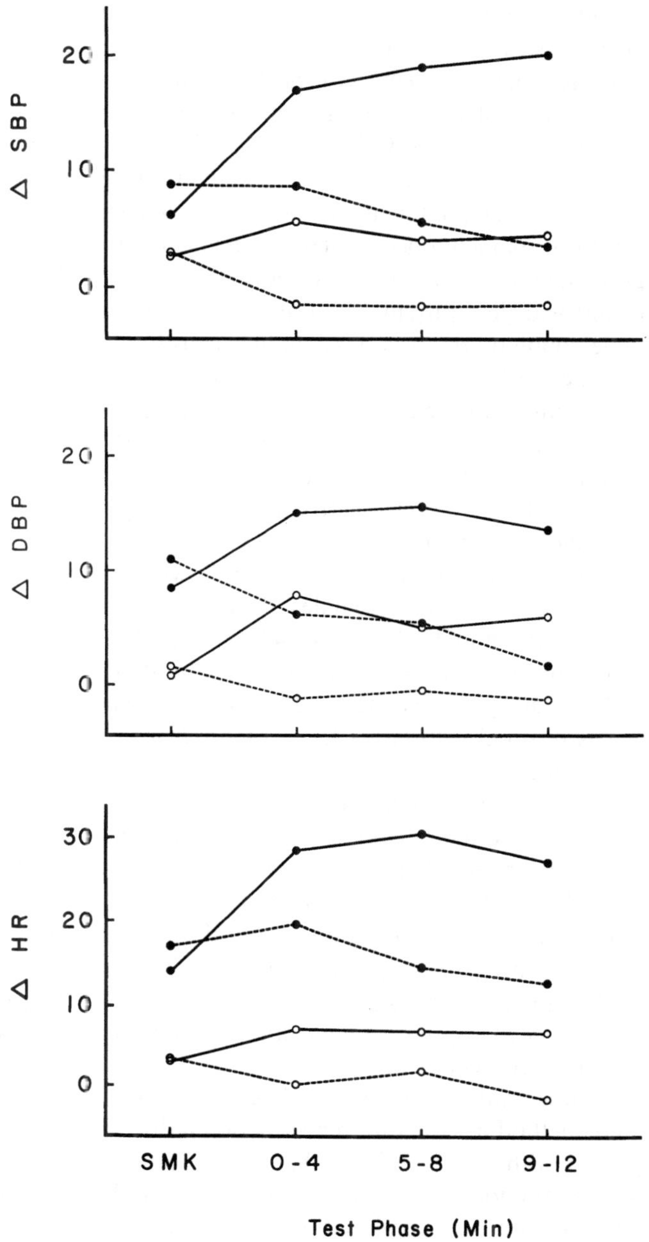

Fig. 2. BP and HR changes for all experimental groups during paced smoking and during beginning, middle, and end of stress test period. O – – – O, no smoke/no stress; O——O, no smoke/stress; ● – – – ●, smoke/no stress; ●——●, smoke/stress

Inspection of the baseline data and reactivity levels induced by the initial test game revealed that the experimental groups, by and large, were statistically homogeneous. The mean overall baseline levels were SBP = 109.1 mmHg, DBP = 70.8 mmHg, and HR = 72 bpm.

In Fig. 2 delta values are presented for SBP, DBP, and HR for all experimental groups. One can see that smoking produced the expected increase in physiological arousal that is typically found in the literature (Cryer et al. 1976). In contrast to our previous study of young males, in which the stress and smoking combination produced basically additive effects with only some suggestive data indicative of synergistic action, the present findings clearly showed synergistic or interactive effects of stress and smoking on SBP and HR in these young women (Fig. 2). Although there were methodological differences between the two studies, our current thinking is that the different findings may very well reflect significant differences in the manner in which males and females respond physiologically to the stress and smoking combination. As mentioned earlier, Frankenhaeuser (1983) and her associates in programmatic research have repeatedly demonstrated the tendency for women to respond with less physiological arousal during stressful situations relative to their male counterparts. It is possible that constitutional differences between the sexes might contribute to this tendency, but other evidence suggests that women may be less prone than men to become competitively involved in challenging situations (MacDougall et al. 1981; Frankenhaeuser 1983). If such is the case, the fundamental difference between the sexes could account for the primarily additive effects in males and the synergistic effects on physiological response induced by the stress and smoking combination in females.

In this connection, consider the following findings for the mean delta SBP response of males and females during the sham smoke and stress condition: Males = 14.3 mmHg; Females = 4.7 mmHg; $P < 0.02$. Next, consider the same reactions in the smoke and stress condition: Males = 22.9 mmHg; Females = 18.7 mmHg; P = NS. These data support the hypothesis that males relative to females respond with larger levels of *psychologically* induced reactivity, perhaps by virtue of their greater competitive involvement, thereby creating more of a ceiling effect that mitigates against a synergistic effect during the smoking and stress situation. In short, males compared with females may have less reactivity "room," because they respond to challenge with physiological levels closer to their maximum level. In contrast, because women respond with significantly less physiological response than men to the same sorts of psychological challenges, the addition of smoking during the stressful activity produces a greater amount of reactivity relative to the situation of not smoking during stress. In this regard, it is noteworthy that the physiological response of men and women during the stress and smoking condition was not significantly different.

These findings were derived from slightly less than 100 subjects. Moreover, there were methodological differences between the two studies. Although the data are in accord with the hypothesis that males respond to psychological challenge with greater physiological response than females and thus mask synergistic effects of the stress and smoking combination, a larger-scale, more methodologically sound study is needed to address the issue properly.

A larger-scale study is also needed to replicate and extend additional interesting findings uncovered in the present studies. For example, both studies found significant correlations between physiological response induced by the initial test game and cardiovascular reactions produced by cigarette smoking. These findings suggest that physiological hyperreactors may show exaggerated cardiovascular reactions in response to both psychological challenge and nicotine stimulation. However, a note of caution is in order here. The time interval between the initial video game and the smoking episode was only a few minutes. Before it can be concluded that "hot" reactors are hyperresponsive to both smoking and psychological (and perhaps physical) challenges, a longer time period between the different stimuli is needed to evaluate the hypothesis. This, too, could be accomplished in a larger-scale study.

Turning now to stable psychological or person variables in this line of research, we found in two earlier studies that women who scored high in hostility scores were significantly more likely to smoke cigarettes relative to those women who were low on the hostility dimension (MacDougall et al. 1981). These findings were replicated and extended in the present study of women smokers. Specifically, we found, once again, that women who smoked cigarettes scored significantly higher in hostility than nonsmoking women. Moreover, strength of addiction, as assessed by length of time of smoking and number of cigarettes typically smoked in a day, were significantly associated with hostility scores within the smoking group. In addition, both strength of addiction and hostility scores correlated with level of physiological response induced by the initial test videogame before the smoking manipulation was performed. These findings are extremely intriguing and may lead to new data bearing on personality, addiction, physiological reactivity, and the reinforcing properties of the smoking habit.

Finally, recall that, in addition to the video game stressor, we also administered the Rosenman Type A SI. As anticipated, subjects who smoked prior to the mildly stressful interview evidenced significantly greater elevations in BP and HR than those who sham smoked prior to the SI. The major purpose of this phase of the experiment, however, did not lie in evaluating the magnitude of the cardiovascular reactions induced by the stress and smoking combination. Instead, we were interested in determining whether the central and peripheral stimulating effects of nicotine would affect the subject's speech mannerisms during the course of the SI. The rationale for this study derived from previous research in the United States and Europe suggesting that administration of beta-blocking medication prior to the SI actually reduces in magnitude the verbal stylistic behaviors of speech - loudness, explosiveness, acceleration, and latency - which are the primary basis for designating an individual as Type A (coronary prone) or Type B (noncoronary prone) (Krantz et al. 1982; Schmieder et al. 1983). The implication of such research is that these noncontent verbal stylistics could be providing a rough index of elevated autonomic nervous system (ANS) activity or reactivity, which may be the mechanism linking the Type A/B designation to increased risk of coronary heart disease (CHD). Thus, persons who, for whatever reasons (perhaps constitutional), are readily or more profoundly aroused physiologically by interpersonal exchanges may show these exaggerated verbal stylistics, and at the same time their greater arousal serves to enhance pathogenic processes involved in CHD (Dembroski et al. 1984).

In the context of the present study, we reasoned that if this hypothesis was correct, then the excitatory effects of nicotine should result in exaggerated speech stylistics in those subjects who actually smoked prior to the SI, compared with those subjects who sham smoked. To test this, each interview was tape-recorded and later individually scored by both authors, who were blind to the smoking condition of the subjects. The scoring procedure has been explained in detail elsewhere (Dembroski and MacDougall 1983). Briefly, in addition to a global Type A designation, the auditor assigns a 1-5 rating for each of the following dimensions: speech *Loud-*

Table 1. Means and standard deviations for SI components for smoking, sham smoking, and nonsmoking female college students

Interview variable	Smoke ($n=22$)		Sham smoke ($n=19$)		Nonsmoke ($n=56$)	
	x	SD	x	SD	x	SD
Type A rating	2.54[a]	0.86	1.63[b]	0.76	2.18[a]	0.96
Loudness	3.39[a]	0.83	2.61[b]	0.81	not available	
Explosiveness	3.25[a]	0.77	2.39[b]	0.61	2.86[a]	1.09
Rapidity and Acceleration	3.27[a]	0.86	2.74[b]	0.70	3.10	0.93
Latency of Response	3.30	0.50	3.00	0.53	3.25	0.82
Potential for Hostility	2.84	0.88	2.79	0.86	2.39	0.76
Anger-In	2.55	1.12	3.00	1.07	not available	
Verbal competitiveness	1.73	0.70	1.82	0.85	1.93	0.81

[a] Significant differences were observed for the Type A through Rapidity/Acceleration dimensions.
[b] Means with different superscripts differ by $P < 0.05$ or greater.

ness, speech *Explosiveness,* speech *Rapidity* and *Acceleration, Latency of Response, Potential for Hostility, Anger-In* (anger suppression), and *Verbal Competitiveness.*

The results of the smoking manipulation were striking. As indicated in Table 1, relative to sham smokers, those subjects who smoked one moderate nicotine cigarette immediately prior to the SI were rated as significantly more Type A and showed significantly higher levels of Speech Loudness, Explosiveness, and Acceleration. Interestingly, comparison of the mean values for these dimensions for both groups with comparable data for similar-age nonsmokers suggested that the differences were arising largely from a tendency for the *sham smokers* (who were thus nicotine deprived) to show abnormally low average values for the overall Type A rating and for the various stylistic dimensions. By contrast, the mean values for the subjects who smoked prior to the SI were slightly, but not significantly, higher than the averages for the nonsmoking reference subjects.

While intriguing, the interpretation of these findings is not totally clear. Ideally, the smoke vs. sham smoke comparisons should be carried out on a within-subject basis, perhaps with a baseline provided by the subject after *substantial* abstinence from smoking. In any case, it appears from these data that the short-term abstinence from cigarettes may significantly *depress* the vocal mannerisms and, perhaps, the SNS functioning of smokers. If replicated with adult male subjects, these results would have important implications for those epidemiological studies that have assessed Type A using the SI, without controlling for the immediate smoking status of the participants (Rosenman et al. 1964; Multiple Risk Factor Intervention Trial Group 1979).

In summary, both the additive and synergistic physiological effects produced by the stress and smoking combination, and the influence of nicotine deprivation on verbal stylistics of subjects suggest very demanding tasks for future research. Certainly the two categories of risk factors, i.e., the traditional and the stress-related forms of coronary-prone behaviors, are not as separate as was previously thought. Rather, it appears likely that there are very complex and dynamic interactions among traditional risk factors, stress-related risk factors, personality attributes, environmental challenges, physiological reactivity, and pathophysiological mechanisms in CHD. Sorting out these complex interrelationships will be very difficult, but should prove very valuable in furthering the understanding, prediction, and control of CHD.

Acknowledgments. Preparation of this paper was supported by Research Grant HL-22809, awarded to the authors by the National Heart, Lung, and Blood Institute of the National Institute of Health, and by Research Grant AG-503, awarded by the American Heart Association, Suncoast Affiliate.

References

Aronow WS, Cassidy J, Vangrow JS, March H, Kern J, Goldsmith JR, Khentza M, Pagno J, Vawler M (1974) Effect of cigarette smoking and breathing carbon monoxide on cardiovascular hemodynamics in anginal patients. Circulation 50: 340-347

Auerbach O, Carter HW, Garfinkel L, Hammond EC (1976) Cigarette smoking and coronary artery disease. Chest 70: 697-705

Bekheit S, Fletcher E (1976) The effects of cigarette smoking on myocardial conduction in the human heart. Am Heart J 91: 712-720

Bellet S, DeGuzman NT, Kostis JB, Roman L, Fleischman D (1972) The effect of inhalation of cigarette smoke on ventricular fibrillation threshold in normal dogs and dogs with acute myocardial infarction. Am Heart J 83: 67-76

Chesebro JH, Fuster V, Elveback LR, Frye RL (1982) Strong family history and cigarette smoking as risk factors of coronary artery disease in young adults. Br Heart J 47: 78-83

Conway TL, Vickers RR, Ward HW, Rahe RH (1981) Occupational stress and variation in cigarette, coffee, and alcohol consumption. J Health Soc Behav 22: 155-165

Cryer PE, Haymond MW, Santiago JV, Shah SD (1976) Norepinephrine and epinephrine release and adrenergic mediation of smoking-associated hemodynamic and metabolic events. N Engl J Med 295: 573-577

Cryer PE, Haymond MW, Santiago JV, Shah SD (1977) Smoking, catecholamines, and coronary heart disease. Cardiovasc Med 471-474

Dembroski TM, MacDougall JM (1982) Coronary-prone behavior, social psychophysiology, and coronary heart disease. In: Eiser JR (ed) Social psychology and behavioral medicine. Wiley, Chichester

Dembroski TM, MacDougall JM (1983) Behavioral and psychophysiological perspectives on coronary-prone behavior. In: Dembroski TM, Schmidt TH, Blümchen G (eds) Biobehavioral bases of coronary heart disease. Karger, New York, pp 106-129

Dembroski TM, MacDougall JM, Musante L (1984) Desirability of control versus locus of control: relationship to paralinguistics in the Type A interview. Health Psychol 3 (1): 15-26

Doyle JT (1972) Cigarette smoking and coronary atherosclerosis. In: Likoff W, Segal B, Insull W (eds) Atherosclerosis and coronary heart disease. Grune and Stratton, New York, pp 35-39

Ferguson D (1973) Smoking, drinking, and non-narcotic analgesic habits in an occupational group. Med J Aust 1: 1271-1274

Frankenhaeuser M (1983) The sympathetic-adrenal and pituitary-adrenal response to challenge: comparison between the sexes. In: Dembroski TM, Schmidt T, Blümchen G (eds) Biobehavioral bases of coronary heart disease. Karger, New York

Frankenhaeuser M, Dunne E, Lundberg U (1976) Sex differences in sympathetic-adrenal medullary reactions induced by different stressors. Psychopharmacology 47: 1-5

Frankenhaeuser M, Rauste von Wright M, Collins A, et al. (1978) Sex differences in psychoendocrine reactions to examination stress. Psychosom Med 40: 334-341

Freestone S, Ramsay LE (1982) Effect of coffee and cigarette smoking on the blood pressure of untreated and diuretic-treated hypertensive patients. Am J Med 73: 348-353

Friedman G, Fireman BH, Petitti DB, Siegelaub AB, Ury HK, Klatsky AL (1983) Psychological questionnaire score, cigarette smoking, and myocardial infarction: a continuing enigma. Prev Med 12: 533-540

Fuller RGD, Forrest DW (1977) Cigarette smoking under relaxation and stress. Ir J Psychol 3: 165-180
Gilbert DG, Hagan RL (1980) The effects of nicotine and extraversion on self-report, skin conductance, electromyographic, and heart responses to emotional stimuli. Addict Behav 5: 247-257
Golding J, Mangan GL (1982) Arousing and dearousing effects of cigarette smoking under conditions of stress and mild sensory isolation. Psychophysiology 19: 449-456
Gordon T, Kannel WB, McGee D, Dawber TR (1974) Death and coronary attacks in men after giving up cigarette smoking: a report from the Framingham study. Lancet 2: 1345-1348
Grossarth-Maticek R (1980) Synergetic effects of cigarette smoking, systolic blood pressure, and psychosocial risk factors for lung cancer, cardiac infarct, and apoplexy cerebri. Psychother Psychosom 34: 267-272
Hatch JP, Bierner SM, Fisher JG (1983) The effects of smoking and cigarette nicotine content on smokers' preparation and performance of a psychosocially stressful task. J Behav Med 6: 207-217
Hartz AJ, Barboriak PN, Anderson AJ, Hoffmann RG, Barboriak JJ (1981) Smoking, coronary artery occlusion, and nonfatal myocardial infarction. JAMA 246: 851-853
Hennekens CH, Lown B, Rosner B, Grufferman S, Dalen J (1980) Ventricular premature beats and coronary risk factors. Am J Epidemiol 112: 93-99
Herbert WH (1975) Cigarette smoking and arteriographically demonstrable coronary artery disease. Chest 67: 49-52
Heyden S, Heiss G, Manegold C, Tyroler HA, Hames CG, Bartel A, Cooper T (1979) The combined effect of smoking and coffee drinking on LDL and HDL cholesterol. Circulation 60: 21-25
Jarvik (1970) The role of nicotine in the smoking habit. In: Hunt WA (ed) Learning mechanisms in smoking. Aldine, Chicago, pp 155-190
Koch A, Hoffmann K, Steck W, Horsch A, Hengen N, Morl H, Harenberg J, Spohr U, Weber E (1980) Acute cardiovascular reactions after cigarette smoking. Atherosclerosis 35: 67-75
Krantz DS, Durel L, Davia J, et al. (1982) Propranolol medication among coronary patients: Relationship to Type A behavior and cardiovascular response. J Human Stress 3: 4-12
MacDougall JM, Dembroski TM, Krantz DS (1981) Effects of types of challenge on pressor and heart rate responses in Type A and B women. Psychophysiology 18: 1-9
MacDougall JM, Dembroski TM, Slaats S, Herd JA, Eliot RS (1983) Selective cardiovascular effects of stress and cigarette smoking. J Human Stress 9: 13-21
Mann JI, Doll R, Thorogood M, et al. (1976) Risk factors for myocardial infarction in young women. Br J Prev Med 30: 94-106
Matazarro JD, Saslow G (1960) Psychological and related characteristics of smokers and non-smokers. Psychol Bull 57: 493-513
McKenna WJ, Chew CYC, Oakley CM (1980) Myocardial infarction with normal coronary angiogram: Possible mechanism of smoking risk in coronary artery disease. Br Heart J 43: 493-498
Multiple Risk Factor Intervention Trial Group (1979) The MRFIT behavior pattern study: I. study design, procedures, and the reproducibility of behavior pattern judgments. J Chronic Dis 32: 293-305
Nesbitt PD (1963) Smoking, physiological arousal, and emotional response. J Pers Soc Psychol 25: 137-144
Pomerleau OF, Pomerleau CS (1984) Neuroregulators and reinforcement of smoking: towards a biobehavioral explanation. Neurosci Biobehav Rev 8: 503-513
Rosenman RH, Friedman M, Straus R, Wurm M, Kositchek R, Hahn W, Werthessen NT (1964) A predictive study of coronary heart disease: the Western Collaborative Group Study. JAMA 189: 103-110
Schmieder R, Friedrich G, Neus H, Ruddel H, Von Eiff AW (1983) Effect of B-blockers on Type A coronary-prone behavior. Psychosom Med 45: 417-423
Slone D, Shapiro S, Rosenberg L, Kaufman DW, Hartz SC, Rossi AC, Stolley PD, Miettinen OS (1978) Relation of cigarette smoking to myocardial infarction in young women. N Engl J Med 298: 1273-1276
Talbott E, Kuller LH, Perper J, Murphy PA (1981) Sudden unexpected death in women. Am J Epidemiol 114: 671-682
Trap-Jensen J, Carlsen JE, Svendsen TL, Christensen NJ (1979) Cardiovascular and adrenergic ef-

fects of cigarette smoking during immediate non-selective and selective beta adrenoceptor blockade in humans. Eur J Clin Invest 9: 181-183
Schachter S (1978) Pharmacological and psychological determinants of smoking. Ann Intern Med 88: 104-114
Vlietstra RE, Frye RL, Kronmal RA, et al. (1980) Risk factors and angiographic coronary artery disease; a report from the Coronary Artery Surgery Study (CASS). Circulation 62: 254-261
Willett WC, Hennekens CH, Bain C, Rosner B, Speizer FE (1981) Cigarette smoking and non-fatal myocardial infarction in women. Am J Epidemiol 113: 575-582
Zalokar JB, Richard JL, Claude JR (1981) Leukocyte count, smoking, and myocardial infarction. N Engl J Med 304: 465-468

Anger, Aerobics and Autonomic Reactivity

N. Schneiderman, N. Tischenkel, and R. Nelesen[1]

Anger is commonly believed to be involved in the development of hypertension, atherosclerosis, coronary heart disease (CHD), and sudden cardiac death. In contrast, a program of moderate, sustained aerobic exercise is thought to retard this development. The paradox is that both the expression of anger and aerobic exercise are both known to elicit enhanced sympathetic nervous system (SNS) and cardiovascular activity. Therefore, in the present chapter we shall review the evidence that anger/hostility and aerobic activity can modulate autonomic functions and/or cardiovascular disease. We shall also discuss some of the biobehavioral variables associated with anger and hostility that might contribute towards cardiovascular disorders and explore some of the variables associated with aerobic activity that might improve cardiovascular functioning and/or retard cardiovascular disease processes.

Anger, Hostility, and Aggression

Anger and Related Constructs

One issue of concern in attempts to relate anger expression to cardiovascular reactivity or disease is that concepts such as anger, hostility, and aggression are often defined ambiguously. Consistent with the usage of Buss (1961), we shall consider anger to be an emotional state that consists of negative feelings varying in intensity from mild annoyance to blind rage. Hostility shall be considered a longstanding attitude of ill will and negative evaluations of other individuals, events, or circumstances. Aggression shall be considered an action that is intended to harm another (hostile aggression) or to coerce an individual to give up a possession (instrumental aggression). When the aggressive act is persistent and committed primarily to intimidate, it can be defined as harassment.

A number of psychometric assessment devices have been developed that not only assess anger and hostility per se, but also the manner in which they are expressed. Thus, in terms of anger, for example, there are psychometric scales that assess state and trait anger (Spielberger et al. 1983), cognitive and somatic aspects of anger (Krantz 1985, personal communication), and anger-in versus anger-out (Harburg et al. 1973b; Haynes et al. 1980). Care must be taken when using these proposed distinctions because the same labels may be applied to different concepts. Consider the oft used distinction between anger-in versus anger-out. Anger-in may be used to describe self-blaming behavior, an unwillingness to display anger, an inability to show it, or the perception that when one is angry others are unlikely to notice

1 Department of Psychology, University of Miami, Coral Gables, FL 33124, USA

Biological and Psychological Factors
in Cardiovascular Disease
Ed. by T. H. Schmidt, T. M. Dembroski, and G. Blümchen

(Averill 1982; Funkenstein et al. 1954; MacDougall et al. 1985; Spielberger et al. 1984; Tavris 1982). Conversely, anger-out may be used to describe a tendency to blame others, a low threshold for outwardly expressing anger, or the perception that when one is angry others are likely to notice. It should therefore be apparent from this discussion that, when relating personality characteristics to cardiovascular functioning or disease processes, the personality characteristics must be specified rigorously.

The assessment of anger or hostility may be based on self-report measures such as questionnaires, or they may be based on direct behavioral observations in structured situations. Among the most frequently used self-report questionnaires have been the Anger Self-Report Inventory (Zelin et al. 1972), the Buss-Durkee Hostility Inventory (Buss and Durkee 1957), the Cook-Medley Hostility Scale (Cook and Medley 1954), the Framingham Anger Scale (Haynes et al. 1980), the Harburg Anger-In/Anger-Out Scale (Harburg et al. 1973b), the Hostility and Direction of Hostility Questionnaire (Caine et al. 1967), the Multidimensional Anger Inventory (Siegal 1984), the Novaco Anger Inventory (Novaco 1975), and the State-Trait Anger Scales (Spielberger et al. 1983). Although the reliability and validity of some of the instruments are unknown, the reliability of several of these instruments, such as the Buss-Durkee Hostility Inventory and the Cook-Medley Hostility Scale, is greater than $r = 0.80$ even after several years (Biaggio et al. 1981; Shekelle et al. 1983). Interestingly, high levels of hostility, as assessed by the Cook-Medley Scale, have also been related prospectively to long-term CHD incidence (Barefoot et al. 1983; Shekelle et al. 1983).

Assessment of anger or hostility can be made on the basis of direct observation as well as by self-report questionnaires. This can be done by having raters evaluate behavioral responses during a well-standardized, challenging interview or some other highly controlled experimental situation. Studies that have related behavioral observations to the severity of atherosclerosis or to the incidence of CHD have done so within the context of the type A Structured Interview (SI). Jenkins et al. (1966) component analyzed the responses to the SI of 25 men diagnosed as having a silent myocardial infarction (MI) upon intake into the Western Collaborative Group Study. The responses of these men were matched with 25 men without diagnosed CHD who were of comparable age and occupation and with 25 men without diagnosed CHD who were of comparable age, occupation, and A-B classification. Of the six major components rated (i.e., competitive involvement, hostility, past achievements, present drive, time urgency, and type A behavior), only the hostility component distinguished men with silent infarcts from the age- and occupation-matched controls. Other component analyses of the SI, using somewhat different categories, have related observed anger or hostility to the severity of atherosclerosis (Dembroski et al. 1985; MacDougall et al. 1985) or to the occurrence of CHD (Matthews et al. 1977).

Association of Anger/Hostility with Cardiovascular Status

Atherosclerosis and CHD. High levels of self-reported hostility have been prospectively linked to an increased incidence of major CHD events in two separate studies (Barefoot et al. 1983; Shekelle et al. 1983). Both studies assessed hostility by using the Cook-Medley Hostility Scale, which is derived from the Minnesota Multi-Phasic Inventory (MMPI). In one of these studies, which was a 25-year follow-up of 255 medical students who had completed the MMPI while in medical school, high hostility scores on the Cook-Medley scale were predictive of both CHD incidence and total mortality rate (Barefoot et al. 1983). These relationships were independent of age, hypertension, smoking status, or family history of hypertension. In the other study, which was a 20-year follow-up of over 1900 men working at Western Electric, high hostility scores on the Cook-Medley scale were also found to be predictive of increases in both CHD and total mortality (Shekelle et al. 1983). These relationships were shown to be independent of alcohol use, blood pressure, cholesterol level, or smoking status.

An association has also been reported between scores on the Cook-Medley scale and the severity of atherosclerosis as detected by coronary angiography (Williams et al. 1980). Associations between anger/hostility and severity of atherosclerosis assessed by coronary angiography have also been reported in two studies that used component scoring of the type A SI (Dembroski et al. 1985; MacDougall et al. 1985). In both studies, subjects rated high in hostility during the SI who also stated an unwillingness to express anger (anger-in) had the most severe atherosclerosis. Hostility was rated in terms of the subjects' use of harsh generalizations, obscenity, emotionally laden words (e.g., "hate"), rudeness, argumentativeness, surliness, etc. Anger-in was assessed by questioning the subjects during the SI as to whether others know when they are angry or annoyed and whether, when resentful of another's tardiness, they would say something about it to the person. In both of the studies that related high hostility and anger-in to the severity of atherosclerosis, the relationship held even when global type A was not predictive of coronary artery disease severity.

Hypertension. Early psychodynamic studies of hypertension used interview methods. These studies were rather consistent in their emphasis on the role of anger and hostility in hypertension. Alexander (1939), for instance, believed that a central conflict existed in hypertensives between hostile impulses and passive-dependent needs. He believed that this hostility was always accompanied by anxiety that was incompletely repressed and incapable of adequate expression. Saul (1939) reported on the psychoanalysis of seven hypertensives. In most instances, the central issue involved was chronic, intense, inhibited hostility.

In a series of papers based on an epidemiologic survey dealing with the contribution of stress and heredity to differences in hypertension between blacks and whites living in Detroit, Harburg and his associates focused on suppressed anger (Esler et al. 1977; Gentry 1972; Gentry et al. 1982; Harburg et al. 1973b; Harburg et al. 1979). Differences between anger-in as opposed to anger-out coping styles were investigated using the subjects' responses to imaginary anger-provoking situations. For each situation, persons who said they would not get angry or annoyed or who said they would get angry but would suppress their anger were classified as anger-in subjects. In contrast, those who said that they would get angry and show their anger were classified as anger-out subjects. The findings by Harburg and his collaborators established that individuals having anger-in coping styles had higher mean diastolic blood pressures (DBP) and more evidence of documented hypertension. The anger-in profile interacted with being black, being male, and living in a high stress/crime area in contributing to hypertension. Suppressed anger was particularly characteristic of young males with borderline hypertension who had biochemical indices of enhanced sympathetic tone (Esler et al. 1977).

In an attempt to determine whether the suppressed anger/hostility seen in hypertensives was a result of the elevated pressure, Sullivan et al. (1981) compared the psychological profiles of patients with secondary neurogenic hypertension (i.e., resulting from pheochromocytoma), patients with primary hypertension, and normotensive volunteers. Patients with primary hypertension had significantly more suppressed anger and guilt as assessed by the Harburg scale and more trait anxiety as detected by the Spielberger Trait Anxiety Scale (Spielberger et al. 1970) than either the normotensive subjects or the patients with pheochromocytoma. These results suggest that the suppressed anger seen in hypertensive patients is not a consequence of the elevated BP.

Agonistic Behavior and the Progression of Atherosclerosis

Although studies conducted on humans have suggested the existence of positive associations between hostility and the severity of coronary atherosclerosis (Dembroski et al. 1985; MacDougall et al. 1985), hostility and the incidence of CHD (Barefoot et al. 1983; Shekelle et al. 1983), and suppressed anger and the prevalence of hypertension (Esler et al. 1977; Gentry et al. 1973; Harburg et al. 1973b; Harburg et al. 1979), it is neither feasible nor ethically permissible to demonstrate these relationships experimentally in humans. In contrast, animal behavior experiments can be used to document experimental relationships between behavior and disease processes.

In an important experiment conducted by Kaplan et al. (1982), 30 male cynomolgus monkeys were assigned to six groups of five members each. All of these monkeys were fed a moderately atherogenic diet for 22 months. For 15 monkeys placed in an *unstable social condition,* group memberships were changed periodically. The remaining 15 monkeys were placed in a *stable social condition* in which group membership was fixed throughout the experiment. Behaviorally, in the unstable condition, dominant monkeys tended to engage in more frequent and severe forms of contact aggression and subordinates in more extreme forms of submission such as cowering and fleeing than did dominant and subordinate monkeys in the stable social groups. At the completion of the study, the animals were necropsied and their coronary arteries examined for severity of atherosclerosis. The results indicated that the dominant animals in the unstable condition had significantly greater coronary atherosclerosis than the dominant animals in the stable condition or the subordinate animals in either condition.

In a similar experiment conducted upon cynomolgus monkeys given a nonatherogenic diet, Kaplan et al. (1983) found behavioral findings that were similar to those in the previous studies. Although the animals in the unstable social condition had reliably more extensive coronary atherosclerosis than the animals in the stable social condition, the extent of the atherosclerosis was in fact very small in each condition. Taken together, the two studies just discussed are consistent with the findings from many other studies indicating that the interaction of behavior with other variables (e.g., genetic background, diet) is far more powerful than behavioral manipulations alone in producing cardiovascular pathology (see Schneiderman 1983).

The experiments by Kaplan et al. (1982, 1983) provide strong evidence that behavior can contribute to the progression of atherosclerosis in primates and suggestive evidence that agonistic behavior is involved. Two other experiments, also conducted upon nonhuman primates, may provide additional clues concerning relationships between agonistic behavior and the development of atherosclerosis. In one of these studies, Coelho and Bramblett (1981) used an ethogram of more than 100 separate behaviors in the baboon (e.g., barking, biting, chasing) and dimensionalized them into five major categories: tension, threat, attack, subordination, and affiliation. Coelho and Bramblett reported that baboons that were high not only in the threat, attack, and tension, but also in the subordination dimensions had the highest levels of serum cholesterol of any subgroup of subjects.

At least to some extent, the relationship between the baboon behavior and its relationship to elevated serum cholesterol are reminiscent of the conceptualizations of type A by Friedman and Rosenman (1959). Thus, like their type A human counterparts, the baboons described by Coelho and Bramblett (1981) (a) engaged more or less unsuccessfully in a struggle to gain control over their environment and (b) had increased levels of serum cholesterol, which could promote atherogenesis.

Another study that may provide a clue concerning the relationship between agonistic behavior and atherosclerosis was conducted by Manuck et al. (1983). Cynomolgus monkeys that had been placed on an atherogenic diet for 20 months were fitted with electrocardiographic telemetry devices. The experimenter subsequently displayed prominently and threateningly before each target animal a large glove usually used in the capture and handling of the animal. The animals were then divided into high and low heart rate reactors on the basis of their responses to the gloved experimenter. At necropsy, it was found that the high heart rate reactors revealed significantly more coronary artery atherosclerosis than the low heart rate reactors. Although the study was retrospective in nature, it is suggestive with regard to atherosclerotic CHD in humans because, relative to type B individuals, type A persons reveal more (a) heart rate reactivity in some experimental situations and (b) coronary atherosclerosis either when studied at autopsy (Friedman et al. 1968) or in some (but not all) coronary angiography studies (Blumenthal et al. 1978; Krantz et al. 1979).

Anger and Hostility in Psychophysiologic Studies of Normotensives

Hokanson (1961) found that subjects who were harassed and frustrated while performing arithmetic computations revealed increased systolic blood pressure (SBP). When these subjects were permitted to deliver electric shocks to the experimenter as a form of counteraggression, the subjects' BP decreased. Subsequently, Hokanson and Burgess (1962) determined that both harassment and blocked goal attainment led to SBP and heart rate increases relative to a no-frustration condition. Opportunities for counteraggression reduced these elevations when the experimenter was presented as being of low status, but did not do so in the presence of a high-status experimenter.

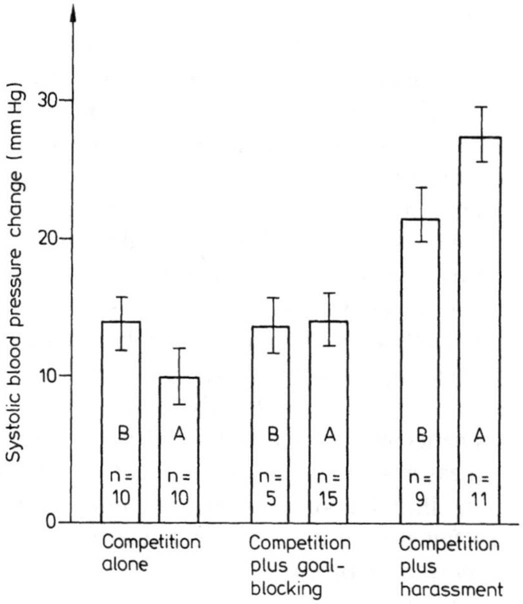

Fig. 1. Change in systolic blood pressure from baseline during a competitive two-person Super-Pong video game for interview-defined type A ($n=36$) and type B ($n=24$) subjects during three experimental conditions (from Diamond et al. 1984)

The frustration/harassment procedure was also used by Gambaro and Rabin (1969) to study the recovery of DBP in subjects classified as high or low in guilt associated with aggression as assessed by a sentence completion task (Mosher 1961). Subjects scoring high on guilt showed slower rates of recovery than subjects scoring low on guilt.

Van Egeren (1979) harassed half of their subjects while these subjects solved anagrams. Each subject subsequently interacted with a confederate on a mixed-motive computer-controlled game while BP, heart rate, digital pulse volume, and pulse transit time were measured. Van Egeren and colleagues found that the previously harassed subjects expressed more anger and revealed more cardiovascular reactivity than the previously nonharassed subjects.

Glass et al. (1980) have also used a frustration/harassment procedure to study BP, heart rate, and plasma catecholamine reactivity. They examined these responses as a function of the type A behavior pattern based on the SI. Glass et al. had their subjects play a computerized video game against an opponent who pretended to be another subject. In a no-harassment condition, the confederate merely played against the subject; in the harassment condition, he also delivered a series of preprogrammed harassing comments such as "I don't understand why you're having so much trouble hitting the ball!"

Glass et al. (1980) found that competition elicited significant increases in heart rate, BP, and plasma catecholamines, which were comparable in type A and B men during the no-harassment condition. In type A but not type B subjects the presence of a harassing opponent led to further significant increases in heart rate, SBP, and plasma epinephrine.

In a subsequent experiment, Diamond et al. (1984) used procedures similar to those used by Glass et al. (1980) to elicit cardiovascular reactivity but also attempted to distinguish the effects of frustration from those of harassment. Thus, in a goal-blocking (frustration) condition, a programmed series of distractions was delivered in order to impede the subject in his effort to compete successfully. In contrast, during a harassment condition, the confederate delivered eight derogatory comments to the subject, such as "Christ, can't you keep your eye on the ball?" In addition to comparing the effects of competition alone or in conjunction with goal-blocking or harassment, Diamond et al. attempted to assess the role that observed and self-reported hostility might have in cardiovascular reactivity.

Diamond et al. (1984) confirmed the findings of Glass et al. (1980) that competition elicited significant increases in heart rate and SBP that were comparable for type A or type B subjects unless harassment occurred (see Fig. 1). Both type A *and* B individuals showed increases in SBP and heart rate with the harassment condition that were significantly greater than those seen with the other two conditions; type A subjects revealed significantly greater reactivity than type B subjects only in the harassment condtion and only for SBP. Exploratory analyses correlating anger/hostility measures and cardiovascular reactivity indicated that only subjects scoring high on the Buss-Durkee Hostility Inventory showed significantly elevated SBP activity as a function of the type A behavior pattern, rated hostility during the type A SI, or outward expression of anger as assessed by the Framingham Anger-In versus Anger-Out Scale.

Anger and Hostility in Psychophysiologic Studies of Hypertension

Patients with hypertension exhibit more pronounced cardiovascular responses to many emotional stressors in the laboratory than do normotensive controls. The first well-designed experiment demonstrating this effect was provided by Brod et al. (1959). Patients with either mild or severe hypertension showed greater cardiovascular responsiveness to the stress of performing arithmetic computations than did normotensive controls. Results in patients with severe hypertension are difficult to interpret, however, because peripheral arteriolar hypertrophy may lead to exaggerated increases in BP responses that are not specifically due to exaggerated SNS arousal. In patients with borderline or mild hypertension, the vasculature is not hypertrophic, and subjects tend to have normal BP responsiveness to such challenges as dynamic exercise (Julius and Conway 1968), static exercise (Sannerstedt and Julius 1972), or the cold pressor test (Cuddy et al. 1966; Drummond 1983).

In contrast to the findings usually seen when physical stressors are used, larger cardiovascular responses have been reported for hypertensive patients than for normotensive controls during stressful behavioral tasks (e.g., Bauman et al. 1973; Drummond 1983; Nestel 1969), experimentally elicited fear and anger (Schachter 1957) or conflict-laden interviews (McKegney and Williams 1967). There is also some limited evidence that hypertensives may show greater pressor responses than normotensives when engaged in tasks involving active coping (e.g., video games) as opposed to passive coping (e.g., watching a distressful film) (Steptoe et al. 1984).

Although the research literature suggests that borderline and mild hypertensives respond excessively to emotionally relevant stimuli as opposed to purely physical stimuli, this is sometimes hard to assess. Thus, for example, responses to tasks such as the cold pressor test may be influenced by instructions and the subject's perceptions of the experimenter or laboratory situation. Weiner et al. (1962) suggested that the physiologic responses of hypertensives, in particular, should be interpreted within the context of their psychological functioning. Weiner et al. suggested that hypertensives habitually protect themselves against interpersonal closeness and vulnerability and that any form of perceived threat could evoke exaggerated pressor responses during any task.

The exaggerated psychophysiologic responsiveness of hypertensives may be constitutional in nature. This is suggested by the results of a series of studies conducted on the normotensive children of hypertensive parents. Thus, when compared with the normotensive children of normotensive parents, the progeny of hypertensive parents tend to show more cardiovascular reactivity to emotional stressors (Falkner et al. 1979; Hastrup et al. 1982; Light et al. 1983; Manuck and Proietti 1982). The experiment by Light et al. is of particular interest because of the finding that, while performing competitive mental tasks, the sodium and fluid excreted by a group of young men who were hypertensive or had two hypertensive parents was reduced in comparison with a group of young men who were normotensive and had normotensive parents. In the former group, the degree of sodium and fluid retention was directly related to the magnitude of heart rate during the stressful task.

Brod et al. (1959) suggested that patients with hypertension exhibit a hemodynamic pattern reminiscent of the acute "defense reaction" (Abrahams et al. 1960; Hess 1957). This suggests that such individuals may have a personality that is prone to increased alertness with frequent increases in central autonomic arousal. The best evidence for autonomic involvement in human essential hypertension occurs in so-called "hyperkinetic" borderline or mild hypertension, in which patients reveal tachycardia and an elevated cardiac output (Eich et al. 1962; Frohlich et al. 1969; Julius and Conway 1968). The elevation of cardiac output is neurogenic and can be abolished by autonomic blockade of the heart. When the elevated cardiac output is reduced, however, peripheral vascular resistance increases, and the BP remains elevated (Julius et al. 1971). When alpha-adrenergic blockade is then used to determine whether the increase in resistance is neurogenic, this has indeed been found to be the case in borderline hypertensive patients with elevated plasma renin activity (Esler et al. 1975).

Three alternative hypotheses could be proposed to account for the relationships among increased SNS activity, elevated plasma renin, and borderline or mild hypertension (Esler et al. 1977). The first hypothesis is that activation of the renin-angiotensin system triggers the SNS hyperreactivity. A second hypothesis is that arterial baroceptor insensitivity in hypertensives with elevated renin mediates the BP elevation. The final hypothesis is that SNS overactivity is associated with behavioral variables, such as suppressed hostility, and that the SNS overreactivity stimulates the renin release.

In order to test these hypotheses, Esler et al. examined hemodynamic functions in young males who were either normotensive or mildly hypertensive with normal or high renin values. Baroreceptor function was evaluated, SNS activity was assessed using pharmacologic blockades, and psychological variables were examined using the Buss-Durkee Hostility Inventory (Buss 1961), the Anger-In/Anger-Out Scale (Harburg et al. 1973b), the 16 Personality Factor (PF) Questionnaire (Cattell et al. 1970), and the IPAT Anxiety Scale (Cattell et al. 1970).

Esler et al. (1977) found that pharmacologic suppression of renin levels by oral administration of propranolol in high-renin hypertensives failed to lower resting plasma norepinephrine, indicating that the renin-angiotensin system did not evoke the SNS hyperreactivity. Baroreceptor function as measured by the reflexive heart rate slowing induced by the acute pharmacologic elevation of BP did not reveal differences between the high- and normal-renin groups. Thus, the first two hypotheses to account for the relationships among increased SNS activity, elevated plasma renin, and mild hypertension were not confirmed. In contrast, the psychological data indicated that the high-renin hypertensives tended to be submissive, guilt-prone individuals having a high level of unexpressed anger. Esler et al. (1977) concluded that "the pathogenesis of the blood pressure in these patients with elevated plasma renin activity may involve suppression of hostility as a persistent reaction pattern leading to chronic elevation of the sympathetic nervous system" (p. 410).

Esler et al. (1977) reported that, compared with patients with normal plasma renin values, those patients with elevated plasma renin also revealed elevated plasma norepinephrine values, heart rate, and cardiac output. The BP of the patients with elevated renin and elevated norepinephrine levels also fell to normal values after autonomic blockade. Thus, the findings of Esler and his collaborators suggest a basis for obtaining more homogeneous subsets of patients with "neurogenic" and "non-neurogenic" hypertension from the heterogenous population having essential hypertension. It appears that suppressed hostility may play a role in the development of neurogenic hypertension, although more research is needed before any firm conclusions can be drawn.

Physiologic Changes Associated with Aversive Behavior

The animal behavior literature indicates that mammals confronted with an acute, aversive situation tend to reveal one pattern of autonomic activity if fight, flight, or other appropriate active coping responses are being attempted, but another pattern if active coping responses seem unavailable. The first pattern, sometimes referred to as the "defense reaction" (Abrahams et al. 1960; Hess 1957) is characterized by increases in movement, heart rate, cardiac output, and vasodilation in skeletal muscle. The second pattern, which occurs in aversive situations in which an active coping response does not seem available, is characterized by extreme vigilance, an inhibition of movement, muscle vasoconstriction, an increase in SNS activity, but also a vagally mediated decrease in heart rate (Von Holst 1972). Both patterns are characterized by increases in BP and plasma catecholamines.

In human psychophysiologic experiments, a pattern similar to the defense reaction can be seen during such tasks as arithmetic computations (Brod et al. 1959), competitive videogames (Glass et al. 1980), and shock avoidance (Obrist 1976). Also in humans, a pattern similar to the passive coping or vigilance reaction can be seen during such tasks as a reaction time test (Williams et al. 1982), watching a pornographic movie (Obrist et al. 1978), or reading words projected upside down and out of focus (Williams 1975). These two patterns of autonomic responses do not necessarily require an obvious aversive contingency to be manifested in humans. The pattern similar to the defense reaction, for example, can be elicited by a competitive video game without harassment; the passive coping or vigilance pattern can be evoked by reading words that are presented upside down and out of focus.

Similar response patterns are seen during competition using a video game whether the player is harassed or not (Glass et al. 1980; Diamond et al. 1984). The difference appears to be in terms of the magnitude of the response rather than in the pattern. This is not as surprising as it first appears when one considers that: (a) hemodynamic adjustments subserve the physiologic needs of the organism; (b) the central nervous system is organized to produce integrated patterns of response rather than changes in single, isolated variables; and (c) the repertoire of patterned cardiovascular responses is not very large.

At present, the psychophysiologic concomitants of anger and hostility have not gone very far beyond observations that acute expressions of anger typically elicit patterns of SNS arousal. Most anger inductions in the laboratory have elicited patterns of response that are reminiscent of the defense reaction. Whether hostility in its more chronic manifestations is accompanied by cardiovascular and hormonal changes akin to the defense reaction or to the passive coping (hypervigilance) pattern is not presently known. Studies that intend to examine the correlates of long-term anger and hostility need to look not only at cardiovascular activity, but also at neuroendocrines substances, including epinephrine, cortisol, prolactin, testosterone, and the endogenous opiates.

Aerobic Exercise

Just as anger and hostility have been implicated in the development of hypertension, atherosclerosis and CHD, programs of moderately intense, sustained aerobic exercise have been thought to retard this development and promote health. Much of this positive benefit is thought to be mediated by improved physiologic functioning and the modification of risk factors for disease. Although the research literature suggests that an active lifestyle is healthier than a sedentary lifestyle and that being moderately fit is healthier than being totally unfit, precise causal relationships between a sedentary lifestyle and poor health and between poor aerobic fitness and disease remain obscure.

In examining the experimental findings concerning aerobic fitness and lifestyle, it is important to distinguish between them. This is particularly important because: (a) many of the epidemiologic studies that have linked sedentary lifestyle to increased health risk have not assessed cardiorespiratory fitness and (b) studies that have linked cardiorespiratory fitness to improved health risk profiles have frequently used insufficiently large population samples to assess adequately the impact of fitness on morbidity and mortality.

Epidemiologic Data

Epidemiologic studies suggest that there is an inverse relationship between physical activity and CHD. Prior to 1970, most of this evidence came from retrospective case-control studies (Frank et al. 1966; Shapiro et al. 1969) and from retrospective cross-sectional investigations comparing the incidence of CHD in reportedly active as opposed to sedentary people (e.g., Kahn 1963; Morris et al. 1953, 1956; Taylor et al. 1962; Zukel et al. 1959). Since 1970, approximately 15 prospective population studies have been reported.

Most of the early studies considered only job activities, and these were inferred from job titles. London bus drivers, for example, were found to have lower CHD and mortality rates than conductors (Morris 1953, 1956), railway switchmen lower CHD morbidity rates than railway clerks or executives (Taylor et al. 1962), and mail carriers lower mortality rates than postal clerks (Kahn 1963). Although the early retrospective studies suggested that there is a relationship between physical inactivity and CHD, they are hardly definitive since they did not consider: (a) physical fitness, (b) leisure time activities, (c) selection factors that might influence entry into or transfer between job categories, and/or (d) differences in job demands other than physical activity.

The prospective Framingham Study found that CHD incidence and mortality rate were positively related to self-reports of physical inactivity in men but not women (Kannel and Sorlie 1979). This relationship between physical inactivity and CHD, which was observed in men, was independent of age, BP, smoking, or cholesterol levels. The magnitude of the relationship between physical inactivity and CHD was smaller than that found for these other risk factors.

The limited correlation between physical inactivity and CHD in men, and the absence of this correlation in women, may have occurred because most of the Framingham population was sedentary, with women having an even smaller gradient of physical activity than men (Rigotti et al. 1983). This view is supported by the results of a Finnish study in which a larger physical gradient was observed in both men and women (Salonen et al. 1982). In the Finnish study, low activity, as assessed by job classification, was associated with a 1.5-fold risk of myocardial infarction in men and a 2.4-fold risk in women over a 7-year period, even after adjustment for other risk factors (Salonen et al. 1982).

The strongest evidence for the protective role of job-related physical activity comes from a 22-year prospective study of more than 3000 San Francisco longshoremen conducted by Paffenbarger and his colleagues (Brand et al. 1979; Paffenbarger et al. 1970; Paffenbarger and Hale 1975; Paffenbarger et al. 1977; Paffenbarger et al. 1978a). Those men whose work activity required an energy expenditure of over 8500 kcal per week were at significantly lower risk of myocardial infarction and sudden death, even after correction for known risk factors. Direct measurement of oxygen consumption, and concerted efforts to reclassify workers annually in terms of transfers to new jobs added strength to the research design. The large differences in work activity level observed between the least and most active job classification maximized the opportunity to detect differences. Positive findings reported in this study suggest that high levels of physical activity on the job may protect against CHD. Selection bias may have occurred, since people who were unable to perform strenuous activity would be more likely to transfer to less strenuous jobs (Froelicher and Oberman 1982). This bias was reduced somewhat by the fact that longshoremen entering the study all had to do heavy work for at least 5 years.

In a study that took into account both work and leisure activities, Paffenbarger et al. (1978b, 1984) studied the relationship between activity level and CHD risk among Harvard University alumni. The original college archives of 16,936 Harvard alumni who entered college between 1916 and 1950 were analyzed in conjunction with questionnaire data obtained in 1962 or 1966 on postcollege physical exercise, other elements of life style and health status. Surviving alumni reported in 1972 on physician-diagnosed CHD and other diseases. The time and causes of deaths from 1962 to 1978 were recorded from official death certificates.

Paffenbarger et al. (1984) found that habitual postcollege exercise, rather than student participation in sports during college, predicted low CHD risk. Sedentary alumni, including ex-varsity athletes who subsequently did not exercise, had a high risk. Those sedentary students who became habitually physically active after college acquired a low risk. The benefits of exercise were evident even after adjustment for other known risk factors. According to Paffenbarger and his colleagues, inadequate exercise is the strongest predictor of CHD incidence on a community basis, although hypertension is the strongest individual predictor clinically.

Although physical inactivity may increase the risk of CHD, the time spent exercising may itself be associated with an increase in risk. Siscovick et al. (1984) examined this question by comparing the time that had been devoted to exercise by men who had died suddenly with the time devoted to exercise by a comparable group of men who remained healthy. Then, by taking into account overall community mortality statistics, Siscovick and his coworkers were able to conclude that, while the risk of cardiac arrest is transiently increased during vigorous exercise, habitual exercise is associated with an overall decreased risk of cardiac arrest.

In summary, the epidemiologic evidence clearly indicates that there is an inverse relationship between habitual physical activity and CHD. The basis of this association is still not entirely clear, however, since studies demonstrating the relationship have had difficulty: (a) adequately quantifying levels of activity actually performed and (b) determining the extent to which self-selection of a sedentary lifestyle is chosen by less healthy individuals.

Biological Effects of Aerobic Exercise

Aerobic exercise that increases heart rate above 70% of capacity for approximately 30 min three to five times per week produces a training effect (Fox and Matthews 1981; Fox et al. 1972a; Pollock et al. 1969). Thus, aerobic training enhances metabolic efficiency by augmenting the number and size of mitochondria, the myoglobin content in muscle tissue, and the concentration of enzymes involved in the Krebs cycle and electron transport system (Gollnick et al. 1972; Benzie et al. 1975). Other effects include increases in cardiac size and stroke volume and decreases in heart rate and DBP (Fox and Matthews 1981). Increases in coronary blood flow occur as a result of longer diastolic phases of the cardiac cycle (Frick 1976), and decreases in SNS sensitivity take place owing to reductions in plasma catecholamine concentrations (Cooksey et al. 1978) and beta-adrenoceptor densities (Butler et al. 1982). Changes are also seen in lipid and carbohydrate metabolism, including an increase in high-density lipoprotein (HDL) cholesterol (Lennon et al. 1983) and a decrease in fasting blood sugar and plasma insulin levels (Leon et al. 1979).

Maximal Oxygen Uptake (MVO). This is the greatest amount of oxygen a person can consume during physical exercise and is a measure of the maximal capacity of the individual to transport oxygen to the tissues of the body (Mitchell and Blomqvist 1971). When young college students were first subjected to bed rest and then placed in a 2-month training program, MVO increased from 2.43 to 3.91 l/min (Saltin et al. 1968). This compares with the MVO of 5.38 l/min found in some Olympic athletes (Blomqvist et al. 1969). The difference in MVO between the students and Olympic athletes presumably reflects the more prolonged, more intensive training of the athletes, but may also partly reflect differences in genetic background (Klissouras 1971; Komi et al. 1977). Improvements in MVO as a function of aerobic training appear to depend upon achieving increased stroke volume and cardiac output during exercise (Blomqvist and Saltin 1983). This increased stroke volume may be associated with a modest increase in cardiac dimensions in the absense of a pronounced change in intrinsic contractile performance. The increase in cardiac dimensions is also associated with a decrease in maximum systemic peripheral resistance during maximal exercise.

Myocardium and Myocardial Performance. Although an increase in MVO is associated with a modest increase in cardiac dimensions, training effects have been demonstrated in the absence of such changes in dimensions. Thus, subsequent to endurance training, young (Frick 1976) or middle-aged (Saltin et al. 1969) individuals have shown relative decreases in exercising heart rate accompanied by increases in stroke volume in the absence of changes in heart volume.

In general, however, even when formerly sedentary individuals are given endurance training over a fairly prolonged period of time, changes in stroke volume are associated with changes in heart volume (Archie 1975). Thus, the heart appears to grow to match the work load placed upon it. This contrasts with the situation in hypertrophic cardiomyopathy, in which the heart becomes enlarged, but both stroke volume and ventricular cavity size decrease.

The increase in stroke volume that occurs as a function of endurance training permits the individual to have the same cardiac output at a lower heart rate. This, in turn, reduces myocardial oxygen requirements. Since the physiologic mediator of CHD is an unfavorable oxygen supply/demand balance, the decreased heart work that occurs as a function of aerobic training may be considered protective.

Extramyocardial Hemodynamic Factors. Coronary blood flow is linearly related to myocardial work during intensive exercise (Holmberg et al. 1971; Jorgenson et al. 1977). Endurance training increases the size of the coronary vascular bed, thereby increasing the coronary reserve (Muntz et al. 1981; Scheuer and Tipton 1977; Wyatt and Mitchell 1978). The changes in coronary flow patterns become evident relatively soon after an exercise program is initiated (Stone 1977, 1980).

Preload also increases as a function of endurance training. Changes in physical activity and MVO are accompanied by small but significant changes in total blood volume. After 8-10 days of aerobic training, blood volume increases by approximately 0.5 l (Convertino et al. 1980; Nadel 1985). This increase in central circulating blood volume results in increased stroke volume and increased maximal cardiac output. It reduces heart rate at moderate cardiac outputs, thereby reducing the metabolic requirement of the heart muscle. Besides providing for an increase in aerobic power, the increase in blood volume also improves an individual's ability to maintain a high skin blood flow in potentially compromising situations (Nadel 1985).

Thus, the increase in blood flow to the skin permits greater heat transport to occur from the body core toward the skin during vigorous exertion in the heat.

Another component of the cardiovascular adaptation to exercise training is a decrease in afterload. Trained athletes can generate a cardiac output of about 40 l/min as compared to 20 l/min generated by sedentary individuals during maximal exercise. Under these circumstances, arterial pressure would be twice as high in the trained athlete, if peripheral systemic resistance did not decrease. It should be noted that the potential gain in stroke volume induced by training would be negated by the increased afterload, unless training also led to a decrease in systemic resistance.

Although endurance training has little effect upon the resting BP of normotensives, it can produce a moderate reduction in BP in both adolescent and adult hypertensives (Boyer et al. 1970; Hagberg et al. 1983; Krotkiewski et al. 1979; Roman et al. 1981). In many instances, the BP of hypertensives is not reduced to the normal range, but a significant reduction is nevertheless achieved. It would thus appear that aerobic fitness can be considered a tool for the long-term maintenance of normal BP.

Autonomic Reactivity. The heart rate response to exercise is normally a function of vagal withdrawal and increased beta-adrenergic activity (Robinson et al. 1966). Aerobic training induces significant changes in resting heart rate and in the autonomic responses to exercise. The resting bradycardia that occurs as a function of training involves increased parasympathetic activity (Scheuer and Tipton 1977), but a significant decrease in intrinsic sinus node rate has also been observed (Lewis et al. 1980a, 1980b).

Plasma levels of epinephrine and norepinephrine in normal subjects at rest do not appear to change as a function of endurance training (Christensen et al. 1979; Cousineau et al. 1977; Peronnet et al. 1981); whereas, plasma concentrations of these catecholamines become lower at any absolute submaximal work load. As might be expected from the relative bradycardia and decreased vasoconstrictor tone of the trained athlete, post-training plasma levels at any particular absolute level of energy expenditure are lower following training. In CHD patients, a program of regular exercise has been reported to reduce plasma catecholamines, heart rate, and BP both at rest and during treadmill exercise (Cooksey et al. 1978).

Lipids and Carbohydrates

Moderate, sustained, high-intensity exercise programs have resulted in changed lipid and cholesterol profiles in healthy individuals (Brownell et al. 1982; Frey et al. 1982; Harting et al. 1980; Haskell 1984; Lehtonen and Viikari 1978; Lennon et al. 1983; Lopez et al. 1974; Rothis et al. 1982). In general, these changes tend to be more pronounced in males than in females. In males, there is usually an increase in HDL cholesterol, a decrease in low-density lipoprotein (LDL) cholesterol, and a decrease in plasma triglycerides. Thus, training improves the body's capacity to eliminate cholesterol from peripheral stores by increasing the HDL fraction, which carries cholesterol away from such sites.

Weight

A regular program of aerobic exercise appears to interact synergistically with diet in controlling body weight. Weight loss is more likely to occur (Epstein and Wing 1980) and is better maintained when diet is combined with increased exercise than when changes occur only through diet (Dahlkoetter et al. 1979). Exercise appears to influence weight loss not only by burning up calories per se, but also by offsetting decreases in the metabolic rate associated with caloric restriction (Wooley et al. 1979) and by suppressing appetite (Mayer 1956).

Hormones. Exercise in diabetic individuals improves glucose tolerance and reduces insulin requirements, presumably by increasing insulin binding in skeletal muscle (Pederson et al. 1980; Vranic and Berger 1979). Similarly, endurance training has been shown to decrease insulin and plasma glycerol in obese individuals even when glucose levels do not change (Bjornstorp et al. 1977), suggesting that these individuals develop increased peripheral sensitivity to insulin.

Comment. The studies just cited suggest that a program of moderate, sustained aerobic exercise can decrease heart work, increase cardiac dimension and MVO, increase preload and decrease afterload during exercise, decrease SNS drive upon the sinoatrial node, and lower plasma catecholamine levels at submaximal work loads. In addition, aerobic exercise programs, particularly in males, can improve LDL/HDL ratios and reduce plasma triglycerides. Aerobic exercise also appears to work synergistically with diet in controlling weight and can reduce insulin requirements in diabetic and obese individuals. Thus, the physiologic effects of exercise should facilitate good cardiovascular functioning and produce a profile consistent with decreased CHD risk.

Combined Exercise and Emotional Stress

Steady-state exercise (Astrand and Rodal 1977) and acute emotional stress (Brod et al. 1959; DeBusk et al. 1979; Schiffer et al. 1976) can both lead to increases in heart rate and BP. The results of combining emotional stressors and aerobic exercise have only recently begun to receive attention. Studies conducted on healthy women (Garber et al. 1983) and on CHD patients (Siconolfi et al. 1984) have shown that superimposing a behaviorally challenging task on an exercise task leads to further elevations in heart rate and BP, but without a sustained increase in oxygen uptake.

In the study by Siconolfi et al. (1984), CHD patients were exercised on a treadmill at 60% of the subject's maximum heart rate. Then, a Stroop color-word conflict test was superimposed on this task after the subject reached a steady-state physiologic response to exercise. Superimposing the emotional stressor on the steady-state exercise for 11 min resulted in significant increases in heart rate, SBP, and DBP, and in the rate-pressure product (the product of heart rate and SBP). In contrast, oxygen uptake increased only briefly during the initial 2 min of the Stroop test and then returned to the steady-state exercise level. The increased hemodynamic activity without a concomitant change in oxygen uptake may have implications for the conditioning of CHD patients, since the emotional aspects of competition could combine with the demands of exercise to increase heart rate and BP without a concomitant increase in total oxygen consumption.

Aerobic Fitness, Morale, and Reactivity to Stressors

Although many committed exercisers are convinced that aerobic fitness results in decreased stress and activity as well as an improvement in coping resources, there is relatively little hard data to support these beliefs. In this regard, one may ask whether aerobic fitness per se leads to improved morale and whether fitness leads to decreased heart rate and BP responses to emotional stressors.

Morale

Many people believe that a regular program of sustained exercise improves emotional well-being. One survey of physicians, for instance, found that 98% believed that running improves psychological as well as physical health (Byrd 1963).

Several studies have looked at the immediate effects of acute exercise on anxiety. Low-level exercise has been reported to have a small beneficial effect (Morgan et al. 1971; Sime 1977); vigorous exercise has been found to lead to a larger decrease in electromyographic activity than that induced by administration of the anxiolytic agent Meprobamate (DeVries and Adams 1972). In contrast, when Bahrke and Morgan (1978) assigned regular exercisers randomly to a session of exercise, meditation, or quiet reading, all had about the same effect in reducing anxiety.

Folkins (1976) assigned subjects to an exercise or to a control group, paying careful attention in each group to issues of compliance. Both groups met three times per week for a period of 12 weeks. The exercise group subsequently reported significantly less anxiety and depression than the control group.

The issue of compliance is important in studies of exercise. In one study in which each running subject jogged with a therapist, a running program was found to be roughly equivalent to time-limited psychotherapy in improving depression (Greist et al. 1979). When the investigators attempted to replicate these findings with a larger sample by having groups of patients jog with an individual therapist, 75% of the subjects in the running group dropped out (Greist et al. 1981). After these investigators switched back to the one-on-one patient-therapist relationship, the drop-out rate improved markedly. It would thus appear that studies comparing depression in studies of joggers as opposed to nonjoggers must take into account the possibility that depressed individuals may be less likely to participate in a regular program of exercise than would be the case for less depressed individuals.

A regular program of exercise has been reported to modify type A behavior (Blumenthal et al. 1980; Lobitz et al. 1983). Moreover, Lobitz found that exercise was more effective than anxiety management training in reducing type A characteristics. Although such studies are provocative, it is not clear what factors are responsible for the behavior change. McPhearson et al. (1965), for example, compared the reported well-being of men assigned to graduated aerobic exercise or to recreational swimming. After 24 weeks, both groups reported pronounced but equal increases in their sense of well-being, despite the fact that the recreational swimmers had not significantly improved their physical fitness.

The incorporation of exercise into cardiac rehabilitation programs has been reported to lessen depression, but this appears to be less correlated with improved aerobic fitness than with compliance to the program (Kavanaugh 1977). Although short-term benefits of exercise on the morale of patients who have suffered myocardial infarctions have been reported, few attempts have been made to examine long-term consequences. The National Exercise and Heart Disease Project, which did attempt to do so, was unable to demonstrate a sustained improvement of morale among exercisers over a 2-year period (Stern et al. 1982).

In summary, people who exercise may be somewhat less anxious and depressed then those who do not, but it is not clear from the available data that any enhanced well-being or improvement in self-concept can be convincingly attributed to an increase in aerobic fitness. There is even less evidence suggesting that an improvement in aerobic fitness per se causes a sustained decrease in anxiety or depression over the long term. Self-selection factors, an improved sense of self-mastery, and group process variables, make such evaluations exceedingly difficult.

Reactivity to Stressors

The cardiovascular adaptations to an aerobic fitness training program include a reduction of heart rate both at rest and during exercise. During exercise, the fit person can do more myocardial work with greater efficiency than the sedentary individual. These adaptations are protective when the individual is confronted with sudden exertional demands. Are these cardiovascular adaptations also protective when the individual is confronted by a sudden emotional challenge? To the extent that the aerobically fit individual may have a lower resting heart rate than a less fit individual, as well as an enhanced margin of increase to maximal heart rate and an improved ability to extract oxygen from the blood, even equivalent increases in heart rate and BP to an emotional stressor would favor the fit individual. Beyond this, the question of whether increases in cardiac dimensions and blood volume could lead the aerobically fit individual to respond to stressors with reduced catecholamine release, a less pronounced heart rate increase, and an increased stroke volume response needs to be addressed. As yet, there is insufficient experimental information to answer definitively these important questions.

Several studies conducted on animals used forced-exercise procedures such as treadmill running or swimming as a countermeasure to stress-induced increases in serum cholesterol and other measures (Farris et al. 1971; Hanson et al. 1967; Kenealy et al. 1977). The inconsistent results observed in these studies may be related to the emotional stress associated with the exercise procedure. More recently, Starzac et al. (1983) subjected rats to 30 daily sessions of unavoidable-controllable or predictable-controllable shocks. Experimental animals were given access to a running wheel for 3 h following each stress session; control animals were not. The major findings of the study were that (a) all animals given access to running wheels chose to run and (b) runners had lower corticosterone and cholesterol levels than nonrunners for all stress treatments.

Keller and Seraganian (1984) randomly assigned human subjects to a 10-week program of either aerobic exercise, meditation, or listening to music. Whereas at the outset of the study, each group showed the same fluctuations in electrodermal activity in response to psychological stressors in the laboratory, by the 6th week of training, the exercise group revealed less electrodermal activity in response to the laboratory stressors. This study suggests that the exercise group showed less sympathetic arousal in response to the laboratory stressors than did the other groups, but neither hemodynamic nor hormonal measures were obtained.

Cox et al. (1979), noted that heart rate responses to WAIS and Stroop tests did not differ in magnitude between trained and untrained subjects, but that the trained subjects' heart rate returned to baseline more quickly. More recently, Sinyor et al. (1983) subjected groups of aerobically trained and untrained students to mental arithmetic, a quiz, and the Stroop color-word conflict test. Heart rate and levels of plasma epinephrine, norepinephrine, cortisol, and prolactin were measured. Subjective arousal level and state anxiety were also assessed. In agreement with the findings of Cox and colleagues, there was a significantly faster return to baseline heart rate values following stress in the aerobically trained students. State anxiety (Spielberger et al. 1970) scores were similar in trained and untrained students prior to the stress tasks, but lower anxiety scores were reported for the trained students during recovery. Sinyor and colleagues also found that norepinephrine peaked earlier in the trained than in the untrained subjects.

Hull et al. (1984) studied subjects differing in aerobic fitness, and examined their heart rate, BP, and catecholamine responses to viewing a stressful movie, performing a Stroop test, and performing a graded maximal exercise test. As expected, norepinephrine was lower in fit than in less fit subjects during submaximal exercise, but was higher in fit subjects after exhaustion reflecting greater work output. Relative DBP but not SBP responses to the film, Stroop task, and exercise were smaller in fit subjects over 40 years of age than in less fit subjects of the same age group. Absolute heart rates were lower in fit subjects at most times except during and after maximal exercise, but no differences in heart rate changes from baseline occurred between fit and less fit individuals as a function of the emotional stressors.

In our laboratory, Lake et al. (1985) subjected both highly fit varsity athletes and less fit students who preferred a sedentary life style to the type A SI, being confronted by a boa constrictor, mental arithmetic, a cold pressor test, and a competitive card game. Neither degree of fitness nor type A classification affected the magnitude of the heart rate or BP changes from baseline after viewing the boa constrictor, performing mental arithmetic, or being subjected to the cold pressor test.

During the type A SI, however, both SBP and DBP were significantly higher for type A than for type B subjects, and for sedentary than for fit subjects. Of particular interest in this study was the finding that sedentary type A subjects revealed significantly greater SBP increases than fit type A, fit type B, or sedentary type B individuals (see Fig. 2). Contrasting with the responses elicited by the type A SI were those elicited by the highly competitive card game. Physically fit type A subjects showed reliably greater SBP and DBP increases than the sedentary type A, sedentary type B, or fit type B subjects.

Since the physically fit subjects were almost exclusively varsity athletes and the sedentary subjects were college students who reported following a sedentary life-

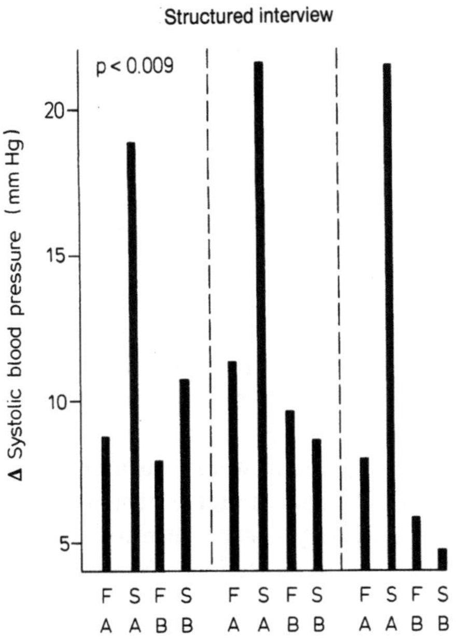

Fig. 2. Systolic blood pressure changes from baseline (delta values) during three successive 5-minute segments of the SI for fit type A (FA), sedentary type A (SA), fit type B (FB), and sedentary type B (SB) subjects (adapted from Lake et al. 1985)

style, the differences between sedentary and fit groups may have been due either to differences in aerobic fitness or to the improved ability of competitive athletes or those engaged in a program of fitness training to match arousal level to task requirements. In terms of the latter hypothesis, the paradoxical fitness by A-B interactions found during the competitive game as opposed to the type A SI may be explicable in terms of differences in the two types of challenge. One might hypothesize that the interview is prototypical of the interpersonal exchanges that confront individuals daily. As such, the increased BP reactivity of the sedentary type A subjects during routine interpersonal confrontations could reflect processes leading to increased coronary risk. In contrast, the increased BP reactivity of fit type A subjects during highly competitive tasks, particularly under the conditions of harassment that occurred during the competitive game, could be adaptive in situations requiring a mobilization of energy for maximum effort.

The preceding hypotheses, of course, are highly speculative. The findings themselves, however, have important implications for future research, since they indicate that A-B differences and fitness differences in cardiovascular reactivity may depend on the type of tasks used and the manner in which they are presented. The difficulties of sorting out differences in fitness per se from associated differences in training experience must also be taken into account.

Summary and Conclusions

The available evidence suggests that hostility may be linked to the severity of atherosclerosis (Dembroski et al., to be published; MacDougall et al. 1985; Williams et al. 1980) and to an increased incidence of CHD (Barefoot et al. 1983; Shekelle et al.

1983). A number of studies have also associated an increased prevalence of hypertension with suppressed anger (Esler et al. 1977; Harburg et al. 1973b, 1979; Sullivan et al. 1981). Whereas a high level of hostility appears to be associated with an increased prevalence of hypertension and an increased incidence of CHD, engaging in habitual physical activity has been associated with the lowering of BP in hypertensives (Boyer et al. 1970; Hagberg et al. 1983; Krotkiewski et al. 1979; Roman et al. 1981) and decreased CHD morbidity and mortality (Paffenbarger et al. 1978a; Paffenbarger et al. 1984; Salonen et al. 1982). The population studies just cited suggest that hostility is associated with an increased risk and habitual exercise with a decreased risk of CHD. Although these studies demonstrate interesting correlational relationships, such correlations do not in themselves imply causality.

The animal behavior studies conducted by Kaplan et al. (1982, 1983), in which diet and social conditions were manipulated in groups of cynomolgus monkeys represent important steps in providing the basis for a causal link between agonistic behavior and the progression of atherosclerosis. A number of other animal behavior experiments previously reviewed (Schneiderman 1983) have also implicated aversive behavioral factors in the development of both arteriosclerosis (Henry et al. 1971; Ratcliffe and Snyder 1967) and atherosclerosis (Bassett and Cairncross 1975, 1977; Lang 1967; Pare et al. 1973; Uhley and Friedman 1959).

The human psychophysiologic studies that we have described in this chapter suggest clues as to how hostility and aversive behavior might contribute toward the pathogenesis of CHD. In these experiments, a pattern similar to the defense reaction (Abrahams et al. 1960; Hess 1957) has been observed during tasks such as mental arithmetic (Brod et al. 1959) or a competitive video game (Glass et al. 1980). The magnitude of the cardiovascular responses to these challenges has been related to harassment, type A behavior, and hostility (Diamond et al. 1984).

The preceding evidence would seem to implicate the sympathoadrenomedullary system in the relationship between hostility and CHD. Emotional behavior, presumably related to SNS activation, has of course been previously related to angina pectoris (Nestel et al. 1967), arrhythmias (Lown et al. 1973), atherosclerosis (Kaplan et al. 1983), hypertension (Graham 1945) myocardial ischemia and infarction (Raab 1966; Russek 1973), sudden death (Lown 1979), and thrombosis (Haft and Fani 1973). Even modest injections of catecholamines have been shown to produce atherosclerosis (Friedman et al. 1955), arrhythmias (Guideri et al. 1975), and myocardial ischemia (Rona et al. 1959).

There are many ways in which heightened SNS activity might mediate relationships between anger, hostility, and harassment on the one hand and CHD on the other. As a precipitating cause in individuals with markedly compromised circulations, the increased SNS activity might: (a) precipitate life-threatening arrhythmias; (b) induce cardiac ischemia owing to an increased need for myocardial oxygenation in conjunction with atherosclerotic stenosis of the coronary arteries; (c) increase cardiac work by causing the heart to pump blood in the face of elevated arterial pressure; or (d) facilitate plaque rupture, which in turn could produce thrombosis and myocardial infarction. As a predisposing cause of cardiovascular pathology, increases in SNS activity could: (a) decrease excretion of sodium and water; (b) increase resistance of blood flow through the arterioles; (c) increase cardiac work by causing the heart to pump blood in the face of higher arterial pressure; (d) insult the coronary endothelium; and (e) facilitate the necrosis and calcification of coronary artery plaques as well as foster the deposition of thromboembolitic components of the blood.

Just as anger, hostility, and harassment have been implicated in CHD, programs of sustained aerobic exercise of moderate intensity have been thought to retard this development by improving cardiovascular efficiency and improving risk profiles. The cardiovascular changes include: (a) decreased heart work, increased cardiac dimensions, increased MVO, increased preload and decreased afterload during exercise; and (b) decreased SNS drive on the sinoatrial node and lower plasma catecholamine levels at submaximal work loads. Risk profiles are improved by the achievement of more favorable LDL/HDL ratios, reduced plasma triglyceride, levels, and improved maintenance of weight and BP.

An interesting paradox to consider is how anger and hostility could promote and habitual exercise retard CHD, when both the expression of anger and aerobic exercise are both known to elicit enhanced SNS and cardiovascular activity. There are many variables involved, and at least a few of them deserve to be highlighted here. Although both emotional stress and aerobic exercise initiate a chain of activities, including increased SNS activation, catecholamine release, lipid mobilization, and the release of free fatty acids, the manner in which the lipids are utilized is different. In the case of aerobic exercise, free fatty acids are rapidly metabolized as an energy source. This contrasts with the metabolism that occurs during episodes of anger and hostility not having an exertional component. In the latter situation, intermediate-density lipoproteins are not utilized as rapidly and consequently have more time to be cycled through the liver. Here, they ultimately become converted to LDL cholesterol, which is suitable for deposition in arterial walls.

During vigorous exercise as opposed to aversive situations not involving movement, more blood tends to be shunted to muscle, and in the case of running, blood also pools in the legs. The result is that the afterload on the heart tends to be less during exercise than during acute episodes of anger and hostility. Still other factors to consider are differences in the processing of sodium and water that occur during emotional stress as opposed to exercise as well as differences in autonomic function that occur in the aftermath of exercise in contrast to sedentary hostile situations.

A final issue to consider in this chapter is the role that aerobic fitness may play in preparing individuals to cope better with emotional stress. At present, there is insufficient evidence to draw strong conclusions. People who exercise may be somewhat less anxious and depressed than those who do not, but self-selection factors and other uncontrolled variables make most findings in this area suspect.

The cardiovascular adaptations to an aerobic fitness training program include a reduction in resting heart rate, an enhanced margin of increase to maximal heart rate, increased cardiac dimensions, and improved ability to extract oxygen from the blood. To the extent that emotional stressors elicit no greater changes from baseline in hemodynamic response, equivalent responses would favor the more fit individual. How meaningful such differences are is not known, but they are likely to vary as a function of age and health status. The findings by Siconolfi et al. (1984) regarding combined exercise and emotional stress suggest that the level of aerobic fitness could be very meaningful in situations involving combined exercise and emotional stress.

Although evidence that aerobic fitness training alters responses to emotional stressors is rather sparse, there is at least some evidence that the magnitude of BP responses to some stressors may be attenuated (Hull et al. 1984; Lake et al. 1985), heart rate recovery may be more rapid (Cox et al. 1979; Sinyor et al. 1983), and type A behavior may interact with variables related to aerobic training to increase hemodynamic reactivity, depending on the task (Lake et al. 1985). The implications of these findings in terms of health are not yet known, but the issues raised deserve further attention.

References

Abrahams VC, Hilton SM, Zbrozyna A (1960) Active muscle vasodilation produced by stimulation of the brain stem: its significance in the defense reaction. J Physiol 154: 491-513

Alexander F (1939) Emotional factors in essential hypertension. Psychosom Med 1: 175-179

Archie JP Jr (1975) Intramyocardial pressure: effect of preload on transmural distribution of systolic coronary blood flow. Am J Cardiol 35: 904-911

Astrand PO, Rodahl K (1977) Textbook of work physiology, 2nd edn. McGraw-Hill, New York

Averill JR (1982) Anger and aggression: an essay on emotion. Springer, New York Berlin Heidelberg Tokyo

Bahrke M, Morgan W (1978) Anxiety reduction following exercise and meditation. Cogn Ther Res 2: 323-334

Barefoot JC, Dahlstrom WG, Williams RB (1983) Hostility, CHD incidence, and total mortality: a 25-year follow-up study of 255 physicians. Psychosom Med 45: 59-63

Bassett JR, Cairncross KD (1975) Morphological changes induced in rats following prolonged exposure to stress. Pharmacol Biochem and Behav 6: 411-429

Bassett JR, Cairncross KD (1977) Changes in the coronary vascular system following prolonged exposure to stress. Pharmacol Biochem and Behav 6: 311-318

Bauman R, Ziprian H, Godicke W, Hartrode W, Nauman E, Lauter J (1973) The influence of acute psychic stress situations of biochemical and vegetative parameters of essential hypertensives at the early stage of the disease. Psychother Psychosom 22: 131-140

Benzie G, Panceri P, DeBernardi M, Villa R, Arcelli E, d'Angelo L, Arrigoni E, Berte F (1975) Mitochondrial enzymatic adaptation of skeletal muscle to endurance training. J Appl Physiol 38 (4): 565-569

Biaggio MK, Supplee K, Curtis N (1981) Reliability and validity of four anger scales. J Pers Assess 45: 639-648

Bjorntorp P, Holm G, Jacobson B, Schiller-de Jounge K, Lundberg PA, Sjostrom L, Smith U, Sullivan L (1977) Physical training in human hyperplastic obesity. IV. Effects on the hormonal status. Metabolism 76: 319-328

Blomqvist G, Johnson RL Jr, Saltin B (1969) Pulmonary diffusing capacity limiting human performance at altitude. Acta Physiol Scand 76: 284-287

Blomqvist CG, Saltin B (1983) Cardiovascular adaptation to physical training. Annu Rev Physiol 45: 169-190

Blumenthal JA, Williams RB, Kong Y, Schanberg SM, Thompson LW (1978) type A behavior and angiographically documented coronary disease. Circulation 58: 634-639

Blumenthal JA, Williams S, Williams RB, Wallace AG (1980) Effects of exercise on the type A (coronary prone) behavior pattern. Psychosom Med 42 (2): 289-296

Boyer JL, Kasch FW (1970) Exercise therapy in hypertensive men. JAMA 211: 1668-1671

Brand RJ, Paffenbarger RS, Sholtz RI, Kampert JB (1979) Work activity and fatal heart attack studied by multiple logistic risk analysis. Am J Epidemiol 110: 52-62

Brod J, Fencl VZ, Hejl Z, Jirka J (1959) Circulatory changes underlying blood pressure elevations during acute emotional stress (mental arithmetic) in normotensive and hypertensive subjects. Clin Sci Mol Med 18: 269-279

Brownell KD, Bachorik PS, Ayerle RS (1982) Changes in plasma lipid and lipoprotein levels in men and women after a program of moderate exercise. Circulation 65: 477-484

Buss AH (1961) The psychology of aggression. Wiley, New York
Buss AH, Durkee A (1957) An inventory for assessing different kinds of hostility. J Consult Psychol 21: 343-349
Butler J, O'Brian M, O'Malley K, Kelly JC (1982) Relationship of beta-adrenoreceptor density to fitness in athletes. Nature 298: 60-62
Byrd OE (1963) The relief of tension by exercise: a survey of medical viewpoints and practices. J Sch Health 33: 238-239
Caine TM, Foulds GA, Hope K (1967) Manual of the hostility and direction of hostility questionnaire. University of London Press, London
Cattell RB, Eber HW, Tatsuoka MM (1970) Handbook for the sixteen personality factor questionnarie. Institute for Personality and Ability Testing, Champaign, IL
Christensen NJ, Galbo H, Hansen JF, Hesse B, Richter EA, Trap-Jensen J (1979) Catecholamines and exercise. Diabetes 28 [Suppl 1]: 58-62
Coehlo AM Jr, Bramblett CA (1981) Interobserver agreement on a molecularethogram of the genus Papio. Anim Behav 29: 443-448
Convertino VA, Greenleaf JE, Bernauer EM (1980) Role of thermal and exercise factors in the mechanism of hypervolemia. J Appl Physiol 48: 657-664
Cook WW, Medley DM (1954) Proposed hostility and pharisaic virtue scales for the MMPI. J Appl Psychol 38: 414-418
Cooksey JD, Reilly P, Brown S, Bomze H, Cryer P (1978) Exercise training and plasma catecholamines in patients with ischemic heart disease. Am J Cardiol 42: 372-376
Cousineau D, Ferguson RJ, DeChamplain J, Gauthier P, Cote P, Bourassa M (1977) Catecholamines in coronary sinus during exercise in man before and after training. J Appl Physiol 43: 801-806
Cox JP, Evans JF, Jamieson JL (1979) Aerobic power and tonic heart rate responses to psychosocial stressors. Pers Soc Psychol Bull 5: 160-163
Cuddy RP, Shulyan H, Keighley JF, Markson CR, Eich RH (1966) Hemodynamics and catecholamine changes during a standard cold pressor test. Am Heart J 71: 446-454
Dahlkoetter J, Callahan EJ, Linton J (1979) Obesity and the unbalanced energy equation: exercise versus eating habit change. J Consult Clin Psychol 47: 898-905
DeBusk RG, Taylor GB, Agras WS (1979) Comparison of treadmill exercise testing and psychological stress testing soon after myocardial infarction. Am J Cardiol 43: 907-914
Dembroski TM, MacDougall JM, Williams RB, Haney TL, Blumenthal JA (1985) Components of type A, hostility and anger-in: relationship to angiographic findings. Psychosom Med 47: 219-223
DeVries H, Adams G (1972) Electromyographic comparison of single dose of exercise and meprobamate as to effects on muscular relaxation. Am J Phys Med 51: 130-141
Diamond EL, Schneiderman N, Schwartz D, Smith JC, Vorp R, Pasin RD (1984) Harassment, hostility, and type A as determinants of cardiovascular reactivity during competition. J Behav Med 7 (2): 171-189
Drummond PD (1983) Cardiovascular reactivity in mild hypertension. J Psychosom Res 27 (1): 291-297
Eich RH, Peters RJ, Cuddy RP, Smulyn H, Lyons RH (1962) The hemodynamics in labile hypertension. Am Heart J 63: 188-195
Epstein LH, Wing RR (1980) Aerobic exercise and weight. Addict Behav 5: 371-388
Esler MD, Julius S, Randall OS, Ellis CN, Kashima T (1975) Relation of renin status to neurogenic vascular resistance in borderline hypertension. Am J Cardiol 36: 708-715
Esler M et al. (1977) Mild high-renin hypertension: neurogenic human hypertension? N Engl J Med 296: 405-414
Falkner B, Onesti G, Angelakos ET, Fernandes M, Langman C (1979) Cardiovascular response to mental stress in normal adolescents with hypertensive parents. Hypertension 1: 23-30
Farris AW, Browning FM, Ibach JD (1971) The effect of physical training upon the total serum cholesterol levels and arterial distensibility of male white rats. Sports Med 11: 24-27
Folkins C (1976) Effects of physical training on mood. J Clin Psychol 32: 385-388
Fox EL, Matthews DR (1981) The physiological basis of physical education and athletics. Saunders, Philadelphia
Fox SM, Naughton JP, Gorman PA (1972a) Physical activity and cardiovascular health. II. The exercise prescription: intensity and duration. Mod Concepts Cardiovasc Dis 61: 21-24

Fox SM, Naughton JP, Gorman PA (1972b) Physical activity and cardiovascular health. III. The exercise prescription: frequency and type of activity. Mod Concepts Cardiovasc Dis 61: 25-30
Frank CW, Weinblatt E, Shapiro S, Sager RV (1966) Physical inactivity as a lethal factor in myocardial infarction among men. Circulation 34: 1022-1032
Frey MAB, Doerr BM, Laubach LL, Mann BL, Glueck CJ (1982) Exercise does not change high-density lipoprotein cholesterol in women after ten weeks of training. Metabolism 31: 1142-1146
Frick MH (1976) Long-term excess physical activity and central haemodynamics in man. Adv Cardiol 18: 136-143
Friedman M, Rosenman RH (1959) Association of specific overt behavior pattern with blood and cardiovascular findings. JAMA 169: 1286-1296
Friedman B, Oester YT, Davis OF (1955) The effect of arterenol and epinephrine on experimental arteriopathy. Arch Int Pharmacodyn Ther 102: 226-234
Friedman, M., Rosenman, R.H., Straus, R., Wurm, M., Kositchek R (1968) The relationship of behavior pattern A to the state of the coronary vasculature: a study of 51 autopsied subjects. Am J Med 44: 525-538
Froelicher VF, Oberman A (1972) Analysis of epidemiologic studies of physical inactivity as a risk factor for coronary artery disease. Prog Cardiovasc Dis 15: 41-65
Frolich ED, Tarazi RC, Dustan HP (1969) Hyperdynamic beta-adrenergic circulatory state: increased beta-receptor responsiveness. Arch Intern Med 123: 1-7
Funkenstein DH, King SH, Drolette ME (1954) The direction of anger during a laboratory stress-inducing situation. Psychosom Med 16: 404-413
Gambaro S, Rabia A (1962) Diastolic blood pressure responses following direct and displaced aggression after anger arousal in high- and low-guilt subjects. J Pers Soc Psychol 12: 87-94
Garber CE, Siconolfi SF, Morton MC, Carleton RA (1983) Hemodynamic effects of mental stress during exercise (abstract). Med Sci Sports Exerc 15: 183
Gentry WD (1972) Biracial aggression. I. Effect of verbal attack and sex of victim. J Soc Psychol 88: 75-82
Gentry WD, Chesney AP, Gary HG, Hall RP, Harburg E (1982) Habitual anger-coping styles. I. Effect on mean blood pressure and risk for essential hypertension. Psychosom Med 44: 195-202
Glass DC, Krakoff LW, Contrada R, Hilton WF, Kehoe K, Manucci EG, Collins C, Snow B, Elting E (1980) Effect of harassment and competition on cardiovascular and plasma catecholamine responses in type A and type B individuals. Psychophysiology 17: 453-454
Gollnick P, Armstrong R, Saubert C, Piehl K, Saltin B (1972) Enzyme activity and fiber composition in skeletal muscle of untrained and trained men. J Appl Physiol 33 (3): 312-319
Graham JDP (1945) High blood pressure after battle. Lancet 1: 239-240
Greist J, Eischens R, Klein M, Gurman A, Morgan W (1979) Running as a treatment for depression. Comp Psychiatr 20: 41-54
Greist J, Eischens R, Klein M (1981) Addendum to running through your mind. In: Sacks MH, Sachs ML (eds) Psychology of running. Human Kinetics, Champaign, IL
Guideri G, Barletta M, Chau R, Green M, Lehr D (1975) Method for the production of severe ventricular dysrhythmias in small laboratory animals. In: Roy P, Rona G (eds) The metabolism of contraction. University Park Press, Baltimore
Haft HI, Fani K (1973) Intravascular platelet aggregation in the heart induced by stress. Circulation 48: 164-169
Hagberg JM, Goldring D, Ehsam AA, Heath GW, Hernandez A, Schechtman K, Holloszy JO (1983) Effects of exercise training on the blood pressure and hemodynamic features of hypertensive adolescents. Am J Cardiol 52: 763-768
Hanson DL, Lorenzen JA, Morris AE, Ahrens RA, Wilson JE (1967) Effects of fat intake and exercise on serum cholesterol and body composition. Am J Physiol 213: 347-352
Harburg E, Erfurt JC, Chape C, Schull W, Schork MA (1973a) Socio-ecological stressor areas and black-white blood pressure: Detroit. J Chronic Dis 26: 596-611
Harburg E, Erfurt JC, Hauenstein LS, Chape C, Schull WJ, Schork MA (1973b) Socio-ecological stress, suppressed hostility, skin color, and black-white male blood pressure: Detroit. Psychosom Med 35: 276-296
Harburg E, Blakelock EH, Roeper PJ (1979) Resentful and reflective coping with arbitrary authority and blood pressure: Detroit. Psychosom Med 3: 189-202
Harting GH, Foreyt JP, Mitchell RF, Vlasek I, Gotto AM (1980) Relation of diet to high-density-

lipoprotein cholesterol in middle-age marathon runners, joggers, and inactive men. N Engl J Med 302: 357-361
Haskell WL (1984) Exercise-induced changes in plasma lipids and lipoproteins. Prev Med 13: 23-36
Hastrup JL, Light KC, Obrist PA (1982) Parental hypertension and cardiovascular response to stress in healthy young adults. Psychophysiology 19: 615-622
Haynes SG, Feinleib M, Kannel WB (1980) The relationship of psychosocial factors to coronary heart disease in the Framingham study. Am J Epidemiol 111: 37-58
Henry JP, Ely DL, Stephens PM, Ratcliffe HL, Santisteban GA, Shapiro AP (1971) The role of psychosocial factors in the development of atherosclerosis in CBA mice. Atherosclerosis 14: 203-218
Hess WR (1957) Functional organization of the diencephalon. Grune and Stratton, New York
Hokanson JE (1961) Vascular and psychogalvanic effects of experimentally aroused anger. J Pers 29: 30-39
Hokanson JE, Burgess M (1962) The effect of status, type of frustration, and aggression on vascular processes. J Abnorm Soc Psychol 65: 232-237
Holmberg S, Serzysko W, Varnauskas E (1971) Coronary circulation during heavy exercise in control subjects and patients with coronary heart disease. Acta Med Scand 190: 465-480
Hull EM, Young SH, Ziegler MG (1984) Aerobic fitness affects cardiovascular and catecholamine responses to stressors. Psychophysiology 21 (3): 353-360
Jenkins CD, Rosenman RH, Friedman M (1966) Components of the coronary-prone behavior pattern. J Chronic Dis 19: 599-609
Jorgensen CR, Gobel FL, Taylor HL, Wang Y (1977) Myocardial blood flow and oxygen consumption during exercise. Ann NY Acad Sci 301: 213-223
Julius S, Conway J (1968) Hemodynamic studies in patients with borderline blood pressure elevation. Circulation 38: 282-288
Julius S, Pascual AV, Sannerstedt R, Mitchell C (1971) Relationship between cardiac output and peripheral resistance in borderline hypertension. Circulation 43: 382-390
Kahn HA (1963) The relationship of reported coronary heart disease mortality to physical activity of work. Am J Public Health 53: 1058-1067
Kannel WB, Sorlie P (1979) Some health benefits of physical activity: The Framingham study. Arch Intern Med 139: 857-861
Kaplan JR, Manuck SB (1981) Stress-induced heart rate reactivity and atherosclerosis in monkeys. Psychosom Med 43: 189
Kaplan JR, Manuck SB, Clarkson TB, Lusso FM, Taub DM (1982) Social status, environment and atherosclerosis in cynomolgus monkeys. Arteriosclerosis 2: 359
Kaplan JR, Manuck SB, Clarkson TB, Lusso FM, Taub DM, Miller EW (1983) Social stress in normocholesterolemic monkeys. Science 220: 733
Kavanagh T, Shepard R, Tuck J, Qureshi S (1977) Depression following myocardial infarction: the effect of distance running. Ann NY Acad Sci 301: 1029-1038
Keller S, Seraganian P (1984) Physical fitness level and autonomic reactivity to psychosocial stress. J Psychosom Med 28: 279-287
Kenealy MD, Jacobson NL, Wiggers KD (1977) The effects of supplemental dietary cholesterol and exercise on blood cholesterol and atherosclerosis in the goat. Atherosclerosis 27: 65-70
Klissouras V (1971) Heritability of adaptive variation. J Appl Physiol 31: 338-344
Komi PV, Viitasalo JH, Havu M, Thorstensson A, Sjodin B, Karlsson J (1977) Skeletal muscle fibers and muscle enzyme activities in monozygous and dizygous twins of both sexes. Acta Physiol Scand 100: 385-392
Krantz DS, Sanmarco MI, Selvester RH, Matthews KA (1979) Psychological correlates of progression of atherosclerosis in men. Psychosom Med 41: 467-475
Krotkiewski M, Mandroukas K, Sjostran L, Sullivan L, Wetterquist H, Bjorntorp P (1979) Effects of long-term physical training on body fat, metabolism, and blood pressure in obesity. Metabolism 28: 650-658
Lake BW, Suarez EC, Schneiderman N, Tocci N (1985) type A behavior pattern, physical fitness, and psychophysiological reactivity. J Health Psychol 4: 169-187
Lang CM (1967) Effects of psychic stress on atherosclerosis in the squirrel monkey (Saimiri sciureus). Proc Soc Exp Biol Med 126: 30-34

Lehtonen A, Viikari J (1978) Serum triglycerides and cholesterol and serum high-density lipoprotein cholesterol in highly physically active men. Acta Med Scand 204: 111-119

Lennon DLF, Stratman FW, Shrago E, Nagie FJ, Hanson PG, Madden M, Spennettaa T (1983) Total cholesterol and HDL-cholesterol changes during acute, moderate-intensity exercise in men and women. Metabolism 32: 244-249

Leon AS, Conrad J, Hunningbake DB, Serfass R (1979) Effects of a vigorous walking program on body composition and carbohydrates and lipid metabolism of obese young men. Am J Clin Nutr 32: 1776-1787

Lewis SF, Nylander E, Gad P, Areskog NH (1980a) Non-autonomic component in bradycardia of endurance-trained men at rest and during exercise. Acta Physiol Scand 109: 297-305

Lewis S, Thompson P, Areskog NH, Marconyak M, Vodak P, DeBusk R, Haskell WL (1980b). Endurance training and heart rate control studied by combined parasympathetic and beta-adrenergic blockade. Int J Sports Med 1: 42-49

Light KC, Koepke JP, Obrist PA, Willis PW IV (1983) Psychological stress induces sodium and fluid retention in men at high risk for hypertension. Science 220: 429

Lobitz C, Brammel H, Stoll S, Nicolli A (1983) Physical exercise and anxiety management training for cardiac stress management in a nonpatient population. J Card Rehabil 3: 683-688

Lopez SA, Vial R, Balart L, Arroyave G (1974) Effect of exercise and physical fitness on serum lipids and lipoproteins. Atherosclerosis 20: 1-9

Lown B (1979) Sudden cardiac death: the major challenge confronting contemporary cardiology. Am J Cardiol 43: 313-319

Lown B, Tykocinski M, Garfein A, Brooks P (1973) Sleep and ventricular premature beats. Circulation 48: 691

MacDougall JM, Dembroski TM, Dimsdale JE, Hacket TP (1985) Components of type A, hostility and anger in: Further relationships to angiographic findings. Health Psychol 4: 137-142

Manuck SB, Proietti J (1982) Parental hypertension and cardiovascular response to cognitive and isometric challenge. Psychophysiology 19: 481-489

Manuck SB, Kaplan JR, Clarkson TB (1983) Behaviorally induced heart rate reactivity and atherosclerosis in Eynomolgus monkeys. Psychosom Med 45 (2): 95-108

Matthews KA, Glass DC, Rosenman RH, Bortner RW (1977) Competitive drive, pattern A, and coronary heart disease: a further analysis of some data from the Western Collaborative Group Study. J Chronic Dis 30: 489-498

Mayer J (1956) Regulation of energy intake and body weight: the glucostatic theory and the lipostatic hypothesis. Ann NY Acad Sci 63: 15-43

McKegney FP, Williams RB (1967) Psychological aspects of hypertension: II. The differential influence of interview variables on blood pressure. Am J Psychiatry 123: 1539-1545

McPhearson B, Paivio A, Yuhasz M, Rechnitzer P, Pickard H, Lefroe N (1965) Psychological effects of an exercise program for post infarct and normal adult men. J Sports Med Phys Fitness 8: 95-102

Mitchell JH, Blomqvist GB (1971) Maximal oxygen uptake. N Engl J Med 971: 1018-1022

Morgan WP, Roberts JA, Feinerman AD (1971) Psychologic effect of acute physical activity. Arch Phys Med Rehabil 52: 422-425

Morris JN, Heady JA, Raffle PAB, Roberts CG, Parks JW (1953) Coronary heart disease and physical activity of work. Lancet 2: 1053-1057, 1111-1120

Morris JN, Heady JA, Raffle PAB (1956) Physique of London busmen: epidemiology of uniforms. Lancet 2: 569-570

Mosher DL (1961) The development and validation of a sentence-completion measure of guilt. Unpublished doctoral dissertation, Ohio State University

Muntz KW, Gonyea WJ, Mitchell JH (1981) Cardiac hypertrophy in response to an isometric training program in the cat. Circ Res 49: 1092-1101

Nadel E (1985) Recent advances in temperature regulation during exercise in humans. Fed Proc 44: 2286-2292

Nestel PS (1969) Blood pressure and catecholamine excretion after mental stress in labile hypertension. Lancet 1: 692-694

Nestel PS, Verghese A, Level RRH (1967) Catecholamine secretion and sympathetic nervous responses to emotion in men with and without angina pectoris. Am Heart J 73: 227-234

Novaco RW (1975) Anger Control. Heath, Lexington, MA

Obrist PA, Gaebelein CJ, Teller ES, Langer AW, Grignolo A, Light KC, McCubbin JA (1978) The relationship among heart rate, carotid dp/dt and blood pressure in humans as a function of the type of stress. Psychophysiology 15: 102-115

Paffenbarger RS, Hale WE (1975) Work activity and coronary heart mortality. N Engl J Med 292: 545-550

Paffenbarger RS, Laughlin ME, Gima AS (1970) Work activity of longshoremen as related to death from coronary heart disease and stroke. N Engl J Med 282: 1109-1114

Paffenbarger RS, Hale WE, Brand RJ, Hyde RT (1977) Work-energy level, personal characteristics, and fatal heart attack: a birth-cohort effect. Am J Epidemiol 105: 200-213

Paffenbarger RS, Brand RJ, Scholtz RI, Jung DL (1978a) Energy expenditure, cigarette smoking, and blood pressure level as related to death from specific diseases. Am J Epidemiol 108: 12-18

Paffenbarger RS, Wing AL, Hyde RT (1978b) Physical activity as an index of heart attack risk in college alumni. Am J Epidemiol 108: 161-175

Paffenbarger RS, Hyde RT, Wing AL, Steinmetz CH (1984) A natural history of athleticism and cardiovascular health. JAMA 252 (4): 491-495

Pare WP, Rothfeld B, Isom KE et al. (1973) Cholesterol synthesis and metabolism as a function of unpredictable shock stimulation. Physiol Behav 11: 107-110

Pederson O, Beck-Nielsen H, Hedings L (1980) Increased insulin receptors after exercise in patients with insulin-dependent diabetes mellitus. N Engl J Med 302: 886-892

Peronnet F, Ferguson RJ, Perrault H, Ricci G, Lajoie D (1981) Echocardiography and the athlete's heart. Physiol Sports Med 9: 102-112

Pollock ML, Cureton TK, Greninger L (1969) Effects of frequency of training on working capacity, cardiovascular function and body composition in young men. Med Sci Sports 1: 10-17

Raab W (1966) Emotional and sensory stress factors in myocardial pathology. Am Heart J 72: 538-564

Ratcliffe HL, Snyder RL (1967) Arteriosclerotic stenosis of the intramural coronary arteries of chickens: further evidence of a relation to social factors. Penrose Research Laboratory, Zoological Society of Philadelphia, and Department of Pathology, University of Pennsylvania, pp 357-365

Rigotti NA, Thomas GS, Leaf A (1983) Exercise and coronary heart disease. Ann Rev Med 34: 391-412

Robinson BF, Epstein SE, Kahler RL, Braunwald E (1966) Circulatory effects of acute expansion of blood volume: studies during maximal exercise at rest. Circ Res 19: 26-32

Roman O, Camuzzi AL, Villalon E, Klenner C (1981) Physical training program in arterial hypertension: a long-term prospective follow-up. Angiology 67: 230-243

Rona G, Chappel CI, Balsay T, Caudry R (1959) An infarct-like myocardial lesion and other toxic manifestations produced by isoproterenol in the rat. Arch Pathol 67: 443-455

Rothis TC, Cote R, Coyle E, Wilmore JH (1982) Relationship between high-density lipoprotein cholesterol and weekly running mileage. J Card Rehabil 2: 109-112

Russek HI (1973) Emotional stress as a cause of coronary heart disease. J Am Coll Health Assoc 22: 120-123

Salonen JT, Puska P, Tuomilehto I (1982) Physical activity and risk of myocardial infarction, cerebral stroke and death. Am J Epidemiol 115: 526-537

Saltin B, Blomqvist G, Mitchell JH Jr, Wildenthal K, Chapman CB (1968) Response to exercise after bed rest and after training. Circulation 38 [Suppl 7]: 1-78

Saltin B, Hartley LH, Kilbom A, Astrand I (1969) Physical training in sedentary middle-aged and older men. II. Oxygen uptake, heart rate, and blood lactate concentration at submaximal and maximal exercise. Scand J Clin Lab Invest 24: 323-334

Sannerstedt R, Julius S (1972) Systemic haemodynamics in borderline arterial hypertension: response to static exercise before and under the influence of propranolol. Cardiovasc Res 6: 398-403

Saul L (1939) Hostility in cases of essential hypertension. Psychosom Med 1: 153-161

Schachter J (1957) Pain, fear, and anger in hypertensives and normotensives. Psychosom Med 19: 17-29

Scheuer J, Tipton CM (1977) Cardiovascular adaptations to physical training. Ann Rev Physiol 39: 221-251

Schiffer F, Hartley LH, Schulman CL, Abelmann W (1976) The quiz electrocardiogram: a new diagnostic and research technique for evaluating the relation between emotional stress and ischemic heart disease. Am J Cardiol 37: 41-47

Schneiderman N (1983) Behavior, autonomic function and animal models of cardiovascular pathology. In: Dembroski TM, Schmidt TH, Blumchen G (eds) Biological basis of coronary-prone behavior: behavioral approaches to a 20th century epidemic. Karger, Basle

Shapiro S, Weinblatt E, Frank C, Sager RV (1969) Incidence of coronary heart disease in a population insured for medical care (HIP). Am J Public Health 59: 1-101

Shekelle R, Gale M, Ostfeld A, et al. (1983) Hostility, risk of coronary heart disease and mortality. Psychosom Med 45: 109-114

Siconolfi SF, Garber CE, Baptist GD, Cooper FS, Careton RA (1984) Circulatory effects of mental stress during exercise in coronary artery disease patients. Clin Cardiol 7: 441-444

Siegal JM (1984) Multidimensional anger inventory. In: Chesney MA, Rosenman RH, Goldston SE (eds) Anger and hostility in behavioral medicine. Hemisphere, New York

Sime W (1977) A comparison of exercise and meditation in reducing physiological response to stress. Med Sci Sports 9: 55-59

Sinyor D, Schwartz SG, Peronnet F, Brisson G, Seraganian P (1983) Aerobic fitness level and reactivity to psychosocial stress: physiological, biochemical and subjective measures. Psychosom Med 45 (3): 205-217

Siscovick DS, Weiss NA, Fletcher RH, Laskey T (1984) The incidence of primary cardiac arrest during vigorous exercise. N Engl J Med 311: 874-877

Spielberger CD, Gorsuch RL, Luschene RE (1970) Manual for the state-trait anxiety inventory (revised). Consulting Psychologists, Palo Alto, CA

Spielberger CD, Jacobs G, Russell S, Crane R (1983) Assessment of anger: the State-trait anger scale. In: Butcher JN, Spielberger CD (eds) Advances in personality assessment, (vol 2). Lawrence Erlbaum, Hillsdale, NJ

Spielberger CD, Johnson EH, Russell SF, Crane RJ, Jacobs GA, Worden TJ (1984) The experience and expression of anger. In: Chesney MA, Goldston E, Rosenman RH (eds) Anger and hostility in behavioral medicine. Hemisphere/McGraw-Hill, New York

Starzac JJ, Berger DF, Hesse R (1983) Effects of stress and exercise on plasma corticosterone, plasma cholesterol, and aortic cholesterol levels in rats. Psychosom Med 45 (3): 219-226

Steptoe A, Melville D, Ross A (1984) Behavioral response demands, cardiovascular reactivity and essential hypertension. Psychosom Med 46 (1): 33-48

Stern M, Cleary P (1982) National exercise and heart disease project: long-term psychosocial outcome. Arch Intern Med 142: 1093-1097

Stone HL (1977) Cardiac function and exercise training in conscious dogs. J Appl Physiol 42: 824-832

Stone HL (1980) Coronary flow, myocardial oxygen consumption, and exercise training in dogs. J Appl Physiol 49: 759-768

Sullivan PP, Procci WR, DeQuatro V, Shoentgen S, Levine D, VanDerMuelen J, Bornheimer JF (1981) Anger, anxiety, guilt and increased basal and stress induced neurogenic tone: causes or effects in primary hypertension. Clin Sci 61: 389S-392S

Tavris C (1982) Anger, the Misunderstood emotion. Simon and Schuster, New York

Taylor HL, Klepetar E, Keys A, Parlin W, Blackburn H, Puchner T (1962) Death rates among physically active and sedentary employees of the railroad industry. Am J Public Health 52: 1697-1707

Uhley HN, Friedman M (1959) Blood lipids, clotting time, and coronary atherosclerosis in rats exposed to a particular form of stress. Am J Physiol 197: 396-398

Van Egeren LF (1979) Cardiovascular changes during social competition in mixed motive game. J Pers Soc Psychol 37: 858-864

Von Holst D (1972) Renal failure as the cause of death in Tupaia belangeri (tree shrews) exposed to persistent social stress. J Comp Physiol 78: 236-273

Vranic M, Berger M (1979) Exercise and diabetes mellitus. Diabetes 28: 147-167

Weiner H, Singer MT, Reiser MF (1962) Cardiovascular responses and their psychological correlates. Psychosom Med 24: 477-498

Williams RB Jr (1975) Physiological mechanisms underlying the association between psychosocial factors and coronary disease. In: Gentry WD, Williams RB Jr (eds) Psychologic aspects of myocardial infarction and coronary care. CV Mosby, St Louis, MO, pp 37-50

Williams RB, Haney TL, Lee KL, Kong Y, Blumenthal JA, Whalen RE (1980) type A behavior, hostility, and coronary atherosclerosis. Psychosom Med 42: 539-549

Williams RB Jr, Lane JD, Kuhn CM, Melosh W, White AD, Schandberg SM (1982) type A behavior and elevated physiological and neuroendocrine responses to cognitive tasks. Science 218: 483

Wooley SR, Wooley OW, Dyrenforth SR (1979) Theoretical, practical, and social issues in behavioral treatments of obesity. J Appl Behav Anal 12: 3-25

Wyatt HL, Mitchell JH (1978) Influences of physical conditioning and deconditioning on coronary vasculature of dogs. J Appl Physiol 45: 619-625

Zelin ML, Adler G, Myerson PG (1972) Anger self-report: an objective questionnaire for the measurement of aggression. J Consult Clin Psychol 39: 340

Zukel WJ, Lewis RH, Enterline MA, Painter RC, Ralston LS, Fawcett RM, Meredith AF, Peterson B (1959) A short-term community study of the epidemiology of coronary heart disease: a preliminary report on the North Dakota study. Am J Public Health 49: 1630-1639

Psychophysiological Responses to Mental Stress in Type A and Type B Subjects With and Without a Family History of Hypertension

C. PERINI, F. B. MÜLLER, and F. R. BÜHLER[1]

Introduction

Prospective association of the Type A behavior pattern (TABP) with an increased incidence of coronary heart disease (CHD) is well established (Cooper et al. 1981). Type A individuals are more likely than Type B individuals to develop arteriographically documented atherosclerosis (Zyzanski et al. 1976; Blumenthal et al. 1978; Frank et al. 1978), to experience either a symptomatic or an unrecognized myocardial infarction (Rosenman and Chesney 1981), and to suffer re-infarction (Jenkins et al. 1976), and sudden death (Friedman et al. 1973). They are described as hard-driving, ambitious, competitive, hostile, impatient, and hyperalert, whereas Type B individuals are defined by the relative absence of Type A attributes and are described as more relaxed, easygoing, satisfied, and unhurried (Rosenman et al. 1981). This Type A behavior pattern, which occurs in response to environmental stressors, contributes to CHD through mechanisms other than traditional risk factors such as hypertension, cholesterol, and smoking.

There is considerable evidence that physiological differences exist between Type A and Type B subjects, which could be important in mediating the relationship between behavior pattern and CHD. In previous studies Type A individuals have been found to respond to various challenging situations with larger increases in systolic (Manuck et al. 1978; Dembroski et al. 1978, 1979a, 1979b; Manuck and Garland 1979; Glass et al. 1980; Corse et al. 1982) and diastolic blood pressure (Dembroski et al. 1979a; Glass et al. 1980; Corse et al. 1982), heart rate (Dembroski et al. 1978, 1979b; Van Egeren 1979; Glass et al. 1980; Holmes et al. 1982; Perkins 1984), plasma catecholamines (Friedman et al. 1975; Glass et al. 1980; Williams et al. 1982a), and plasma cortisol (Williams et al. 1982a).

These biochemical and cardiovascular responses exhibited by Type A individuals are indicative of enhanced sympathetic nervous system and adrenocortical activities. There is also some evidence of sympathetic nervous system hyperactivity in progeny of hypertensive parents (Falkner et al. 1979). A positive family history of hypertension might aggravate the adrenergic hyperactivity of Type A subjects and thus permit identification of a particularly high-risk subgroup of Type A individuals.

The present investigation was undertaken to corroborate the findings of physiological differences between Type A and Type B subjects and to elucidate the influence of a positive family history of hypertension on the magnitude of physiological responses in Type A individuals. Thus, subjects both with and without a family his-

1 Division of Cardiology, University Hospital, Kantonsspital, 4031 Basel, Switzerland (Correspondence should be addressed to the second author)

Biological and Psychological Factors
in Cardiovascular Disease
Ed. by T. H. Schmidt, T. M. Dembroski, and G. Blümchen

tory of hypertension were screened for Type A and Type B behavior using the Bortner scale (Bortner 1969), and were compared in their cardiovascular and neuroendocrine responses to cognitive stressors. Plasma adrenaline and noradrenaline served as markers for the sympathetic nervous system involvement and plasma cortisol for the participation of the adrenocortical system.

Method

Subjects

The study population of 99 healthy young subjects aged 16–24 years comprised 48 unselected offspring of hypertensive patients from our outpatient clinic and 51 subjects recruited by advertisement, who were without a family history of hypertension. They had blood pressure measurements below 140/90 mmHg on repeated occasions. Blood pressures of all parents were checked.

Behavior Pattern Classification

Each subject completed a German translation of the Bortner short rating scale (Bortner 1969). This questionnaire has 14 items, each comprising two contrary statements separated by a horizontal line of 1.5 in. Type A and B responses are represented at opposite ends of the line. The subject is required to indicate for each item his position between both extremes. Scores are computed for each item by measuring the distance of the selected position from the "B" end (in sixteenth of an inch). The total Bortner score is derived by adding the scores of all 14 items.

The Bortner scale has been validated against the structured interview both in the Western Collaborative Group Study (Bortner 1969) and the Belgian Heart Disease Prevention Project (Rustin et al. 1976), correctly classifying 70% and 75% of the subjects, respectively. The Belgian study showed that the Bortner score is significantly associated with the incidence of CHD (Lellouch and Kornitzer 1982).

In a population of 137 young subjects, the relationship between the Bortner scale and the six scales of the Giessen test (Beckmann and Richter 1975), a German personality inventory, was examined. The only statistically significant correlation was an association between the Bortner score and the Giessen scale "Dominance" ($r=0.33$, $P<0.001$), which tallies with aggressiveness as one of the most important characteristics of the TABP.

Subjects who scored in the top third of the distribution were selected as Type A (Bortner score $\geqslant 181$ for those with hypertensive parents and $\geqslant 188$ for those without hypertensive parents). Subjects who scored in the bottom third were selected as Type B (Bortner score $\leqslant 153$ for those with hypertensive parents and $\leqslant 155$ for those without hypertensive parents). The cut-off points are very similar to the mean scores in the Belgian study, which were 186 for Type A and 149 for Type B. In our study, the mean scores for Type A were 203 ± 25 (SD) for subjects with, and 211 ± 17 (SD) for subjects without hypertensive parents. The mean scores for Type B were 129 ± 19 (SD) for subjects with, and 133 ± 17 (SD) for subjects without hypertensive parents, respectively.

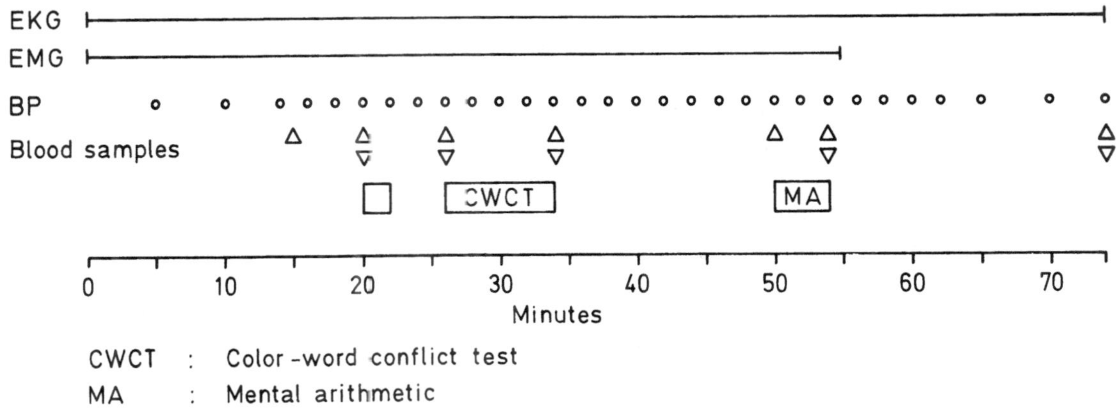

Fig. 1. Mental stress testing in Type A and Type B behavior patterns

Cognitive Stress Tests

1. *Stroop color-word conflict test* (Stroop 1935): In this version of the test, four color words (red, green, blue, yellow) written in alternative colors are presented on slides. The subject is further distracted by hearing the name of a third incongruous color. The task of the subjects is to state first the name of the color in which the word is written, secondly the name of the written color and thirdly the name of the color they hear.

2. *Mental arithmetic:* Two problems of the type $8-2+3=?$ were projected for 5–8 s on each of 30 slides. The subject was asked to give the difference between the two arithmetical problems.

Physiological Measurements

Measurements of blood pressure were obtained with an automatic monitor. Korotkoff sounds were detected by a microphone placed over the brachial artery. Manual blood pressure readings were taken with a stethoscope and sphygmomanometer at the beginning of the experimental session to ensure that the microphone was accurately located. Diastolic pressure was defined by Korotkoff V. Heart rate was measured by ECG. Blood samples for measurement of plasma catecholamines and cortisol were collected by a venous catheter into chilled glass tubes containing lithium heparin and then placed on ice. Immediately after the session samples were centrifuged at 3500 rpm for 15 min. The plasma was stored at $-20\,°C$. Adrenaline and noradrenaline were measured within 4 weeks by the radioenzymatic method of Da Prada and Zürcher (1976), and cortisol was measured by a specific radioimmunoassay with a commercial kit (Travenol, Boston, Mass. USA).

Procedures

Physiological testing was conducted 1–2 weeks after completion of the Bortner scale. Subjects were tested individually between 10 a.m. and 12 a.m. by the same experimenter, who was unaware of the subject's Type A/B classification. All subjects abstained from smoking, coffee, and alcohol for at least 12 h before being tested. Subjects were first handed a German translation (Laux et al. 1981) of the State-Trait Anxiety Inventory (Spielberger et al. 1970). Subsequently, a venflow was inserted in an antecubital vein, electrodes for ECG were fixed, and the blood pressure cuff including a microphone was attached.

The experimental session, as depicted in Fig. 1, was divided into seven periods: pretask baseline (20 min), exercise phase (=pilot phase) of the Stroop test (2 min), interval (4 min), Stroop test (8 min), interval (16 min), mental arithmetic (4 min), and relaxation baseline (20 min). Written instructions for the Stroop test and mental arithmetic were given 2 min before each task.

Measurements of heart rate were made continuously while recordings of blood pressure were made intermittently throughout the experimental session. Blood samples were taken 5 minutes before the pilot phase of the Stroop test (in the anticipatory waiting period), immediately before the pilot phase of the Stroop test, before and during (the last 30 seconds of) the Stroop test, and before and during mental arithmetic. A final sample was drawn after 20 minutes of supine rest.

Results

Table 1 presents some characteristics of the four groups. Age, Quetelet-index, sodium excretion of a 24-h urine collection, and state- and trait-anxiety were similar. Sex distribution was unequal in the groups with a positive family history of hypertension.

Table 1. Some biological and psychological characteristics of the subjects (means ± SD)

	Type A −FHH	Type B −FHH	Type A +FHH	Type B +FHH
Men	8	8	11	7
Women	9	9	5	9
Age, years	21 ± 2.42	21 ± 1.99	19 ± 2.23	20 ± 2.40
Quetelet-index	2.10 ± 0.23	2.07 ± 0.16	2.07 ± 0.23	2.08 ± 0.17
Sodium excretion, mEq/24 h	155 ± 90	166 ± 60	162 ± 57	157 ± 74
State-Anxiety	35 ± 5.25	36 ± 8.00	36 ± 6.40	36 ± 6.04
Trait-Anxiety	36 ± 8.73	33 ± 8.84	33 ± 4.22	34 ± 7.05

−FHH, negative family history of hypertension; +FHH, positive family history of hypertension.

Fig. 2. Heart rate responses to mental stressors in Type A and Type B subjects with hypertensive parents ▷

Fig. 3. Heart rate responses to mental stressors in Type A and Type B subjects without hypertensive parents

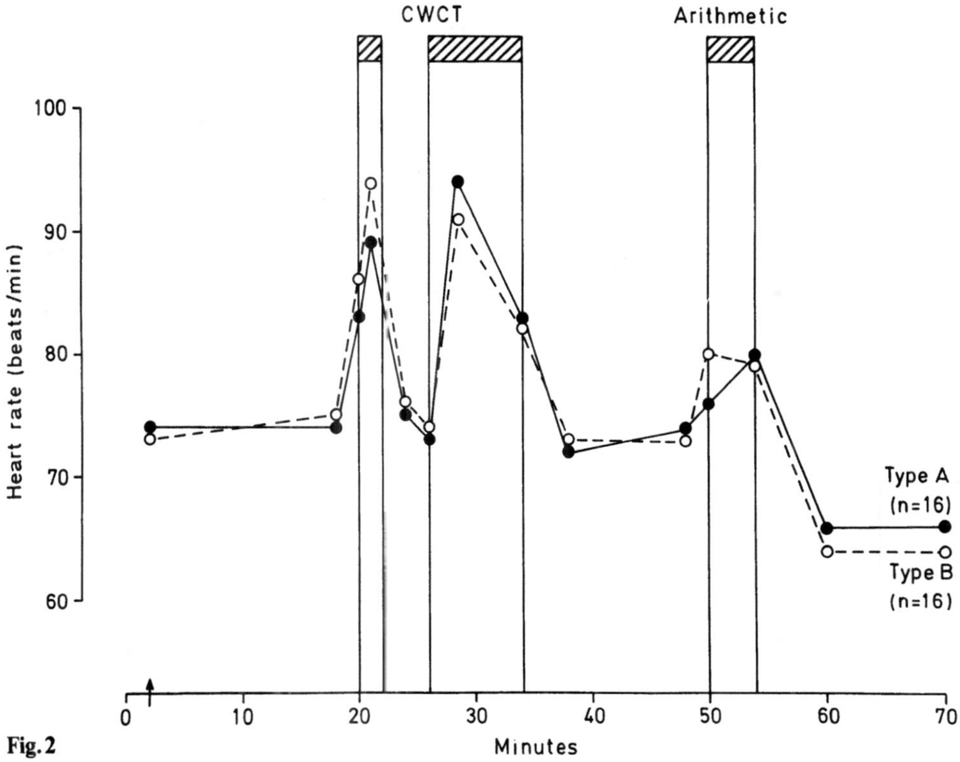
CWCT
Arithmetic
Heart rate (beats/min)
100
90
80
70
60
Type A
(n=16)
Type B
(n=16)
0
10
20
30
40
50
60
70
Minutes

Fig. 2

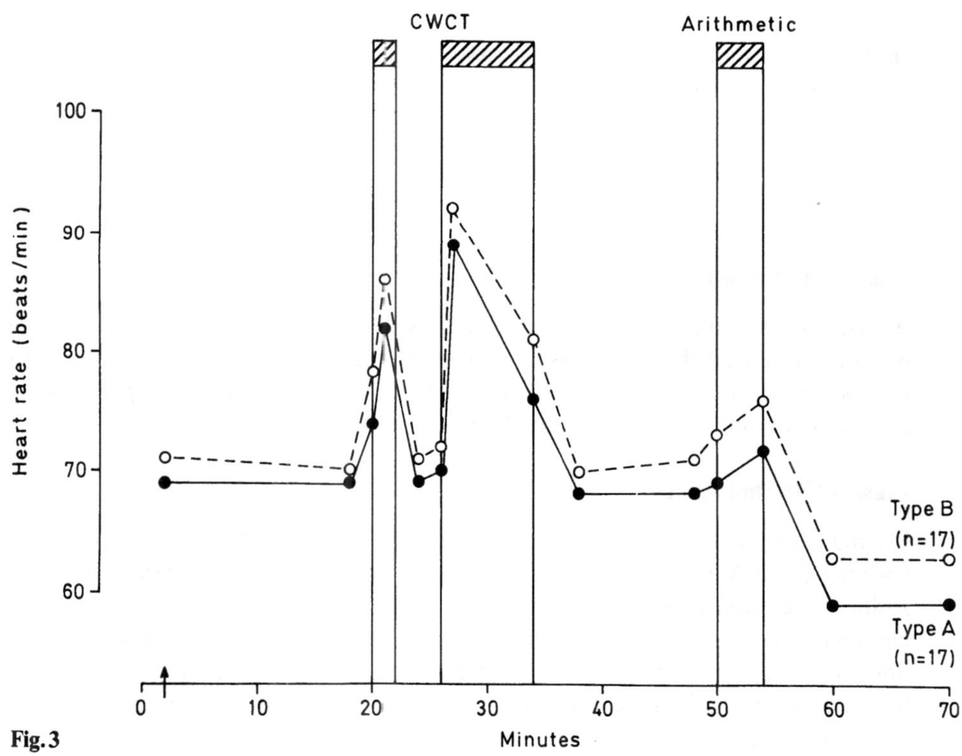
CWCT
Arithmetic
Heart rate (beats/min)
100
90
80
70
60
Type B
(n=17)
Type A
(n=17)
0
10
20
30
40
50
60
70
Minutes

Fig. 3

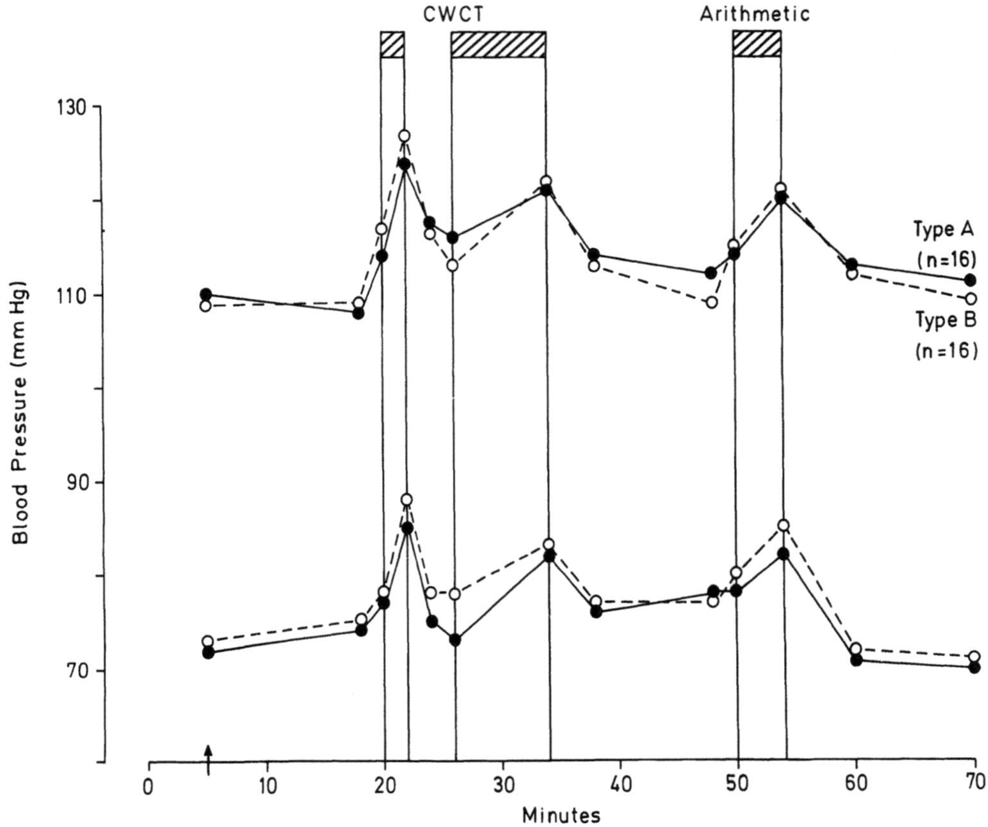

Fig. 4. Blood pressure responses to mental stressors in Type A and Type B subjects with hypertensive parents

Heart Rate and Blood Pressure

A repeated measures analysis of variance (ANOVA) with TYPE and SEX as factors was performed on the cardiovascular data. No reliable main effect or interaction was observed in any of these ANOVAs. Mean heart rate and blood pressure differed only minimally between Type A and Type B groups (Figs. 2–5).

Plasma Catecholamines

Plasma catecholamines were analyzed by 2 × 2 (TYPE × SEX) factorial analysis of variance (ANOVA). To eliminate the influence of Quetelet-index, state-anxiety and sodium excretion upon the sympathetic nervous system, these variables were included as covariates in all analyses reported below. Analyses of changes from baseline (Δ scores), i.e., subtraction of the relaxation baseline value from the responses before and during the stressful stimuli, were performed using the baseline as additional covariate.

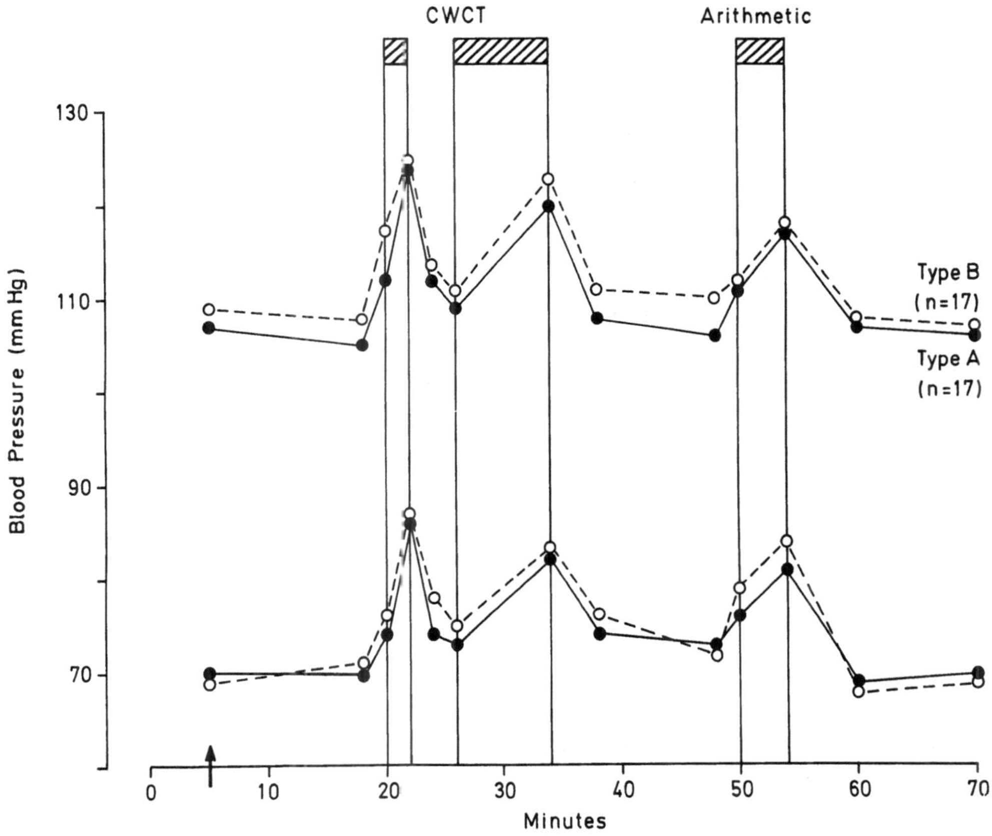

Fig. 5. Blood pressure responses tc mental stressors in Type A and Type B subjects without hypertensive parents

Adrenaline in Subjects With Hypertensive Parents

There were reliable main effects for TYPE before the exercise phase of the Stroop test ($F=5.01$; $P=0.036$), before ($F=4.40$; $P=0.049$), and during mental arithmetic ($F=9.56$; $P=0.006$), and a reliable effect for SEX 5 min before the exercise phase of the Stroop test ($F=4.32$; $P=0.05$). Adrenaline elevations were greater for Type A than for Type B subjects (Fig. 6), and the level was greater in males than females for a few minutes before the stressful stimuli only. No other main or interaction effect involving TYPE and SEX was reliable. Analysis of adrenaline Δ scores (Table 2) yielded a reliable TYPE main effect during mental arithmetic ($F=6.16$; $P=0.023$), reflecting greater reactivity of Type A compared with Type B subjects. No other main effects or interactions were significant.

Adrenaline in Subjects Without Hypertensive Parents

The ANOVA revealed a main effect for TYPE before mental arithmetic ($F=8.94$; $P=0.006$), reflecting the higher adrenaline level of Type B compared with Type A individuals (Fig. 7). The analysis also revealed a main effect for SEX before the exercise phase of the Stroop test ($F=4.59$; $P=0.042$). Males exhibited a higher adren-

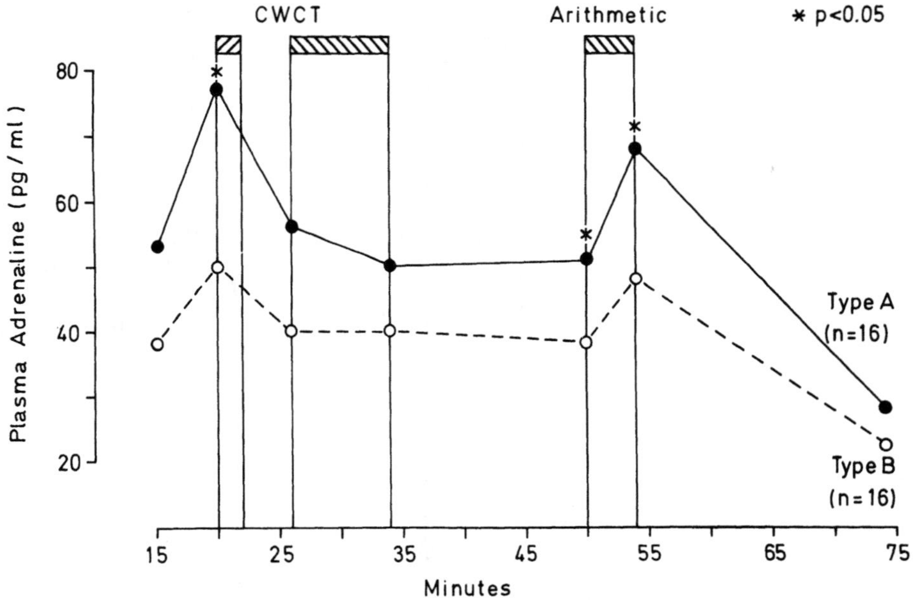

Fig. 6. Adrenaline responses to mental stressors in Type A and Type B subjects with hypertensive parents

Table 2. Means ± SEM (pg/ml) of adrenaline changes from baseline (Δ scores)

	Type A −FHH	Type B −FHH	Type A +FHH	Type B +FHH
Before pilot	17.47 ± 5.26	19.57 ± 4.59	49.18 ± 12.78	28.06 ± 5.30
Before Stroop test	17.41 ± 4.96	20.57 ± 4.11	27.93 ± 5.02	19.33 ± 3.66
During Stroop test	20.52 ± 4.62	24.92 ± 4.71	22.06 ± 4.29	19.0 ± 3.20
Before mental arithmetic	11.94 ± 4.62	20.0 ± 3.22[a]	23.43 ± 4.30	16.93 ± 4.0
During mental arithmetic	23.52 ± 6.34	26.85 ± 4.91	40.43 ± 4.79[b]	26.73 ± 3.07

[a] $P < 0.01$; [b] $P < 0.05$ Type A vs. Type B subjects.
− FHH, negative family history of hypertension; + FHH, positive family history of hypertension.

aline concentration than females. Analysis of variance of Δ scores (Table 2) revealed a TYPE main effect ($F = 10.45$; $P = 0.004$) and SEX effect ($F = 8.92$; $P = 0.007$) before mental arithmetic, which indicates the greater adrenaline reactivity in Type B subjects and among males.

Noradrenaline in Subjects With Hypertensive Parents

There was a main effect for TYPE 5 min before the exercise phase of the Stroop test ($F = 4.35$; $P = 0.049$). Reliable TYPE × SEX interactions were revealed before the exercise phase of the Stroop test ($F = 6.57$; $P = 0.018$), before the Stroop test ($F = 4.54$; $P = 0.046$), and during mental arithmetic ($F = 11.75$; $P = 0.003$). Analysis of variance of Δ scores (Table 3) revealed reliable TYPE main effects: 5 min before the exercise phase of the Stroop test ($F = 4.99$; $P = 0.037$) and before the Stroop test

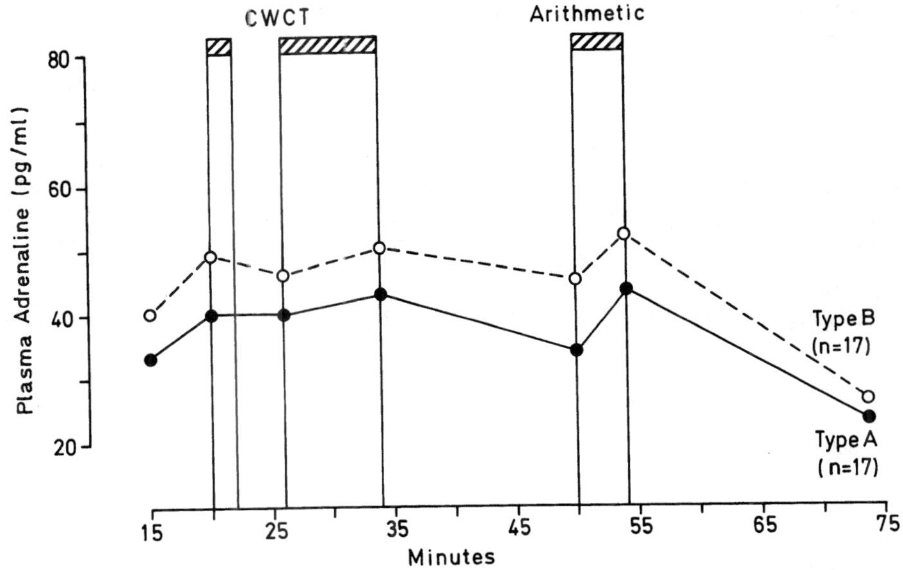

Fig. 7. Adrenaline responses to mental stressors in Type A and Type B subjects without hypertensive parents

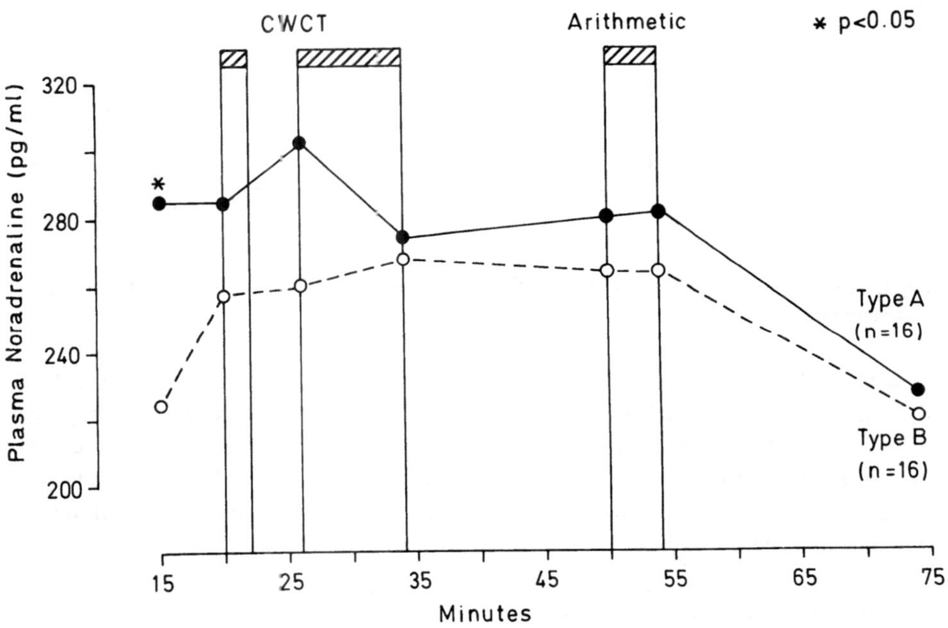

Fig. 8. Noradrenaline responses to mental stressors in Type A and Type B subjects with hypertensive parents

Table 3. Means ± SEM (pg/ml) of noradrenaline changes from baseline (Δ scores)

	Type A −FHH	Type B −FHH	Type A +FHH	Type B +FHH
Before pilot	29.64 ± 21.55	16.92 ± 22.62	56.75 ± 18.53	37.42 ± 23.73
Before } Stroop test	44.11 ± 16.74	38.21 ± 25.32	74.62 ± 12.25[a]	48.20 ± 14.07
During } Stroop test	73.35 ± 17.24	51.28 ± 29.70	46.93 ± 17.14	56.80 ± 18.80
Before } mental arithmetic	51.82 ± 21.19	41.57 ± 20.16	52.37 ± 16.96	51.80 ± 19.75
During } mental arithmetic	42.41 ± 16.84	35.14 ± 24.74	53.25 ± 22.31	52.20 ± 20.43

[a] $P < 0.05$ Type A vs. Type B subjects.
− FHH, negative family history of hypertension; + FHH, positive family history of hypertension.

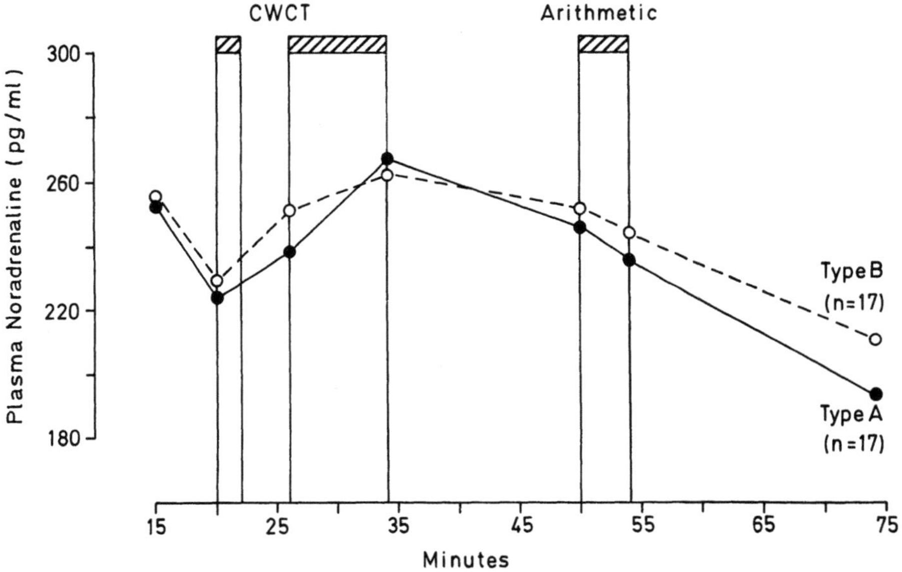

Fig. 9. Noradrenaline responses to mental stressors in Type A and Type B subjects without hypertensive parents

($F = 4.97$; $P = 0.038$). There were also interactions between TYPE and SEX before the exercise phase of the Stroop test ($F = 4.65$; $P = 0.044$) and before the Stroop test ($F = 4.94$; $P = 0.039$). Noradrenaline elevation was higher (Fig. 8), and reactivity greater (Table 3) for Type A than for Type B subjects. Amongst Type A individuals females had higher noradrenaline concentrations and greater reactivity than males, whereas in Type B individuals the reverse applied.

Noradrenaline in Subjects Without Hypertensive Parents

The analysis of variance did not reveal a reliable TYPE effect (Fig. 9). However, a significant SEX effect was found before the exercise phase of the Stroop test ($F = 8.06$; $P = 0.009$), reflecting a higher noradrenaline concentration for males than for females. The analysis of Δ scores revealed a SEX effect before the exercise phase of the Stroop test ($F = 6.34$; $P = 0.019$), indicating a greater reactivity among males.

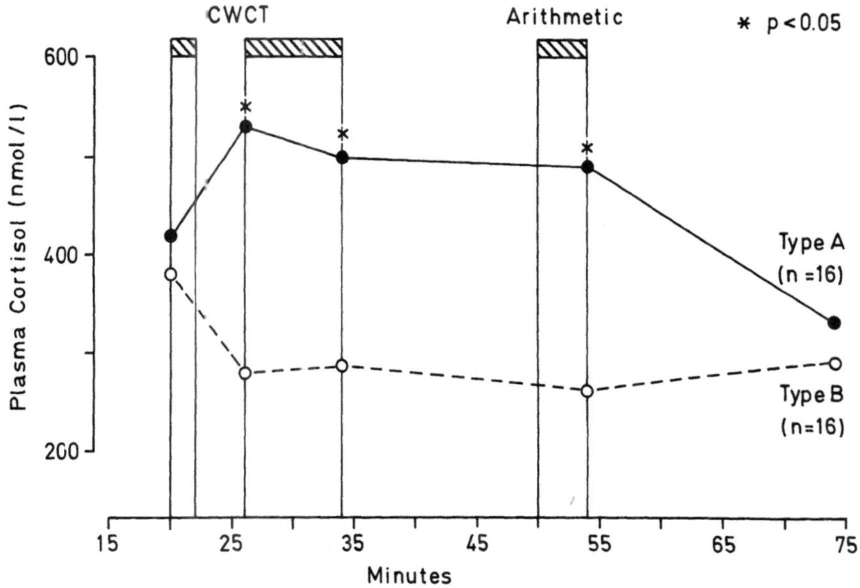

Fig. 10. Cortisol responses to mental stressors in Type A and Type B subjects with hypertensive parents

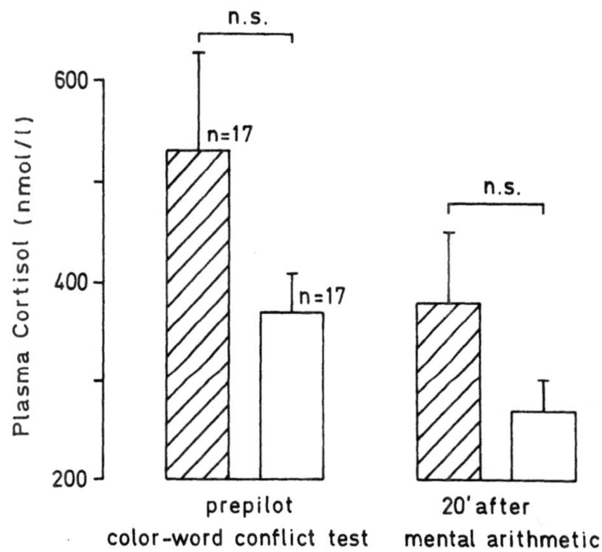

Fig. 11. Cortisol in Type A ▨ and Type B ☐ subjects without hypertensive parents

Plasma Cortisol

Plasma cortisol was analyzed by 2 × 2 (TYPE × SEX) factorial analysis of variance (ANOVA).

Cortisol in Subjects With Hypertensive Parents

ANOVA revealed a statistically reliable main effect for TYPE before ($F=7.70$; $P=0.018$) and during the Stroop test ($F=5.06$; $P=0.046$), and during mental arithmetic ($F=4.81$; $P=0.05$). Cortisol concentrations in Type A subjects were greater than in Type B subjects (Fig. 10). No other main or interaction effect involving TYPE and SEX was reliable.

Cortisol in Subjects Without Hypertensive Parents

Although cortisol concentrations before the exercise phase of the Stroop test (prepilot) and at rest (20 min after mental arithmetic) tended to be higher in Type A than in Type B, this difference was not significant (Fig. 11). Cortisol levels before and during the Stroop test and during mental arithmetic were not measured in this subject group.

Discussion

In subjects with TABP, substantially greater cardiovascular, catecholamine, and cortisol responses during cognitive and psychomotor challenges as compared with Type B subjects were observed in some but not all studies.

The data presented herein do not support a general hyperresponsiveness of Type A subjects to environmental challenge, at least as measured by the Bortner scale. However, the results corroborate the predicted notion of a positive family history of hypertension as an additional factor influencing the physiological reactions to cognitive stressors. Type A subjects with hypertensive parents responded to cognitive stressful stimuli with enhanced physiological arousal, as reflected by the higher plasma adrenaline and cortisol concentrations relative to those in Type B counterparts. Type A subjects without hypertensive parents either did not differ from Type B subjects or tended to be less reactive, as seen in the adrenaline responses. Our results confirm the findings of Lane et al. (1984) and Williams et al. (1982b), whereby a positive family history of cardiovascular disease was shown to be an important modulating factor for increased physiological arousal in Type A subjects.

Sex differences may confound A/B differences and make it necessary to take the sex of the subjects into account (Houston 1983). Although we found some sex differences and SEX by Type A/B interactions, our main results were not influenced by sex differences.

We were unable to demonstrate a difference in cardiovascular response between Type A and Type B subjects. These results are consistent with data reported by Williams et al. (1982a), Diamond et al. (1980), and Lovallo and Pishkin (1980), but disagree with other studies (Dembroski et al. 1978, 1979a, b; Manuck et al. 1978; Manuck and Garland 1979; Van Egeren 1979; Glass et al. 1980; Corse et al. 1982; Holmes et al. 1982; Perkins 1984). The lack of Type A vs. B differences in heart rate and blood pressure could be due to using the Bortner scale as the method for assessing the behavior pattern. Since the type and presentation of the stressful stimuli seem to be important for demonstrating differences in psychophysiological responses (Houston 1983), an alternative explanation for data discrepancies might arise from use of the Stroop color-word conflict test and mental arithmetic as stressors. Perhaps these types of stressors lacked incentive and competition and therefore were unable to elicit increased cardiovascular reactivity.

Both the sympathetic adrenal medullary (Raab 1963) and the adrenal cortical system (Troxler et al. 1977; Henry 1983) have been related to biological processes which have pathogenic relevance to CHD and sudden death. Catecholamines facilitate lipid mobilization (Havel and Goldfien 1959; Dimsdale et al. 1983), which results in endothelial injury (Ross and Glomset 1976), enhances intravascular platelet aggregation (Mills and Roberts 1967; Haft 1974; Simpson et al. 1974), thereby releasing a platelet derived growth factor thus promoting proliferation of smooth muscle cells (Ross and Glomset 1976). Catecholamines are also associated with myocardial lesions (Haft 1974; Eliot and Buell 1983) and ventricular arrhythmias (Lown et al. 1977). Glucocorticoids also enhance lipid mobilization (Adlersberg et al. 1951), and an association between cortisol and cholesterol has been found in subjects with coronary artery disease (Schwertner et al. 1984). In addition, interactions exist between catecholamines and glucocorticoids. Catecholamines stimulate adrenocortical activity (Tilders et al. 1982), whereas glucocorticoids regulate catecholamine biosynthesis in the adrenal medulla (Wurtman and Axelrod 1966; Axelrod and Reisine 1984). Catecholamine-induced lipid mobilization is dependent upon intact adrenal function. Thus, hypercholesterolemia may be partly due to the accompanying hyperactivity of the adrenal medulla and adrenal cortex (Shafrir and Steinberg 1960). Metabolic cardiotoxity (Raab 1968) and development of atherosclerosis (Herd 1983) have been ascribed to combined catecholamine and glucocorticoid hyperactivity.

At present, any significance of our findings must be based on the assumption that neurohormonal arousal is related to incidence of CHD. Nevertheless, the interaction of both factors, a parental history of hypertension, and Type A behavior, might increase the risk for CHD. Both Type A behavior (Rosenman et al. 1975) and a parental history of cardiovascular disease (Sholtz et al. 1975) are significantly associated with the incidence of CHD in the Western Collaborative Group Study. Thus, the present study suggests that a subgroup of Type A subjects may be identified which is especially coronary prone.

Acknowledgment. This research was supported by the Fritz Hoffman-La Roche Foundation.

References

Adlersberg D, Schaefer LE, Drachman SR (1951) Studies on hormonal control of serum lipid partition in man. J Clin Endocrinol 11: 67-83

Axelrod J, Reisine TD (1984) Stress hormones: their interaction and regulation. Science 224: 452-459

Beckmann D, Richter H-E (1975) Giessen-Test. Huber, Bern

Blumenthal JA, Williams RB, Kong Y, Schanberg SM, Thompson LW (1978) Type A behavior pattern and coronary atherosclerosis. Circulation 58: 634-639

Bortner RW (1969) A short rating scale as a potential measure of pattern A behavior. J Chronic Dis 22: 87-91

Cooper T, Detre T, Weiss SC (eds) (1981) Coronary-prone behavior and coronary heart disease: a critical review. Circulation 63: 1199-1215

Corse CD, Manuck SB, Cantwell JD, Giordani B, Matthews KA (1982) Coronary-prone behavior pattern and cardiovascular response in persons with and without coronary heart disease. Psychosom Med 44: 449-459

Da Prada M, Zürcher G (1976) Simultaneous radioenzymatic determination of plasma and tissue adrenaline, noradrenaline and dopamine within the femtomole range. Life Sci 19: 1161-1174

Dembroski TM, MacDougall JM, Shields JL, Petitto J, Lushene R (1978) Components of the Type A coronary-prone behavior pattern and cardiovascular responses to psychomotor performance challenge. J Behav Med 1: 159-176
Dembroski TM, MacDougall JM, Lushene R (1979 a) Interpersonal interaction and cardiovascular response in type A subjects and coronary patients. J Human Stress 5: 28-36
Dembroski TM, MacDougall JM, Herd AL, Shields JL (1979 b) Effect of level of challenge on pressor and heart rate responses in Type A and B subjects. J Appl Soc Psychol 9: 209-228
Diamond EL, Carver CS (1980) Sensory processing, cardiovascular reactivity, and the Type A coronary-prone behavior pattern. Biol Psychol 10: 265-275
Dimsdale JE, Herd AJ, Hartley H (1983) Epinephrine mediated increases in plasma cholesterol. Psychosom Med 45: 227-232
Eliot RS, Buell JC (1983) Role of the central nervous system in sudden cardiac death. In: Dembroski T, Schmidt T, Blümchen G (eds) Biobehavioral bases of coronary heart disease. Karger, Basel, pp 257-270
Falkner B, Onesti G, Angelakos ET, Fernandes M, Langman C (1979) Cardiovascular response to mental stress in normal adolescents with hypertensive parents. Hypertension 1: 23-30
Frank KA, Heller SS, Kornfeld DS, Sporn AA, Weiss MB (1978) Type A behavior pattern and coronary angiographic findings. JAMA 240: 761-763
Friedman M, Manwaring JH, Rosenman RH, Donlon G, Ortega P, Grube SM (1973) Instantaneous and sudden deaths: Clinical and pathological differentiation in coronary artery disease. JAMA 225: 1319-1328
Friedman M, Byers SO, Diamant J, Rosenman RH (1975) Plasma catecholamine response of coronary-prone subjects (Type A) to a specific challenge. Metabolism 24: 205-210
Glass DC, Krakoff LR, Contrada R, Hilton WF, Kehoe K, Mannucci EG, Collins C, Snow B, Elting E (1980) Effect of harassment and competition upon cardiovascular and plasma catecholamine responses in Type A and Type B individuals. Psychophysiology 17: 453-463
Haft JI (1974) Cardiovascular injury induced by sympathetic catecholamines. Prog Cardiovasc Dis 17: 73-86
Havel RJ, Goldfien A (1959) The role of the sympathetic nervous system in the metabolism of free fatty acids. J Lipid Res 1: 102-108
Henry JP (1983) Coronary heart disease and arousal of the adrenal cortical axis. In: Dembroski T, Schmidt T, Blümchen G (eds) Biobehavioral bases of coronary heart disease. Karger, Basel, pp 365-381
Herd AJ (1983) Physiological basis for behavioral influences in arteriosclerosis. In: Dembroski T, Schmidt T, Blümchen G (eds) Biobehavioral bases of coronary heart disease. Karger, Basel, pp 248-256
Holmes DS, Solomon S, Rump BS (1982) Cardiac and subjective response to cognitive challenge and to controlled physical exercise by male and female coronary prone (Type A) and non-coronary prone persons. J Psychosom Res 26: 309-316
Houston KB (1983) Psychophysiological responsivity and the Type A behavior pattern. J Res Personal 17: 22-39
Lelloch J, Kornitzer M (1982) Ischemic heart disease and psychological patterns. Adv Cardiol 29: 25-31
Jenkins DC, Zyzanski SJ, Rosenman RH (1976) Risk of new myocardial infarction in middle-aged men with manifest coronary heart disease. Circulation 53: 342-347
Lane JD, White AD, Williams RB (1984) Cardiovascular effects of mental arithmetic in Type A and Type B females. Psychophysiology 21: 39-46
Laux L, Glanzmann P, Schaffner P, Spielberger CD (1981) State-Trait-Angstinventar. Beltz, Weinheim
Lovallo WR, Pishkin V (1980) A psychophysiological comparison of Type A and B men exposed to failure and uncontrollable noise. Psychophysiology 17: 29-36
Lown B, Verrier RL, Rabinowitz SH (1977) Neural and psychologic mechanisms and the problem of sudden cardiac death. Am J Cardiol 39: 890-902
Manuck SB, Craft S, Gold KJ (1978) Coronary-prone behavior pattern and cardiovascular response. Psychophysiology 15: 403-411
Manuck SB, Garland FN (1979) Coronary-prone behavior pattern, task incentive, and cardiovascular response. Psychophysiology 16: 136-142

Mills DCB, Roberts GCK (1967) Effects of adrenaline on human blood platelets. J Physiol 193: 443-453

Perkins KA (1984) Heart rate change in Type A and Type B males as a function of response cost and task difficulty. Psychophysiology 21: 14-21

Raab W (1963) Neurogenic multifocal destruction of myocardial tissue. Rev Can Biol 22: 217-239

Raab W (1968) Correlated cardiovascular adrenergic and adrenocortical responses to sensory and mental annoyances in man. Psychosom Med 30: 809-818

Rosenman RH, Brand RJ, Jenkins DC, Friedman M, Straus R, Wurm M (1975) Coronary heart disease in the Western Collaborative Group Study: final follow-up experience of 8½ years. JAMA 233: 872-877

Rosenman RH, Chesney MA (1981) The relationship of Type A behavior pattern to coronary heart disease. Act Nerv Super (Praha) 22: 1-45

Ross R, Glomset JA (1976) The pathogenesis of atherosclerosis. N Engl J Med 295: 369-377, 420-425

Rustin RM, Dramaix M, Kittel F, Degré C, Kornitzer M, Thilly C, De Backer G (1976) Validation de techniques d'évaluation du profil comportemental 'A' utilisées dans le 'Projet belge de prévention des affections cardio-vasculaires'. Rev Epidemiol Sante Publique 24: 497-507

Schwertner HA, Troxler RG, Uhl GS, Jackson WG (1984) Relationship between cortisol and cholesterol in men with coronary artery disease and Type A behavior. Arteriosclerosis 4: 59-64

Shafrir E, Steinberg D (1960) The essential role of the adrenal cortex in the response of plasma free fatty acids, cholesterol, and phospholipids to epinephrine injection. J Clin Invest 39: 310-319

Sholtz RI, Rosenman RH, Brand RJ (1975) The relationship of reported parental history to the incidence of coronary heart disease in the Western Collaborative Group Study. Am J Epidemiol 102: 350-356

Simpson MT, Olewine DA, Jenkins DC, Ramsey FH, Zyzanski SJ, Thomas G, Hames CG (1974) Exercise-induced catecholamines and platelet aggregation in the coronary-prone behavior pattern. Psychosom Med 36: 476-487

Spielberger CD, Porsuch RL, Lushene RH (1970) State-Trait Anxiety Inventory. Consulting Psychologists, Palo Alto

Stroop JR (1935) Interference in serial verbal reactions. J Exp Psychol 18: 643-666

Tilders FJH, Berkenbosch F, Smelik PG (1982) Adrenergic mechanisms involved in the control of pituitary-adrenal activity in the rat: a beta-adrenergic stimulatory mechanism. Endocrinology 110: 114-120

Troxler RG, Sprague EA, Albanese RA, Fuchs R, Thompson AJ (1977) The association of elevated plasma cortisol and early atherosclerosis as demonstrated by coronary angiography. Atherosclerosis 26: 151-162

Van Egeren LF (1979) Cardiovascular changes during social competition in a mixed-motive game. J Pers Soc Psychol 37: 858-864

Williams RB, Lane JD, Kuhn CM, Melosh W, White AD, Schanberg SM (1982a) Type A behavior and elevated physiological and neuroendocrine responses to cognitive tasks. Science 218: 483-485

Williams RB, Lane JD, White AD, Kuhn CM, Schanberg SM (1982b) Gender and family history of cardiovascular disease modulate the expression of cardiovascular and neuroendocrine hyperreactivity to behavioral challenges among Type A persons. Psychosom Med 44: 129 (abstract)

Wurtman RJ, Axelrod J (1966) Control of enzymatic synthesis of adrenaline in the adrenal medulla by adrenal cortical steroids. J Biol Chem 241: 2301-2305

Zyzanski SJ, Jenkins DC, Ryan TJ, Flessas A, Everist M (1976) Psychological correlates of coronary angiographic findings. Arch Intern Med 136: 1234-1237

Vigilance Performance and Psychophysiologic Reactions of Type A and Vitally Exhausted Persons

W. Riedel[1] and R. Lulofs[2]

Introduction

Type A Behavior and Inactivity

In previous research in our laboratory, attempts were made to reproduce results in which type A subjects would show higher physiologic reactivity to challenging situations, as numerous studies had demonstrated earlier. Friedman et al. (1970), Glass (1977), and Glass et al. (1980a, b) observed higher physiologic and neurohormonal responses in task situations by type B subjects and in rest situations by type A subjects. In fact, higher levels of urinary catecholamine excretion were found in type B subjects during reaction time tasks, while, after watching a nonengaging movie, type A individuals excreted more urinary catecholamines (Van der Molen 1982).

Lundberg and Forsman (1979) reported a study in which male type A subjects had heightened cortisol excretion in a monotonous vigilance task. Within the same framework of studies, Frankenhaeuser et al. (1980) demonstrated that type A individuals were more aroused and felt more distressed than type B when they were deprived of work. In the work situation on the other hand, they found higher catecholamine and cortisol excretion in type B individuals. These results were explained in terms of active coping; the authors alleged that, as long as type A persons have the possibility of choosing their own work pace, they will work more effectively than type B subjects and choose higher work loads, thus not showing any signs of distress or higher physiologic and hormonal reactivity. When type A individuals are forced to inactivity, they display an inability to relax, showing more signs of distress and physiologic and hormonal reactivity than type B subjects. In many cases, the higher reactivity of type A persons can be explained, as illustrated by Glass (1977), in terms of the controllability of a situation. When no control over the environment is possible or when feedback about performance is lacking, type A individuals tend to give up earlier and feel more distressed.

We wanted to explore this effect in more detail, simulating the aspects described above by presenting subjects with a very monotonous auditory vigilance task. Earlier experience with this type of task (Riedel 1982) disclosed clear-cut differences in the physiologic reactions of good performers as opposed to poor performers; i.e., subjects who displayed an increasing performance deterioration over time also showed signs of drowsiness in their EEG recordings and an increase in heart rate variability (HRV), especially in the 10-s rhythm as a function of time on task. All the effects disappeared after a short rest break. Subjects who did not undergo a perfor-

1 Institute for Drugs, Safety and Behavior, State University of Limburg, P.O. Box 616, 6200 MD Maastricht, The Netherlands

2 Department of Medical Psychology, State University of Limburg, Maastricht, The Netherlands

Biological and Psychological Factors in Cardiovascular Disease
Ed. by T.H. Schmidt, T.M. Dembroski, and G. Blümchen

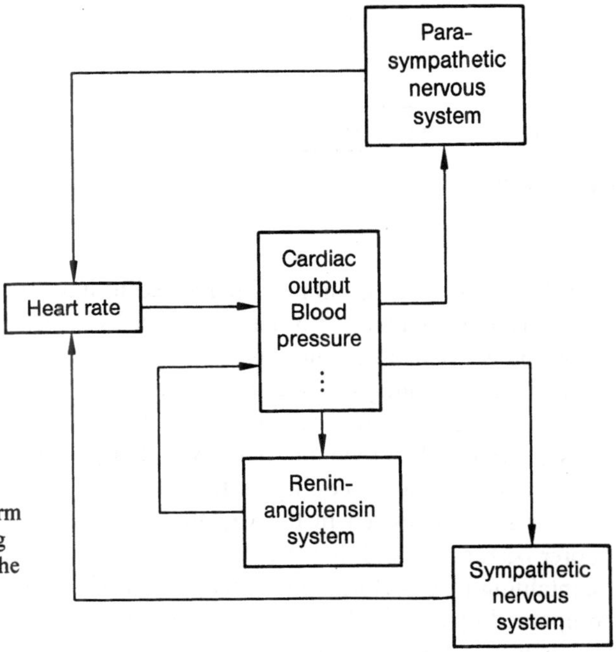

Fig. 1. Block diagram of short-term cardiovascular control illustrating primary independent actions of the parasympathetic, β-sympathetic, and renin-angiotensin systems. (From Axelrod et al. 1981)

mance drop over time neither showed signs of drowsiness in their EEG, nor did they have an increase in HRV over time. Neither group differed in terms of heart rate.

Mulder (1980) and Mulder and Mulder (1981) demonstrated that a decrease in HRV, especially in the 10-s rhythm, is a sensitive indicator of mental effort. They assumed that effort is determined either by task-induced mental load (i.e., by varying the number of decisions to be made in a fixed time) or by emotional load (e.g., a marked decrease in the 10-s rhythm HRV observed just before and during dental treatment). The mechanisms underlying HRV have also been described by Axelrod et al. (1981) and are summarized in Fig. 1. Sympathetic and renin-angiotensin influences on HRV are only reflected in the low-frequency band ranging from 0.02–0.06 Hz. Parasympathetic influences originating from the blood pressure control system are reflected in the 10-s rhythm ranging from 0.07–0.14 Hz. Respiratory sinus arrhythmia, usually within the 0.15–0.50-Hz range, also reflects parasympathetic activity (Grossman 1983).

In a series of studies on the effects of monotonous work, O'Hanlon (1981) reported that poor work performers became bored and irritated more easily than others, displayed more hostility, and were more likely to develop psychosomatic disease, even though they invested more effort in trying to sustain their performance level. Furthermore, he identified two underlying physiologic factors: habituation initiated by monotonous stimulation, which thus inhibits sympathetic activity originating from the mesencephalic reticular formation, and effort, an unrewarding voluntary compensatory process elicited to restore arousal to an optimal level for task performance. Effort also tends to extinguish over time. The relation of these two factors to task performance is illustrated in Fig. 2.

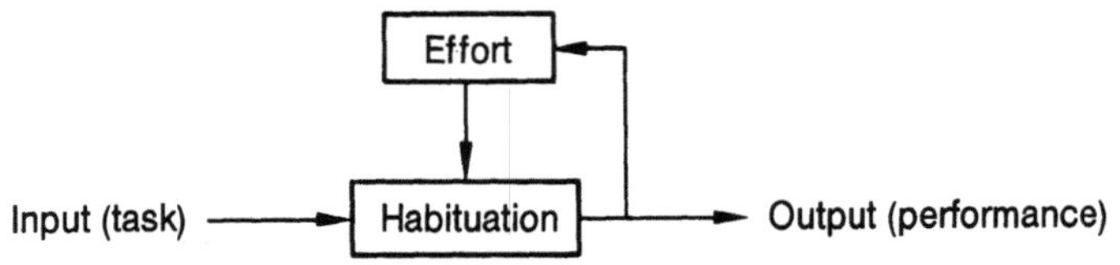

Fig. 2. Simple model of habituation and effort explaining vigilance performance

When performance failure is perceived to have punishing consequences, subjects can counteract the performance decline by investing voluntary effort. Thus, the critical objective in a vigilance task is not only attending to the stimuli but, more importantly, maintaining an optimal arousal level. As Matthews (1979) pointed out, type A subjects tend to focus on central tasks and more or less ignore peripheral tasks, as well as their own internal physical or physiologic state. In a vigilance task, this would be the worst coping strategy.

It was hypothesized in the vigilance study that type A individuals would be poorer performers and that they would invest less effort than type B individuals in maintaining task performance. This pattern of performance decline would be accompanied by an initial decrease in HRV in the 0.07-0.14-Hz region, followed by an increase in HRV as a function of time on task.

Alternatively, we hypothesized that type A subjects would invest more effort and would become more distressed. The pattern exhibited by type A would consist of a decrease in HRV in the 0.07-0.14-Hz region throughout the task and elevated levels of adrenaline and noradrenaline when compared with type B subjects.

Vital Exhaustion and Platelet Aggregation

A second purpose of the study was to explain different physiologic and neurohormonal response patterns in terms of the concept of vital exhaustion.

The syndrome of vital exhaustion, which consists of self-reported feelings of depression and diminished energy and can be measured with the Maastricht Questionnaire (MQ), differentiates individuals with and without cardiovascular complaints and is predictive for the development of myocardial infarction (MI) (Appels et al. 1979). This syndrome manifests itself more often after exposure to stressful life events and is more common in middle-aged persons who show predominantly type A behavior (Falger and Appels 1982).

One of the possible pathologic mechanisms that lead to MI is heightened platelet activity. When platelets are activated, they adhere to one another, forming microaggregates. Further activation leads to the release of a number of substances that accelerate the aggregation process and cause vasoconstriction. This combination of effects can lead to partial or total occlusion of coronary arteries and thus to MI. Apart from evaluating the direct effects of catecholamines and glucocorticoids on myocardial pathology, a few studies describe the effects of these hormones on blood platelets (Steptoe 1981).

Conflicting results exist between in vitro and in vivo studies regarding the effects of catecholamines, particularly adrenaline. In vitro studies show a potentiating effect of epinephrine (Scrutton and Wallis 1981), but in vivo studies seem to indicate

Table 1. Mean MQ scores of fit and exhausted type A and B subjects

	Exhausted		Fit		Total	
	Score	Subjects (*n*)	Score	Subjects (*n*)	Score	Subjects (*n*)
Type A	100	8	58	4	86	12
Type B	82	4	60	8	67	12
	94	12	59	12	77	24

that stress leads to diminished platelet sensitivity (Arkel et al. 1982). Information relating to the pituitary-adrenocortical influence on platelet activity is scarce. We found one study in which infusion of adrenocorticotropic hormone (ACTH) led to an increase in thrombus formation (Warner et al. 1967).

In an earlier study in our laboratory (Lulofs et al., to be published), no differences between fit and exhausted persons were found during a task situation, while, after watching a nonengaging movie, exhausted persons showed greater aggregation of blood platelets and higher urinary excretion of cortisol.

Platelet sensitivity was assessed by determining the speed of aggregation through the reactivity of the blood plasma to a trigger substance, collagen, which was added in vitro. However, because this method does not control for the total number of platelets present in the blood sample, a somewhat different method used in the vigilance study will be described in the section to follow.

Subjects and Methods

A group of 24 healthy men without medication, aged 38–42 years, participated as subjects in the experiment. They were selected as follows: initial inquiries were sent by the medical psychology unit to 2000 men, aged 38–42, whose addresses were provided by the city council of Maastricht. Of these, 1300 men consented to participate. The Dutch version of the Jenkins Activity Survey (Appels et al. 1982) was sent to a subsample of 800 men, of whom 650 returned the questionnaire. From the highest and lowest scoring quartiles, two samples were drawn: 12 subjects were classified as type A, and 12 subjects as type B.

All subjects were also administered the MQ. The MQ score ranging from 50 (fit) to 150 (exhausted) was used in the analysis either as a continuous variable or as a dichotomous variable by using the median of a known population (Appels 1980) as a cut-off point. By doing so, two categories consisting of 12 fit and 12 exhausted subjects were obtained Table 1 shows that type A subjects were more exhausted than type B subjects. This is in agreement with the positive correlation (0.38) of JAS with MQ scores previously reported by Appels (1981).

Vigilance Tasks

The tasks presented to the subjects comprised four auditory vigilance tasks lasting 25 min, followed by a short break and a 5-min reference task. The tasks were signal detection tasks in which event rate and signal rate varied. Subjects had to attend to a series of clicks in which the signals that required a response were somewhat weaker clicks within a sequence of clicks that were equally loud. The event rate was one click every 2 or 6 s. The signal rate was one weaker signal for every 5 or 15 clicks on average, but was held constant within every 5-min period during the vigilance task. The duration and pitch of each click were 2 ms and 1000 Hz respectively. Prior to each session, the sound level was set at 40 dB above hearing threshold, and the difference between signal and nonsignal was adjusted individually, so that in a 5-min training period, a performance of 90% correct detection was achieved by each subject. The behavioral dependent variables were reaction time (RT), errors of omission (misses), and errors of commission (false alarms).

Physiologic Recordings

Heart rate was measured using three Ag/AgCl electrodes that were fed into a Schmitt-trigger circuit, which was in turn fed into a PDP 11/04 MINC computer. A time series of heart beats was stored on line. In later analyses, average interbeat intervals (IBI) per 5-min period were calculated, and spectral analysis of the IBI time series was performed using the INSPAN program (Mulder 1979). The INSPAN program yields HRV split up over specific frequency bands defined as temperature band (0.02-0.06 Hz), blood pressure band (0.07-0.14 Hz), and respiration band (0.15-0.50 Hz). Spectral power values of these bands were also obtained for every 5-min analysis period.

Blood Samples

Within a 20-s interval after every vigilance task or video film, venous blood samples were drawn from a syringe coupled to an indwelling catheter placed in the antecubal vein of the subject. In the meantime, the catheter was kept free of coagulation by very slowly infusing isotonic fluid.

Every blood sample was divided into three subsamples: one tube for determining cortisol levels, one tube for determining adrenaline and noradrenaline levels, and four tubes for determining platelet aggregation. The first two tubes were transported to the Department of Pharmacology, where levels of adrenaline, noradrenaline, and cortisol were determined through radioenzymatic assay.

Platelet aggregation was determined as follows: blood was divided between two tubes containing ethylenediaminetetra-acetic acid (EDTA) and two tubes containing EDTA and formalin. In the first two tubes, it was assumed that platelet aggregates would disintegrate, while in the remaining two tubes, it was assumed that platelet aggregates would be conserved intact. All four tubes were centrifuged for 10 min at 180 g. Next, after diluting the platelet-rich plasma 10000-fold the number of particles in each tube of 0.50-ml solution was counted using a Coulter counter with detection threshold set to 7 μ and 70 μ. With this method, an estimation of the total number of platelets (n) was obtained for the first two tubes and an estimation of the total number of platelets minus the number of platelets adhering together in microaggregates $(n-a)$ was obtained for the remaining tubes. The ratio of $(n-a)$ to n yields a measure of platelet aggregation. Values of 1 indicate no aggregation, whereas a value of 0.8 indicates 20% aggregation. This method is described in detail by Wu and Hoak (1974) and Deshmukh et al. (1976).

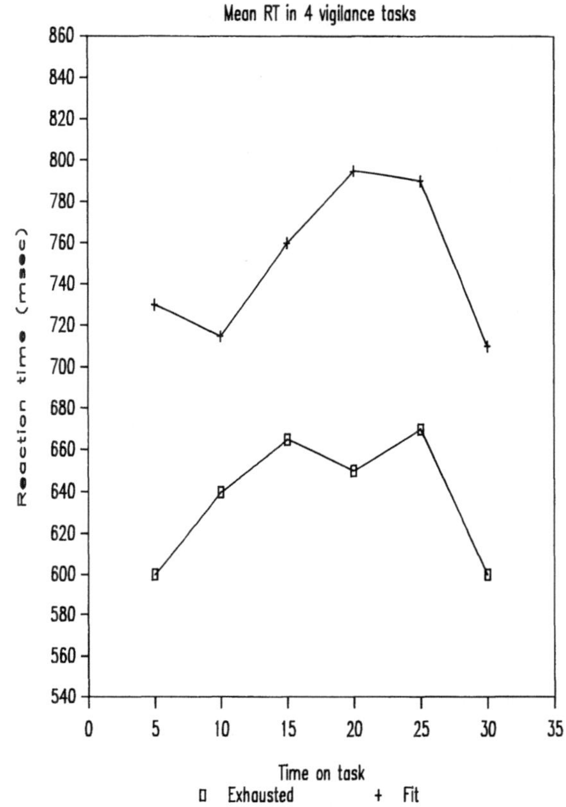

Fig. 3. Reaction time in ms increased in the course of four vigilance tasks and two reference tasks. The points on the abscissa refer to the following events: *0*, 3-min rest period; *5–25*, 25-min vigilance task; *30*, 5-min reference task; *35*, 3-min rest period

Procedure

Every subject participated in three experimental sessions, two of which were task sessions and one of which was a rest session in which, instead of two vigilance tasks, two nonengaging documentary movies were presented. Task order, film order, and session order were balanced for both type A and type B. The time course in minutes of a task session was as follows:

rest	vigilance task	reference task	rest	vigilance task	reference task	rest
3	25	5	3	25	5	3

When the subject entered the laboratory, ECG leads were attached, and the physician on duty inserted an indwelling venous catheter via venous puncture. The subjects were trained in the task until performance criteria were met, after which the experimental session started. Initially, the subjects were asked to rest with their eyes closed for approximately 3 min. Then, they were instructed to perform the vigilance task as well as possible by reacting as quickly as they could without making errors. They were told the task would last at least 30 min.

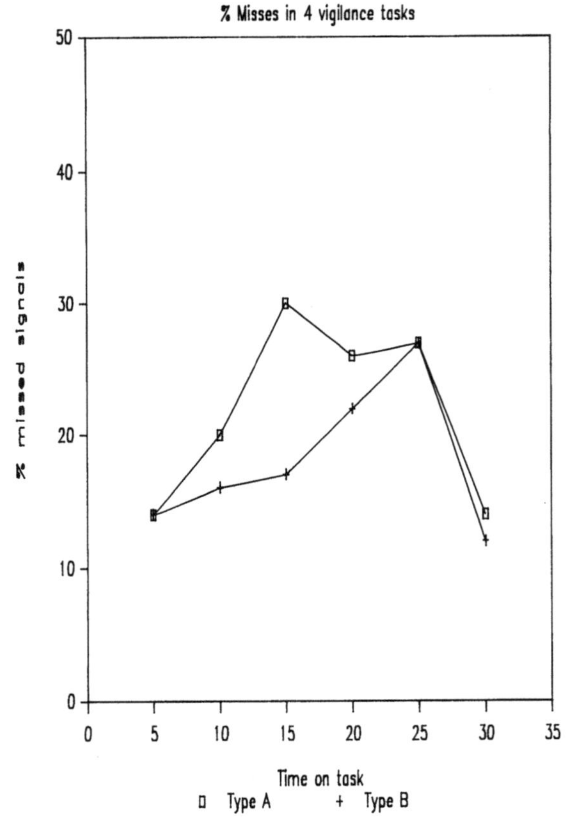

Fig. 4. Percentage of missed signals increased significantly in the course of four vigilance tasks *(5–25)* and reference tasks *(30)*

Results

For all four vigilance tasks, there was a clear-cut time-on-task effect (Fig. 3). RT latency increased as time-on-task increased. After the break following the 5-min reference task, RT latency returned to the same level as in the first 5 min of the vigilance task ($F = 6.78$; $P = 0.0001$). RT during tasks with a low event rate were about 100 ms longer; this was an overall effect ($F = 20.13$; $P = 0.001$). There was no effect of signal rate.

There was no effect of type A/B on RT. However, there was an interesting tendency of the exhausted subjects to respond more slowly in all task conditions independently of time on task ($F = 2.72$; $P = 0.10$; see Fig. 3). This effect can be regarded as an external validation of the MQ, as a high score on this questionnaire indicates difficulties in processing information rapidly.

The percentage of missed signals also increased over time in all tasks ($F = 18.53$; $P = 0.0001$; see Fig. 4). There was no effect of event rate or signal rate. However, as can be seen in Fig. 4, there was a significant interaction of type A/B with time on task, indicating that type A subjects had more difficulties in sustaining their attention than type B individuals ($F = 2.22$; $P = 0.05$).

Analyzing the number of false alarms was not possible, because the distribution was severely pathologic in statistical terms.

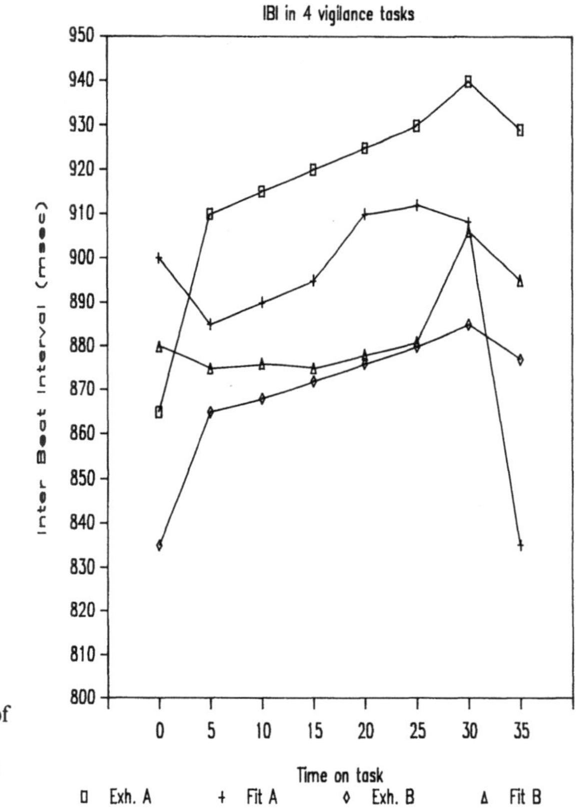

Fig. 5. Interbeat intervals increased during the testing period consisting of four vigilance *(5–25)* and reference *(30)* tasks (with pre- *(0)* and post-task *(35)* rest intervals)

There was an effect on time on task for IBI length. However, the observed increase in IBI continued during the reference tasks, and surprisingly, there was a decrease in IBI during the last rest period. Although type B persons had shorter IBI during task conditions, this effect was not significant. A more interesting question would be the effect of the decrease in IBI for fit subjects at task onset as opposed to the increase in IBI for exhausted subjects at task onset (see Fig. 5).

HRV plotted over time across the four vigilance tasks revealed significant effects of event rate (F=10.04; P=0.01). Little HRV in high event rate tasks indicated that the latter impose a somewhat greater mental load on the subjects, a phenomenon that is also reflected in the shorter RT latency. There was also an interaction between type A/B and time on task that was not found in the control condition (F=2.92; P=0.01; see Fig. 6). By splitting up the HRV into frequency bands, it can be seen that the effect of time on task is mainly found in the low-frequency band and that the effect of task onset after the rest period is mainly found in the so-called 0.10-Hz band with exhausted type A subjects. The latter finding indicates decreased vagal tone prior to the experiment and increasing vagal tone during task performance.

Type A subjects produced slightly more noradrenaline (Table 2), but the effect failed to reach significance (F=2.28; P=0.14).

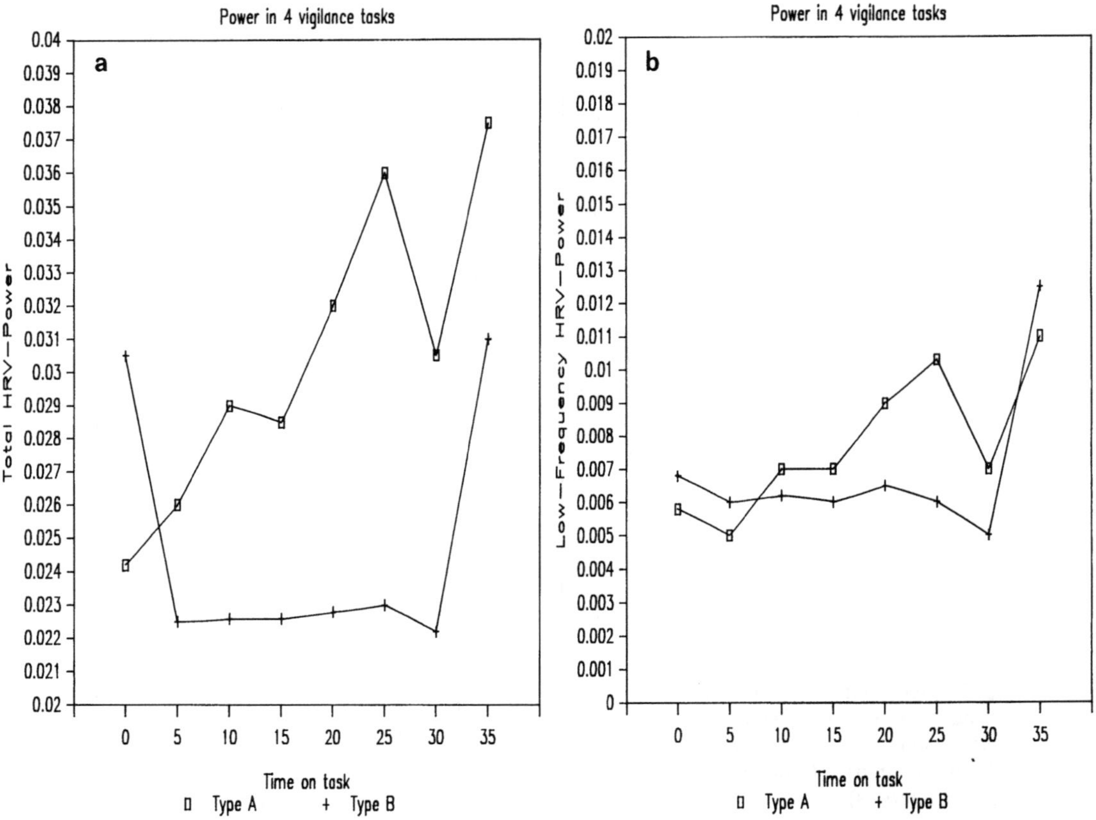

Fig. 6a–d. HRV increased during the testing period consisting of four vigilance *(5–25)* and reference *(30)* tasks (with pre- *(0)* and post-task *(35)* rest intervals). **a** Total HRV power. **b** HRV in the temperature frequency range of 0.02–0.06 Hz. **c** HRV in the blood pressure frequency range of 0.07–0.14 Hz. **d** HRV in the respiration frequency range of 0.14–0.50 Hz

There were positive correlations between the amount of circulating noradrenaline and MQ scores in all three sessions (high event rate tasks: $r=0.44$; $P=0.01$; low event rate tasks: $r=0.30$; $P=0.08$; film: $r=0.47$; $P=0.01$).

The range for circulating adrenaline levels was slightly higher, although not significantly so, for low event rate tasks ($F=2.15$; $P=0.13$). There was an interaction between type A/B and the fit/exhausted groups ($F=3.63$; $P=0.07$) that was dependent on task condition as opposed to film condition (Table 3).

There was also an interaction effect (Table 4) of type A/B with the fit/exhausted categories for cortisol levels, independently of task or film condition ($F=6.51$; $P=0.01$).

Only in task sessions were there positive correlations of adrenaline with cortisol levels (high event rate tasks: $r=0.37$; $P=0.05$; low event rate tasks: $r=0.32$; $P=0.06$).

A marginal interaction effect of type A/B with the fit/exhausted groups was found for platelet aggregation ratios during task conditions only ($F=2.88$; $P=0.10$). This means that exhausted type A and fit type B subjects have slightly more platelet aggregation during task performance (Table 5).

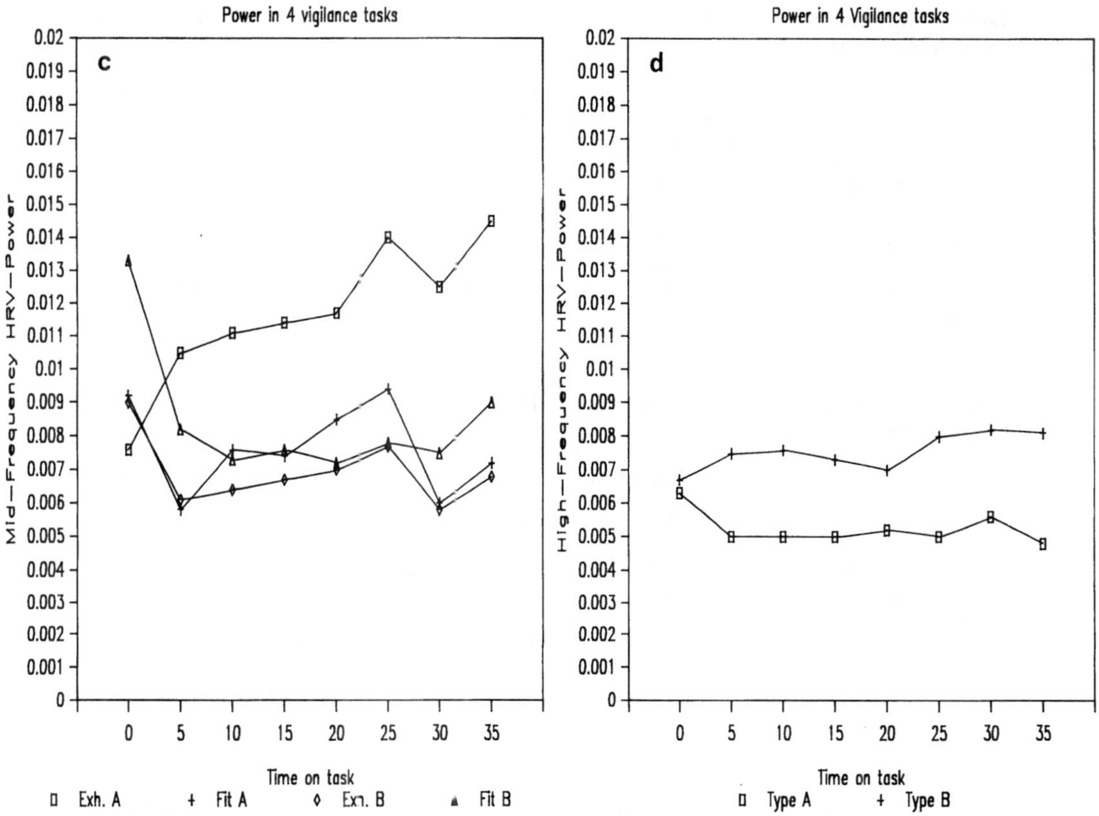

Table 2. Mean values and standard deviations (SD) of noradrenaline levels[a] for fit and exhausted type A and type B subjects

		High event rate task		Low event rate task		Film		(n)
		Mean	SD	Mean	SD	Mean	SD	
Type A	exhausted	453	191	421	135	479	277	8
	fit	307	83	373	172	339	145	4
Type B	exhausted	374	51	308	100	303	143	4
	fit	326	136	335	124	336	122	8

[a] Values of noradrenaline are in pg/ml.

Table 3. Mean values and standard deviations (SD) of adrenaline levels[a] for fit and exhausted type A and type B subjects

		High event rate task		Low event rate task		Film		(n)
		Mean	SD	Mean	SD	Mean	SD	
Type A	exhausted	56	23	86	93	72	49	8
	fit	39	20	47	20	57	42	4
Type B	exhausted	56	31	52	12	112	36	4
	fit	63	27	101	87	74	35	8

[a] Values of adrenaline are in pg/ml.

Table 4. Mean values and standard deviations (SD) of cortisol levels[a] for fit and exhausted type A and type B subjects

		High event rate task		Low event rate task		Film		(n)
		Mean	SD	Mean	SD	Mean	SD	
Type A	exhausted	309	93	310	109	301	177	8
	fit	195	38	235	121	177	49	4
Type B	exhausted	245	83	231	80	184	66	4
	fit	353	143	351	157	350	154	8

[a] Values of cortisol are in μg/l.

Table 5. Mean values[a] and standard deviations (SD) of platelet aggregation ratios for fit and exhausted type A and type B subjects

		High event rate task		Low event rate task		Film		(n)
		Mean	SD	Mean	SD	Mean	SD	
Type A	exhausted	79.9	12.0	78.8	16.0	87.8	14.2	8
	fit	81.3	15.2	81.0	9.6	82.3	12.3	4
Type B	exhausted	89.8	7.4	84.8	6.9	88.3	8.7	4
	fit	80.6	12.7	72.8	13.0	87.4	15.0	8

[a] Values are the number of nonaggregated platelets divided by the total number of platelets times 100

Negative correlations of platelet aggregation ratios with noradrenaline levels were apparent during task conditions, whereas the opposite relation was found during rest condition (high event rate tasks: $r=-0.46$, $P=0.01$; low event rate tasks: $r=-0.34$, $P=0.05$; film: $r=0.47$, $P=0.01$). This striking result indicates that high levels of noradrenaline during stress are related to increased platelet aggregation, whereas during rest, high levels of noradrenaline are related to decreased platelet aggregation. It was also found that, in the low event rate tasks, high levels of adrenaline were associated with lower total numbers of platelets ($r=-0.25$; $P=0.10$), while high levels of noradrenaline were associated with higher numbers of platelets ($r=0.38$; $P=0.05$).

Discussion

We concluded that the type A/B hypothesis was supported by the performance data (i.e., percentage of missed signals) and by the HRV data. It was interesting to note that this was especially true of exhausted type A persons. As they seem to be the main risk group for MI, it is tempting to formulate a better explanation for these effects. As Grossman (1983) pointed out, the control of parasympathetic nervous system activity seems to be as important as that of sympathetic activity in the development of myocardial pathology.

The increase in low-frequency HRV in type A subjects might be explained by the somewhat higher levels of noradrenaline excretion in type A persons, which can produce an increase in low-frequency HRV, as Kleinjans (1983) has demonstrated.

Concerning the neurohormonal data, the picture is not entirely clear, for the significance of the effects is simply not sufficient to draw firm conclusions. On the other hand, the correlational analyses provided some evidence to support the conclusion that exhausted individuals, as compared with fit individuals, displayed higher levels of noradrenaline on all three experimental occasions. Consecutively, higher levels of noradrenaline were correlated with increased platelet aggregation only during task conditions, whereas during rest conditions, higher norepinephrine levels were correlated with decreased platelet aggregation. However, we failed to obtain a direct association of MQ scores with platelet aggregation.

Summary

Type A/B differences were found in a study of 24 middle-aged male subjects performing a vigilance task. Type A subjects showed a somewhat poorer signal detection performance as a function of time on task. As a function of time on task, type A individuals also showed an increased amount of HRV indicating higher parasympathetic nervous system activity. Contrary to challenging task situations where type A persons perform better and show greater physiologic and neurohormonal responses, type A subjects tend to give up their efforts in a typical nonchallenging vigilance task.

In another aspect of the study, it was found that persons with higher scores on a vital exhaustion scale predictive of MI were typically slow reactors and tended to have higher levels of circulating noradrenaline in all three experimental sessions. High levels of circulating noradrenaline and a high degree of platelet aggregation were found to correlate in vivo under task conditions, whereas during rest sessions, high circulating noradrenaline levels were correlated with a low degree of platelet aggregation.

References

Appels A (1980) Het jaar voor het hartinfarct. Internal report. Department of Medical Psychology, State University of Limburg

Appels A (1981) Het jaar voor het hartinfarct. Hart Bull 6: 123-127

Appels A, Pool J, Lubsen J, van der Does E (1979) Psychological prodromata of myocardial infarction. J Psychosom Res 23: 405-421

Appels A, Jenkins CD, Rosenman RH (1982) Coronary-prone behavior in the Netherlands: a cross-cultural validation study. J Behav Med 5: 83-90

Arkel YS, Haft J, Buxton M, Sheppard H, Burghardt G, Williams R (1982) Emotional arousal and platelet physiology: a review and some original contributions. J Human Stress 3: 19-27

Axelrod S, Gordon D, Ubel FA, Shannon DC, Barger AC, Cohen RJ (1981) Power spectrum analysis of heart rate fluctuations: a quantitative probe of beat-to-beat cardiovascular control. Science 213 (10 July): 220-222

Deshmukh SV, Meyer JS, Mouche RJ (1976) Platelet dysfunction in migraine: effect of self-medication with aspirin. Thromb Haemost 36: 319-325

Falger PF, Appels A (1982) Psychological risk factors over the life course of myocardial infarction patients. Adv Cardiol 29: 132-139

Frankenhaeuser M, Lundberg U, Forsman L (1980) Note on arousing type A persons by depriving them of work. J Psychosom Res 24: 45-47

Friedman M, Byers SL, Rosenman RH, Elevitch FR (1970) Coronary-prone individuals (type A): Some biochemical characteristics. JAMA 212: 1030-1037

Glass DC (1977) Behavior patterns, stress and coronary disease. Wiley, New York

Glass DC, Krakoff LR, Finkelman J, Snow B, Contrada R, Kehoe K, Manucci EG, Isecke W, Collins C, Hilton WF, Elting E (1980a) Effect of task overload upon cardiovascular and plasma catecholamine responses upon type A and type B individuals. Basic Appl Soc Psychol 1 (3): 199-218

Glass DC, Krakoff LR, Finkelman J, Snow B, Contrada R, Kehoe M, Manucci EG, Isecke W, Collins C, Hilton WF, Elting E (1980b) Effect of harassment and competition upon cardiovascular and plasma catecholamine responses in type A and type B individuals. Psychophysiology 17 (5): 453-464

Grossman P (1983) Respiration, stress and cardiovascular function. Psychophysiology 20 (3): 284-300

Lulofs R, Molen MG, Bevers E, Hornstra G, Tangelder GJ (to be published) Blood platelet activity in vitally exhausted persons. Proceedings of the NATO symposium on cardiovascular psychophysiology. June 1983, Noordwijkerhout, The Netherlands

Lundberg U, Forsman L (1979) Adrenal-medullary and adrenal-cortical responses to understimulation and overstimulation: comparison between type A and type B persons. Biol Psychol 9: 79-89

Matthews KA, Brunson BI (1979) Allocation of attention and the type A coronary-prone behavior pattern. J of Pers Soc Psychol 37 (11): 2081-2090

Mulder G (1980) The heart of mental effort. Dissertation, State University of Groningen

Mulder G, Mulder LJM (1981) Information processing and cardiovascular control. Psychophysiology 18 (4): 392-402

Mulder LJM (1979) INSPAN. Internal report 79-HB-439 RP. State University of Groningen

Kleinhans SJ (1983) Stimulation of renal adrenergic mechanisms as a model for the development of hypertension. Dissertation, State University of Limburg, Maastricht, The Netherlands

O'Hanlon JF (1981) Boredom: practical consequences and a theory. Acta Psychol 49: 53-82

Riedel WJ (1982) Vigilantie na trauma capitis. Internal report. Department of Neuropsychology, State University of Groningen

Scrutton MC, Wallis RB (1981) Catecholamine receptors. In: Gordon JL (ed) Platelets in biology and pathology. Elsevier-North Holland, Amsterdam

Steptoe A (1981) Psychological risk factors in cardiovascular disorders. Academic, New York

Van der Molen MG (1982) Psychofysiologische stressreacties bij personen met een verhoogd risico op coronaire afwijkingen (type A). Internal report. Department of Medical Psychology, State University of Limburg

Warner ED, Hoak JC, Connor WE (1967) In: Platelets, their role in haemostasis and thrombosis. 249-259

Wu K, Hoak JC (1974) A new method for the quantitative detection of platelet aggregates in patients with arterial insufficiency. Lancet 2: 924

Psychophysiologic Testing of Cardiovascular Responses to Physiologic and Psychological Challenge: Analysis of Intraindividual Stability

M. Horvath, E. Frantik, and A. Slaby[1]

Introduction

Clinical, experimental, and epidemiologic evidence provides many supporting arguments for the assumption that reactions to various types of functional load may participate in the pathogenesis of some chronic disease states. This may occur in a variety of ways: such reactions may function as precipitating agents in states of acute failure, through a mechanism whereby misregulations become fixed, or as a source of cumulative organic microinjuries. When these processes are in play, the originally adaptive reaction may become a part of the pathologic process, which, in turn, may modify reactions to stress, thus closing the vicious circle. If this conception is valid, consistent qualitative or quantitative peculiarities in the nature of these reactions represent one of the sources of individually differing risk for disease.

This conceptual framework has undergone periodic "inflows" and "outflows" of ideas. At the present time, attempts to analyze physiologic mechanisms are beginning to prevail over the descriptive statistical approach.

Similar trends have influenced the development and systematic use of physiologic functional tests, helping to bring about methodological improvements and standardization, so that these tests can serve not only in the analysis of possible pathogenetic mechanisms, but also tentatively to supplement individual diagnosis and prognosis and to suggest proper measures of intervention, especially in borderline states and in primary or secondary preventive health care programs (Horvath et al. 1983).

If the above assumptions are true for reactions to physiologic stress, their validity is even more important in investigating the role of psychological stress factors, particularly those that include a potent emotional component. Here, cardiovascular reactions are even more intense, and truly pathologic pictures, in fact, can occur in clinically healthy subjects. These changes persist for a longer time and undergo greater inter- and intraindividual variation. A proposal for a universally efficient test in this field is, of course, more difficult, since the relationship of any particular psychological stimulus to cardiovascular reactions is mediated through as yet insufficiently understood psychophysiologic mechanisms.

The aim of adding to the complex of physiologic functional tests a model of emotionally provoking situations is to deepen our insight into regulation mechanisms and, possibly, into pathogenetic mechanisms. According to psychophysiologic conceptions, several components are in play, including psychosocial components (i.e., the total quantity of frustrating influences from the psychosocial environment, which is, of course, reciprocally influenced by the behavior of the individual), psy-

1 Institute of Hygiene and Epidemiology, Prague, Czechoslovakia

Biological and Psychological Factors in Cardiovascular Disease
Ed. by T. H. Schmidt, T. M. Dembroski, and G. Blümchen

chological components (e.g., behavioral patterns defined as a set of typical reactions to current working and life situations), psychophysiologic components, and other components (characteristic patterns of homeostatic cardiovascular reactions).

The models of psychogenic stress used thus far are a mixture of mental effort and frustration due to an actual conflict or stress induced by the use of recall techniques. Experience indicates that the interpretation of data obtained through such methods is made more meaningful through the simultaneous use of a model situation which utilizes emotional stimuli specific to the individual. These can include conversation on topics selected on the basis of previous psychological examinations, questionnaires, or interviews, the recall of frustrating situations, and a test eliciting a standard amount of frustration (conflict tasks such as the Stroop test, etc.).

The model of moderate emotional stress should possess several characteristics:
1. It should induce marked cardiovascular responses minimally dependent on habituation and occupation.
2. The test should have a considerable degree of reliability in the sense of intraindividual stability.
3. It should have validity in relation to the health risk.

Apart from these general demands, there are some specific circumstances which are important. The idea of the physiologic adequacy of rhythmical activity and the resulting hypothesis that unfavorable health effects are caused by continuous and habitually maintained activation, underscores the importance of investigating not only the intensity and proportionality of reactions to a model load, but also their dynamics, with special emphasis on persistence.

Testing Procedure

Laboratory examination of cardiovascular reactivity (heart rate, blood pressure, forearm blood flow) to standard physical and emotional stimuli was performed with the use of three standard physiologic stimuli, including the orthostatic and cold pressor tests and Valsalva's maneuver, and a psychological challenge, including the Stroop test and the numerical square test (Fig. 1).

The subjects were in a semisupine position in a quiet room. The recording instruments were located away from the subject. Heart rate was continually monitored by a cardiotachometer, blood pressure was measured by an indirect method (Physiomat), and forearm blood flow was measured by means of occlusion plethysmography according to Dohn (1965). Basal values were recorded six times at the end of a 20-min rest period. Individual functional tests were separated by rest periods sufficiently long to ensure the return to initial values. The Czech version (Horvath et al. 1980) of the Mood Adjective Checklist according to McNair et al. (1971) and the tension rating scale were administered twice, i.e., after the rest period and after the emotional test.

The psychological challenge was induced by the color-word naming component of the Stroop Interference Test for a period of 3 min, immediately followed by ranking of three-digit numbers, arranged in a numerical square. The latter task lasted 7 min. Both tests were presented in printed form or were shown on slides.

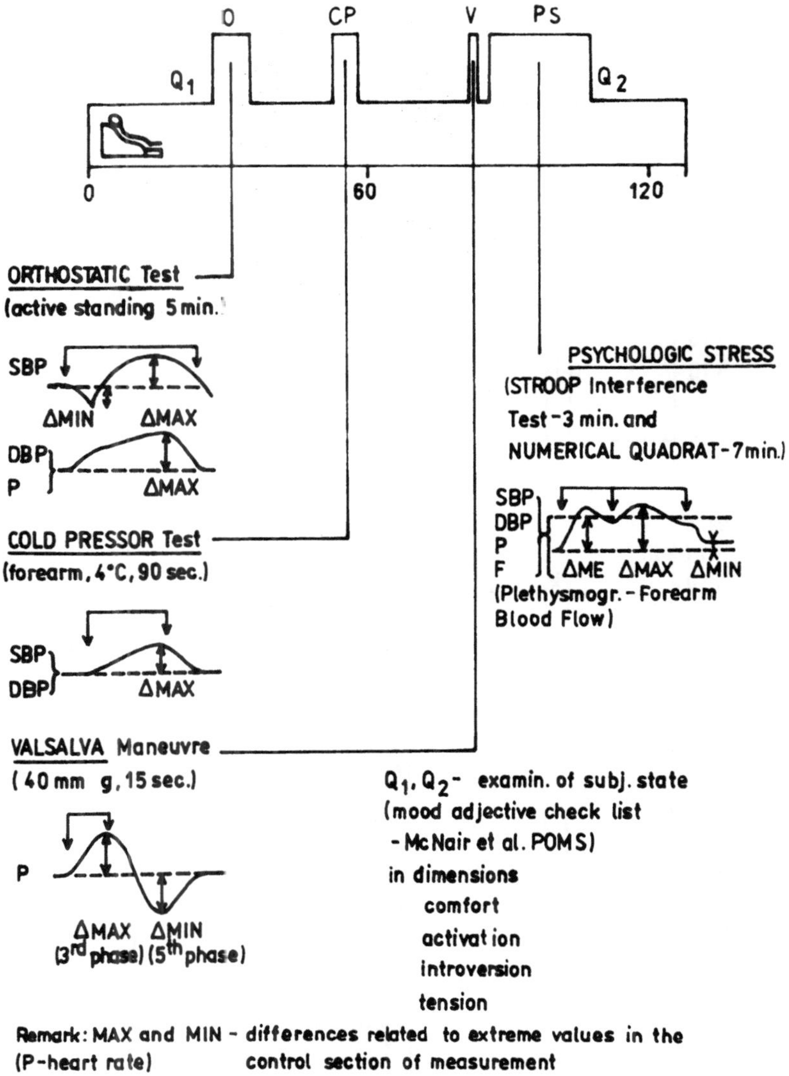

Fig. 1. Physical and emotional stimuli used to test cardiovascular reactivity (heart rate, blood pressure, forearm blood flow) to physiologic and psychological challenges. (*O*, orthostatic test; *CP*, cold pressor test; *V*, Valsalva's maneuver; *PS*, psychological stress; Q_1, Q_2, examination of subjective state; *SBP*, systolic blood pressure; *DBP*, diastolic blood pressure; *P*, heart rate; *F*, forearm blood flow)

The names of colors in the Stroop table are printed in colors other than the ones the words designate, and the respondent is requested not to read the words, but to name the colors, which causes a conflict between the two deeply automatized abilities of recognizing the colors and globally reading the words. In the numerical square task, the subject ranked three-digit numbers, read from right to left, according to their sequence, and looked for the numbers marked by the symbol "-". The subject was given the first number in a series and was blamed for errors. Before the psychological stress test, subjects received both written and oral instructions.

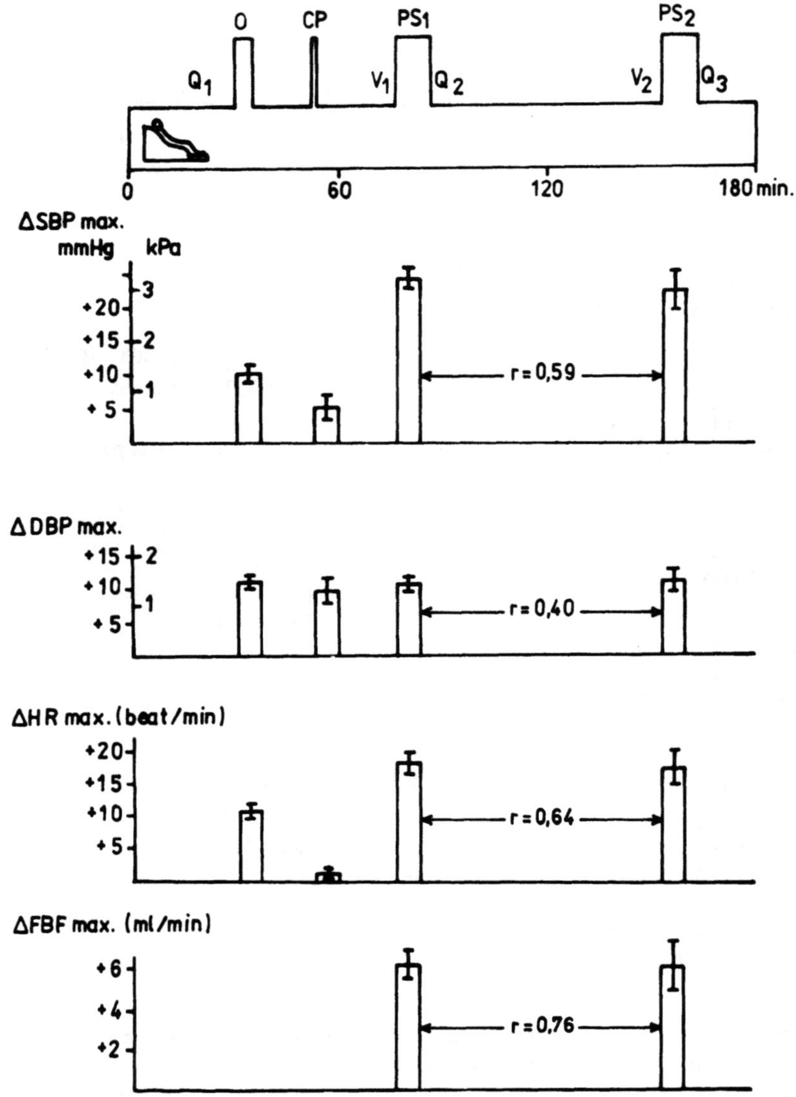

Fig. 2. Mean cardiovascular responses to physiologic challenge (orthostatic and cold pressor tests) and psychological stress (Stroop and number ranking tests). *FBF*, forearm blood flow; for definitions of other abbreviations, see Fig. 1

Both parts of the test elicit approximately the same elevation in diastolic and systolic blood pressure, heart rate, and forearm blood flow and are therefore administered without interruption as one test and evaluated together. After the end of the emotional test, return to initial values was monitored for at least 10 min.

A great advantage of these tasks is the negligible habituation of circulatory responses during repetition. This agrees with findings cited by Jensen (1966) concerning the stability of the classic parameter of performance time. Another advantage is the low age dependence of the performance criterion for the range of 13–65 years, as described by Comalli et al. (for a discussion, see Jensen and Rohwer 1966). Color

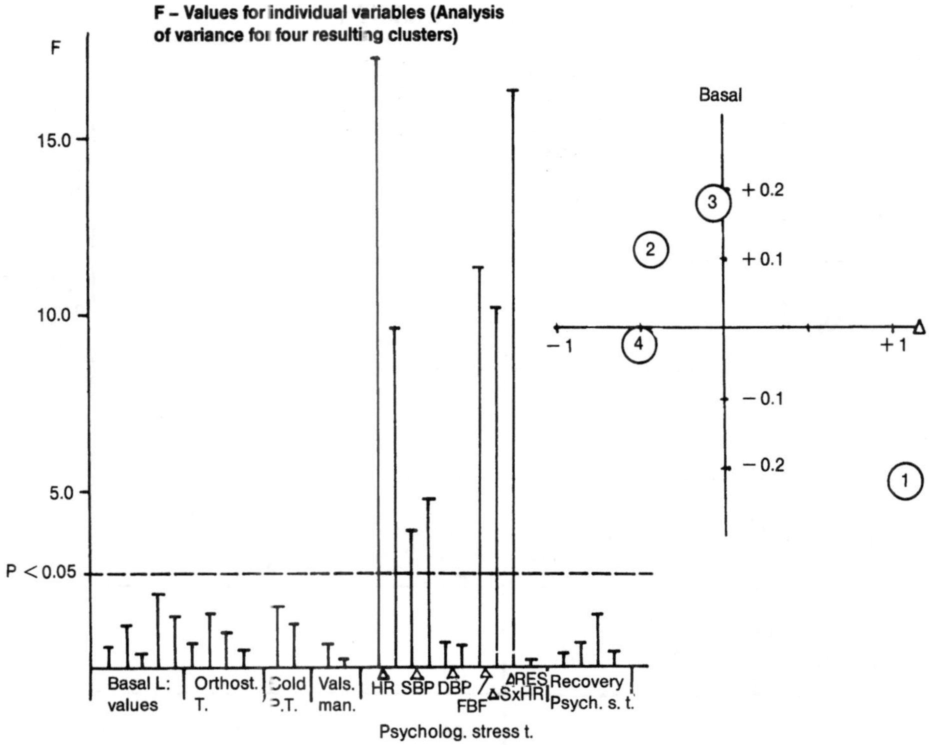

Fig. 3. Cluster analysis of cardiovascular reactions of test subjects distinguishes four categories of responses *(right: 1–4)*. The significantly differentiating variable is response to psychological stress test. *x*-axis, mean standard change in the psychological stress test; *y*-axis, mean standard basal line values; for definitions of abbreviations, see Fig. 1

naming and ranking of three-digit numbers are not dependent on sociocultural background. The latter is less dependent on occupational skills than the frequently used mental arithmetic tasks.

The experimental design described here has proved satisfactory in a number of individual studies. A series of mutually independent parameters were chosen, which show very satisfactory short-term and long-term intraindividual stability.

The importance of introducing the model of emotional stress into the examination set is underscored by the fact that it has not proved possible to predict reliably the response to emotional stimuli on the basis of responses to physiologic stress, psychological characteristics, or a combination of the two.

Analysis of Results

For this paper, a total of 240 examinations performed on 106 respondents, all of whom were research workers, were evaluated (Horvath and Frantik 1982; 1983). Mean responses are given in Fig. 2.

Cluster analysis using all measured circulatory characteristics divided the respondents into four categories, with the significantly differentiating variable being

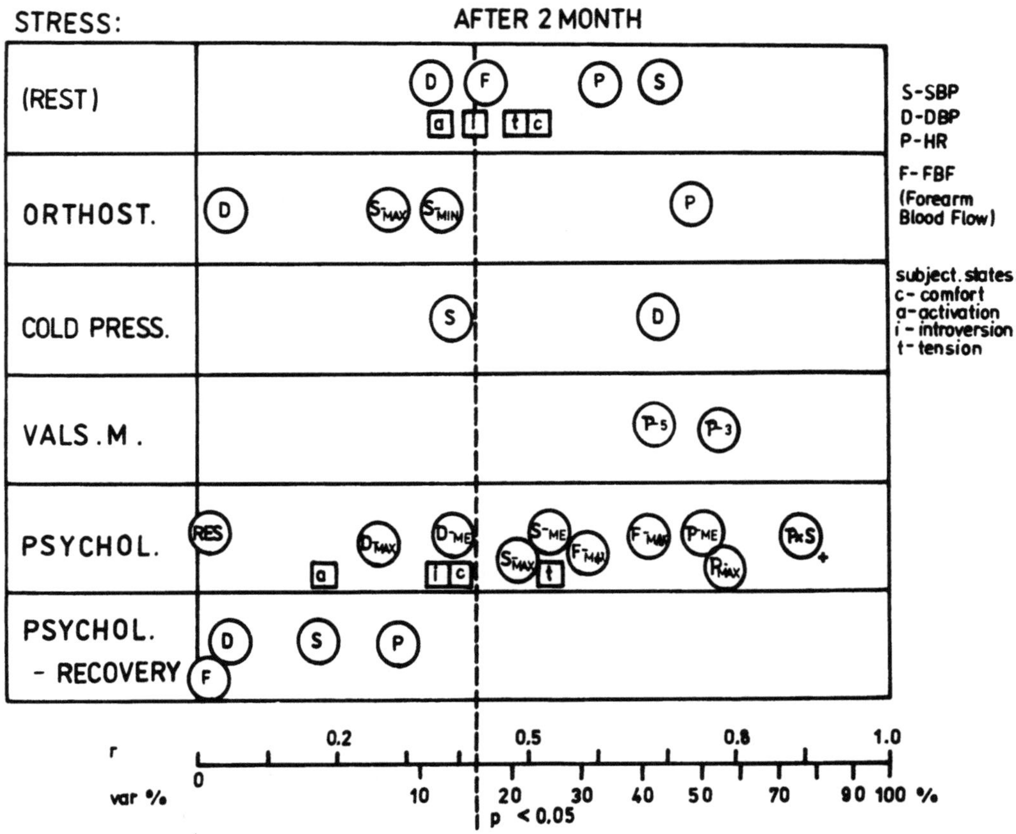

Fig. 4. Intraindividual correlations of results of stress tests, with retest carried out 2 months after initial test

the response to the psychological stress test. The left part of Fig. 3 contains the variables entered into the cluster analysis. The F-values on the y-axis characterize the ability of the variables to discriminate between the four resulting clusters.

The right part of Fig. 3 illustrates schematically the position of the four clusters in relation to two complex variables. On the x-axis, cardiovascular responses to the psychological stress test are plotted; the resting values of these responses are plotted on the y-axis. The first group shown in the cluster analysis has an abnormally high reaction to psychological stress at a low basal level of blood pressure, heart rate, and vascular resistance. The third group responded with a reaction of medium intensity at high basal values. In groups two and four, low-intensity reactions were observed, the latter group having the smallest increase in forearm blood flow and the highest basal vascular resistance.

The intraindividual stability of reactions to psychological stress at retest is shown in Fig. 2. In Figs. 4 and 5, intrasubjective correlations of results of stress tests performed at 2-month and 1-year intervals are given. On the x-axis of the upper scale, the values of correlation coefficients are shown, and the bottom scale shows the percentage of common variability at retest for individual cardiovascular re-

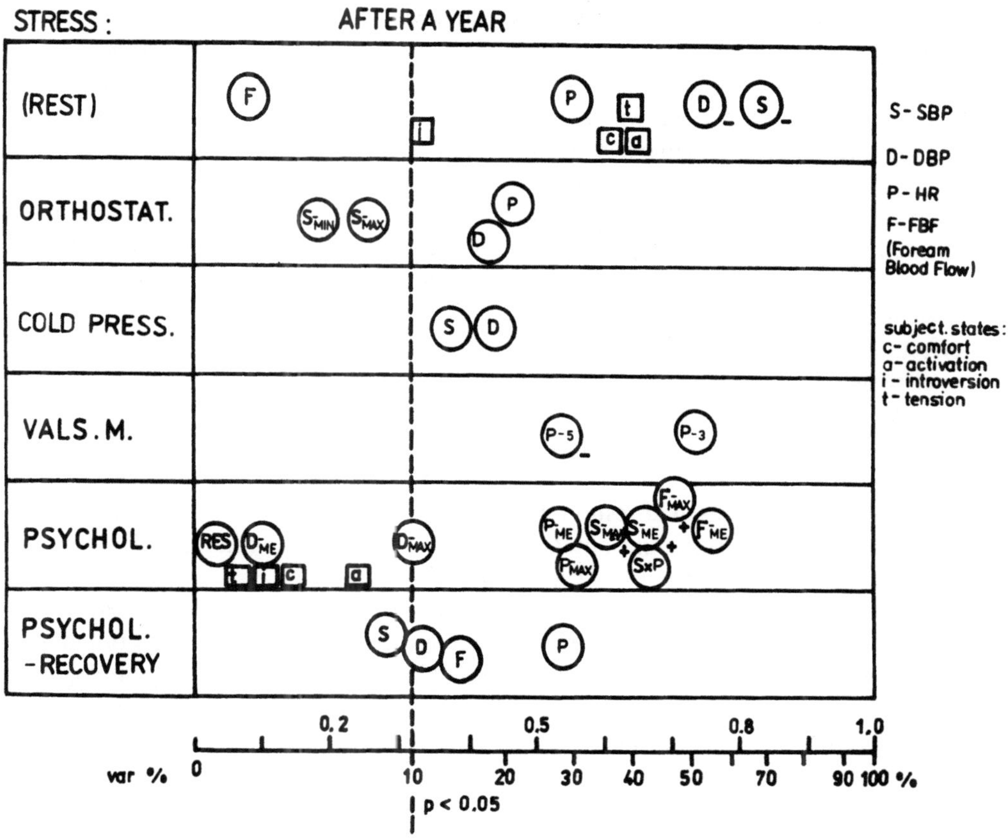

Fig. 5. Intraindividual correlations between results of initial stress test and retest administered 1 year later

sponses to tests presented in corresponding lines. The vertical dotted line illustrates the limit of statistical significance of the correlation coefficients at the 5% level.

Cardiovascular reactions to psychological stress were generally more stable than those to orthostatic and cold pressor tests. The responses to repeated tests have a satisfactorily high ratio of common variability sources; e.g., for repetition at 1-year intervals, common variability lies between 40% and 70%.

Stress-induced heart rate changes were generally more stable than so-called rest values of heart rate. This confirms the well-known fact that it is difficult to define basal conditions when pulse frequency is measured. The reverse was true for blood pressure: reactions of diastolic pressure under stress conditions showed only low reproducibility. The characteristics measured in recovery after the stress test generally exhibited low stability and were predominantly determined by the noise factor. For this reason, the evaluation of the recovery characteristics needs to be improved.

As far as validity with respect to risk is concerned, final evaluation will be possible only when sufficiently long-term follow-up data are available. However, several implications may be deduced on the basis of a relationship with genetic factors. Subjects with a positive family history of hypertension showed greater increases in systolic blood pressure during the psychological stress test and smaller increases in heart rate in the third phase of Valsalva's maneuver. The latter finding suggests less effective vagal regulation in these subjects. A similar difference in the response of systolic blood pressure to psychological stress was found to relate to a family history of coronary heart disease, with subjects having a positive family history responding with greater increases in heart rate and forearm blood flow (Slaby et al. 1984).

Greater responses were also associated with a number of social and personality characteristics. Those research workers with a high proportion of managerial duties showed greater increases in diastolic blood pressure during the cold pressor test. Subjects with a high degree of occupational responsibility showed greater increases in heart rate during both the orthostatic and the psychological stress tests. All these effects were controlled for in the analysis of covariance, which excluded the influence of age.

Using the JAS questionnaire to assess type A/B behavior, we found greater increases in heart rate and diastolic blood pressure during the emotional stress test in subjects with high type A scores. On the other hand, we were unable to discern any differences in cardiovascular response related to the results of the type A structured interview. These results in our population-based sample are at variance with several studies using clear-cut type A (A 1) subjects.

In summary, one can conclude that a multistage examination set of adequate psychological psychophysiologic, and physiologic measurements would permit assessment of the role that individual levels of regulation play in normal or pathologic reactions of the cardiovascular system. As a step following psychological screening, the described procedure could contribute to estimates of individual risk and to identifying targets of intervention.

Acknowledgements. We thank M. Nosek and M. Sugarova for technical assistance and E. Holoubkova for assistance in statistical processing.

References

Dohn K (1965) Plethysmography during functional states for investigation of the peripheral circulation. Proceedings of the 2nd international congress of physical medicine. Copenhagen, p 51

Horvath M, Frantik E (1982) Behavioral and personality characteristics in R and D personnel: occupational and health correlations. Activ Nerv Sup [Suppl 3]: 212

Horvath M, Frantik E (1983) Testing the psychophysiological reactivity of subjects with coronary-prone behavior pattern in a multifactorial preventive study. In: Rosenmann RH (ed) Psychosomatic risk factors and coronary heart disease: Indications for specific preventive therapy. Huber, Berne, p 55

Horvath M, Frantik E, Josifko K (1980) Vigilance impairing drugs: Analysis of subjective responses. Activ Nerv Sup 22: 188

Horvath M, Frantik E, Slaby A (1983) Psychophysiological risk factors of ischaemic heart disease: a primary preventive study in Czechoslovakia. In: Dembroski T, Schmidt T, Blümchen G (eds) Biobehavioral bases of coronary heart disease. Karger, Basel, p 228

Jensen AR, Rohwer WD (1966) The Stroop color-word test: a review. Acta Psychol 25: 36

McNair DM, Lorr M, Droppleman LF (1971) Profiles of mood states (POMS) Educational and Industrial Testing Service, Inc., San Diego, California

Slaby A, Frantik M, Horvath M, Josifko M, Kozena L (1984) Cardiovascular responses to emotional stress as related to genetic and environmental characteristics. Activ Nerv Sup 26 (3): 215–217

Psychobiological Markers of Stress in Surgeons and Anaesthetists

R. L. PAYNE[1] and J. T. RICK[2]

Introduction

Recent theorizing about the relationship between environmental stress and psychophysiological strain has suggested that the simple direct relationship between the two may be moderated by two other variables. Karasek and various co-authors (Karasek 1979; Karasek et al. 1982) have demonstrated that the degree of control the person has over his environment affects the degree to which he may experience strain. The most stressful occupational environments are those that have high demands combined with low ability to control the situation. In a study of cases of coronary heart disease carefully matched with controls, Alfredsson et al. (1982) showed that CHD was higher among those who had been employed in jobs with these sorts of characteristics. Other investigators have demonstrated that the level of social support available to the person can buffer the person from experiencing the worst effects of environmental stressors (Pinneau 1975; La Rocco et al. 1980). Payne (1979) has proposed that the degree of environmental stress can only be estimated when the three variables od demands, supports and constraints (i. e. control) are measured simultaneously. It is possible to construe support as a means of increasing control: the more help one has, the more one can control both the situational demands and therefore one's own reactions to them. The advantage of making this assumption for present purposes is that it reduces the model to two variables - demands and control - and permits us to utilize the theorizing of Karasek et al. (1982), who have most thoroughly related environmental stress situations to physiological responses.

Karasek et al. propose that high-strain situations are caused by the combination of high demands and low control. The physiological response to this combination of conditions is high output of epinephrine and cortisol. When demands are high, but control is also high, then only epinephrine is elevated. The situation of high demand and high control is described as an "active situation" and is hypothezised to produce the following physiological responses: increased serum high-density/low-density lipoprotein ratio, lower average baseline serum cortisol and normal serum catecholamine responses, a more rapid return to baseline levels following acute stressor exposure, and subsequent lower average heart rate and blood pressure. The evidence for the physiological pattern associated with high demand and low control is the most securely established, and the authors remark that "links between these phenomena and the 'active' environmental situations (high demand-high control occupational conditions) must still be further explored".

1 MRC/ESRC Social and Applied Psychology Unit, University of Sheffield, Sheffield S10 2TN, UK
2 Department of Psychology, University of Sheffield, Sheffield S10 2TN, UK

Biological and Psychological Factors
in Cardiovascular Disease
Ed. by T. H. Schmidt, T. M. Dembroski, and G. Blümchen

While the evidence for the association between high demands, low discretion and poorer physical and mental health is quite good, much less is known about what Karasek calls "active" jobs, though these are characterized by high job demands. Because high discretion is part of many highly responsible and professional occupations, it seems unlikely that high discretion alone permits the occupants of such demanding jobs to avoid physical and mental stress totally. The purpose of this study was to evaluate levels of stress in jobs which are highly demanding both in terms of skill and the number of hours worked, but which also entail high levels of discretion. The first occupation chosen was that of cardiothoracic surgery. The results from this study proved surprising in terms of theory, and the study was extended to include anaesthetists who worked with the cardiothoracic team. While studying these anaesthetists, it was also possible to replicate the more interesting findings from the surgeons (e.g. urine analyses and subjective reports of stress).

Study 1: Cardiothoracic Surgeons

The first study described the psychological and physiological responses of a team of people who have an "active" job: The team included all the medically qualified members of a group performing cardiothoracic surgery. Their job is demanding, not only in the technical skills and knowledge required to perform it, but also in the long hours of work (10 or more h a day, with frequent night and weekend work). The long professional training, on the other hand, gives the surgeons much discretion in their everyday lives.

Some Previous Research on Stress in Surgeons

In a study of heart rate among eight general surgeons while operating, Foster et al. (1978) found a mean heart rate of 121 bpm and maximum heart rates of over 150 bpm. They further found that type of operation did not affect heart rate, and that observers were not able to detect stress even when tachycardia was present. These levels of heart rate are high compared to many other occupations: teachers while teaching (93 bpm; Leonard 1983), trawlermen fishing (112 bpm; Rodahl and Vokac 1977), physicians during ward rounds (97 bpm), and cardiologists doing cardiac catheterization (104 bpm; Ira et al. 1962). However, Taggart et al. (1969) found that racing drivers, while competing, experience even higher rates (180 bpm). Foster et al. suggested that such high heart rates would be associated with increased heart disease but note that the incidence of ischaemic heart disease is actually lower among surgeons than other doctors. An alternative interpretation of their results might be that heart rate alone is not an adequate indicator of occupational stress. The present study employed different measures of both acute and chronic stress.

Method

All the members of a cardiothoracic team were studied. The eight members ranged in rank from house officer to consultant. Two were females. Measurements were taken for 12 × 24-h periods over 3 months, and different days of the normal working week were sampled. The data recorded were as follows:

1. Recordings of the ECG were made using a miniature body-borne tape-recorder, the ECG signal being detected by two chest electrodes. A single person was studied on 11 of the 12 24-h periods, and the apparatus was worn for the full 24 h. Three persons were studied on two occasions. A record of concomitant activities was made by observers.
2. A questionnaire was designed to assess the nature and severity of *job demands*. These included demands from patients, colleagues, relatives, demands on knowledge/skills, together with demands on physical capacities. The same questionnaire asked whether the doctors felt they had the *authority* necessary to meet the demands made upon them. It also contained questions about the *support* given by colleagues and their *satisfaction* with the way things had gone. Questionnaires were administered to every doctor at least once per day and up to three times a day (i.e. separate questionnaires could be completed for the morning, the afternoon and the night).
3. A second questionnaire simply asked whether the person had felt stressed during the period studied. If they replied positively, they were asked to rate (a) how severe the stress was on a five-point scale, where the categories ranged from "very mild" to "very severe"; and (b) how long the stress lasted, the extreme categories of the five-point scale being "a few minutes" to "all the period and continued afterwards."
4. Urine samples were collected for each 24-h period (8.30 a.m. to 8.30 a.m.). These were assayed in the hospital laboratory. VMA was measured, as a marker for catecholamine levels, using a modification of Pisano's method (1962), and cortisol by the Amerlex Radioimmunoassay.[3]

Results

Perceptions of Stress

The nature and severity of the demands reported by the surgical team are shown in Table 1. Demands on medical and surgical knowledge and physical demands (fatigue) are the two most frequently rated as stressors, but, on average, even these only score between 1 and 2 (i.e., between "coping without any help" and "sometimes feeling one needs help"). As others have shown, hospital doctors tend to describe even the more stressful events they encounter as only "moderately stressful". The answers to the second questionnaire tell a slightly different story.

This questionnaire simply asked whether the person had felt stressed. A positive reply was given to this question 35 times out of 74. On 15 of these occasions the

3 Amerlex RIA, Amersham International Ltd., Amersham, UK.

Table 1. Frequency distribution and mean scores for self-reports on job demands and pressures

Item	Score					Mean
	0	1	2	3	4	
Demands on knowledge	0	60	39	9	0	1.53
Physical demands	0	76	26	6	0	1.35
Colleagues	1	88	15	3	1	1.21
Skills	7	76	23	2	0	1.19
Other departments	5	83	15	4	1	1.19
Patients	19	83	6	0	0	0.88
Relatives	31	66	10	1	0	0.82

Total of responses = 108 for each item. Scale: 0 = not applicable; 1 = dealt with demand/pressure without needing help; 2 = dealt with but felt needed help sometimes; 3 = dealt with problems but only by getting help; 4 = failed to deal with problems even with help. Only responses 2-4 are considered indications of felt stress.

Table 2. % of waking time at various bpm levels of heart rate in bpm

Subject	<60	60-80	80-100	100-120	120>	Maximum	Minimum	Total waking time in min
1A	1.0	59.7	38.7	0.3		104	40	881
2A	36.5	57.4	6.7			98	35	885
1B		7.9	61.2	30.1	0.2	122	60	950
2B		20.3	75.4	4.2		155	64	900
1C	13.3	60.5	22.5	2.7	1.0	173	48	1008
2C	16.0	63.9	18.7	1.0	0.4	130	53	1008
4D		2.8	46.0	47.9	3.2	140	68	845
5E		33.7	61.0	5.3		120	80	1090
6F		11.5	43.4	37.7	7.5	150	64	1280
7G	8.9	17.2	46.0	27.3	0.6	128	40	900
8H		2.5	29.4	61.0	7.5	164	68	1037

stress was reported to have lasted several hours or longer, and on 12 of the 15 the stress was rated as "severe" or "quite severe". These doctors experience regular acute stress, which they describe as "moderate" on most occasions. The category "very severe", for example, was never used, but this moderate stress is reported almost daily.

The answers to other parts of the questionnaire partly explain why the stress is less severe than might be expected from a job which has two of the characteristics of stressful jobs: responsibility for people and long, unsocial hours. When asked if they felt they lacked the authority necessary to meet their job demands, the members of the team reported feeling this lack on only 16 occasions out of 108. The level of occupational support they received from colleagues was extremely good, as it was reported as lacking on only 2 out of 108 occasions. Finally, they had very high levels of satisfaction and expressed dissatisfaction with the way things had gone on only 13 occasions. By most standards surgery is a demanding job, but its overall

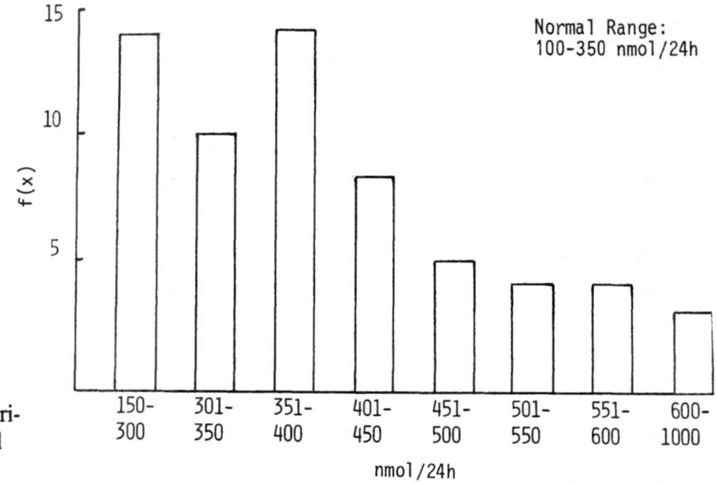

Fig. 1. Frequency distribution of 24-h cortisol levels

stress is much moderated by the high discretion, support, and satisfaction the job entails. This pattern of results also justifies the classification of this job as "active" according to Karasek's model.

Heart Rate. Table 2 contains summary data on heart rate for each doctor. Doctors A, B, and C were monitored on two days, and two sets of data appear for each of them. These data were abstracted from the paper tape records by hand so they are not exact, but there is no reason to assume consistent forms of bias. The paper record enables one to measure time accurately to the minute, but the record of the heart rate itself is likely to be accurate to only about 5 bpm. Since only the absolute level of heart rate in bpm is of interest, this level of accuracy is quite acceptable. Table 2 shows that the percentage of time various levels of heart rate were recorded as a proportion of the time they were awake. This includes times when they were not working. The table also shows the maximum bpm recorded during the waking period, the minimum and the total number of minutes they were awake.

One of the most striking things in Table 2 is the large individual differences. Person A rarely has more than 100 bpm whilst persons D and H have heart rates of over 100 bpm for more than half of their waking time. There is no evidence of age or experience being related to these average levels. The overall average is about 85 bpm which is slightly higher than managers (Hennigan and Wortham 1975) and much lower than trawlermen who had mean heart rates of 112 bpm whilst working and 88 bpm whilst resting but awake (Rodahl and Vokac 1977).

Since the doctors were all followed whilst wearing the equipment used to monitor their heart rate activity and their actions recorded, it was possible to relate changes in heart rate to their activities. Tables 3, 4 and 5 illustrate some of the activities related to heart rate levels for a less experienced, moderately experienced and experienced surgeon respectively. Things worth noting from these tables are that scrubbing up raises heart rate by about 10 bpm, which is similar to the increase caused by walking between wards. It is possible to interpret this rise as due to pre-operating anxiety or to the physical effort involved in scrubbing up. Discussions

Table 3. Events changing heart rate in less experienced surgeons

Increases in bpm		Decreases in bpm	
100–110	scrubbing up	120– 80	arrival of registrar who was phoned for help
90–140	brisk trot to childrens' ward	100– 80	tea
100–125	taking blood from 2-year-old	110– 90	end of operating to writing notes
100–120	talking to relatives	100– 80	checking around POITU
100–120	assisting senior surgeon (day)	130–100	call to senior for advice
80– 90	assisting a registrar (evening)		

Table 4. Events changing heart rate in moderately experienced surgeon

Increases in bpm		Decreases in bpm	
100–110	scrubbing up	100–80	stitching (X 2)
100–115	coffee	80–60	phoning senior for advice
90–100	walk to 2 B	80–60	big X mean drop in heart rate when senior arrived at 9 p. m.
80–100	finish operation and taking patient to POITU		
50– 65	getting potassium measure		
60– 80	playing pool		
70– 90	watching very ill patient		

Table 5. Events changing heart rate in experienced surgeon

Increases in bpm		Decreases in bpm	
95–100	scrubbing up	100–80	looking at angiograms
100–110	patient dies	100–95	end of operation
100–120	waiting to lecture	100–90	work to coffee break
100–120	driving		
90–110	operating (day)		
110–125	operating (late evening)		

about this with the doctors indicated individual differences: some were aware of being slightly anxious and others were not. What is also evident is the powerful effect of having the support of more senior people when things are going wrong. Simply phoning a senior or having him arrive on the scene is related to considerable falls in heart rate. This is physiological support for the effects of social support in alleviating the effects of environmental stressors which has been shown in several correlational studies where the data are all self-reported (La Rocco et al. 1980) (Tables 3, 4 and 5).

Since a major part of a surgeon's job is to operate it is interesting to examine heart rate during this activity. Foster et al. (1978) recorded mean heart rates of 120 bpm on eight surgeons whilst they were operating. Eccles (1969) reports mean heart rates for dentists of 85 bpm. The mean heart rate for the eight surgeons, studied by Foster and his colleagues, was 92 bpm whilst they were working in a busy clinic. The large individual differences shown in Table 2 indicate that it is not particularly meaningful to give average heart rates, and it is perhaps more sensible to compare within individuals. Even for individuals the mean heart rate whilst operating varies across different operating sessions. The rate for surgeon F, for example, fluctuated between 100 and 120 bpm whilst assisting the senior registrar in the morning, but this dropped to 80-90 bpm whilst assisting a registrar in the evening of the same day. Below are the ranges of heart rates for various surgeons compared with their heart rates when driving their cars:

Surgeon	*Operating*	*Driving Car*
A	80- 90	45-70
B	90-110	85-95
C	60- 80	70-80
E	80-100	70-85

Car driving is a useful comparison because it has been studied by others and in town is a task which requires attention with potential serious consequences if the attention lapses. Hunt and Marcus (1966) found the mean heart rate for bus drivers to be 90 bpm, and a study by CIBA in 1972 found that businessmen driving on motorways had a mean heart rate of 93 bpm. Doing ward rounds and general patient care showed an average drop in heart rate for the surgeons studied here of 10-15 bpm compared to operating suggesting that operating is more stressful. For most of the surgeons, however, the noticeable thing about operating compared to other activities is that the heart rate is usually less variable. It has been shown that heart rate is less variable when concentration is required by the task (Kalsbeck 1971).

It is clear from these data that these surgeons as a whole have mean rates somewhat lower than the 120 bpm reported by Foster et al. (1978), but it is nevertheless an activity which raises their heart rate above that of most other routine activities they perform. The mean heart rate in this group is about 100 bpm, but for surgeon A it is about 80 bpm and surgeon D about 110. On being hauled out of bed at 4 a.m. for a cardiac arrest, Surgeon C's heart rate went to 175 bpm.

VMA and Cortisol

The levels of VMA are consistent with the perceived stress data and substantiate the findings of one other study of surgeons. Frequent acute stress of some severity would be expected to lead to elevated levels of VMA, but the levels were above normal for only 6% of the 62 measures taken. The cortisol results present a very different picture.

Figure 1 shows the histogram for cortisol levels. The first two bars of the histogram show those measures that lie within the normal range; 72% of the observations were outside the normal range. Because cortisol is regarded as an indicator of chronic stress, it was hypothesized that those who had been engaged in surgery the

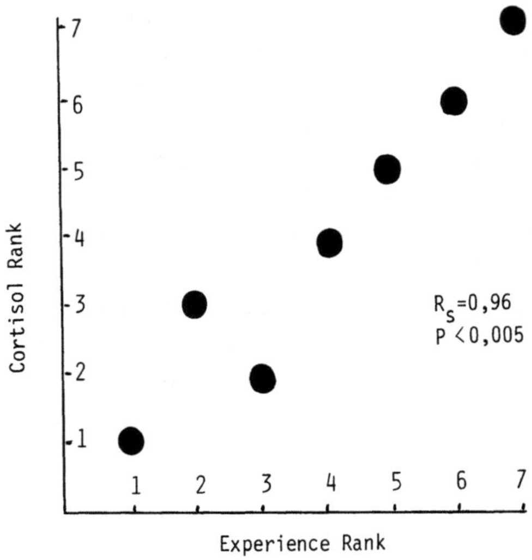

Fig. 2. Rank-order correlation between length of experience and mean cortisol for seven surgeons

longest would have higher levels. This proposition assumes that the length of exposure to the stresses of the job increases the level of cortisol. The hypothesis was tested by ranking seven of the team according to the length of time they had been practising surgery. One subject was excluded because creatinine levels in several urine samples were less than expected over a 24-h period. The mean level of cortisol for each person was calculated and the means ranked. Figure 2 plots these two rankings against each other. Higher rankings represent greater ammounts on both axes. Spearman rank-order correlation reached 0.96 ($P < 0.005$). The more time a person has been exposed to the practice of surgery, the higher the mean level of cortisol.

The final set of analyses involved relating the psychological measures to the biochemical markers. No relationship was found between the measures of subjective stress and VMA, but a relationship was found with cortisol levels. On those days when individuals reported having experienced stress, they also produced levels of cortisol above average for themselves. The 2×2 contingency table of these data produced a chi-square of 5.5, $P < 0.025$, one-tailed test. These data show a pattern of results where cortisol is chronically high, where it is higher for those who have the longest exposure, and where it is higher on days when the doctors report they have experienced stress.

Summary

The mean heart rate of these cardiothoracic surgeons while operating was lower than that of general surgeons, though Becker et al.'s study (1983) of ten general surgeons found almost exactly the same mean heart rate (99.4 bpm) as the present study. While these rates are not dramatically higher than for other occupations, they are higher than many others; operating is the main cause of the higher rates. In this respect, surgery is different from other occupations with high heart rates such as airline pilots and racing drivers. Occupants in both jobs have higher rates at particular times (landing and taking off, racing) but the periods are shorter and less frequently experienced. On the other hand, increases in heart rate can arise from increases in rate of breathing due to even minor exertion and/or to increased temperatures. When controlling for changes in oxygen consumption and other environmental conditions, however, it has been shown that a heart rate of 100 bpm leaves "little evidence of strain resulting from the psychological stress of operating" (Becker et al. 1983). The subjective reports of stress, however, do show regular acute episodes of moderate severity.

The high cortisol levels also suggest there may be a long-term physiological cost of which the surgeons are not necessarily aware. The relationship between level of cortisol and length of experience at surgery emphasizes this possibility.

The study has failed to support the notion of Karasek and his colleagues concerning the physiological reactions to "active" jobs. They predicted that active jobs would produce low levels of cortisol and lower than average heart rates, but neither of these predictions was upheld. Given the small number of subjects these results clearly warranted replication and extension to other professional groups. Study 2 achieves both these goals.

Study 2: Cardiothoracic Anaesthetists

The results of study 1 suggested two lines for further research. First, comparative data on the same measures would be useful, as the psychological measures, in particular, were designed specifically to meet the situation. Secondly, as the high levels of cortisol were not predicted from current theorizing, it would be desirable to attempt a replication. This goal is best achieved by studying a group of people working in the same, or a similar environment. Several groups would potentially fit this demand, such as nursing staff, technical staff and anaesthetists. The last group are the most suitable, as they are also qualified medical personnel with similar career patterns and terms of employment. They are predominantly male and also, like the surgeons, spend much of their work time in operating theatres and on intensive care wards. We were able to establish the similarity of the working conditions even more rigorously by studying only those anaesthetists engaged in cardiothoracic surgical cases. Thus, the subjects of the study worked in exactly the same environments, and with the same senior personnel as in study 1. During this study, the surgeons also agreed to assist us in seeing whether the cortisol results would be replicated by providing 24-h urine samples and by completing the shorter of the subjective stress questionnaires. This questionnaire asked whether the surgeons had felt stress at all during the day of the study, and if they had, they were further asked to indicate its severity and duration.

Method

The design was the same as that used in study 1, except that some additional measures were employed to attempt to study acute stressors. These consisted of short questionnaires to measure current mood states combined with the assessment of potassium and sodium from saliva. These last data are not reported here. Otherwise the same procedure was followed as in study 1. One person wore an ECG monitor and was observed throughout the working day. The demands, authority, support, and satisfaction questionnaires were completed by all anaesthetists connected with cardiothoracic surgery on each day of the study. Each anaesthetist also completed the subjective stress questionnaire determining presence, severity and duration of stressful episodes. Urine samples were collected for each 24-h period from all anaesthetists and as many surgeons as practically possible. As for the surgeons, observations and measurements were made on 12 separate days, and different weekdays were sampled to cover the different levels of activity occurring on different days of the week.

Subjects

Surgeons

Three of the surgeons were the same individuals as in study 1. These were the three most senior people, although, as the study took place 1 year later, two of them had changed status. The senior registrar had become a consultant, and the most senior of the registrars had become the senior registrar. This involved more responsibility for both of them, and enabled the senior consultant to share some of his responsibilities with his newly promoted colleague. This might not have reduced his workload much, however, because the unit increased the number of cases it handled. Data were collected from the remaining registrars and senior house officiers. There were two each of these, making a total of seven in all. However, because of holidays and other absences, as well as the practical difficulties of keeping track of so many people, it was rare for us to be able to get seven urine samples.

Anaesthetists

The structure of training in anaesthetics is different from that in surgery. The senior registrar was near the end of his training and was spending his final period of specialist training in cardiothoracic anaesthetics. He was present throughout the study. There were three consultants attached to cardiothoracic theatres and each of them was on 24-h call on different days of the week. It was not possible, therefore, to study the same consultant each week as we had been able to do with the surgeons. Each consultant and other anaesthetists were studied on at least three separate occasions. The same variation applied to the registrars and senior house officers because their training period in cardiothoracic anaesthetics lasted 6 weeks; thus, during the study different people occupied these roles. On a typical day we would be able to study one consultant, one senior registrar and two registrars/senior house officers. On each day we studied as many anaesthetists as we could, provided they were doing cardiothoracic work. Altogether nine anaesthetists were studied. Three were consultants, one a senior registrar, four registrars and one a senior house officer. Among these subjects the actual experience of cardiothoracic anaesthetics differed considerably. All the subjects except one registrar were male.

The Anaesthetist's Role

The day before the patient is to have an operation the anaesthetist will visit him/her and describe what will happen up to the point at which the patient becomes unconscious. The anaesthetist's day starts between 7.45 and 8.15 a.m., when he meets the patient in the suite outside the operating theatre. The patient will have had some premedication to reduce the level of anxiety. The anaesthetist's immediate task is to insert catheters into the wrist and neck to allow the monitoring of pressures while the operation is in progress. The senior registrar will almost always be present for this, and the consultant and a registrar or senior house officer are usually also present. The consultant may perform the catheterization or may supervise or train more junior staff. When this part of the process is complete and the patient is stable, he/she is taken into the operating theatre and anaesthetized. The anaesthetist then places a tube down the patient's throat to enable the breathing to be maintained by a ventilator. This intubation, the process of putting the patient into a strate of unconsciousness, and catheterization are all potentially dangerous/stressful points for both patient and anaesthetist. Once the patient is asleep the anaesthetist's job is to keep a careful eye on the various monitoring devices and to use drugs to support the patient if necessary. He also has to keep records of drugs administered, the patient's progress, and to organize tests of blood samples at regular points throughout the operation. There are always at least two anaesthetists available, although one may give the other a break if the operation is at a routine stage. Once the operation is under way, and particularly if the patient is having open heart surgery where the function of lungs and heart are performed by machines, then the anaesthetist may have a quiet period lasting 2 or 3 h, although close monitoring continues throughout. The next physically active phase, which is again potentially stressful, is waking the patient from the operation and transferring him/her to the intensive care ward where he/she has to be reconnected to essential monitoring equipment and the ventilator. The anaesthetist completes this with the surgical staff and nursing staff. When this is complete, the anaesthetist prepares the next patient. In a typical day, two or three operations may take place. Anaesthetists not on night duty usually finish between 5.00 and 7.00 p.m., but emergencies or cases which have to be taken back into theatre can make it much later. Unlike the junior surgeons, however, the anaesthetists are not directly responsible for those patients remaining in intensive care, so they manage to get a little more sleep than the surgeons (on 27% of occasions surgeons had obtained less than 5 h of sleep during the night prior to the study, while this occurred only 10% of the time for anaesthetists). Being junior doctors, however, they still work long hours compared with most occupations. The registrars and senior house officers will be on call several times a week and perhaps one weekend in three, and during this time they may give anaesthetics on their own, as well as dealing with emergencies and routine work on other wards in the hospital. The consultants have administrative roles in addition to their clinical responsibilities and the training and teaching that goes on continually. They, too, are on call one night in four and one weekend in four.

Table 6. Frequency distribution (percentages) of severity and duration of stress

	Frequencies of stress severity					
	Very severe	Severe	Quite severe	Mild	Very mild	*n*
Surgeons *t*1		20	60	20		35
Surgeons *t*2	4	8	18	63		27
Anaesthetists	11		27	53	9	45
	Frequencies of duration of stress					
	Not more than few min	About 1 h	Several hours	Whole period	Whole period and afterwards	*n*
Surgeons *t*1	11	46	29	8	6	35
Surgeons *t*2	27	30	33		10	27
Anaesthetists	69	25	2	2	2	45

*t*1, time one; *t*2, time two

Results[4]

Perceptions of Stress

The only psychological variable measured on both occasions for the surgeons and the anaesthetists was whether they had experienced any stress or strain during the period under review. If they gave a positive answer they were then asked to rate the severity of the stress and the duration of the stress. In study 1 the surgeons reported stress on 35 occasions out of 74 (47%) and in study 2, 27 occasions out of 46 (58%). The anaesthetist reported stress 45 times out of 89 occasions (51%), so there is close similarity in the frequency with which stress is reported. Table 6 shows percentages of severity and duration for those occasions on which stress was reported. In terms of severity the surgeons reported more severe stress at time 1 than they did at time 2. Their reported severity at time 2 is concurrent with and very similar to that of the anaesthetists although the latter are slightly more inclined to use the "very severe" category.

The patterns for duration of stress were similar at times 1 and 2 for the surgeons but somewhat different for the anaesthetists. The latter are more likely to report stress which was short lived; only 6% of their responses were for periods longer than 1 h, and nearly 70% were for no more than a few minutes. Over 40% of the surgeons' experiences of stress lasted several hours or more.

Perceptions of Job Demands

Because the job demands data were not collected from surgeons at time 2, it is only possible to compare the surgeons at time 1 with the anaesthetists. The surgeons reported less severe stress at time 2, although they actually reported stress slightly

4 Results of ECG date not yet available.

Table 7. Mean scores for job demands of surgeons ($t1$) and anaesthetists

Item	Surgeons	Anaesthetists
Demands on knowledge	1.53	1.15
Physical demands	1.35	1.17
Colleagues' demands	1.21	0.96
Demands on skills	1.19	1.11
Demands from other departments	1.19	0.92
Demands from patients	0.88	0.69
Demands from relatives of patients	0.82	0.15
	$n=108$	$n=89$

$t1$, time 1.

Table 8. Frequency distribution (percentages) of perceptions of authority, support and satisfaction

	Feeling you did not have necessary authority to make the decisions needed				
	NA	Did not happen	Happened once	Happened twice	Happened more than twice
Surgeons $t1$ ($n=108$)	4	81	13	2	
Anaesthetists ($n=89$)	6	85	8	1	
	Feelings about support from colleagues/coworkers				
	NA	Gave all support needed	Support good most of time	Support sometimes lacking	Support lacking lot of time
Surgeons $t1$ ($n=108$)	3	83	11	2	
Anaesthetists ($n=89$)	9	76	12	3	
	Satisfaction with way things went				
	NA	Very satisfied	Quite satisfied	Slightly dissatisfied	Very dissatisfied
Surgeons $t1$ ($n=108$)		47	40	9	3
Anaesthetists ($n=89$)		53	31	15	1

$t1$, time one; NA, not applicable

more frequently. The comparison supports the data in the previous paragraph, suggesting longer lasting stress among the surgeons. Table 7 presents the means and standard deviations for the job demands items and shows that the surgeons reported higher demands on all seven items directly assessing job demands variables. The item asking about pressures from people outside of work showed no difference (1.18 vs. 1.20). These differences are consistent with our own observations of people performing these two different functions. Both groups regularly encounter problems that have severe implications for the patients, but the anaesthetists are usually in control quickly or not at all. The surgeons often have more time, because there

Table 9. Means of mean levels of VMA for surgeons and anaesthetists

Surgeons $t1$		Surgeons $t2$		Anaesthetists		Normal range
$\bar{x}$	SD	$\bar{x}$	SD	$\bar{x}$	SD	
59	10	59	8	47	7	15–85

Surgeons $t2$ vs. anaesthetists: $P < 0.01$ (two-tailed tests). $t1$, time one; $t2$, time two

Table 10. Means of individual mean levels of cortisol for surgeons and anaesthetists

Surgeons $t1$		Surgeons $t2$		Anaesthetists		Normal range
$\bar{x}$	SD	$\bar{x}$	SD	$\bar{x}$	SD	
389	83	449	34	364	80	100–350

Surgeons $t2$ vs. anaesthetists: $P < 0.025$ (two-tailed tests). $t1$, time one; $t2$, time two

are alternative surgical procedures, but they also live with the uncertainty of the outcome for a much longer period.

Perceptions of Authority, Support and Satisfaction

Table 8 shows the frequency distributions for these three variables as percentages. The data show clearly that the feelings of the two groups were very similar. They rarely lacked authority to make the decisions they feel they need to make, support is felt to be good nearly all the time, and they report dissatisfaction on about 15% of the occasions on which they were asked. In terms of the hours they work and the responsibilities they carry, both groups have demanding jobs, although the surgeons see theirs as slightly more demanding. Both groups have high discretion and good support from colleagues. Both groups are highly satisfied with their jobs. In Karasek's terms both are classifiable as "active" jobs on the basis of these data.

Vanillylmandelic Acid

The means, standard deviations and confidence limits for comparisons for the means are presented in Table 9. The distributions of VMA were within normal limits virtually all of the time. There was no difference between the means for the surgeons on the two occasions. The surgeons scored significantly higher than the anaesthetists ($P < 0.01$), which perhaps reflects the longer periods of acute stress reported above.

Cortisol

Table 10 contains the descriptive statistics for the surgeons at times 1 and 2, and for the anaesthetists, as well as normative data. The high levels of cortisol among surgeons were replicated. They were significantly higher than the norms quoted for the technique of assay used here (Amerlex method), and its norms compare well with norms for other techniques (Gough and Ellis 1981) and for data from larger samples (Nakamura and Yakata 1983). The surgeons demonstrated significantly higher

Table 11. Self-reports of stress for each surgeon at time 1 ($t1$) and time 2 ($t2$)

Reports of stress for consultant

	$t1$		$t2$	
	Yes	No	Yes	no
Felt stress	7	2	3	3
Mean severity } of stress	1.00		0.66	
Mean duration } of stress	1.80		0.66	

Reports of stress for senior registrar becoming a consultant

	$t1$		$t2$	
	Yes	No	Yes	No
Felt stress	0	5	4	1
Mean severity } of stress	0.0		1.00	
Mean duration } of stress	0.0		1.60	

Reports of stress for registrar becoming a senior registrar

	$t1$		$t2$	
	Yes	No	Yes	No
Felt stress	6	3	7	2
Mean severity } of stress	1.00		1.33	
Mean duration } of stress	0.66		1.33	

levels than the anaesthetists, suggesting again that they experience stress more chronically. The anaesthetists showed significantly higher levels of cortisol than the normal population: 54% of their scores were outside the normal range, compared with 86% for the surgeons.

Length of Experience and the Biochemical Markers

As in the first study, there was no relationship between length of experience and VMA. The strong rank-order correlation between length of experience and mean cortisol level found among the surgeons was not replicated amongst the surgeons at time 2, nor was there any evidence for a relationship between these two variables amongst the anaesthetists.

Subjective Stress and Biochemical Indices

Another relationship not replicated was that between reports of stress on a day and higher than average levels of cortisol for the individual on the same day. As with the first study, there was no evidence of any relationship between subjective data and VMA in either the data from the surgeons or the anaesthetists.

Table 12. Cortisol and VMA levels for three surgeons at time 1 ($t1$) and time 2 ($t2$)

	Senior consultant		Senior registrar →consultant		Registrar→ senior registrar	
	$t1$	$t2$	$t1$	$t2$	$t1$	$t2$
Cortisol	562	507	359	423[a]	370	417[a]
VMA	62	56	55	68[a]	65	51

[a] $P<0.05$

Comparisons of the Same Surgeons at Two Points in Time

As indicated earlier, three of the surgeons were studied at two different points in time, and two of them had been promoted in the interim. This not only had implications for themselves, but also for the senior consultant, who up to that time had been on call continuously and had done all the work of building up the unit. The appointment of another consultant allowed him to be off duty every other night and every other weekend, as well as to share other responsibilities. Given these changes it is possible to test the sensitivity of the measures used as indicators of stress by making predictions for each of the three individuals.

We predicted that the senior consultant would report less stress and show lowered cortisol. We expected the newly appointed consultant to experience more subjective stress and show higher cortisol. The registrar appointed to senior registrar was expected to show the same trends, although perhaps not quite so strongly, as he still had two consultants above him who were ultimately responsible for treatment, diagnosis and decisions. The numbers of observations were small, of course, but still quite impressive. Table 11 shows the self-reports of stress with mean ratings of severity and duration for each surgeon at times 1 and 2. In all three cases, the predictions were substantiated. The senior consultant's stress was lower and those of the other two were higher in frequency, severity and duration. Table 12 shows the data for cortisol and VMA. The predictions are once again reasonably well supported. The senior consultant's cortisol and VMA levels dropped, while the newly appointed consultant's cortisol and VMA were significantly higher and the senior registrar's cortisol level was higher. These results seem supportive of the value of both the subjective ratings and cortisol in detecting the consequences of relatively long-term changes in roles and responsibilities.

Summary and Discussion

Put at its simplest, the relationship of coronary heart disease to occupational stress is complex. Theories differentiating "at risk" employment are invariably *post hoc,* so that medical practice is variously described as a "low-strain occupation" (Kauppinen-Toropainen et al. 1983) or an "active job" (Karasek et al. 1982). The practice of medicine is generally perceived as being severely stressful (Krakowski 1982a; Bates 1982), even though in terms of standardized mortality ratios relating to death from all causes and for cardiovascular diseases in particular, physicians and surgeons fare far better than the general population (Doll and Peto 1979), and surgeons fare better than physicians. Cardiac surgery for the surgeon, and presumably the anaesthetist, has been described as "periods of prolonged boredom interspersed with anticipated, or even worse, unanticipated episodes of sheer terror" (Norman 1980), and a behavioural study of general anaesthetists contained self-reports of high levels of stress and fatigue at the end of the day (Branton and Oborne 1979). Much of their work is carried on outside the operating theatre in the intensive care unit, and Gentry and Parkes (1982) and Friedman (1982) both highlight the continual presence of psychological and emotional stress in such units.

In our studies, if episodes of sheer terror did occur, the subjects could only have been adding to their stress by disguising the occurrence most successfully. More often than not, we only became aware of the severity of the stress they had experienced on receiving their own reports. Typically, stress occurred on over 50% of working days (see Table 6), and perceived job demands were significantly higher in the surgeons than in the anaesthetists (see Table 7). How such demand loads compare, either qualitatively or quantitatively, with other medical or non-medical occupations is at present unknown. The overall impression we were left with, after more than 200 h of observations, was that our subjects experienced physical and/or psychological stress during the majority of their working days. Krakowski (1982b) has associated stress in medical practice with greater than normal mental and emotional maladaption in private life. In our study, with only 20 subjects, this could not meaningfully be assessed. However, on each occasion when job demands were monitored, the subjects were asked to rate external demands (as for other items in Table 1). It is interesting to note that the two groups were almost equal (1.20 vs. 1.18) on perceived demands in their private lives. Also, it can be noted from Table 4 that in terms of control, support and job satisfaction both groups do extremely well with very similar profiles. Thus, any differences that we found between the surgeons and anaesthetists on the psychobiological markers are likely to reflect differing levels of stress.

It has already been noted that the surgeons perceived significantly higher overall job demands than the anaesthetists (see Table 7), and this psychosocial measure of stress was consistent with the measures taken of VMA and cortisol excretion in the urine. Over 24 h, on average, the VMA measures (see Table 9) were within the normal range for all the subjects, but the surgeons did have significantly higher levels of VMA excretion (59 ± 8 vs. 47 ± 7; $P < 0.01$). Only 10% of the measures taken were outside the normal range (15-85 nmoles/24 h), and, although the anaesthetists' average excretion was lower than that of the surgeons, as individuals they were significantly more labile (16.8 ± 6.3 vs. 25.6 ± 8.2; $P < 0.5$). This could be a ceiling effect, reflecting the more chronic aspects of the surgeon's job. A disappointing finding in both studies was that the fluctuations in VMA scores did not match the self-reports of stress or job demands. It may well be that direct measures of urinary adrenaline and noradrenaline would have proved more successful for relating catecholamine activity to perceived stress.

The levels of cortisol (see Table 10) found among surgeons and anaesthetists in these studies were clearly chronically high, particularly in the surgeons, compared with those found in normal populations (Gough and Ellis 1981; Nakamura and Yakata 1983). The levels found, however, were still well below or above those found in patients with identifiable illnesses such as Cushing's disease or hypopituitarism

(Nakamura and Yakata 1983). The fact that these high levels in surgeons were replicated over a 1-year period and that the anaesthetists working in the same environment also had levels above average does indicate a stable, chronic condition. Furthermore, the changes in subjective stress and biochemical markers associated with changes in the job responsibilities of individual surgeons (see Tables 11 and 12) suggest that more responsibilities can lead to more felt stress and to increased biochemical activity to cope with the stress. This appears to take place over time, as we found little support for a day-to-day relationship between subjective stress and levels of these two biochemical markers. Others have shown an increase in catecholamines in response to acute real-life stress (Dimsdale and Moss 1980) over much shorter periods. Questions remain, however, concerning the meaning of these chronically elevated levels of cortisol: are they clinically significant?

Cortisol levels have been hypothesized by several writers to indicate stress in a person, but their interpretations are not totally consistent. Selye (1956) argued that chronic exposure to stresses will eventually lead to the exhaustion of the endocrine system and result in low levels of cortisol. Caplan et al. (1979) pursued this hypothesis in a occupational setting. They studied 200 employees in administrative, engineering and scientific jobs involved in the NASA organization. They found no support for an association between high workload and low cortisol levels. Their findings did suggest that high workload might lead to lowered cortisol levels early-in the morning, but levels over 24 h were no lower among those with a higher workload.

More recently, researchers have interpreted *high* levels of cortisol to indicate stress (e.g. Frankenhaeuser and Johansson 1982; Karasek et al. 1982). The former authors hypothesized that different conditions produce different endocrine responses. A state of active effort (similar to Karasek's notion of a "strained" job) produces high catecholamine and high cortisol excretion. A passive, helpless state, where the person feels low control, is accompanied primarily by increased cortisol. In one study they compared people in what we have called an "active" job (production and planning control) with those in a "strained" job (process monitoring) and showed that the former individuals had increased adrenaline but decreased cortisol. In the "strained" job both adrenaline and cortisol were slightly higher at the workplace than when the person was at home. Unfortunately, absolute levels were not reported, so it is not clear whether they were high relative to those in the normal population. Baker et al. (1984) compared a group of new medical students with an experienced group and found levels of cortisol differed, with those in the new (more anxious) group being significantly higher (470 nmol/litre vs. 362 nmol/litre). However, Schwertner et al. (1984) found no relationship between levels of cortisol and coronary artery disease, as assessed by coronary angiography in a sample of over 600 men.

It seems crucial to distinguish between acute and chronic stress in assessing the meaning of different levels of cortisol. Frankenhaeuser and Johansson have dealt with acute stressors at work that raised cortisol levels, but over 24 h the body may balance out these effects to produce levels within the normal range. This is what we believe we have found with the surgeons: They often report acutely stressful periods, but over 24 h the levels of VMA were normal. For surgeons, however, the small acute stresses appear to occur frequently enough each day to produce a higher level of cortisol. This level, while abnormally high, may not be clinically dangerous. There is no evidence from epidemiological data that hospital specialists have higher standardized mortality ratios. They actually have rates lower than those for general physicians for deaths from heart disease (Doll and Peto 1977), and both are lower than the general population. If the acute stresses experienced by surgeons were even more stressful, and even more frequent, then Selye's prediction of the exhaustion of cortisol leading to excessive levels of noradrenaline and deterioration of the arterial walls may be realized. At present it seems likely that the elevated levels of cortisol result from the body's adaptive response to cope with moderate but bearable levels of job stress. Is cortisol elevation in response to increased stress a physiological adaptation analogous to changes in red blood cell count with changes in altitude and therefore not in any sense pathological?

References

Alfredsson L, Karasek R, Theorell T (1982) Myocardial infarction risk and psychosocial work environment: an analysis of the male Swedish working force. Soc Sci Med 16: 463-467

Baker GH, Byrom NA, Irani MS et al (1984) Stress, cortisol and lymphocyte sub-populations. Lancet I: 574

Bates E (1982) Doctors and their spouses speak: stress in medical practice. Soc Health Illness 4: 25-39

Becker WGE, Ellis H, Goldsmith R, et al (1983) Heart rates of surgeons in theatre. Ergonomics 26: 803-808

Branton P, Oborne DJ (1979) A behavioural study of anaesthetists at work. In: Oborne DJ, Gruneberg MM, Eiser JR (eds) Research in psychology and medicine, vol 1. Academic, London

Caplan RD, Cobb S, French JRP Ur (1979) White collar work load and cortisol: disruption of a circadian rhythm by job stress. J Psychosom Res 23: 181-192

Dimsdale JE, Moss J (1980) Short-term catecholamine response to psychological stress. Psychosom Med 42 (5): 493-497

Doll R, Peto R (1979) Mortality among doctors in different occupations. Br Med J 1: 1433-1436

Foster GE, Evans DF, Hardcastle J (1978) Heart rates of surgeons during operations and other clinical activities and their modification by oxprenolol. Lancet I: 1323-1325

Frankenhaeuser M, Johansson G (1982) Stress at work: psychobiological and psychosocial aspects. 20th International Congress of Applied Psychology, Edinburgh 1982

Friedman EH (1982) Stress and intensive care nursing: a ten year reappraisal. Heart Lung 11: 26-29

Gentry DW, Parkes KR (1982) Psychological stress in intensive care unit and non-intensive care unit nursing. A review of the past decade. Heart Lung 11: 43-47

Gough RM, Ellis G (1981) The radioimmunassay of cortisol in urine: difficulties experienced in the development of an assay, and problems of specificity observed with commercial reagents as supplied as kits. Clin Biochem 14 (2): 74-81

Hennigan JK, Wortham AW (1975) Analysis of workday stresses on industrial managers using heart rate as a criterion. Ergonomics 18 (6): 675-681

Hunt TJ, Marcus P (1966) The investigation of habitual activity in bus crews using SAMI heart-rate integrator. J Physiol 189: 36-37

Ira GH, Bogdonoff MD, Durham NC (1962) Application of radiotelemetry in man for continuous recording of heart rate. JAMA 180 (11): 976-977

Karasek RA (1979) Job demands, job decision latitude and mental strain: implications for job redesign. Admin Sci Q 24: 285-308

Karasek RA, Russell RS, Theorell T (1982) Physiology of stress and regeneration in job related cardiovascular illness. J Human Stress 8: 29-42

Kaupinnen-Toropainen K, Kandolin I, Mutanen P (1983) Job dissatisfaction and work-related exhaustion in male and female work. J Occup Behav 4 (3): 193-207

Krakowski AJ (1982a) Stress and the practice of medicine. J Psychosom Res 26: 91-98

Krakowski AJ (1982b) Stress and the practice of medicine II. Stressors, stresses and strains. Psychother Psychosom 38: 11-23
La Rocco JM, House JS, French JRP Jr (1980) Social support, occupational stress and health. J Health Soc Behav 21: 202-218
Leonard RA (1983) A psychological study of stress in London school-teachers. Ph D Thesis, University of London, London
Nakamura J, Yakata M (1983) Clinical evaluation of the liquid-chromatographic determination of urinary free cortisol. Clin Chem 29/5: 847-851
Norman JC (1980) Histrionics, vignettes and quartets: a syndrome of stress in heart surgeons. Cardiovasc Dis 7: 339-343
Payne RL (1979) Demands, supports, constraints and psychological health. In: Mackay CJ, Cox T (eds) Response to stress: occupational aspects. International Publishing Corporation, London
Pinneau SR Jr (1975) Effects of social support on psychological and physiological stress. Ph D Thesis, University of Michigan, Ann Arbor
Pisano JI, Crout RJ, Abraham D (1962) Determination of 3-methoxy-4-hydroxymandelic acid in urine. Clin Chim Acta 7: 285-291
Rodahl K, Vokac Z (1977) Work stress in Norwegian trawler fishermen. Ergonomics 20 (6): 633-642
Schwertner HA, Troxler EG, Uhl GS, Jackson WG (1984) Relationship between cortisol and cholesterol in men with coronary artery disease and Type A behaviour. Arteriosclerosis 4: 59-64
Selye H (1956) The stress of life. McGraw Hill, New York
Taggart P, Gibbons D, Sommerville W (1969) Some effects of motor-car driving on the normal and abnormal heart. Br Med J 4: 130-134

New Dimensions in Studying Sympathetic Nervous System Responses to Stressors

J. E. Dimsdale[1]

Introduction

One way or another, all theories about the relationship between stress and cardiovascular disease suggest the importance of sympathetic and adrenal medullary responses. These systems may act as crucial pathogenic links between emotion and cardiac events such as sudden death, coronary artery spasm, angina, congestive heart failure, and hypertension. While such a linkage is plausible, it is nonetheless far from established, partly because of the difficulty of studying sympathetic nervous system activity.

In this paper I will review material discussed originally at the 1982 Altenburg Conference on Biobehavioral Bases of Coronary Disease (Dimsdale 1983). Then I will summarize some recent findings observed by our group and others; these developments rely on new techniques for studying this complex area.

Background

Although many speak of the sympathetic nervous system as a homogeneously responding unit, this is a vast oversimplification. At minimum, there are two wings: the sympathetic nervous system, a primarily neural system with transmission via norepinephrine; and the adrenal medullary system, more of a traditional hormonal system with communication occurring mainly via epinephrine. While both sympathetic activity and adrenal activity are increased by stressors, a number of studies suggest that norepinephrine is increased mainly by dynamic exercise, whereas epinephrine is increased by anxiety and other dysphoric states (Leblanc et al. 1979).

In monitoring sympathetic and adrenal activity, one can examine the signal either as it is *emitted* or as it is *received* (Dimsdale 1985). Psychosomatic research has oscillated between valuing one or the other approach. Historically, because the chemical recognition of the signal was so difficult, investigators tracked activity by the end organ response to a received signal. Thus, many early studies examined galvanic skin response, heart rate, or blood pressure, and used them as indices of sympathetic activity. This approach was far from satisfying because of the many other factors regulating such end organ response.

With improved techniques in electrophysiology and biochemistry, examining the emitted signal itself became feasible. It is now even possible to monitor directly the electrical activity of sympathetic nerve endings in the periphery (Wallin 1981).

1 UCSD Medical Center, 225 Dickinson Street (T-004), San Diego, CA 92103, USA

Biological and Psychological Factors
in Cardiovascular Disease
Ed. by T. H. Schmidt, T. M. Dembroski, and G. Blümchen

However, because this technique is somewhat invasive, it has limited utility in human studies of responses to stress.

Because of the brief half-life of plasma catecholamines, their rapid elevation in response to a simple venapuncture, and because of technical problems with early assays for plasma catecholamines, early investigations focused on examining the chemical traces of signal emission as found in urine. These early studies provided considerable groundwork for developing this field (Levi 1965; Frankenhaeuser 1975; Mason 1975). However, examining the urinary catecholamines is decidedly unsatisfactory for clarifying transient, short-term responses to stressors. Given that the signal onset and half-life is on the order of 2 min, it is impossible to obtain appropriate fractional urine samples representing such short-term intervals. For studies which have hypothesized that a given population may be chronically overactive in sympathetic nervous activity, however, such urinary studies may continue to be useful (Baum et al. 1983).

We have focused on plasma catecholamine responses to moderate stressors. This work was facilitated not only by advances in chemical assays, but also by advances in biomedical equipment. The research relies heavily on a portable blood withdrawal pump used in conjunction with a Tedmac-treated catheter system.[2] The special catheter binds heparin to the internal surface wall and thus prevents problems of coagulation in the line. No heparin enters the patient's system nor is any manipulation with a heplock required. Factors for determining the rate of blood withdrawal and the frequency of sample integration were discussed in our paper at the 1982 Altenberg Conference (Dimsdale 1983).

In searching for an appropriate and potent behavioral setting for examining stress, we were struck by the stressfulness of public speaking, particularly for speakers in their early days of medical training. In comparing public speaking with dynamic exercise, we observed that public speaking was usually accompanied by a tripling of epinephrine and a 50% increase of norepinephrine, whereas the exact opposite pattern was observed for dynamic exercise (Dimsdale and Moss 1980a). Furthermore, we observed that the timing of sampling was of major importance in the context of a behavioral stress such as public speaking. Epinephrine increased rapidly in the initial 3 min of speaking. However, by the time the speaker had spoken for 15 min, his epinephrine levels were no longer significantly increased over baseline values. We concluded that one could not be casual about the timing of blood sampling for plasma catecholamines in behavioral interventions (Dimsdale and Moss 1980b).

Our group has continued these research activities from a number of perspectives. I will summarize additional work concerning exercise physiology, pharmacology, theoretical design issues, dietary factors, and novel approaches for examining receptor response.

2 The TEDMAC-treated catheter may be obtained from Cormed, 591 Mahar Street, Medina, New York 14103.

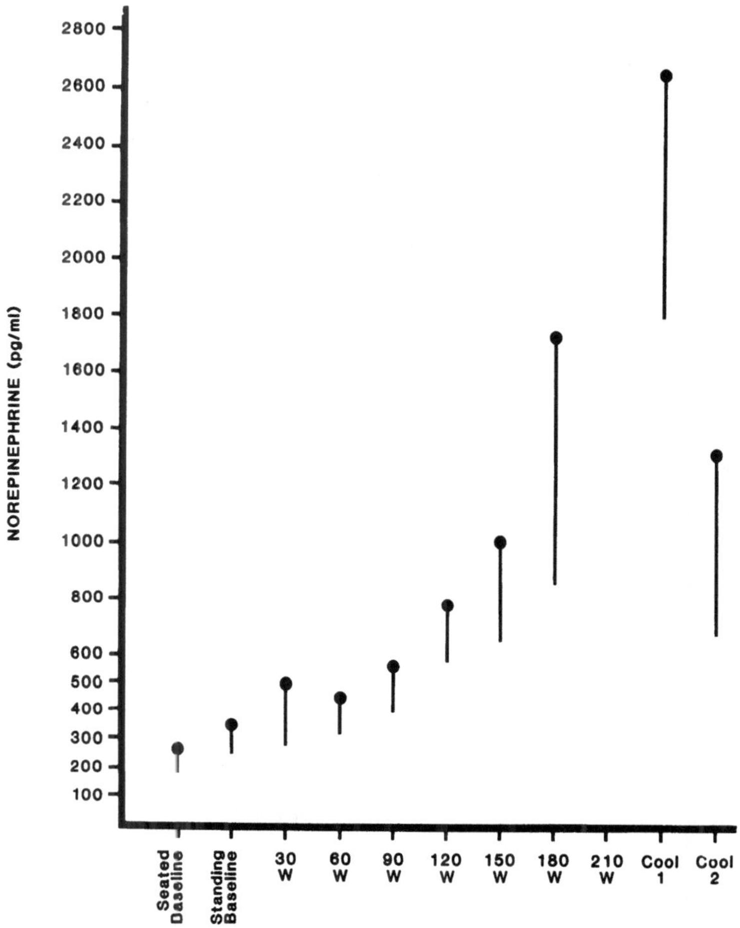

Fig. 1. The effect of increasing work load on plasma norepinephrine (Dimsdale et al. 1984b)

Further Delineation of Exercise Physiology

In our initial studies we used a gross measure of dynamic exercise. Our subjects ran up and down flights of stairs for 3 min. We did not control for the rapidity of the running, the heart rate, or the work load exerted by our subjects. The next natural research direction was to examine plasma catecholamine responses in the context of careful, standardized exercise testing. Again, using the blood withdrawal pump and catheter technique, we examined 11 healthy, young men during a maximal exercise tolerance test on a bicycle ergometer. Subjects began pedaling at a work load of 30 w and increased by 30 w every 3 min until they reached exhaustion.

It is inappropriate to speak of one homogeneous catecholamine response to exercise. Issues of sample timing are important for dynamic exercise, just as they are for psychological stress. Norepinephrine in particular is highly dependent on work load, increasing as the work load increases (Fig. 1). Thus one needs to specify work load when referring to levels of catecholamines.

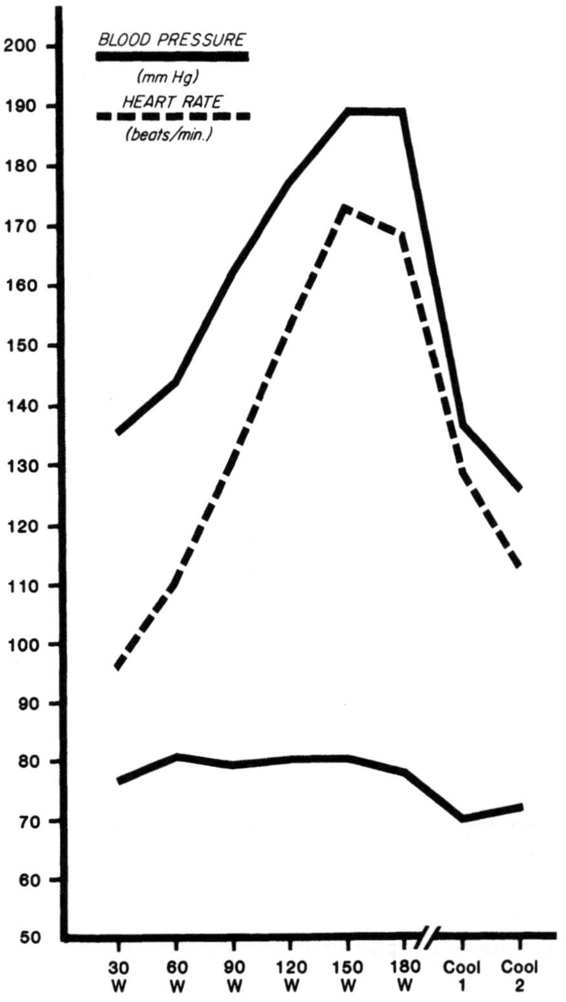

Fig. 2. Heart rate and blood pressure responses to exercise (Dimsdale 1984b)

Our other observation relates to a long-term puzzle, that of post-exercise morbidity and mortality. Dating from antiquity, case reports have accumulated concerning individuals dying suddenly, immediately *after* completing a race. Indeed, the original marathon runner Pheidippedes is purported to have died in 490 B.C. immediately after delivering the news to the Athenians that their forces had triumphed over Darius. (See Dimsdale 1984a for a discussion of the Pheidippides legend.)

Now that jogging has become so popular, it is not uncommon to read of a jogger dying during exercise. Although some of the deaths occur on the course, some occur immediately *after* the race, at a time when the victim was no longer exercising but was in the recovery phase from exercise. Another thread that makes exploration of the post-exercise period interesting comes from the exercise testing laboratory. Many individuals develop arrhythmias or faintness in the immediate recovery period (Ekblom et al. 1979).

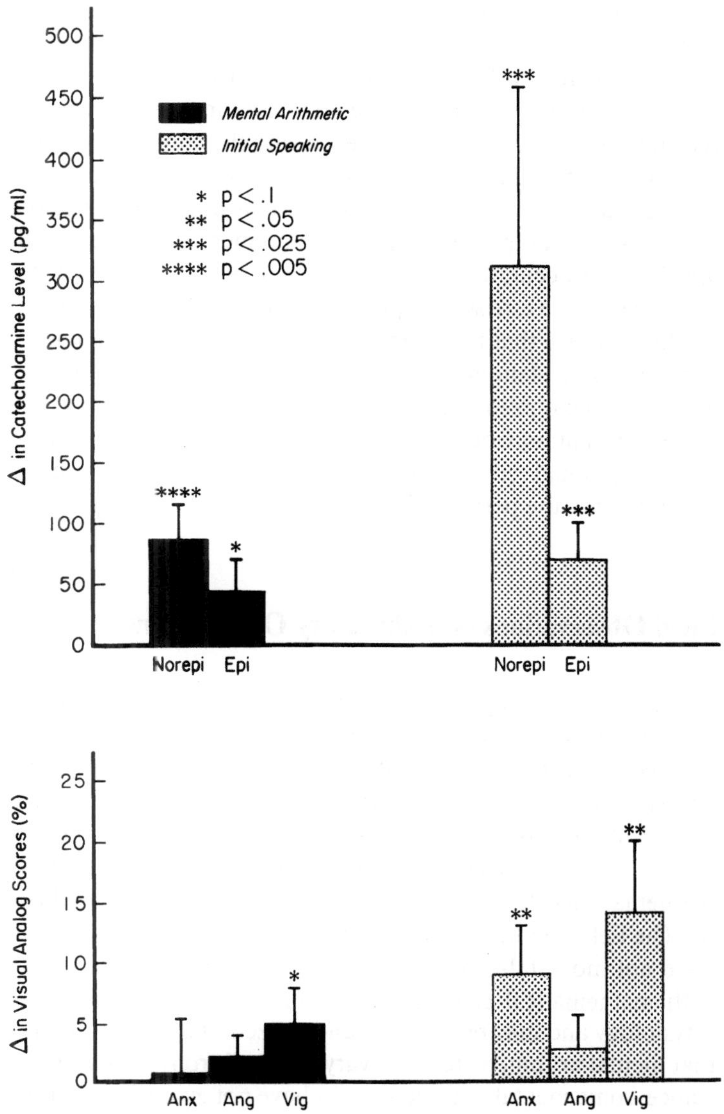

Fig. 3. Differences between observations in the laboratory and the field. *Norepi*, norepinephrine; *Epi*, epinephrine; *Anx*, anxiety; *Ang*, anger; *Vig*, vigilance. (Dimsdale 1985b)

In our recent exercise study (Dimsdale et al. 1984b), we continued to obtain plasma catecholamine samples after each subject had reached his maximum tolerable exercise. We have referred to these time intervals as "cool-down samples": "cool-down 1" refers to the first 3 min following exercise cessation and "cool-down 2" refers to the second 3 min after exercise cessation. Figure 1 demonstrates that norepinephrine continues to increase dramatically even after the exercise is completed. These levels, taken in conjunction with the large stroke volumes occurring after exercise (Cumming 1977), may precipitate arrhythmias, particularly in individuals with preexisting coronary artery disease.

It is difficult to pinpoint a mechanism for these increases; however, some evidence points to a baroreceptor-mediated phenomenon. Figure 2 illustrates the blood pressure and heart rate responses to exercise. Note that the normal systolic response is a progressive increase up to maximal work load, followed by an abrupt return to normal systolic pressures during the cool-down interval. We hypothesize that the abrupt fall in systolic pressure is misperceived by the baroreceptors and interpreted as a signal of impending hypotension; the baroreceptors then call for defense of the blood pressure and trigger an increased secretion of norepinephrine. If this theory is accurate, then the manner in which one terminates exercise may well affect the post-exercise norepinephrine level and the resulting post-exercise peril. We hypothesize that the worst possible strategy for terminating exercise is to stop abruptly while standing in place. Under this circumstance, the venous pooling in the legs is maximized, the drop in blood pressure is maximized, and the stimulus to the baroreceptors would presumably be the strongest. A healthier strategy would call for a gradual reduction of work load by walking after exercise or by lying down. In both cases, the peripheral venous pooling would be minimized.

Field Observations vs. Laboratory Observations

Because behavioral phenomena are so complex, it is helpful to study physiological responses to stressors, both as they occur naturally in the field and in the laboratory. In theory the naturalistic setting would capitalize on observations during truly stressful circumstances which are difficult to standardize; whereas laboratory stressors would be more readily standardizable but might not be as stressful.

We examined a group of individuals in the laboratory as they responded to mathematical calculations, and in the field as they responded while speaking in public. The field conditions were similar to those discussed in our earlier studies; these were not mock talks but were required lectures. We chose to compare this stress with mathematical calculations because math tasks are widely used in psychophysiology and may be readily standardized. It is important to emphasize, however, that mental arithmetic tests do vary in detail from laboratory to laboratory. For instance, some mental arithmetic tasks have not evoked profound increases in plasma catecholamines. Our task was quite demanding, calling for subjects to perform serial 7 subtraction from the number 600. The instructions were delivered by tape-recorder, and the subject was asked to continue the calculations for a 3-min interval. A loud metronome continually reminded the subject of the passing of time. Furthermore, at occasional points the tape-recording reminded the individual that he had a certain amount of time left in his calculation, thus further complicating the subtraction efforts.

Public speaking and mathematical calculations did not lead to the same picture either subjectively or hormonally (Dimsdale 1984b). Mental arithmetic led to increases in vigilance and norepinephrine but did not affect anger, anxiety, or epinephrine (Fig. 3). In contrast, public speaking led to increases in anxiety, vigilance, norepinephrine, and epinephrine. We feel that this data argues for the importance of studying responses to stressors both in the laboratory and in the field.

Table 1. Effects of beta-blockade on plasma catecholamine levels

Reference	Drug	Dose	Subjects	Catecholamine assay	Resting level		Exercise level	
					NE	E	NE	E
Franco-Morselli et al. (1978)	propranolol	chronic	5 hyper.	RE	–	d	i[b]	d[b]
Sjoberg et al. (1979)	propranolol	acute	15 norm.	FL[a]			i	i
Taggart et al. (1973)	oxprenolol	acute	8 norm.	FL			d[c]	–[c]
			7 CAD	FL			d[c]	–[c]
Irving et al. (1974)	oxprenolol	acute	5 norm.	FL	–	–	–	i
	propranolol	acute	5 norm.	FL	–	–	–	i
	pindolol	acute	5 norm.	FL	–	–	–	i
Barontini et al. (1981)	propranolol	chronic	9 norm.	RE	–	–	–	–
	mepindolol	chronic	10 hyper.	RE	–	–	i	–
	propranolol	chronic	6 hyper.	RE	–	–	i	–
Sheehan et al. (1983)	propranolol	chronic	9 norm.	RE	–	–	–[d]	–[d]
	propranolol	chronic	9 norm.	RE			–[e]	i[e]
Franz et al. (1980a)	metoprolol	chronic	7 hyper.	RE	–	–	i	i
Vlachakis et al. (1980)	propranolol	chronic	16 hyper.	RE	i	i	–	–
Galbo et al. (1976)	propranolol	acute	7 norm.	RE	i	–	–	i
Franz et al. (1980b)	metoprolol	chronic	8 hyper.	RE	–	–	i[e]	–[e]
	metoprolol	chronic	8 hyper.	RE			–[d]	–[d]
	pindolol	chronic	8 hyper.	RE	–	–	–[e]	–[e]
	pindolol	chronic	8 hyper.	RE			–[d]	i[d]

RE, radioenzymatic; FL, fluorimetric; CAD, coronary artery disease; i, increased by blocker; d, decreased by blocker; NE, norepinephrine; E, epinephrine; –, not changed by blocker; hyper., hypertensive; NE, maximal exercise; E, submaximal exercise.
[a] urinary assay; [b] response to postural challenge; [c] response to psychological stress; [d] maximal exercise; [e] submaximal exercise.

Drug Effects on Plasma Catecholamines

Beta-blocking agents are widely used after myocardial infarction and for treatment of angina and hypertension. Strictly speaking, these blocking agents might be expected to leave plasma catecholamines unaffected since they act primarily on the receptors. However, one could hypothesize that these agents lead to increases in norepinephrine and/or epinephrine levels because of a feedback reaction to the receptor blockade. Alternatively, one could hypothesize that the beta-blockers lead to a decrease in plasma catecholamine levels, because they break the vicious circle whereby anxiety produces somatic symptoms, and the awareness of such symptoms provokes more anxiety. All three of these hypotheses have been supported in a growing and confusing literature, summarized in Table 1. It is important to highlight certain crucial methodological distinctions in these studies. Foremost, beta-blockers are not homogeneous agents; they differ in terms of their lipophilicity, their specificity and their intrinsic sympathetic activity. Thus, it is possible that they affect

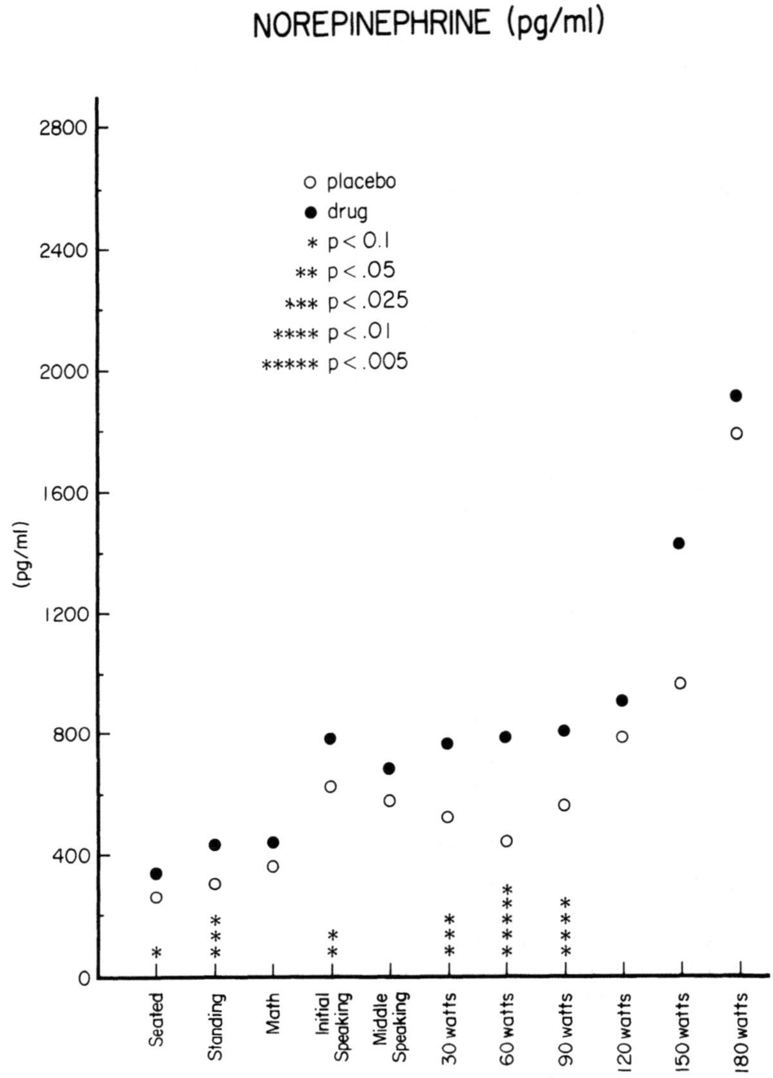

Fig. 4. The effect of metoprolol on plasma norepinephrine. Mean norepinephrine levels for drug and placebo trials are plotted for all experimental conditions. Significance levels are from a repeated measures ANOVA (see text)

plasma levels differently. Many previous studies were neither blinded nor sequence controlled. Given the exquisite sensitivity of sympathetic activity to the behavioral environment, such control is desirable.

We chose to examine responses to a single dose of metroprolol (Lopressor), a moderately lipophilic beta 1 selective blocker. Eleven subjects were investigated in a double-blind study on two occasions, half receiving 50 mg of Lopressor on the initial test occasion, and half receiving placebo on the initial test occasion. Since the sympathetic nervous system may not react uniformly to all types of challenge, we examined the plasma catecholamine response to: baseline conditions, postural stimulation, dynamic exercise, and behavioral stressors. While plasma epinephrine

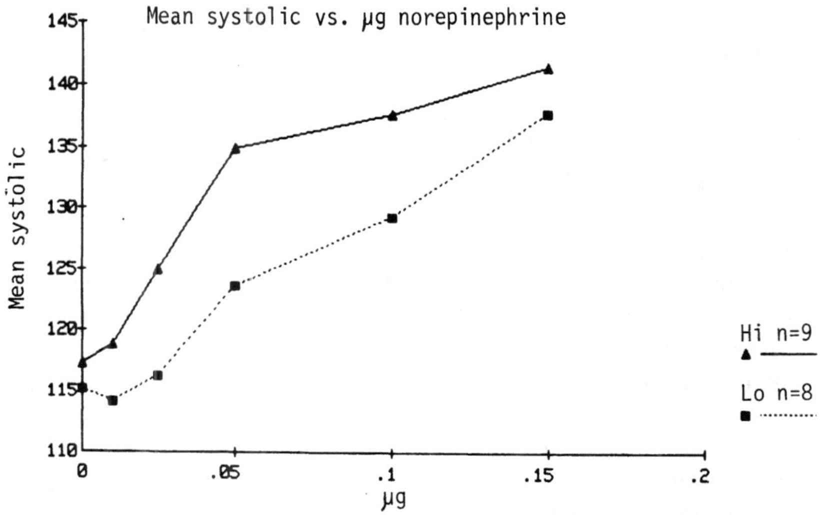

Fig. 5. Effect of high or low salt on blood pressure response to norepinephrine. Intravenous norepinephrine infusions are in micrograms per kilogram per minute

levels were not significantly affected by metroprolol, the drug led consistently to a roughly 30% increase in plasma norepinephrine levels across most observable points (Fig. 4). The increased norepinephrine levels may be a baroreceptor-mediated compensation for reduced heart rate and cardiac output elicited by beta-blockers (Dimsdale et al. 1984a). Given that these drugs have prominent neuroendocrine actions and are used so widely by patients with cardiac disease, one cannot infer anything about such patient's responses to stressors without examining the responses of controls treated with the same medication.

Salt Sensitization of Neuroadrenergic Receptors

In the introduction to this paper, I commented on cycles in research strategy that sometimes favor studies of receptor response and sometimes studies of signal emission. In many ways the field is returning to receptor studies, but they are examining these receptors in a highly sophisticated manner. For example, Anderson (1984) mentioned that there is increasing evidence that salt acts synergistically with behavioral stress to increase both the amplitude and the duration of the blood pressure response to stress (Anderson 1984; Rankin 1981).

We have recently examined this in men studied at two extremes of salt (Na) intake. The subjects were hospitalized and placed on carefully monitored diets, a high-salt diet containing 200 mEq Na per day, and a low-salt diet containing 10 mEq Na per day. After each subject came into salt balance on his respective diet, progressively increasing doses of norepinephrine were administered intravenously, and the blood pressure response to such infusions was examined. As Fig. 5 demonstrates, there appears to be sensitization of the peripheral receptors to norepinephrine in the presence of high salt, although the sample size is small. This type of study suggests that attention to dietary factors may be of increasing importance in future studies of stress physiology.

Studies of Ejection Fraction Responses to Stressors

I would like to end this paper by alluding to some work in progress that may yield different perspectives on sympathetic and adrenal medullary responses to stressors. There are many ways of examining receptor response to sympathoadrenomedullary activation. We can go far beyond monitoring peripheral galvanic skin responses or blood pressure. We can examine biochemically the number and avidity of various receptors in the periphery (Davis and Lefkowitz 1980). We can use infusions to demonstrate a dose-response curve of the sensitivity of receptors. We can even examine aspects of end organ receptor response - cardiac hemodynamics.

Ejection fraction (EF), the percentage of blood ejected from the left ventricle during systole, is of considerable clinical importance. EF is of interest in early essential hypertension, when a hyperdynamic cardiac state is postulated (Julius and Conway 1968). It is also relevant to decompensation in congestive heart failure, which is occasionally emotionally induced.

A fall in EF during exercise is a sensitive measure of ischemia and is today monitored with combined exercise stress testing and gated blood pool scanning. Unfortunately, this technique is unlikely to be useful in behavioral physiology studies. The major theoretical reason is that the gamma camera gated scanner requires a relatively long gating period before sufficient data is gathered for calculating EF. Given the rapidly changing nature of emotional provocations, one would wish for a measure of EF that could be obtained from a shorter scanning period, say on the order of 2 min. A second problem with traditional gated scanners is that they are located in nuclear medicine suites that are frequently crowded, noisy, and thus not suited for the subtleties of behavioral studies.

One can observe EF during angiography, but there the problem is exactly the opposite of the traditional gated scanner. During angiography, one obtains an almost instantaneous measure of EF, but because of limitations in the amount of dye solution that can be safely injected during angiography, one cannot obtain more than one or two glimpses of EF during a catheterization study. Here again, the catheterization suite is hardly the place where one may do undisturbed behavioral physiology studies.

A number of indirect methods have been suggested for measuring EF, including impedance electrocardiography (Miller and Horvath 1978). Most cardiologists, however, rely on the relatively more direct methods of angiographic studies or gated scanning studies for assessing EF.

Recently, my colleagues in nuclear medicine at Massachusetts General Hospital have invented a miniature, gated blood pool scanner that may be worn by ambulatory subjects and that generates repeated, 2-min assessments of EF for up to 8 h. This 5-kg device employs a cadmium telluride detector, portable computer, and power pack. When red blood cells have been previously labelled with technetium and the experimental detector aligned in conjunction with a traditional gamma counter detector, this device may then be used even in field settings (Wilson et al. 1983).

We are currently examining the effects of exercise, cold, high-fat diet, and various psychological stressors on EF, blood pressure, and plasma catecholamines. With careful attention to synchronization, all of these physiological measures may be obtained stimultaneously. Thus, one may be able to observe the effects of behavior on sympathetic nervous system discharge as measured peripherally by plasma catecholamines, and on the receptor response to such discharge as measured by changes in left ventricular contractility.

Conclusion

In this paper I have argued in favor of a research approach that relies closely on a collaboration between behavioral scientists, cardiologists, and physiologists. Such a collaboration is likely to yield considerable information on the pathophysiological links between emotion and cardiovascular disease.

Acknowledgments. This work was supported in part by grants from Ciba-Geigy, the American Heart Association, and from the National Heart, Lung, and Blood Institute (HL 36005).

References

Anderson D (1984) Interactions of stress, salt and blood pressure. Ann Rev Physiol 46: 143-153

Barontini M, Feldstein C, Armando I, Marchezotti A, Levin G, Vilches A, Olivieri A, Burucua J (1981) Sympathetic nervous system response to graded exercise effect of beta blockade. Hypertension 3 [Suppl II]: II-155-II-159

Baum A, Gatchel R, Schaeffer M (1983) Emotional, behavioral and physiological effects of chronic stress at Three Mile Island. J Consult Clin Psychol 5: 565-572

Cumming G (1977) Hemodynamics of supine bicycle exercise in 'normal' children. Am Heart J 93: 617-622

Davis A, Lefkowitz R (1980) Corticosteroid induced differential regulation of beta-adrenergic receptors in circulating human polymorphonuclear leukocytes and mononuclear leukocytes. J Clin Endocrinol Metab 51: 599-605

Dimsdale J (1983) Wet Holter monitoring: techniques for studying plasma responses to stress in ambulatory subjects. In: Dembroski T, Schmidt T, Blumchen G (eds) Biobehavioral bases of coronary heart disease. Karger, Basel

Dimsdale J (1984a) The death of Pheidippides. JAMA 252: 481

Dimsdale J (1984b) Generalizing from laboratory studies to field studies of human stress physiology. Psychosom Med 46: 463-469

Dimsdale J (1985) Measuring human sympathoadrenomedullary responses to stressors. In: Baum A, Singer J (eds) Handbook of psychology and health, vol 5. (to be published)

Dimsdale J, Moss J (1980a) Plasma catecholamines in stress and exercise. JAMA 243: 340-342

Dimsdale J, Moss J (1980b) Short term catecholamine response to psychological stress. Psychosom Med 42: 493-497

Dimsdale J, Hartley L, Ruskin J, Greenblatt D, Sabrie R (1984a) Effect of beta blockade on plasma catecholamine levels during psychological and exercise stress. Am J Cardiol 54: 182-185

Dimsdale J, Hartley L, Griney T, Ruskin J, Greenblatt D (1984b) Post exercise peril; plasma catecholamines and exercise. JAMA 251: 630-632

Ekblom B, Hartley L, Day W (1979) Occurrence and reproducability of exercise induced ventricular ectophy in normal subjects. Am J Cardiol 43: 35-40

Franco-Morselli R, Baudouin-Legros M, Meyer P (1978) Plasma adrenaline and noradrenaline in essential hypertension and after long-term treatment with beta adrenoreceptor blocking agents. Clin Sci Mol Med 55: 97s-100s

Frankenhaeuser M (1975) Experimental approaches to the study of catecholamines and emotion. In: Levi L (ed) Emotions - their parameters and measurement. Raven, New York
Franz I, Lohmann F, Koch G (1980a) Excessive plasma dopamine increase at rest and during exercise after long-term beta adrenoreceptor blockade in hypertensive patients. Br Heart J 44: 25-29
Franz I, Lohmann F, Loch G (1980b) Differential effects of long term cardioselective and nonselective beta-receptor blockade on plasma catecholamines during and after physical exercise in hypertensive patients. J Cardiovasc Pharmacol 2: 35-44
Galbo H, Holst J, Christensen N, Hilsted J (1976) Glucagon and plasma catecholamines during beta receptor blockade in exercising men. J Appl Physiol 40: 855-863
Irving M, Britton B, Wood W, Padgham C, Carruthers M (1974) Effects of beta adrenergic blockade on plasma catecholamines in exercise. Nature 248: 531-533
Julius S, Conway J (1968) Hemodynamic studies in patients with borderline blood pressure elevation Circulation 38: 282-288
Leblanc J, Cote J, Jobin M, Labrie A (1979) Plasma catecholamines and cardiovascular responses to cold and mental activity. J Appl Physiol 47 (6): 1207-1211
Levi L (1965) The urinary output of adrenaline and noradrenaline during pleasant and unpleasant emotional states. Psychosom Med 27: 80-85
Mason J (1975) Emotion as reflected in patterns of endocrine integration. In: Levi L (ed) Emotions - their parameters and measurement. Raven, New York
Miller J, Horvath S (1978) Impedance cardiography. Psychophysiology 15: 80-91
Rankin L (1981) Sodium intake alters the effect of norepinephrine on blood pressure. Hypertension 3: 650-656
Sheehan M, Brammell H, Sable D, Nies A, Horwitz L (1983) Effect of beta-blockade on circulatory catecholamines and dopamine beta hydroxylase activity during exercise in normal subjects. Am Heart J 105: 777-782
Sjoberg H, Frankenhaeuser M, Bjurstedt H (1979) Interactions between heart rate psychomotor performance and perceived effort during physical work as influenced by beta-adrenergic blockade. Biol Psychol 8: 31-43
Taggart P, Carruthers M, Somerville W (1973) Electrocardiogram, plasma catecholamines and lipids, and their modification by oxprenolol when speaking before an audeince. Lancet II: 341-346
Vlachikis N, Aledort L (1980) Hypertension and propranolol therapy: effect on blood pressure, plasma catecholamines and platelet aggregation. Am J Cardiol 45: 321-325
Wallin B (1981) New concepts of sympathetic function in man. In: Stalberg E, Young R (eds) Clinical neurophysiology. Butterworths, London
Wilson R, Sullivan P, Moore R et al (1983) An ambulatory ventricular monitor: validation and preliminary clinical results. Am J Cardiol 52: 601-606

The Measurement of Continuous Finger Arterial Pressure Noninvasively in Stationary Subjects

K. H. Wesseling, J. J. Settels, and B. de Wit[1]

Introduction

In 1967 the Czech physiologist Docent Dr. Jan Peňáz patented a method with which it was possible to measure noninvasive finger arterial pressure as a continuous, calibrated waveform with a true zero reference (Peňáz 1969). Six years later he devoted a brief publication to this method (Peňáz 1973) and he demonstrated the device at the 10th International Conference on Medical and Biological Engineering at Dresden. At the time, we at TNO were in need of a device that would provide us with such a signal to be used as input to a pulse contour cardiac output computer (Wesseling et al. 1983b). In 1976 we started to construct a laboratory model on the basis of the 1973 publication, as none was available commercially. We started on a small scale as we did not understand most of the details of the method. In fact, we did not believe the method would work for various physiological reasons, because there had been no follow-up in the literature, and because we were aware that similar methods had met with little success as reported in the literature at least as far back as 1880. Yet we were struck by the elegance of the Peňáz principle. By 1978 we had a preliminary working model and were encouraged enough by the initial results, and by the response and enthusiasm of a number of clinicians, to start a large-scale development and clinical research effort. This led only recently to a design (prototype 4) which we are convinced is of clinical and experimental usefulness (Wesseling et al. 1982) and commercial viability[2].

This paper is divided into two parts. Part 1 presents evidence for the need of a continuous arterial pressure registration to study a person's short-term blood pressure variability, both spontaneous and evoked, as it is controlled by the baroreflex and cardiopulmonary reflex regulating systems.

Part 2 gives a description of the Peňáz method and results of its clinical validation in various stages of the development together with limitations of its applicability. We have also performed a number of physiologically oriented studies with prototype devices to unravel some of the secrets of baroreflex blood pressure control (Settels et al. 1980a, b, 1982; Goedhard et al. 1984). These studies, of course, have only scratched the surface of the research possibilities with this new method, which are limited only by the imagination of scientists interested in the behavior of the cardiovascular system and its interactions with other organs and systems.

---

1 Research Unit Biomedical Instrumentation TNO, Academic Medical Center, Suite G1-111, Meibergdreef 9, 1105 AZ Amsterdam, The Netherlands

2 The device will be commercially available through Ohmeda (formerly OHIO), 355 Inverness Drive South, Englewood, CO 80112 5810, USA

Biological and Psychological Factors
in Cardiovascular Disease
Ed. by T. H. Schmidt, T. M. Dembroski, and G. Blümchen

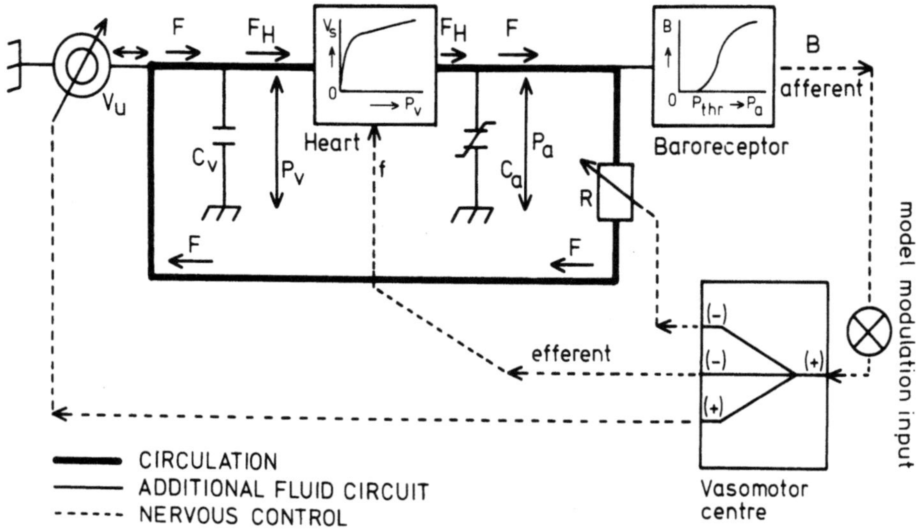

Fig. 1. Model of the closed circulation including baroreflex control of arterial pressure *(P_a)*. The one-ventricle heart is characterized by a venous input pressure/stroke volume relationship. Cardiac output *(F_H)* is the product of the reflex-controlled heart rate *(f)* and stroke volume *(V_s)*. C_a and C_v are the arterial and venous Windkessel compliances. Total peripheral perfusion *(F)* is determined by arterial pressure *(P_a)* and peripheral resistance *(R)*. Venous return *(F)* is accumulated in C_v, building up a pressure *(P_v)*, which controls the filling of the heart. The baroreflex has one baroreceptor feeding afferent impulses into the vasomotor center. There are three effectors, in inverse order of importance: heart rate *(f)* peripheral restistance *(R)* and venomotor tone, controlling venous unstretched volume *(V_u)*. Baromodulation is here placed in the baroreceptor afferent connection with the vasomotor center. *(Pthr, threshold pressure)*

Need For Continuous Blood Pressure Monitoring

Studies of long-term blood pressure regulation have shown that the development of essential hypertension is governed by kidney function (Guyton 1980). However, in the short-term blood pressure regulation during a 24-h day the baroreflex and cardiopulmonary reflex play a dominant role (Folkow and Neil 1971; Guyton 1980). It even has been proposed that short-term blood pressure variability at rest and in stress is mediated through the baroreflex, via the concept of baromodulation (Wesseling and Möller 1983; Wesseling and Settels 1984). The baromodulation hypothesis thereby provides a semiquantitative approach to the influence of higher brain centers on medullary vasomotor regulation.

It is therefore of importance to be able to study aspects of baroreflex blood pressure regulation. However, this poses some formidable problems if such studies are to be performed on subjects in which an invasive blood pressure registration is not indicated, since current noninvasive blood pressure measurement techniques have large systematic and random errors that render them virtually useless for such studies. In addition, current noninvasive methods provide, at best, only intermittent blood pressure readings, of which the systolic and diastolic levels are not even obtained simultaneously, i.e., from the same pulse wave. In view of blood pressure variability, this is a serious defect even if no responses are evoked by interventions.

Furthermore, the study of blood pressure alone is inconclusive, as can be elucidated from Fig. 1. It shows a primitive model of the circulation with the baroreflex. The systemic circulation includes a one-chamber heart, an aortic Windkessel compliance (C_a), a total peripheral resistance (R), and a venous compliance (C_v). A single baroreceptor senses arterial pressure and sends an afferent signal (B), nonlinearly proportional to arterial pressure, to the vasomotor center in the medulla oblongata. Here, signal B is modulated by higher centers in the brain, after which efferent signals vagally modulate heart rate and sympathetically modulate the smooth muscle tone in the arterioles, thereby changing peripheral resistance and, venous volume. In the actual circulation other parameters such as cardiac contractility are also modulated, and heart rate is also sympathetically modulated (not shown in this model). The reasoning behind this model and its justification are more fully given elsewhere (Wesseling et al. 1983 a). At this point it suffices to indicate the decisive but obscured role blood pressure plays in the circulation. On the one hand, blood pressure is the input to the baroreceptor; on the other hand, it is the result of the various factors (rate, resistance, volume) that are controlled by the vasomotor center based upon baroreceptors sensing blood pressure. Blood pressure is thus at the same time cause and effect of regulatory actions. A system of this kind is a control system in which the controlled signal is blood pressure. It is held constant and its measurement gives little or no clues as to the state of the control system itself. However, baroreflex activity can be observed quite explicitly by monitoring its effectors: rate, resistance and volume. In particular, this can effectively be done by eliciting baroreflex responses to known circulatory challenges. Possibilities are (Parati et al. 1983) pharmacological interventions: atropine, beta-blockers, sympaticomimetics (Smyth et al. 1969) etc., and hemodynamic challenges such as caused by Valsalva maneuvers and other breathing exercises, postural changes (Borst et al. 1982; Goedhard et al. 1984), lower body positive and negative pressures, compression and suction transferred to the carotid baroreceptors via neck chambers (Mancia et al. 1977), etc. In all cases one can observe the dynamics of the blood pressure response; however more information can be obtained from the observation of rate, resistance, volume, and cardiac contractility.

The response of heart rate is, in particular, easily studied. A small injection of phenylephrine has been used to measure the momentary association between blood pressure and heart interval changes (Smyth et al. 1969). This has led to the very useful concept of baroreflex sensitivity as the ratio of heart interval to blood pressure increases in millisecond per millimeter of mercury (Sleight et al. 1979). However, only one of the baroreflex effectors, vagal heart rate control, is quantified in this manner. A similar measure for sympathetic control actions is needed. Peripheral resistance is sympathetically controlled and can be computed from mean blood pressure and cardiac output (F in the model of Fig. 1), and both are measurable quantities.

To capture the important dynamics of the baroreflex both mean pressure and cardiac output must be available as beat-to-beat values (Wesseling 1981). Mean pressure, pulse rate and stroke volume, and thus cardiac output and peripheral resistance changes can be obtained from the continuous blood pressure signal in a simple way. This is shown in Fig. 2. Mean pressure is the area under the blood pressure curve (A_1) between consecutive upstrokes divided by the time period (T_{uu}) be-

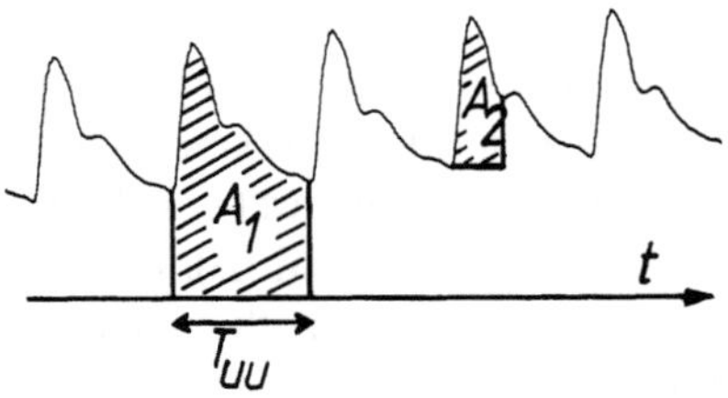

Fig. 2. Arterial pressure registration showing the computation of areas A_1 and A_2 under the pressure contour. Area A_1, when divided by T_{uu} yields mean pressure for that beat. Area A_2 is proportional to left ventricular stroke volume after division by a subject constant Z

tween these instants. Pulse rate is inversely proportional to the time period T_{uu}. Left ventricular stroke volume is proportional to the area under the pressure pulse (A_2) divided by an unknown subject constant. For improved precision the latter computation must be corrected for the effects of mean pressure, pulse rate, and age on the subject constant, as explained by Wesseling et al. (1983b). The product of stroke volume and pulse rate gives cardiac output.

In summary:

$$f_p = 60/T_{uu}\ \text{(bpm)} \qquad F = V_s f_p/1000\ \text{(litres/min)}$$
$$\bar{P} = A_1/T_{uu}\ \text{(mmHg)} \qquad R = \bar{P}/F = 60\bar{P}/(f_p V_s)$$
$$V_s = K\,A_2/Z\ \text{(ml)} \qquad = \bar{P}T_{uu}/V_s\ \text{(mmHg.s/ml)}$$

in which f_p is pulse frequency or pulse rate, T_{uu} is the interval between two consecutive upstrokes, $\bar{P}$ is mean pressure, A_1 is as indicated in Fig. 2, V_s is the left ventricular stroke volume, K is a correction factor, A_2 is as indicated in Fig. 2. Z is an individual subject constant usually adjusted so that resting cardiac output is at a reasonable value such as 5 litres/min (Z is usually quite close to 0.10 mmHg.s/ml). F is cardiac output, and R is peripheral resistance. Thus a single arterial pressure signal may provide information on the effectiveness of the baroreflex and on the sensitivity of both the vagally and sympathetically mediated effectors of baroreflex blood pressure control, which affect rate and resistance, respectively. An example of how this is used to explain orthostatically evoked responses can be found in the literature (Wesseling 1981).

Method of Peñáz

A finger blood pressure device according to Peñáz (1973) consists of the following principal components (Fig. 3):

A rigid, segmented cuff in which a light-plethysmograph is mounted
A proportional valve controlling fluid pressure in the cuff
A manometer reading cuff pressure
A servo system which keeps the plethysmographic output from the finger constant by comparing it to a setpoint value

Operation of the device is basically as follows: Potentiometer C1 is set at a value equivalent to the amount of light seen by the plethysmograph when the venous compartment is collapsed and the arterial compartment under the cuff is compressed to its unstretched size from the outside. Next, when intra-arterial pressure tends to increase, more blood is pressed into the arteries, thus increasing light attenuation and therefore decreasing the plethysmographic output. The difference to

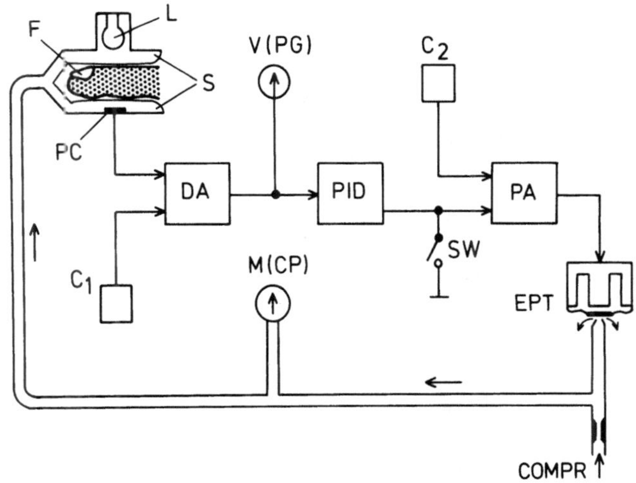

Fig. 3. Original block diagram of the servo-plethysmo-manometer published by Peňáz (1973). Following the *arrows* in the diagram a closed servo loop is traced. A finger *(F)* is shown in a rigid cuff *(S)* illuminated by a lamp *(L)*. The plethysmogram is from a photocell *(PC)*. In closed loop operation, with switch *(SW)* as shown, the output from the photocell is compared with a constant reference level *(C1)*. Any difference is amplified by differential amplifier *(DA)*, and shown on the volume output *(V(PG)*. An electronic controller *(PID)*, followed by power amplifier *(PA)*, drives the electropneumatic transducer *EPT)*. Cuff pressure is read by manometer *M(CP)* supplied by a source of compressed air *(COMPR)*

C1, which now develops, is amplified and controls the proportional valve to increase its output pressure and thereby cuff pressure. Thus cuff pressure follows intra-arterial pressure in a continuous fashion, the artery is clamped at its unstretched volume, provided the servo system acts fast enough. Note that the finger arteries do not collapse. Clearly, the correct setting of potentiometer C1 so that transmural pressure is precisely zero, is of paramount importance and determines the accuracy achievable with this method. Otherwise a positive or negative transmural pressure would remain, giving systematic errors.

The arterial volume at which the transmural pressure is zero and cuff pressure is equal to intra-arterial pressure can be derived from a finger arterial pressure-volume diagram. Figure 4 shows such a diagram obtained from a human finger in vivo. The finger arteries in this subject are seen to collapse when cuff pressure is 5-10 mmHg above intra-arterial pressure, hence at a transmural pressure of −5- −10 mmHg. The artery is fully opened to a volume of 160 arbitrary units at a cuff pressure which is 40-50 mmHg below intra-arterial, hence at a positive transmural pressure of 40-50 mmHg.

Apart from a slight hysteresis, zero transmural pressure occurs at a volume equal to about one-half to one-third of the open volume. When intra-arterial pressure pulsates and cuff pressure is kept constant and in value near mean arterial pressure, the arterial volume changes can be observed dynamically from the plethysmogram, from which the open and the collapsed arterial volumes can be derived. It is then an easy matter to adjust the setpoint, C1, of the servo loop to a proper value about halfway between those extremes. Since the pressure-volume diagram

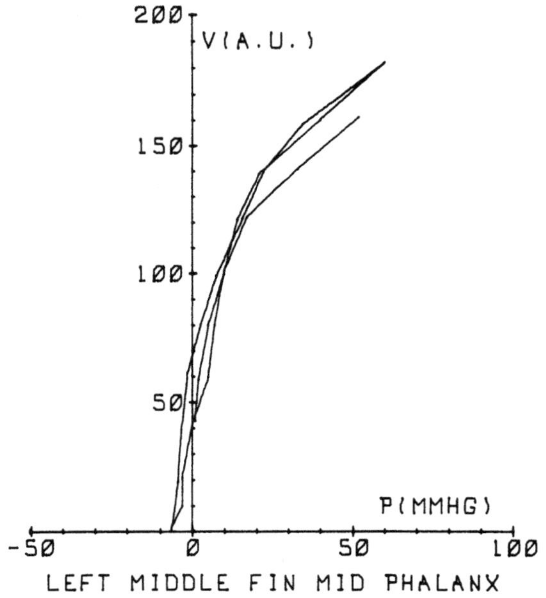

Fig. 4. Pressure-volume diagram of a human finger, as seen by the Peňáz plethysmograph. Note that arterial collapse is steep, i. e. a large volume change is present for a small change in transmural pressure. The pressure axis is calibrated in mmHg. The volume axis is in arbitrary units

is steep near collapse, a substantial error in the volume setpoint produces only a small error in the cuff pressure tracking intra-arterial pressure.

The improvement of the Peňáz method over earlier methods is the separation of instrumentation with which the artery is observed (a light-transmission plethysmograph) from the system with which unloading of the artery to zero transmural pressure is produced (an electropneumatic servo). The light-plethysmograph can thus be made to respond almost exclusively to changes in blood volume within its field of view, not to the total liquid compartment under the cuff. Once the venous system is collapsed and capillary flow blocked, only arterial volume changes are monitored by the plethysmograph. In addition, by limiting the field of view of the light-plethysmograph to a small volume near the middle of the cuff, any cuff-end-effects are effectively reduced.

Implementation

Although the principle of the method is quite simple and the advantages readily understood, implementation of the method to a functioning instrument that is accurate, reliable, and easy to operate in a clinical environment proved to be no easy matter. In our development of the Peňáz method, we did not deviate substantially from the original block diagram. However, we tried to optimize the various components and parts in the system on the basis of experience obtained in our laboratory and in various clinics. In addition, we made the instrument fully automatic, with no manual adjustments or controls. This automatic version has been named FIN.A.PRES for *fin*ger *a*rterial *pres*sure. We will now describe some features of our implementation.

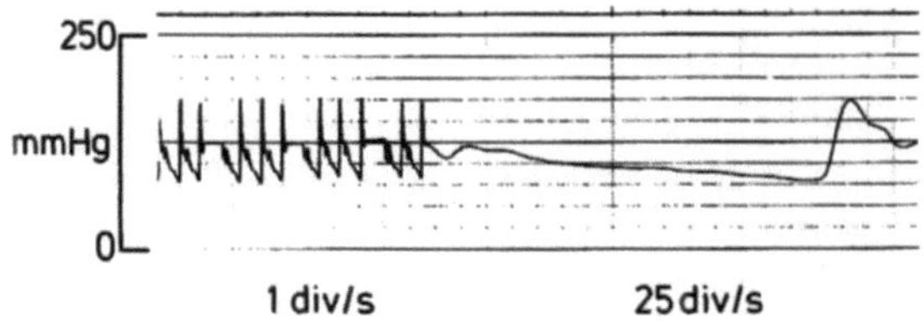

Fig. 5. Left middle finger registration of blood pressure in a young adult female subject. Note the steep pulse upstroke at the right. The interrupted beats are part of the repeated search procedure

Cuff

The cuffs are of a wrap-on variety, built from various layers of plastic. Fixation around the finger is accomplished with a piece of Velcro. The small bladder is heat-sealed from two layers of thin plastic foil. The plethysmograph consists of a miniature infrared light-emitting diode (LED), and the receiver is a photodiode. Both components are mounted inside the cuff and are in direct contact with the skin on opposite sides of the finger. Because infrared LEDs are of high efficiency, power dissipation is negligible, and no burning or warming up of the skin can be felt. The LED is emitting modulated light. A short length of air hose connects the cuff bladder to the pressure control valve. The cuff is of light weight, is practically immune to motion artifact, and is insensitive to ambient light.

Valve

The valve is of a balanced flapper-nozzle type. Because the cuff bladder and connecting air hose volume are small, the valve can also be made small so that it consumes only a small amount of air. A National Semiconductor miniature strain gauge pressure transducer is mounted directly on the pneumatic valve to measure cuff pressure. Valve, pressure transducer, and plethysmographic preamplifier, are mounted in a patient front end box which can be strapped to the patient's hand.

Servo System

A servo system bandwidth of 30 Hz suffices according to Frank (as cited by Stegemann 1956), considering the absence of high-frequency components in the peripherally recorded arterial pressure wave. If the sole purpose is to record proper systolic and diastolic pressure levels, an even smaller bandwidth suffices. However, in some trials we observed pulse pressures of over 200 mmHg (systolic/diastolic = 330/110) and upstrokes with slopes as steep as 4000 mmHg/s peripherally. The latter is more than twice that in the left ventricle. We therefore made a major effort to design a wide bandwidth servo system for which the very fast valve was developed. This resulted in a servo bandwidth of about 100 Hz. The servo system proved stable under practically all conditions found in the laboratory or clinic, with very small residual servo errors. With the improved system, we are indeed able to follow an arterial pressure rate rise of more than 4000 mmHg/s (Fig. 5 is an example) and pressure pulse amplitudes of over 200 mmHg. Pressures from zero to over 300 mmHg can be followed linearly with this system.

Automation

An Intel 8080-based 8- bit microcomputer controls the operation of FIN.A.PRES and performs all necessary functions and several convenience features automatically. Upon pushing the front panel start button, a search procedure for the arterial unstretched volume is performed by stepwise increase of cuff pressure through a range of pressures in search of that plethysmogram at which the artery is seen to collapse. Based on the observed plethysmogram, the servo setpoint (C 1) is established, the proper loopgain is estimated, and the control loop is closed. Depending on the level of the blood pressure and the pulse rate, this process takes from 10 to 20 s to complete. In the case of malfunction the process is stopped and an appropriate error message is displayed. Because the arterial wall shows a certain hysteresis after unloading, with a very long time constant, and since red blood cells trapped in the microcirculation by the increased tissue pressure wash out at a very slow rate (Wesseling et al. 1982), the setpoint has a tendency to drift in the initial minutes after the search procedure. Therefore, an abbreviated search procedure is automatically repeated at intervals to adjust the servo setpoint accordingly.

Even more importantly, the arterial unstretched volume varies under the influence of a changing vascular smooth muscle tone. Such changes may occur at random instants and may be particularly severe when a subject is under cardiovascular stress after substantial blood losses. The search procedure therefore continues to repeat at regular intervals to adapt to such phenomena when they occur. Because this search procedure disturbs the continuity of the waveform registration, which is undesirable if the waveforms must be Fourier analyzed or when acute blood pressure changes must be recorded, the feature can be turned off and on manually.

Clinical Studies

Because we did not - and still do not - fully understand all the intricate physiological details of the Peñáz method and as no results with the Peñáz method were reported in the literature, we decided that clinical trials were of the utmost importance to test this new method. Of course, the case of a method not being fully understood and yet proving to be of of great medical value is not unique by any means. It is true, in fact, for any indirect method used to measure blood pressure. For example, the origin of the various Korotkov sounds is still debated. No agreement exists even now on the optimal dimensions of the ordinary Riva-Rocci cuff. The point of maximal oscillations in an oscillometric method is equated with mean blood pressure without a theoretical basis. However, established methods have been thoroughly compared with each other and with intra-arterial measurements under a range of clinical conditions and on a variety of patients, establishing the accuracy and precision of such methods and determining under which conditions they do not perform properly, so that corrective actions can be anticipated.

The purpose of our clinical trials has been to establish such knowledge for the Peñáz method. Information will be given on FIN.A.PRES performance in 33 hypertensive subjects, in 17 anesthetized subjects undergoing critical heart, vessel, or brain surgery, and in 6 anesthetized subjects in which peripheral vasoconstriction was frequently observed. In these studies FIN.A.PRES pressure was compared with intra-arterial blood pressure. In two further studies, FIN.A.PRES was com-a 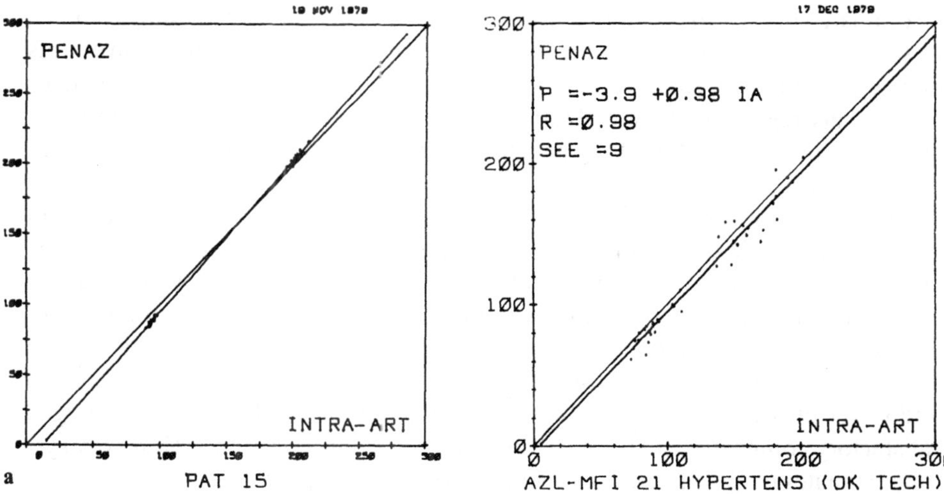 b

Fig. 6. **a** Scattergram of 20 measured systolic and diastolic points of a patient showing typically small "withinpatient" scatter. Finger pressures *(Peñáz)* are compared to intrabrachial pressures *(intra-art)*. **b** Scattergram of 21 systolic and diastolic values; each *point* is an average of up to 20 measurements per patient

pared to standard Riva-Rocci/Korotkov blood pressures in 39 subjects in a general practicioner's office and in another 39 subjects in a retirement home. We were particularly interested in discovering in how many subjects the method would not perform well, and, if so, for what reasons, and what could be done to improve the method. A further point of interest was linearity. Theoretically the method should be perfectly linear, since the nonlinear viscoelastic behavior of the arterial wall is eliminated by keeping it at a constant nonzero, unstretched diameter at all times. Some indirect methods have difficulty in measuring very low pressures as occur in shock or with very highly variable pressures. Theoretically this should be no problem for FIN.A.PRES. Finally we were interested in observing the possible problems a physician unfamiliar with the method might have in applying the cuff to a finger, in operating the instrument, and in accepting the values and waveforms it presents.

Study of 33 Hypertensive Patients

The first clinical study was performed in 1978 and 1979 with 33 awake patients suspected of having (cuff) hypertension. For this study we used our primitive laboratory model, which already included a wrap-on cuff. The fast valve had not yet been developed, but we used one driven by a loudspeaker. The servo system bandwidth was about 25 Hz. Operation of the laboratory model was manual. We expected that the large hypertensive pulse pressures would be a real challenge to the servo system, while, on the other hand, the relatively thick-walled arteries of such patients would present a good sensitivity test for the plethysmograph. This proved to be true.

The reference pressure was obtained via percutaneous right brachial arterial cannulation. Ipsilateral intra-arterial and finger pressures were recorded for about 10–15 min. All patients gave informed consent. In addition, the Leiden University ethical committee expressed no objection. Blood pressures in five patients could not be evaluated because of malfunction of some components in the recording channel. In seven patients it was impossible to obtain correct, undistorted Peñáz waveforms having a sufficiently small residual plethysmogram. In the remaining 21 patients high-quality registrations were obtained. Every 30 s both waveforms were sampled and a one-beat systolic/diastolic pair recorded. Up to 20 sample pairs per patient were taken (Fig. 6 a).

An analysis of variance showed the *within* patient variance in the results to be an order of magnitude smaller than the *between* patient differences. We therefore averaged the results per patient and plotted them as one systolic/diastolic pair in Fig. 6 b. It appeared that both the systolic and the diastolic levels were underestimated by the Peñáz method by 6 mmHg averaged over the 21 patients (range 0-15 mmHg). The standard deviation of the error between intrabrachial (reference) and finger pressures was 7% for the systolic and 6% for the diastolic level, judged satisfactory compared with the best values reported for Riva-Rocci/Korotkov systolic estimates of 5% and diastolic estimates of 10% (Huige 1980).

The 6 mmHg, by which finger pressure underestimates intrabrachial pressure on average, is due to a pressure gradient in the arteries of the hand. If finger pressure is measured in the thumb, which is much closer anatomically to the radial artery, this underestimate almost disappears. Clearly the Peñáz method performed at very high pressures (330 mmHg systolic was observed in one patient both in the brachial artery and in the finger) and on thick arterial walls which showed only very small pulsations. The distorted waveforms taught us that a wider bandwidth pneumatic servo system was necessary. With the new valve incorporated in FIN.A.PRES we have just completed a small study of an additional 31 hypertensive subjects under the same conditions without observing distorted waveforms. For a physicist, the search procedure was quite difficult to perform manually; for a physician, it would have attracted too much attention away from the patient. The need for an automatic search procedure was therefore clearly indicated. The study has been more fully described elsewhere (Molhoek et al. 1984).

Study in 17 Male Surgical Patients

The second study was done in 1980 using 17 anesthetized male surgical patients. Eight of these patients, who underwent a coronary artery bypass graft (CABG) operation, were maintained on a nonpulsatile heart-lung machine and were cooled during a substantial fraction of the total monitoring period. The average duration of the operation was 5 h 24 min, ranging from 2 h 45 min to 7 h 31 min in duration. Two prototypes with a fast servo system were used on the left and the right middle finger and compared with a usually left-sided, intraradial arterial pressure signal. All patients were informed about the additional noninvasive procedures and gave their consent.

One prototype was operated manually on the left hand, while the second prototype had a built-in microcomputer and could be used manually or automatically, with an initial version of an automatic search algorithm. All signals were recorded on an instrumentation tape-recorder. Upon playback, each one of the three pressure signals was fed through a low pass filter to obtain mean pressures. At approximately 160-s intervals samples were taken of the three mean pressure signals: more fre-

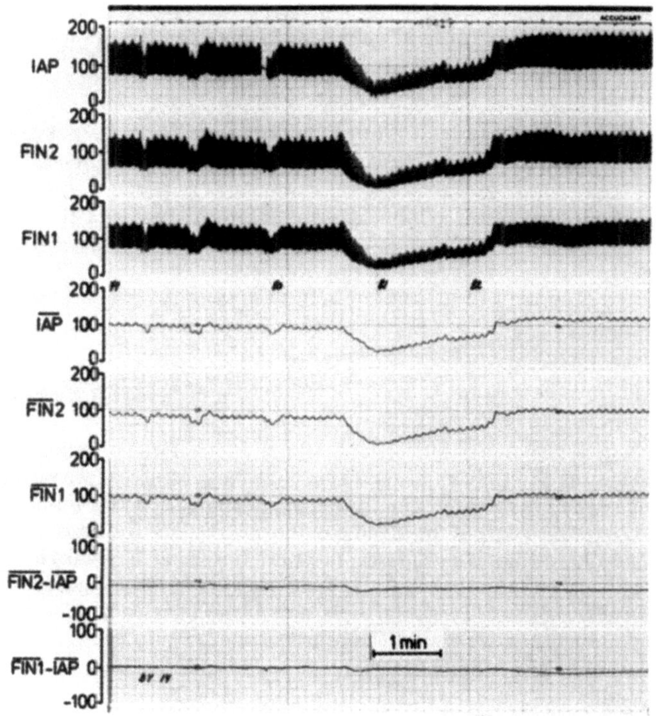

Fig. 7. An 8-min segment of the intraoperative registration in a patient showing good agreement of left *(FIN1)* and right *(FIN2)* finger pressures with left intraradial pressure during embolus recovery in brain surgery. The pressure difference between right and left hand was caused by a difference in hydrostatic height: The left hand had slipped some 20 cm below heart level, recording an erroneously high blood pressure. The three upper traces show pulsatile pressures; the next three traces show mean pressures obtained by feeding the pulsatile signals through three low pass filters; the bottom two traces are zero center difference signals. Vertical sensitivity for all eight channels is 200 mmHg full scale

quent samples were taken during fast blood pressure variations and less frequent ones during periods of stable pressures. About 2800 mean pressure triplets were recorded in total. Average statistics were first computed per patient. Then, the per patient results were again averaged to obtain pooled results. No correction was made for the hydrostatic difference of the finger being positioned about 10 cm below heart level. The offset error for mean pressure averaged at 1 ± 4 mmHg ($m \pm s$). The standard deviation of the error ranged from 4 to 9, with an average of 5 mmHg or 7%. The typically good agreement of finger and intra-arterial pressures can be judged from the registration in Fig. 7, which was obtained during the occurrence of a pulmonary embolus. Both prototypes worked satisfactorily on all patients, but did not do so all of the time. Some samples were lost because of easily correctable technical problems, such as a kinked air hose, representing 2.3% of the monitoring time. These problems have since been solved. Finger arterial smooth muscle activity prevented measurement of finger blood pressure in an additional 5.4% of the time, since the search procedure for the unstretched arterial diameter was not yet auto-

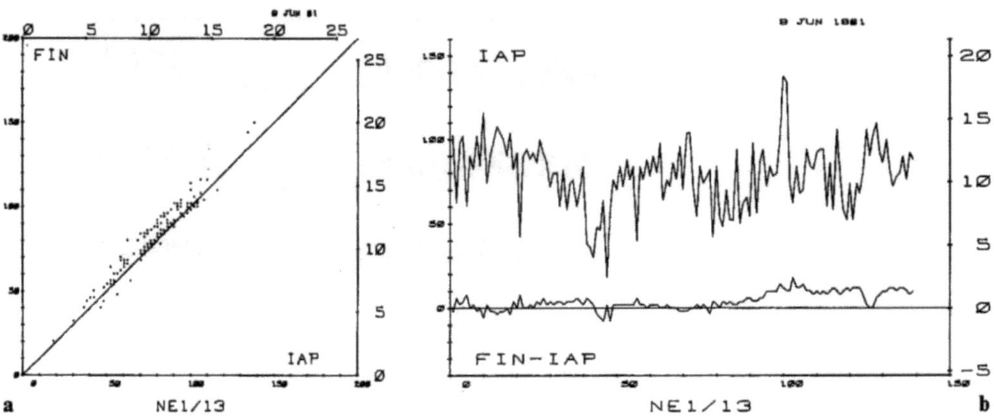

Fig. 8. a Scattergram of intraoperative finger arterial mean pressure *(FIN)* versus intraradial mean pressure *(IAP)* in the contralateral arm. Note the presence of two distinct clouds of points shifted 10 mmHg in a vertical direction. Scales are in mmHg and kPa. **b** Trend chart of the same 140 data but now plotted against the number of the observation. The upper trace is intraradial mean pressure; the lower trace is the difference between finger and intraradial mean pressures. Note from observation 90 onwards that finger pressure reads some 10 mmHg higher with respect to *IAP*, probably caused by vasoconstriction of the arterioles (increased peripheral resistance) in the arm. This trend explains the two distinct clouds seen in **a**

matically repeated in the microcomputer-controlled prototype or manually in the other prototype. (In a new series of such operations, it has been observed that the improved search algorithms solve this problem until the instant of complete arterial spasm occurs, resulting in a much reduced percentage of lost time due to this cause).

The instrument had no difficulty in measuring very low blood pressures, mean pressures ranged from 2(!) to 164 mmHg in the subject pool. The linearity of the method is satisfactory over the full range, as can be judged from Fig. 8a. Fig. 8b shows a trend chart of the same data. Note that finger pressure error shows a systematic trend, as was already suspected from the data of Fig. 8a. We now know that such trends are caused by changes in arm and finger peripheral resistance, increased resistance being associated with relatively higher finger pressures (Wesseling et al. 1985).

Proper performance of the instruments did not seem to be affected by the administration of anaesthetic or other agents; nor by physical factors, such as substantial hemodilution; the absence of pulsations during cardiopulmonary bypass, or return-to-flow or total body cooling; nor by pathological factors, such as shock. The satisfactory performance of the prototypes is particularly significant considering the types of patients and cases that were investigated. Both cases and patients represent those in whom noninvasive blood pressure measurements traditionally have been difficult to obtain. Many of the patients had generalized vascular disease and high vascular reactivity. The operations required intra-arterial pressure (IAP) monitoring and were therefore not routine. Rapid changes in arterial pressure, blood volume, hematocrit, and vascular status were a common occurrence. Nine cases were open-heart, which are painful and stressful operations. There were frequent conditions leading to vasospasm, including hemorrhage, shock, and myocardial failure, requir-

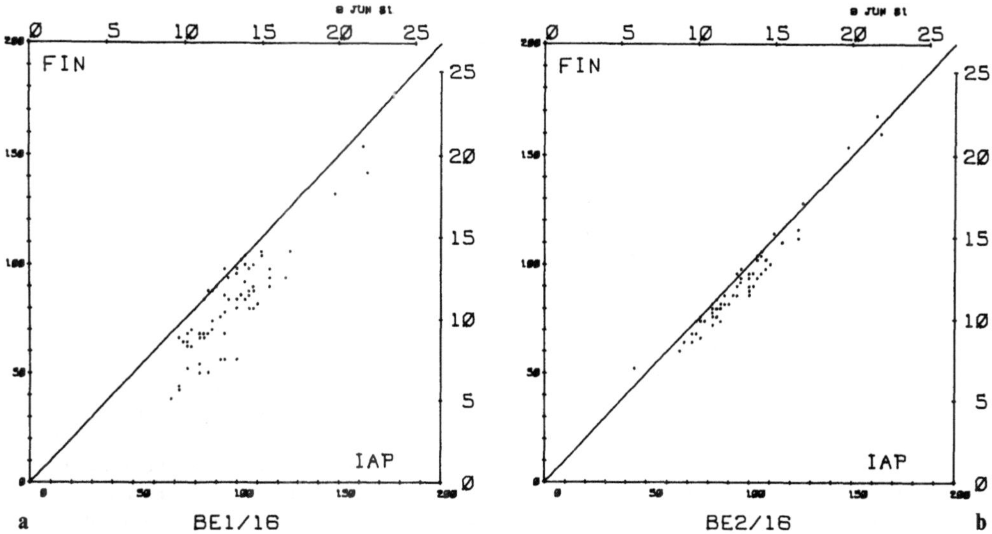

a **b**

Fig. 9. Scattergrams of finger versus radial arterial pressure (similar to Fig. 8) in an anaesthetized patient receiving a carotid-subclavian bypass of an arterial lesion. **a** is on the side of the obstruction. Blood pressures in the finger, distal to the obstruction, are low at first but return to normal after completion of the operation. **b** is on the ipsilateral side of the intraradial measurement and shows good tracking throughout the operation. Intra-arterial obstructions proximal to the finger prevent a good correlation of finger pressure with more central pressures, but the fact can be easily detected from a prolongation of the upstroke of the finger pressure wave. Hemodynamically significant obstructions very seldom occur bilaterally

ing use of a balloon pump, high infusion rates of vasopressors, and hypothermia. In no instance did the finger pressure measurement read normal or high when in fact blood pressure was too low.

Hydrostatic errors occur when the finger arterial wall, which acts as a pressure transducer membrane, is not at the level of the tricuspid valve, the reference level for blood pressure measurements since Stephen Hales first measured blood pressure. In this study, the hand was usually resting on the operating table while the IAP transducer was adjusted at the estimated reference position, thus creating a level difference of nearly 10 cm. This causes a pressure overestimate of 7 mmHg which on average compensates for the radial to finger pressure difference of 6–7 mmHg. Thus care must be used in positioning the finger, the same care as taken in positioning the IAP transducer.

Finger pressures were measured essentially uninterruptedly for the duration of the operations, up to 7½ h; yet no finger morbidity or later patient complaint occurred. The tissue under the cuff lost most of its interstitial edematous liquid after a few hours of monitoring. Swelling of the finger tip distal to the cuff was not seen, although venous congestion was sometimes apparent from a typical bluish discoloration. However, the finger tip often returned to a normal rose color while the patient was under anesthesia, or in other studies, for unexplained reasons, when naturally asleep.

Proximal intra-arterial lesions do prevent proper finger arterial pressure readings. Such lesions were present in the left subclavian region in one patient who re-

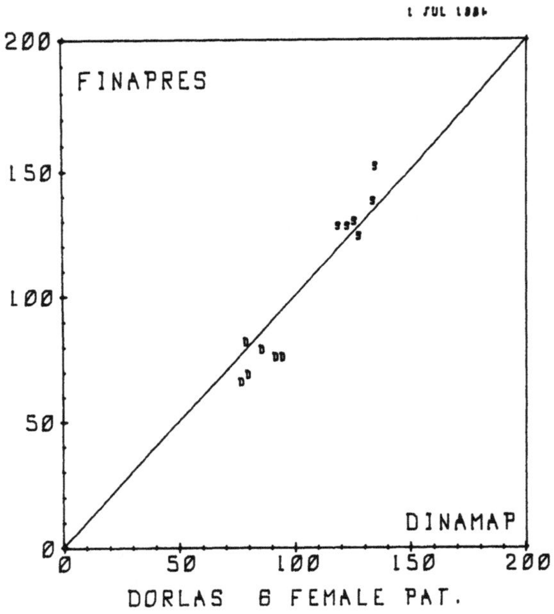

Fig. 10. Scattergram of the average comparisons of finger with oscillometric systolic and diastolic pressures in six subjects undergoing gynecological surgery under general anaesthesia. Each *point* is the average of from 55 to 77 individual comparisons in each patient, taken once every 2 min during the operation

ceived a carotid-subclavian bypass. Figure 9 presents the reductions in mean finger pressure caused by the left subclavian obstruction, and recovery to correct pressure levels after the bypass. Such obstructions, when hemodynamically significant, can be easily recognized from the increased rise time of the upstroke in the finger pressure.

The computerized prototype proved easy to operate, even by novice users, with only cuff application requiring some care and instruction. Setting up and starting a measurement could be done in 3 min. The extended servo bandwidth of the new system proved adequate in all cases. A full report of the study is found in Smith et al. (1985).

Study of Six Female Surgical Patients

Since the previous study was performed under very critical surgical conditions, operations of very long duration in male patients without the automatically repeating search procedure, it was thought desirable to test the Peñáz method under surgical conditions of a lesser degree of severity, during operations that would take at most 2 h to complete. Of course, for these operations, the extra risk of an invasive blood pressure registration was not indicated. Thus, comparisons were made on an intermittent basis with an automated oscillometric technique of good reliability and reasonable precision (Dinamap), applied to the contralateral upper arm. Since Raynaud's phenomenon and cold fingers have a higher frequency of occurrence in the female population, and since such vasoconstrictions were thought to cause the total collapse of finger pressures, it was decided to perform this study in female patients. The Groningen University ethical committee had no objection to this study, and all patients gave informed consent.

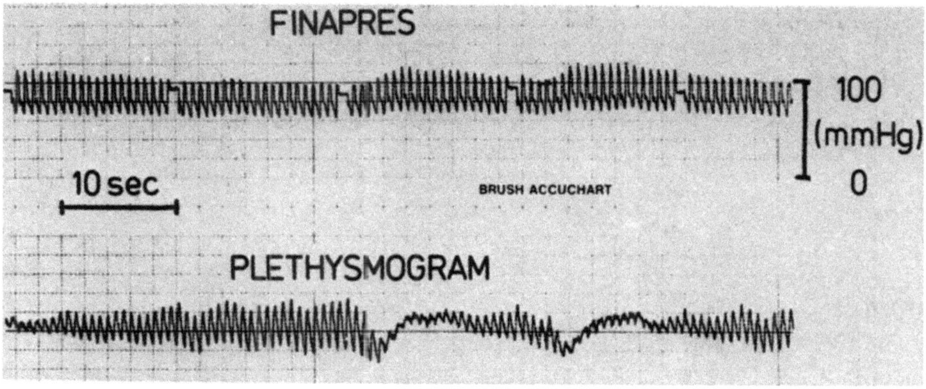

Fig. 11. The upper trace is a FIN.A.PRES continuous blood pressure registration; the lower trace is a finger plethysmogram. Two brief constriction reactions concurrent with a rise in finger pressure can be seen. About 20 such constriction reactions occurred on average per operation, of which 90% had associated increases in finger pressure

Simultaneous systolic, diastolic and mean pressures were compared, and the amplitude of a continuous finger reflection plethysmogram was sampled concurrently to observe peripheral vasoconstriction.

A total of 378 readings was taken in these six patients, one every 2 min. The offset error ranged from −4 to −15 mmHg (average −9.6 mmHg) for mean, from −3.3 to +18 for systolic, and from −18 to +4 for diastolic levels (Fig. 10). The standard deviation of the error ranged from 4% to 11% for all three levels, averaging at 7%, 9% and 8% for mean, systolic, and diastolic levels, respectively. It should be realized that a portion of this error is due to the reference method, which was also indirect. Finger pressures increased with respect to upper arm values when the finger-reflection-plethysmogram decreased in amplitude because of vasoconstriction. A typical blood pressure registration during abrupt vasoconstriction reactions is shown in Fig. 11. Such abrupt constrictions appeared in at least 51% of the sample instants in these subjects. The systolic difference between methods correlated significantly ($P < 0.01$) with the amplitude of the reflection plethysmogram in all patients, with the correlation coefficient ranging from −0.38 to −0.59. In all six patients finger arterial pressure could be measured 100% of the time. This was at least partially due to the automatically repeating search procedure, which performed well and proved essential at anaesthetic induction, when finger arterial smooth muscle tended to relax, and similarly in the waking-up phase, when the tendency was the opposite (see Wesseling et al. 1985 for further details).

Study of 39 Persons in a General Practioners' Office

In November, 1983, a study was performed using 39 volunteer subjects to compare Riva-Rocci/Korotkov with Peñáz finger blood pressures. All subjects had large upper arms, in fact, 12 were body builders. Subjects ranged in age from 22 to 78 years (mean 44 years). Of the subjects 20 were male, 24 subjects rated their health as good, 19 subjects knew their blood pressure was too high, one subject had a "dif-

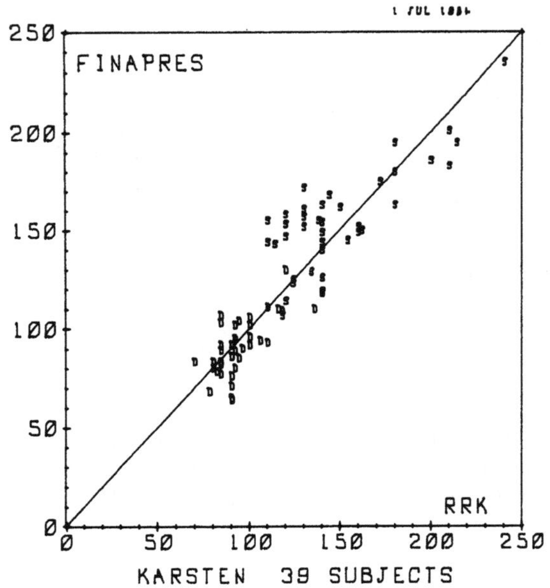

Fig. 12. Scattergram of finger with Riva-Rocci/Korotkov *(RRK)* systolic and diastolic pressures in 39 normal subjects in the office of a general practitioner. The measurements were not simultaneous. The finger systolic overestimates at low systolic pressures occurred in a group of 12 young body builders. Such overestimations are due to an amplification of the pulse wave towards the fingers in young subjects. Correction of systolic finger pressures is simple: subtract 30 mmHg then add half the age. Diastolic pressures need no correction for age. The line of identity (at 45°) and the regression are shown to be in close proximity

ficult" blood pressure (in fact he had arrhythmias), 10 subjects were treated pharmacologically for hypertension, and 3 used drugs for other reasons. Of the body builders, one was a Dutch champion and another a European champion. Riva-Rocci/Korotkov (RRK) blood pressures were measured in erect position by an experienced physician, using the Dutch Heart Foundation (DHF) cuff (bladder dimension 14.5 × 38 cm). The subjects were next transferred to another room for FIN.A.PRES finger pressure registrations, which were taken 5-10 min later.

A finger cuff was wrapped around the left middle finger mid phalanx, except in one subject in which the left index finger was used because of an old shrapnel wound on the middle finger.

The finger was levelled approximately 5 cm below the midpoint of the upper arm cuff and held against the breast. The subjects were seated during testing. The results of the comparison are shown in Fig. 12. RRK systolic pressures ranged from 110 to 240 mmHg, averaging 149 mmHg, while finger pressures ranged from 107 to 235 mmHg, averaging 155 mmHg. RRK diastolic pressures, similarly, ranged from 70 to 136 mmHg, averaging 94 mmHg, and finger pressures ranged from 64 to 130 mmHg, averaging 91 mmHg. Thus, finger systolic pressure overestimated RRK upper arm pressure by 6 mmHg on average, with a standard deviation of 20 mmHg (13%). The systolic overestimates were most notable in the relatively younger subjects. Alternatively, finger diastolic underestimated RRK pressures by 3 mmHg on average, with a standard deviation of 11 mmHg (12%). RRK clearly underestimated

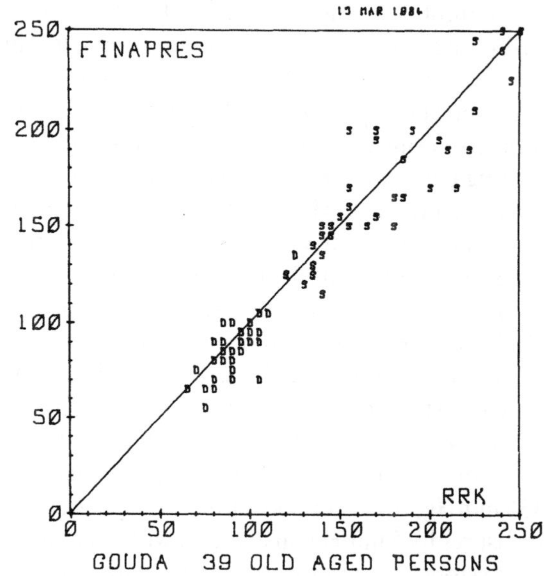

Fig. 13. Scattergram similar to the one in Fig. 12, but now measured in 39 elderly subjects (60–97 years) living in retirement home. The datapoints with large systolic errors are either traceable to errors in the application of the RRK method or to the presence of arrhythmias. Arrhythmias of various etiology were present in 44% of these subjects, causing difficulties in the determination of RRK end points, in particular systolic, and in the reading of the finger pressure signal

diastolic pressures in the body builder subgroup, in which phase IV diastolic might have given a more accurate blood pressure estimate than phase V. On all 39 subjects FIN.A.PRES application was easy and uneventful. No subject had extremely cold hands or white fingers.

None of the blood pressure measurements used in the comparisons were taken simultaneously. A period of 5–10 min elapsed in all cases between the RRK and the finger measurements. This nonsimultaneity adds error to the comparison, since blood pressure is variable. The difference in subject position, erect versus sitting, adds further uncertainty. Also, most upper arms could be considered as large. If a normal-size cuff had been used, most RRK blood pressures would have read too high. The DHF cuff allows for arm sizes as large as 38 cm. Nonetheless, 15 arms had an even larger circumference. Given these circumstances an error standard deviation of almost 20 mmHg for systolic and 11 mmHg for diastolic should be considered acceptable. A typical FIN.A.PRES measurement took about 8 min, of which less than 2 min were used to set up and start the measurement.

Study of 39 Elderly Persons

The applicability of finger pressure measurement in elderly persons was studied in January 1984 with 39 subjects, 10 male, 29 female, living in a retirement home. The subjects were 60–97 years of age, with a mean of 79 years. They were seated with their right arm resting on a table, on which an ordinary mercury column sphygmomanometer was placed. The values recorded with the mercury column were within 2 mmHg of the FIN.A.PRES manometer.

In most cases the right middle finger was used for measurement, in two or three cases the right ring finger was used. After cuff application FIN.A.PRES was started and after 3-5 min a DHF cuff was wrapped around the right upper arm, usually over one layer of clothing. The radial artery was palpated and the arm cuff rapidly inflated to suprasystolic pressures. This caused the distal finger pulse to disappear. During deflation the beginning of phase I sounds was noted as systolic, phase V as diastolic pressure. Here, only one measurement was taken. During the measurement the finger cuff was about 10 cm below mid-arm cuff position. This compensates, on average, for the brachial to finger pressure drop of about 6-7 mmHg.

Figure 13 is a plot of the systolic and diastolic comparisons of the two methods. RRK systolic pressures ranged from 120 to 250 mmHg, averaging 174 mmHg, and finger systolic pressures from 115 to 245 mmHg, averaging 172 mmHg. Finger systolic pressure underestimated RRK values by 3 mmHg on average, with a standard deviation of 19 mmHg or 11%. RRK diastolic pressures ranged from 65 to 125 mmHg, averaging 91 mmHg, and finger diastolic pressures ranged from 55 to 135 mmHg, averaging 86 mmHg. Finger diastolic pressures underestimated RRK pressures by 5 mmHg on average, with a standard deviation of 10 mmHg or 11%.

Systolic pressures were overestimated almost with the same frequence by either method. However, diastolic pressures were overestimated by RRK in 21 cases but underestimated in only 7 of the 39 subjects with respect to finger pressure. This is probably due to poor Korotkov sound generation and poor sound transmission to the stethoscope in elderly subjects, causing RRK diastolic overestimates.

In 17 of the 39 subjects (44%), some form of irregular heart rate was detected, ranging from frequent extra systoles via atrial fibrillation and bi- and trigemini to a probable case of recurrent bursts of supraventricular tachycardia. Even more interesting was the observation that 23 subjects (59%) were so-called cuff responders, who raised their blood pressure by 15-60 mmHg systolic in response to upper arm cuff inflation. As a consequence of the RRK systolic and diastolic overestimates, 18 subjects were classified as hypertensive (pressures greater than 170/100 mmHg), compared with only 9 if the more basal and more accurate finger pressures were used. Seven subjects were hypertensive in both determinations. Therefore, it seems that elderly subjects run a substantial risk of being classified artifactually as hypertensive, thus increasing the chance of subsequent expensive drug treatment with possibly unpleasant side effects. A simple, quick finger arterial pressure measurement prevents cuff responses, provides closer to baseline blood pressures and may detect the presence of pathological arrhythmias, though without giving a firm indication as to their cause. This study showed the possibility that finger arterial pressure measurement is beneficial to those of very old age and has the advantages of the absence of cuff responses and easy detection of most arrhythmias (Wesseling et al. 1984).

Conclusions

It appears that the Peñáz method, as implemented in FIN.A.PRES prototypes, operated with increasing reliability as the prototype hardware (especially the servo system) and software (especially the search and repeated search algorithms) grew

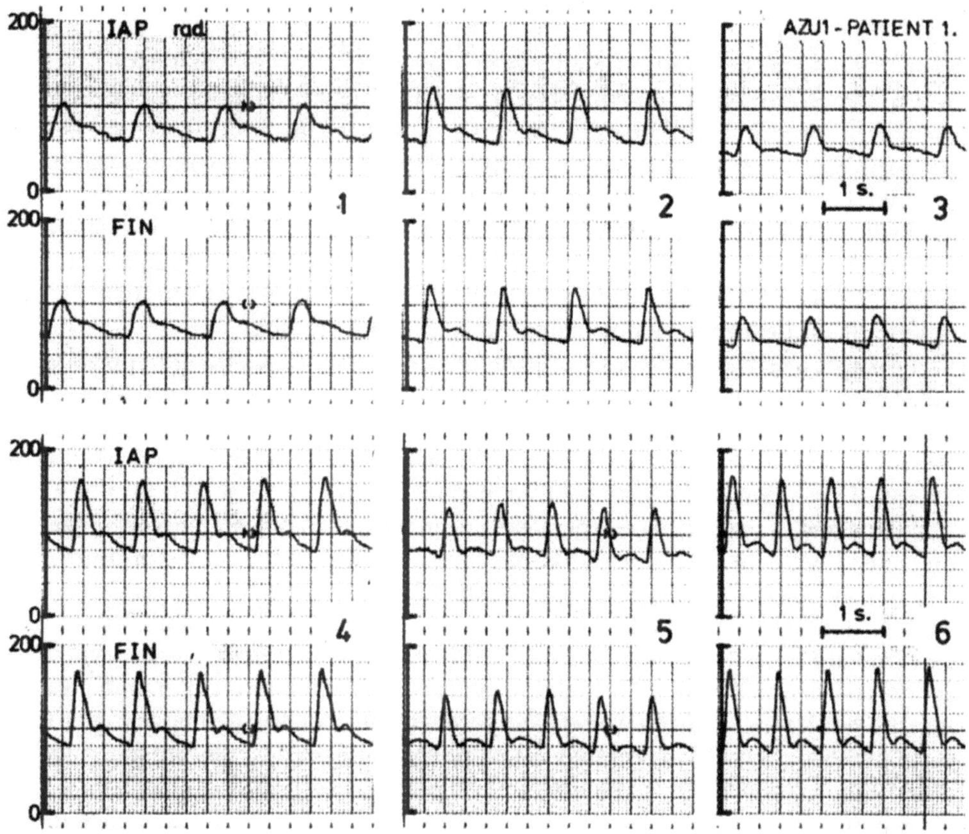

Fig. 14. Registrations in pairs of finger pressure and intraradial pressure in a subject in a CCV. Note the satisfactory correspondence in pressure levels and also in particular in the waveforms recorded with both methods. Episodes 1-6 are taken from a continuous recording of 2-h duration. When displayed on an oscilloscope, noninvasive finger pressures typically coincide with intraradial pressures if care has been taken to level the finger properly at the height of the manometer membrane

more sophisticated. Finger pressures are 6 mmHg below the more central brachial or radial artery pressures on average, ranging from 0 to 15 mmHg. This effect can be compensated for by placing the finger 10 cm below heart level. Possibly, pressure underestimation can also be substantially reduced by using the thumb instead of one of the other fingers for monitoring, but this awaits a systematic study.

The coefficient of variation is the standard deviation of the error of the comparison in proportion to the average pressure level. It appears to be 6%-7% when compared to intra-arterial pressures, which is better than that obtainable with most other indirect methods. The error is 9%-16% in comparison with other noninvasive methods such as oscillometry or the Riva-Rocci/Korotkov method. In other words, finger pressure appears to be more precise when using a better reference method.

Finger pressure monitoring is not only reasonably precise, but shows good linearity over pressures ranging from 0 to 350 mmHg, the lowest and highest pressures that can be measured with FIN.A.PRES. The servo system bandwidth is such that faithful waveform recordings can be made. A particularly nice example of the variability that may occur in the pulse waveform in a single subject in a matter of hours in a coronary care unit (CCU) is shown in Fig. 14. The very large pulse pressures sometimes observed in hypertensive subjects and the steep upstrokes in some young adult subjects under stress present no difficulty to the method. Monitoring can be continued for hours on a single finger. Monitoring of up to 12 h in brain surgery have not caused any harm to the finger. In awake subjects, monitoring has continued for 2-3 h without morbidity or substantial unpleasant effects to the finger or the subject. The vertical height of the finger, with respect to heart level, is important as it is the case for the manometer membrane in invasive monitoring.

Proximal arterial obstructions of hemodynamic significance do not appear to occur very frequently, even in the elderly. When such obstructions are occasionally present they are easily recognized from an increased rise time of the finger pressure upstroke. In that case, monitoring should be switched to the contralateral side for improved precision. During stressful or painful surgery, or in subjects suffering from Raynaud's phenomenon, complete finger arterial spasm may occur. Finger pressure as such can still be measured, but correlation with central blood pressure is reduced and may eventually become zero. The FIN.A.PRES instrument sends out a warning message when serious contractions are observed by the algorithm. In many cases monitoring may be continued on the thumb, since the thumb arteries seem to go into spasm last, if at all. In fact, the advantages of the monitoring of thumb pressure are substantial, so that it would have been recommended at all times except for some problems that need more study. With present cuff designs it is difficult, often impossible, to properly fit a cuff around the thumb.

A periodically repeated search procedure for the finger arterial unstretched diameter appears mandatory, since this diameter varies with the tone of the smooth muscle in the arterial wall at unpredictable intervals. With the frequent readjustment of the setpoint and the gain of the servo loop (see above) such changes are followed and corrected for when they occur, usually without noticeable error in the pressure registration. In normal subjects, the procedure may be turned off for extended periods of time to allow the undisturbed registration of the acute effects of various kinds of intervention, or to allow for the subsequent Fourier analysis of the pressure signal, which also requires an undisturbed waveform.

Acknowledgments. This work has been supported in part by Research Grant 28-491 from "Praeventiefonds," The Hague, The Netherlands. We would gratefully like to thank Prof. dr. A. C. Arntzenius and Dr. H. W. H. Weeda and coworkers of the Leiden Medical Faculty, Dr. N. Ty Smith and colleagues at the Veterans Administration Hospital, San Diego, CA, Prof. dr. J. C. Dorlas and associates of the Groningen Academic Hospital, Dr. M. E. H. Karsten, physician in Haarlem, and Dr. W. J. A. Goedhard, Dept. of Occupational Health TNO, for their fine cooperation in the clinical studies, for sharing our excitement with the method, and for their warm friendship.

Development of FIN.A.PRES has been a true team effort in which 12 technical people at the Institute of Medical Physiscs TNO have cooperated, supported when needed by 9 administrative persons. Of these 21 people we would like to thank W. H. Klawer and Mrs. D. Boom most particularly for their sharing with us the heat of the days and the cold at nights and equally for their friendship.

References

Borst C, Wieling W, van Brederode JFM, Hond A, de Rijk LG, Dunning AJ (1982) Mechanisms of initial heart rate response to postural change. Am J Physiol 243: H676-681

Folkow B, Neil E (1971) Circulations. Oxford University Press, New York

Goedhard WJA, Wesseling KH, Settels JJ (1984) Baroreflex pressure control responding to orthostasis. Changes with age. In: Orlebeke, Mulder, Van Doornen (eds) Psychophysiology of cardiovascular control. Methods, models and data. Plenum, New York

Guyton AC (1980) Arterial pressure and hypertension. Saunders, Philadelphia

Huige MC (1980) Onderzoek naar de betrouwbaarheid van de auscultatoire bloeddrukmeting aan overwegend dikke bovenarmen. Thesis, Leiden

Mancia G, Ferrari A, Gregorini L, Valentini R, Ludbrook J, Zanchetti A (1977) Circulatory reflexes from carotid and extracarotid baroreceptor areas in man. Circ Res 41: 309-315

Molhoek PG, Wesseling KH, Settels JJ, van Vollenhoven E, Weeda HWH, Arntzenius AC (1984) Evaluation of the Peñáz servoplethysmomanometer for the continuous, noninvasive measurement of finger blood pressure. Basic Res Cardiol 79: 598-609

Parati G, Pomidossi G, Ramirez A, Gavazzi C, Bertinieri G, Mancia G (1983) Reproducibility of laboratory tests evaluating neural cardiovascular regulation in man. J Hypertension 1 [Suppl 2]: 88-90

Peñáz J (1969) Patentová Listina, CISLO 133205

Peñáz J (1973) Photoelectric measurement of blood pressure, volume and flow in the finger. In: Digest 10th int conf med biol engng. Dresden, p 104

Settels JJ, Donders JJH, Wesseling KH, Beneken JEW, Rompelman O, Arntzenius AC (1980a) Blood pressure and heart rate fluctuations in normo- and hypertensive man. In: Proc 20th int conf b.e.s. pp 265-268 (Biol Engng Soc, 1980)

Settels JJ, Wesseling KH, Donders JJH, Rompelman O (1980b) Nature of the ten second blood pressure fluctuations in normo- and hypertensive man. In: Rompelman O, Van Duyl W (eds) Oscillatoire verschijnselen in fysiologische systemen. Erasmus University, Rotterdam, pp 37-46

Settels JJ, Wesseling KH, van Esch HJ, Donders JJH (1982) Effects of mental loading on blood pressure and heart rate fluctuations. In: van Beekum T, Eijnsbergen B, Kamp WA (eds) Progress report 8. Institute of Medical Physics TNO, Utrecht, pp 134-143

Sleight P (1979) Reflex control of the heart. Am J Cardiol 44: 889-894

Smith NT, Wesseling KH, de Wit B (1985) Evaluation of two prototype devices producing noninvasive, pulsatile calibrated blood pressure from a finger. J Clin Monit 1: 17-29

Smyth HS, Sleight P, Pickering GW (1969) Reflex regulation of arterial pressure during sleep in man. A quantitative method of assessing baroreflex sensitivity. Circ Res 24: 109-121

Stegemann J (1956) Die fortlaufende, unblutige Blutdruckregistrierung unter Verwendung eines mechanisch-elektrischen Transducers. Pflügers Arch 262: 419-424

Wesseling KH (1981) Physics of the cardiovascular system. In: Greening JR (ed) Medical physics. North Holland, Amsterdam, pp 66-162

Wesseling KH, Möller DPF (1983) Simulationsuntersuchungen zum barorezeptorreflex als Beispiel für die Anwendung derzeitiger Simulationssprachen auf Kleinrechnern. Funkt Biol Med 2: 85-93

Wesseling KH, Settels JJ (1985) Baromodulation explains short term blood pressure variability. In: Orlebeke JF, Mulder G, van Doornen LJP (eds) Psychophysiology of cardiovascular control. Methods, models and data. Plenum, New York

Wesseling KH, Settels JJ, Goedhard WJA (1984) Nieuwe ontwikkelingen in het bloeddrukmeten in het bijzonder bij oudere mensen. In: Goedhard WJA, Knook DL (eds) Bloeddruk en hypertensie op oudere leeftijd. Stafleu, Alphen, pp 37-53

Wesseling KH, Settels JJ, Walstra HG, van Esch HJ, Donders JJH (1983a) Baromodulation as the cause of short term blood pressure variability? In: Alberi G, Bajzer Z, Baxa P (eds) Applications of physics to medicine and biology. World Scientific, Singapore, pp 247-276

Wesseling KH, de Wit B, Settels JJ, Klawer WH (1982) On the indirect registration of finger blood pressure after Peñáz. Funkt Biol Med 1: 245-250

Wesseling KH, de Wit B, Weber JAP, Smith NT (1983b) A simple device for the continuous measurement of cardiac output. Adv Cardiovasc Phys 5: 16-52

Wesseling KH, Settels JJ, van der Hoeven GMA, Nijboer JA, Butijn MWT, Dorlas JC (1985) Effects of peripheral vasoconstriction on the measurement of blood pressure in a finger. Cardiovasc Res 19: 139-145

III. Pathophysiology

Neural Mechanism in Human Cardiovascular Regulation

G. Parati, G. Pomidossi, and G. Mancia[1]

A large number of animal studies have shown that neural factors exert a major control over the cardiovascular system (Kirchheim 1976; Korner 1979) and that derangement of this control may play an important role in the pathophysiology of cardiovascular diseases, such as essential hypertension, angina pectoris, myocardial infarction and sudden death (Folkow 1982). However evaluation of neural factors involved in cardiovascular regulation in human beings is difficult, both because of their complexity and because of the paucity and the limitations of the techniques available for this purpose (Mancia and Mark 1983).

This paper will further emphasize the drawback of such techniques in the light of recent data obtained in our laboratory. However, it will also deal with an experimental approach that has gained popularity in the past few years - the technique of intra-arterial ambulatory blood pressure monitoring - and will describe some of its results and discuss its potential for a better understanding of neural cardiovascular regulation in health and disease.

Traditional Maneuvers for Studying Neural Cardiovascular Control

Over the years a large number of maneuvers have been devised to study excitatory and inhibitory influences of reflex or central origin exerted on the heart and the peripheral circulation. Blood pressure and heart rate responses to these maneuvers have been employed to clarify the extent of the cardiovascular influence of the vagus and the sympathetic divisions of the autonomic nervous system, and to characterize their differences in different individuals and pathophysiological states (Mancia and Mark 1983).

This approach suffers from several limitations, however. One limitation is the poor reproducibility of the responses (Parati et al. 1983). This has been shown by our group in subjects under prolonged intra-arterial blood pressure and heart rate recording in whom a variety of maneuvers involving neural excitatory and inhibitory influences were repeated at regular intervals of 30 min, for a total of six times each, the performance of which had been carefully standardized. As shown in Fig. 1, the average cardiovascular responses always displayed a large variation coefficient. For the blood pressure responses reflexly elicited by alterations in the carotid baroreceptor activity (i. e., inhibitory influences), the average variation coefficient ranged from 10% to 15%. For the heart rate responses reflexly elicited by alterations in baroreceptor activity and for the blood pressure and heart rate responses elicited

1 Cattedra di Semeistica Medica e Centro di Fisiologia Clinica e Ipertensione, Istituto di Clinica Medica IV dell' Università di Milano, Ospedale Maggiore, Via Francesco Sforza, 35-20122 Milan, Italy

Biological and Psychological Factors
in Cardiovascular Disease
Ed. by T. H. Schmidt, T. M. Dembroski, and G. Blümchen

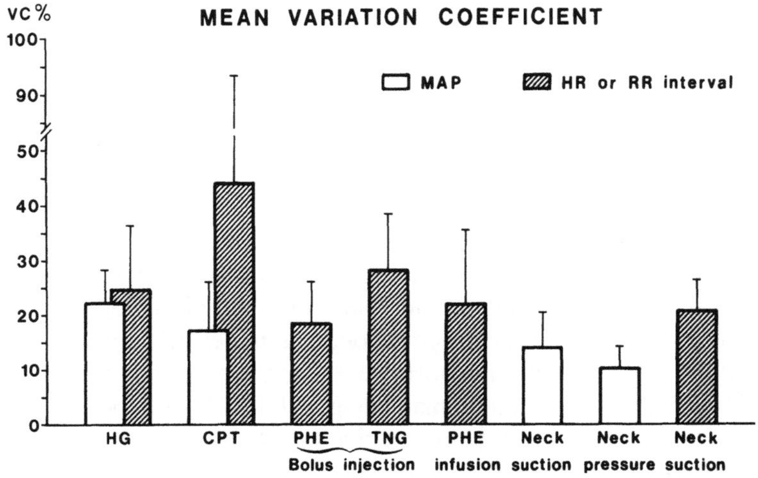

Fig. 1. Variation coefficients (*VC*) of the average hemodynamic responses to maneuvers commonly employed for studying inhibitory and excitatory influences of reflex and/or central nature. In each subject each maneuver was repeated at 30-min intervals up to a total of six times. Variation coefficients were calculated by the standard deviation divided by the average response, times 100. *HG*, hand-grip; *CPT*, cold pressor test; *PHE*, phenylephrine; *TNG*, trinitroglycerine; *MAP*, mean arterial pressure; *HR*, heart rate

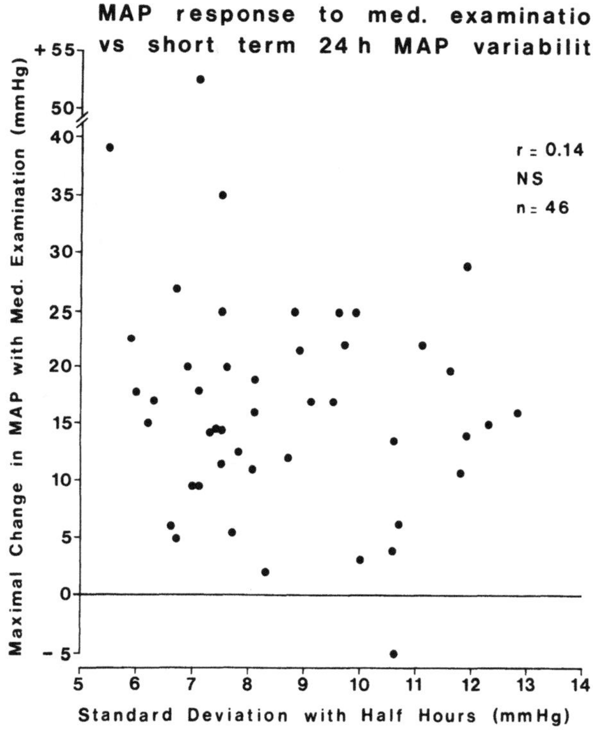

Fig. 2. Lack of correlation between the magnitude of the mean arterial pressure (*MAP*) rise observed during a 10- or 15-min visit by a doctor unknown to the subjects and the variability in MAP assessed in the same subjects by 24-hour intra-arterial blood pressure recording. MAP variability was measured as described in Figs. 6 and 8. Data from 46 subjects are shown

Table 1. Range of the variation coefficients of the average cardiovascular responses to the maneuvers reported in Fig. 1 in the subjects studied

Variation coefficient (%)	Hand-grip ($n=8$)		Cold pressor test ($n=8$)		Phenylephrine bolus test ($n=8$)	Phenylephrine infusion test ($n=8$)
	ΔMAP	HR	MAP	HR	RR/SBP	RR/SBP
Range	12.8-32.3	11.9-49.1	8.2-34.7	18.1-158.1	8.3-28.1	6.7-46.5
Variation coefficient (%)	Trinitroglycerine bolus test ($n=8$)		Neck suction[a] ($n=8$)		Neck pressure[a] ($n=8$)	Neck suction[b] ($n=8$)
	RR/SBP		MAP		MAP	RR
Range	11.1-38.2		4.2-25.6		5.4-17.7	14.1-30.5

[a] The neck chamber method employed was that developed by Ludbrook et al. (1977).
[b] The neck chamber method employed was that developed by Eckberg et al. (1975).
MAP, mean arterial pressure; HR, heart rate; RR, heart interval; SBP, systolic blood pressure. *n* refers to the number of subjects within each group.

by handgrip and cold pressor test (i.e., central and reflex excitatory influences), it was greater than 20% and sometimes greater than 30%. Another constant feature of all these responses was the marked interindividual difference in the magnitude of the variation coefficient (Table 1).

Besides suffering from limitations, the approach that makes use of cardiovascular effects of laboratory tests is based on three assumptions: (1) that the increased cardiovascular responses to laboratory stressors reflect an overall cardiovascular hyperresponsiveness to daily stress, (2) that hyperresponsiveness to stress represents a marker of the subject's tendency to display greater blood pressure oscillations, and (3) that these oscillations increase the risk of developing cardiovascular diseases such as sustained hypertension and coronary events. These assumptions may be incorrect. Indeed, there is evidence that the magnitude of the blood pressure and heart rate responses to tests such as hand-grip, cold pressor test, and mental arithmetic may be poorly interrelated (Parati, Pomidossi, and Mancia 1985, unpublished data). Furthermore, hyperresponsiveness to stress does not correlate with the magnitude of spontaneous blood pressure variability as measured by the standard deviation of the blood pressure values recorded in ambulant subjects over 24 h (Fig. 2). Finally, the importance of phasic blood pressure uses (and that of increased blood pressure variabilities) in the genesis of hypertension and in the production of its target organ damage are not yet clear.

Ambulatory Blood Pressure Recording

In the past few years it has become possible to record blood pressure intra-arterially for 24-48 h without interference or with minimal interference with the subject's lifestyle (Bevan et al. 1969; Littler et al. 1972). This has provided a powerful means of

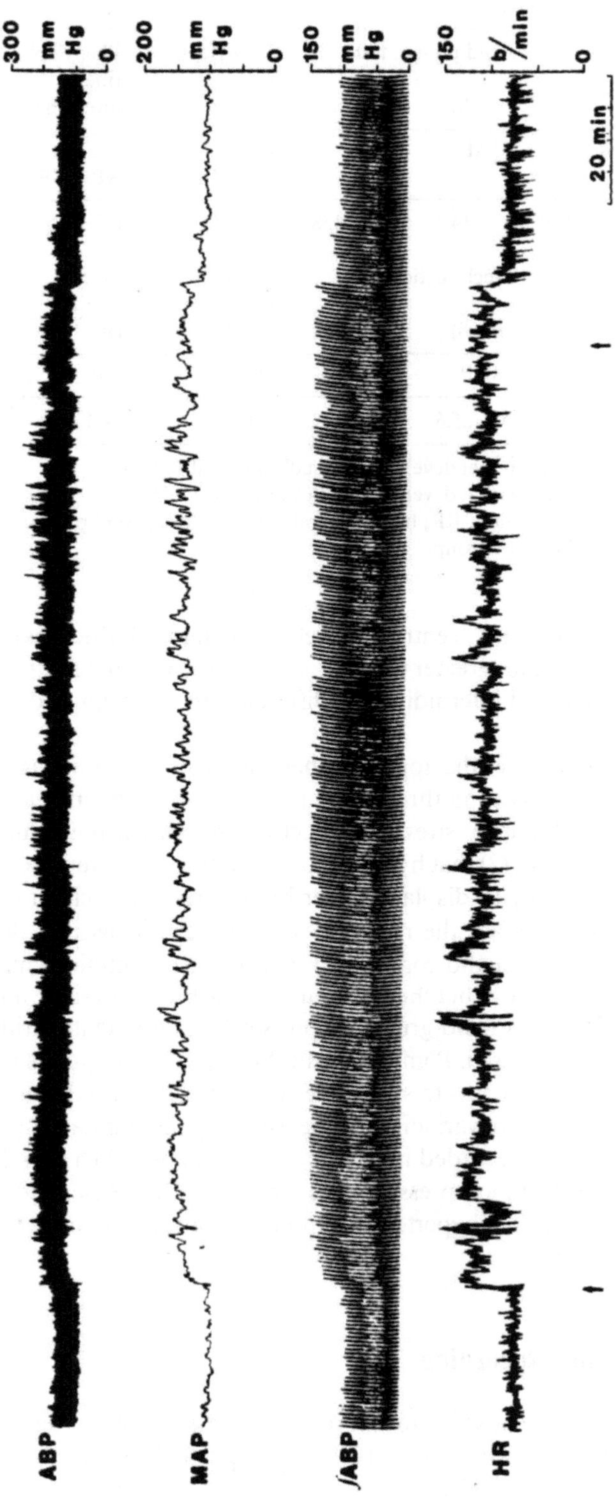

Fig. 3. Blood pressure and heart rate *(HR)* rises during a poker game of several hours duration. Original tracing from one subject under 24-h intra-arterial recording. *ABP*, pulsatile arterial blood pressure; *MAP*, mean arterial pressure; ∫ABP, arterial blood pressure integrated at regular intervals of several seconds

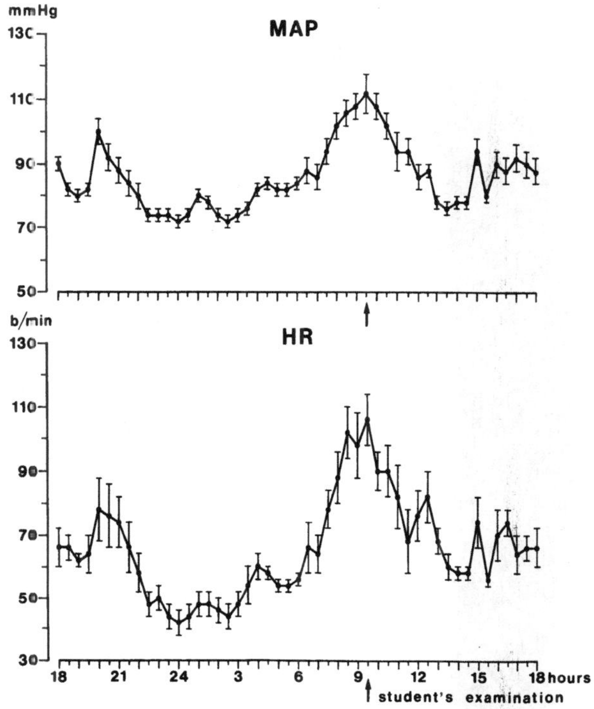

Fig. 4. Mean arterial pressure *(MAP)* and heart rate *(HR)* values throughout a 24-h intra-arterial blood pressure recording performed in a medical student. *Points* and *vertical bars* show the mean and standard deviation values of each 30 min of the recording. The arrow indicates the time of the student's examination by the university board

detecting behavioral effects on blood pressure, and of confirming the extent of central cardiovascular control in an undisputable manner.

Our laboratory has been engaged in intra-arterial 24-h blood pressure recording in human beings since 1976, which has allowed us to collect a large number of examples of the blood pressure responses to stress and additionally, to clarify such complex phenomena as blood pressure variability during day and night.

Figures 3, 4, and 5 show examples of the marked and prolonged effects of stress on blood pressure. It can be seen that situations such as playing poker, examination of a student by a university board, and a medical check-up were all able to raise blood pressure and heart rate markedly, and that these effects persisted throughout the short or relatively more prolonged duration of the events (Mancia et al. 1983 a; Mancia et al. 1983 b). By showing the pronounced cardiovascular effects of emotional behaviors, emphasis is given to the potential importance of central factors in modulating circulation in human beings. The importance of the issue is further shown by the results obtained in studying spontaneous blood pressure and heart rate variability over 24 h in ambulant subjects. When analyzed by a computer, these variabilities showed a close positive relationship to each other both in the whole group and in single subjects, this also being the case for blood pressure and heart rate means (Figs. 6 and 7) (Mancia et al. 1983 b).

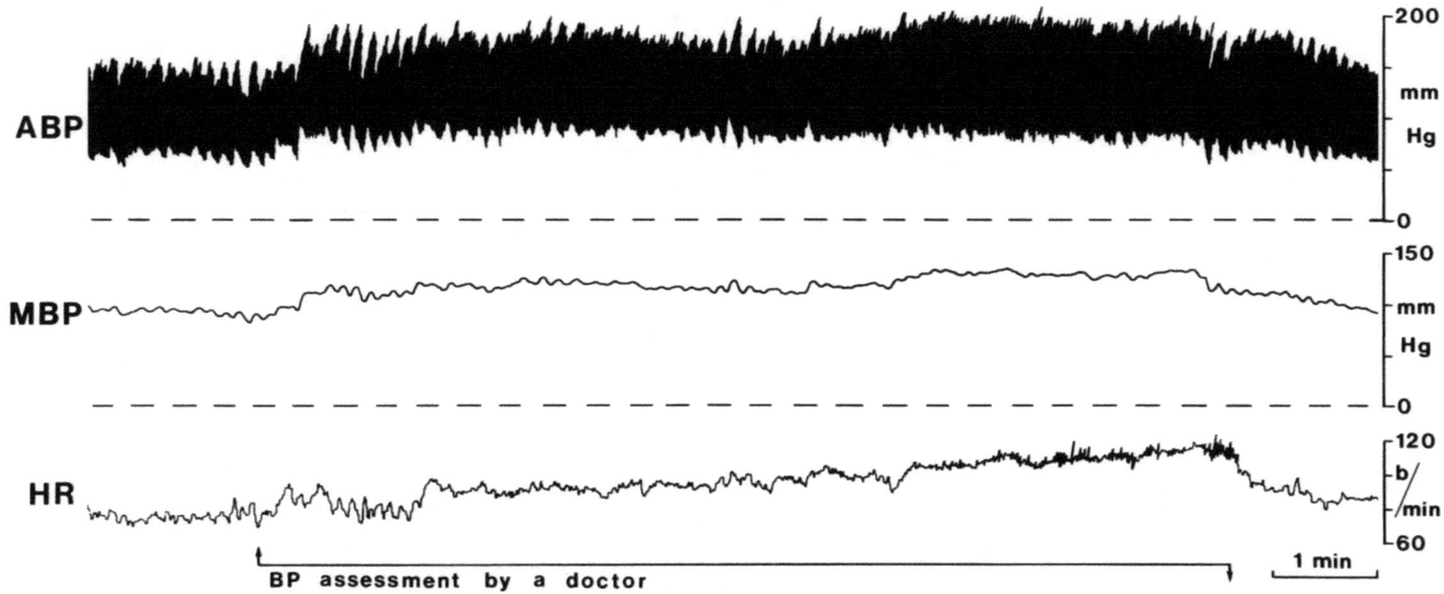

Fig. 5. Blood pressure *(BP)* and heart rate *(HR)* values before, during, and after the visit of a doctor who performed three sphygmomanometric blood pressure measurements on the patient. Original tracing from one subject during 24-h intra-arterial blood pressure recording. The *arrows* mark the beginning and the end of the doctor's visit. *ABP*, pulsatile arterial blood pressure; *MBP*, mean blood pressure

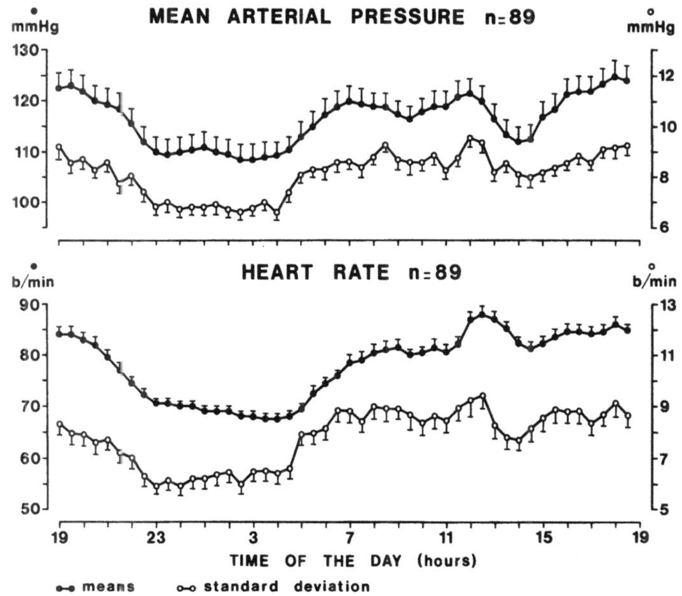

Fig. 6. Blood pressure and heart rate *(HR)* mean values and variabilities during a 24-h period. Data are shown as averages (± SE) for 89 subjects. Variabilities were derived from the standard deviations of each 30 min period of the recording after beat-to-beat analysis of the tracing

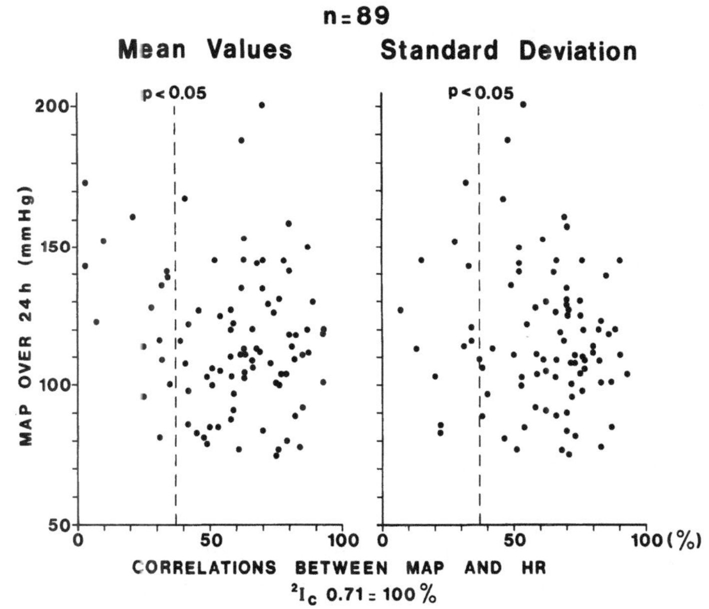

Fig. 7. Correlation between mean arterial pressure *(MAP)* and heart rate *(HR)* values, and between mean arterial pressure and heart rate variabilities in each of the 89 subjects of Fig. 6. The correlation indices (calculated by the nonparametric tests of Smirnoff) are plotted versus the 24-h average mean arterial pressure value. The *dotted line* refers to the value over which the correlation was significant at $P<0.05$

Table 2. Correlation coefficients between mean arterial pressure (MAP) variability and the baroreflex sensitivity as measured by the currently employed techniques

Baroreflex sensitivity during:			MAP variability			
			Standard deviation		Variation coefficient	
			r	P	r	P
Neck suction	$\left(\frac{-\mathrm{MAP}}{-\mathrm{NTP}}\right)$	$n=58$	−0.36	0.01	−0.38	0.01
Neck pressure	$\left(\frac{+\mathrm{MAP}}{+\mathrm{NTP}}\right)$	$n=58$	−0.05	NS	−0.05	NS
PHE bolus injection	$\left(\frac{+\mathrm{RR}}{+\mathrm{SBP}}\right)$	$n=62$	−0.45	0.001	−0.10	NS
TNG bolus injection	$\left(\frac{-\mathrm{RR}}{-\mathrm{SBP}}\right)$	$n=64$	−0.28	0.05	−0.01	NS

PHE, phenylephrine; TNG, trinitroglycerine; NTP, level of pressure exerted on neck tissues; SBP, systolic blood pressure; RR, heart interval; NS, not significant. *n* refers to the number of subjects studied.

These observations indicate that in everyday life, blood pressure and heart rate change concurrently, i. e., that an increase or a reduction in one is accompanied by an increase or a reduction in the other. It is likely that this parallelism reflects the fact that central factors exert a similar influence on the heart and systemic blood vessels and dominate in neural cardiovascular regulation.

A further point of interest is the involvement of baroreflexes in human blood pressure variability. A number of animal studies have shown that arterial baroreceptors exert an important buffering role on blood pressure oscillations. This role can also be seen in man, an inverse relationship existing between blood pressure variability and the sensitivity of the baroreflexes as measured by the currently available techniques (Table 2, Mancia et al. 1986). However, the *r*-value of such relationships is relatively small, which suggests that the importance of this mechanism in buffering the extent of this phenomenon may be limited. This may depend on a species difference in baroreflex function. It may also reflect, however, a reduced ability of the baroreflex to buffer blood pressure variations, which, as discussed above, are largely central in nature (Cowley et al. 1973).

Blood Pressure and Heart Rate Variabilities in Normal and High Blood Pressure

Figure 8 shows the blood pressure and heart rate variabilities (calculated as averages of all 30-min standard deviations obtained during the 24-h recordings) in three groups of subjects, classified as normotensive, moderately hypertensive, and severely hypertensive on the basis of their 24-h average mean arterial pressure value (Mancia et al. 1983 b). The blood pressure variability showed a progressive increase from the normotensive to the severely hypertensive group. However, this increase was proportional to the elevation in the average 24-hour blood pressure, as shown

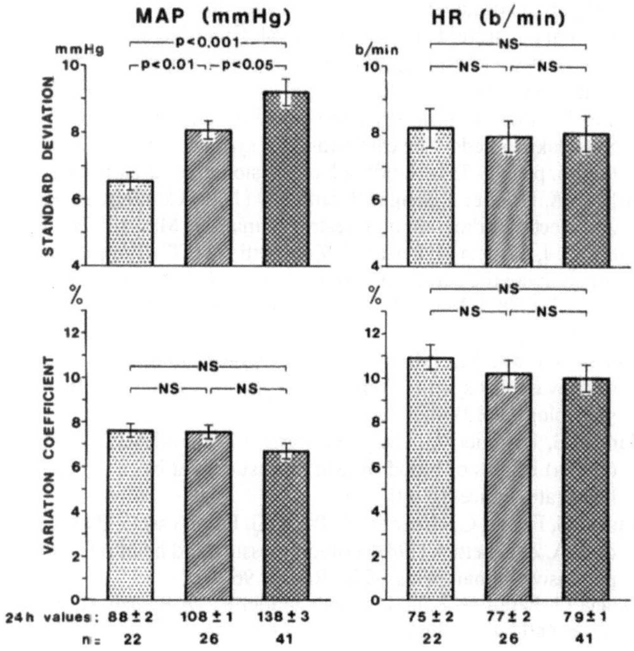

Fig. 8. Mean arterial pressure (*MAP*) and heart rate (*HR*) variabilities in normotensive, moderately and severely essential hypertensive subjects. Data are shown as averages of the 48 30 half hour standard deviations (see Fig. 6) and of the 48 30-min variation coefficients. *n* refers to the number of subjects within each group and *P* to the statistical significance of the differences

by the fact that blood pressure variation coefficients (i.e., percentage variabilities) were similar in the three groups. The standard deviations were also similar in the three groups as were the variation coefficients for heart rate and the average 24-h heart rate values. These data suggest that the variability phenomenon may be substantially unchanged in subjects with high blood pressure, and that central control of the heart and the peripheral circulation may be unaltered in this condition. It should be emphasized that unaltered blood pressure and heart rate variabilities have also been reported in borderline hypertension, a finding that has made the term "labile", previously adopted for this condition, obsolete.

Acknowledgment. The research summarized in this paper has been made possible in part through grants from CNR (Finalized Project on Degenerative Disease, Subproject Hypertension; Finalized Project of Biomedical Technology, Subproject Cardiopulmonary).

References

Bevan AT, Honour AJ, Stott FD (1969) Direct arterial pressure recording in unrestricted man. Clin Sci 36: 329-344

Cowley AW, Liard JF, Guyton AC (1973) Role of the baroreceptor reflex in daily control of arterial blood pressure and other variables in dogs. Circ Res 32: 564-576

Eckberg DL, Cavanaugh RS, Mark AL, Abboud FM (1975) A simplified neck suction device for activation of carotid baroreceptors. J Lab Clin Med 85: 167-173
Folkow B (1982) Physiological aspects of primary hypertension. Physiol Rev 62: 347-504
Kirchheim MR (1976) Systemic arterial baroreceptor reflexes. Physiol Rev 56: 100-176
Korner PI (1979) Central nervous control of autonomic cardiovascular function. In: Berke RM, Sperelakis N (eds) The cardiovascular system. The Heart. American Physiological Society, Bethesda, pp 691-739 (Handbook of physiology, section 1, vol 1, Chapter 20)
Littler WA, Honour J, Sleight P, Stott FD (1972) Continuous recording of direct arterial pressure and electrocardiogram in unrestricted man. Br Med J 3: 76-78
Ludbrook J, Mancia G, Ferrari A, Zanchetti A (1977) The variable pressure neck chamber method for studying the carotid baroreflex in man. Clin Sci Mol Med 53: 165-171
Mancia G (1983) Methods for assessing blood pressure values in humans. Hypertension 5 [Suppl III]: 5-13
Mancia G, Mark AL (1983) Arterial baroreflexes in humans. In: Shepherd J, Abboud F (eds) The cardiovascular system. American Physiological Society, Bethesda, pp 755-794 (Handbook of physiology, vol 3)
Mancia G, Bertinieri G, Grassi G, Parati G, Pomidossi G, Ferrari A, Gregorini L, Zanchetti A (1983 a) Effects of blood pressure measurement by the doctor on patient's blood pressure and heart rate. Lancet II: 695-698
Mancia G, Ferrari G, Gregorini L, Parati G, Pomidossi G, Bertinieri G, Grassi G, Di Rienzo M, Pedotti A, Zanchetti A (1983b) Blood pressure and heart rate variabilities in normotensive and hypertensive human beings. Circ Res 53: 96-104
Mancia G, Parati G, Pomidossi R, Caradei R, Di Rienzo M, Zanchetti A (1986) Arterial baroreflexes and blood pressure and heart rate variabilities in humans. Hypertension 8: 147-153
Parati G, Pomidossi G, Ramirez A, Gavazzi C, Bertinieri G, Mancia G (1983) Reproducibility of laboratory tests evaluating neural cardiovascular regulation in man. J Hypertension 1 [suppl 2]: 88-90

Behavioral Influences on Neuroendocrines and Insulin Sensitivity as Precursors of Coronary Heart Disease

J. A. HERD[1]

Introduction

Risk factors for coronary heart disease have been identified through epidemiological, clinical, and experimental laboratory studies. The association of coronary heart disease with high blood pressure, cigarette smoking, and high total cholesterol concentrations in blood was demonstrated in the Framingham Study more than 20 years ago (Dawber et al. 1957). In addition to the major risk factors, epidemiological studies have also identified other associated characteristics including diabetes mellitus (Stamler and Epstein 1972), obesity (Armstrong et al. 1951), physical inactivity (Jenkins et al. 1974), and the Type A behavior pattern (Jenkins et al. 1974). Also, a decreased risk of coronary heart disease has been demonstrated in association with elevated high-density lipoprotein cholesterol concentrations in blood (Gordon et al. 1977).

Although abnormal concentrations of lipoproteins in blood are often associated with atherosclerosis, the metabolic abnormalities in lipid metabolism are poorly understood. Abnormalities in lipid metabolism have been demonstrated in patients with familial hypercholesterolemia (Fredrickson et al. 1978). Individuals with that disorder were demonstrated to have a decreased or absent cell-surface receptor binding for circulating low-density lipoproteins. The result was abnormal concentrations of low-density lipoprotein cholesterol in blood. However, familial hypercholesterolemia affects less than 5% of the population, and patterns of lipid metabolism in those individuals are not the same as seen in the general population. A more common abnormality in lipid metabolism is that seen in the presence of diabetes mellitus. Epidemiological, clinical, and experimental laboratory studies of insulin and its effects on carhohydrate and lipid metabolism suggest that abnormal circulating insulin levels may be associated with atherosclerosis (Stout 1977 a; Stout 1981; Stout 1982).

Insulin and Coronary Heart Disease

The association between diabetes mellitus and atherosclerosis has been demonstrated in several epidemiological studies. Three prospective studies have provided convincing evidence. These are studies carried out in large communities as part of the Framingham Study (Garcia et al. 1974), the Tecumseh Community Health Study (Ostrander et al. 1965; Epstein 1967 a), and the Bedford Study (Keen et al.

1 Sid W. Richardson Institute for Preventive Medicine, The Methodist Hospital, MS-400, 6565 Fannin Street, Houston, TX 77030, USA

Biological and Psychological Factors
in Cardiovascular Disease
Ed. by T. H. Schmidt, T. M. Dembroski, and G. Blümchen

1965). Analyses of epidemiological data have shown that hyperglycemia is an independent risk factor for atherosclerosis (Epstein 1967a; Garcia et al. 1974).

Studies of insulin and lipid metabolism frequently involve patients with diabetes mellitus or laboratory animals with experimental forms of abnormal glucose metabolism. However, insulin affects lipid metabolism in subjects without overt diabetes mellitus, and elevated insulin levels may be associated with atherosclerosis in the absence of hyperglycemia. Several clinical studies have reported an association between high concentrations of insulin in blood following oral administration of glucose in patients with coronary artery disease (Nikkila et al. 1965; Christiansen et al. 1968; Tzagournis et al. 1968; Kashyap et al. 1970; Malherbe et al. 1970; Gertler et al. 1972). In addition, angiographic studies of patients with coronary disease have shown elevated insulin responses in the absence of complete occlusion of any coronary arteries and in the absence of myocardial infarction (Tzagournis et al. 1968). Apparently high levels of insulin concentration in blood in response to glucose administered orally differentiates subjects with coronary heart disease from those without evidence of vascular disease.

Results of three prospective studies of insulin concentrations in blood with the incidence of myocardial infarction and coronary heart disease have been published (Logan et al. 1978; Pyorala 1979; Ducimetiere et al. 1980). Ducimetiere et al. (1980) demonstrated that the fasting level of insulin concentration in blood and the fasting insulin/glucose ratio were positively associated with risks for myocardial infarction and coronary heart disease mortality independent of all the other risk factors. Logan et al. (1978) reported that elevated levels of insulin concentration in blood had a strong association with development of coronary heart disease over a 5-year period. They also reported a predictive value of responses in the level of insulin concentration in blood following oral administration of glucose that was independent of other risk factors including total cholesterol concentration in blood, level of blood pressure, and glucose concentration in blood. Pyorala (1979) reported that the combination of low glucose and high insulin responses or high glucose and low insulin responses to an oral glucose tolerance test were associated with an increased risk of coronary artery disease. Each of these studies was conducted with individuals who did not have diabetes mellitus.

Ducimetiere et al. (1980) reported that excess insulin concentration in blood for a given glucose concentration was a risk factor for coronary heart disease. They measured serum cholesterol, serum triglycerides, systolic blood pressure, body weight, and height, as well as history of cigarette smoking. In addition, they measured glucose and insulin concentrations in blood before and 2 h after administering 75 g of glucose by the oral route. The population under study was 7246 nondiabetic working men aged 43-54 years who were initially free from heart disease and were followed for 63 months on the average. They demonstrated significant differences for incidence of coronary heart disease in individuals among the highest quintile for fasting levels of insulin concentration in blood and levels of insulin concentration 2 h following the oral glucose load (Fig. 1; West 1978).

When the insulin concentration in blood and other risk factors were kept constant in a multivariate analysis, the fasting insulin/glucose ratio was positively associated with risk for myocardial infarction and coronary heart disease mortality independent of all the other risk factors (Fig. 2; Epstein 1967b). This high insulin

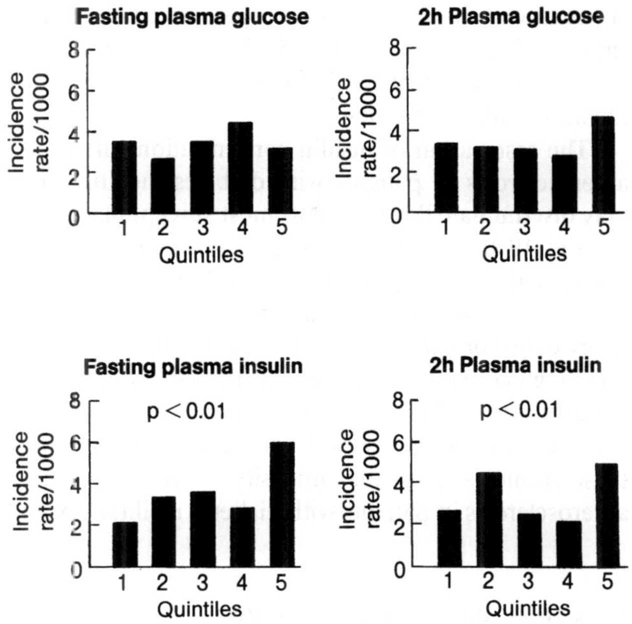

Fig. 1. Mean annual incidence of coronary heart disease complications by quintiles of glucose and insulin concentrations in plasma during fasting and 2 h after an oral glucose load. Note that no significant differences of incidence were observed among quintiles of glucose concentrations in plasma during either fasting or 2 h after an oral glucose load. Significant differences of incidence were observed among quintiles of insulin concentrations in plasma during fasting and 2 h after an oral glucose load

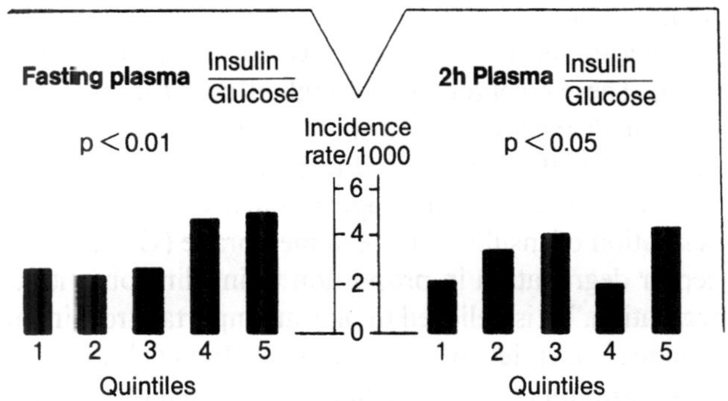

Fig. 2. Mean annual incidence of coronary heart disease complications according to quintiles of ratios for insulin concentration to glucose concentration in plasma during fasting and 2 h after an oral glucose load. Note that significant differences of incidence were observed for the last two quintiles of the ratio between insulin concentration and glucose concentration in plasma during fasting

concentration in blood for a given glucose concentration has been called insulin resistance. These authors concluded that insulin resistance in the fasting state constituted an independent risk factor for coronary heart disease complications in middle-aged nondiabetic men.

The association of insulin concentrations in blood with lipid metabolism and atherosclerosis in patients with diabetes mellitus suggests that insulin resistance may discriminate those patients most susceptible to coronary heart disease (Kashyap et al. 1970; Santen et al. 1972). Kashyap et al. (1970) reported that patients with diabetes mellitus and coronary heart disease had higher levels of insulin concentration in blood in response to an oral load of glucose than patients with diabetes but no evidence of coronary heart disease. Glucose concentrations in blood following an oral glucose load were the same in both groups. Santen et al. (1972) reported that patients with diabetes mellitus who were not receiving insulin had higher insulin/glucose ratios in association with atherosclerosis than in its absence. Results of these studies suggest that intensity of insulin resistance may predict severity of atherosclerosis in patients with diabetes mellitus not treated with insulin.

Receptors and Insulin Resistance

Although insulin exerts a number of effects on cellular metabolism, its influence on glucose transport across cell membranes has been studied most extensively. Consequently, the concept of insulin resistance has developed in connection with glucose metabolism. However, in addition to stimulating glucose and amino acid transport, insulin also influences cell growth and differentiation (Czech 1981). These effects show great variation over a wide range of insulin concentrations and through a wide range of time for activation. Its effects on glucose metabolism depend upon its binding to specific receptors located on cell membranes (Roth 1973; Roth et al. 1975). These receptors have a high affinity for insulin, rapid and saturable binding, and a high specificity for insulin. They are not a static component of a cell but rather have a half-life measured in hours. In addition to rapid turnover, the affinities and numbers of insulin receptors under various conditions are regulated by the concentration of insulin at the cell membrane (Gavin et al. 1974). This mechanism, receptor degradation in proportion to insulin concentration, has been called "down regulation." It is believed to play an important role in the pathogenesis of insulin resistance in a variety of diseased states (Bar et al. 1979). Other modulators of receptor concentration or affinity include dietary maneuvers such as fasting or high carbohydrate diet and exercise. Other regulators of insulin receptor expression include cortisol, growth hormone, ketones, nucleotides, and ions (Merimee et al. 1976; Muggeo et al. 1977; Thomopoulos et al. 1977). In addition to diverse effects of physiological processes on insulin receptor expression, it is likely that resistance to one action of insulin need not necessarily be associated with resistance to other actions. Thus, patients with insulin resistance may have overt diabetes mellitus while others may be normoglycemic with high levels of insulin concentration in blood (Flier 1983).

Cortisol, growth hormone, glucagon, and catecholamines all produce states of insulin resistance (Harrison and Flier 1980). Under some conditions, combinations of hormones may synergize to amplify insulin resistance (Eigler et al. 1979). Furthermore, effects on insulin sensitivity may occur by a variety of mechanisms including influences on substrates such as fatty acids which antagonize insulin action, actions which stimulate hepatic enzymes to mediate gluconeogenesis and glycogenolysis, actions to influence insulin secretion from the pancreas, and direct actions on expression of insulin receptors (Harrison and Flier 1980). Although hormones such as cortisol and catecholamines may affect insulin receptor expression, effects on other metabolic processes may be as important (Beck Nielsen et al. 1980; Yasuda and Kitabchi 1980; Fantus et al. 1981).

Several techniques have been used to quantify insulin resistance. When insulin resistance was first defined, it was measured by determining the level of glucose concentration in blood that occurred after the intravenous administration of insulin (Alford et al. 1971). To avoid the hypoglycemia associated with the insulin tolerance test, patients have been given 50 g of glucose orally followed by 50 g of glucose and regular insulin intravenously (Himsworth and Kerr 1939). Levels of glucose concentration in blood measured during the next hour were plotted as the increment above the initial value, and the increment was used as an estimate of insulin action. Further refinements have been developed to quantitate glucose utilization in response to insulin administration when glucose concentration in blood is held at a predetermined constant level by a constant intravenous infusion (Cherrington et al. 1978). Although each of these techniques has advantages and disadvantages, all demonstrate the ability of insulin to stimulate glucose utilization, and the failure to do so is a measure of insulin resistance.

The most common clinical condition associated with insulin resistance is obesity. Studies of insulin receptors and insulin action in obese human subjects revealed that the concentration of insulin receptors on freshly obtained monocytes, red blood cells, and adipocytes was reduced (Bar et al. 1976; Olefsky 1976). Studies of receptor deficiency and insulin resistance have indicated that insulin receptor deficiency contributes to insulin resistance in all obese subjects studied (Kolterman et al. 1980). However, a postreceptor abnormality may also be present. Hyperglycemia, elevated free fatty acid levels, or insulin deficiency could each be responsible for postreceptor defects.

Cellular Mechanisms in Atherosclerosis

Atherosclerosis is a process in which lipids are deposited in the arterial wall. Through some process not well understood, endothelial cells are lifted from the lining of the artery, and lipids gain access to the intima. In response to the altered intimal composition, vascular smooth muscle cells move into the arterial intima and proliferate. Lipids accumulate in the smooth muscle cells and produce lipid streaks. Later, lipids, fibrous tissue, and other proteoglycan materials are deposited in the extracellular space. Chronic inflammatory cell proliferation, hemorrhage, necrosis, and calcification occur at later stages. Although lipid infiltration into the arterial wall is an important part of atherogenesis, the formation of the atheromatous plaque is initiated by the proliferation of vascular smooth muscle cells. Thus, the pathophysiological mechanisms promoting the primary proliferative process of vascular smooth muscle may be critical for the development of atherosclerosis.

Techniques have been developed to study mechanisms stimulating proliferation of vascular smooth muscle cells. Using a variety of techniques, arterial smooth muscle cells have been obtained from the aorta of human fetuses (Jarvelainen et al. 1982), nonhuman primates (Stout et al. 1975), and explants from the aorta of nonhuman primates maintained continuously in tissue culture (Ross et al. 1974). These techniques provide the opportunity to study the growth and metabolism of vascular smooth muscle cells in detail.

Effect of insulin on the proliferation of cultured primate arterial smooth muscle cells was reported by Stout et al. (1975). Smooth muscle cells were grown from the thoracic aortas of 1-year old monkeys. The effect of insulin on the proliferation of these cells was studied by comparing the growth of cells in culture medium to which insulin had been added in concentrations of 10, 100, 1000, 10000 microunits/ml. There was a significant linear relationship between the logarithm of the insulin dose and cell growth (Ross and Glomset 1973). However, the highest concentration of insulin produced only 50% of the effect seen when the cells were cultured in 5% serum. Results of these experiments suggest that insulin had growth-promoting properties but that it was not the only growth-promoting factor in serum. Both lipoproteins (Ross and Glomset 1973) and platelets (Ross et al. 1974) may also have the potential for stimulating proliferation of vascular smooth muscle cells.

Insulin has also been reported to enhance the incorporation of labeled acetate into sterols in cultured rat arterial smooth muscle cells (Stout 1977b). Insulin also stimulated DNA synthesis in vascular smooth muscle cells (Taggart and Stout 1980). Effects of insulin on lipid metabolism in cultured arterial smooth muscle cells include stimulation of cholesterol synthesis (Stout 1977b). Although the effect of insulin on uptake of lipoproteins by arterial tissue is not known, insulin does increase the cellular binding and degradation of low-density lipoproteins by fibroblasts (Chait et al. 1978). Thus, it can be said that insulin results in proliferation of vascular smooth muscle cells, and synthesis of cholesterol, phospholipids, and triglycerides. These are all effects of insulin which might promote atherogenesis.

The combination of high levels of insulin concentration in blood and high levels of triglyceride concentration may create a vicious cycle with atherogenic potential. Steiner and Vranic (1982) reviewed the evidence that high levels of triglyceride concentration in blood can interfere with metabolic processes involving insulin even without concomitant obesity or diabetes mellitus. Since high levels of insulin concentration in blood can stimulate triglyceride-containing lipids with atherogenic potential, the combination may constitute a vicious cycle.

Endogenous production of triglycerides has been shown to be directly related to level of insulin concentration in blood (Streja et al. 1977). When obese individuals were studied before, during, and after a prolonged fast, increases in insulin concentration in blood were accompanied by increases in the rate of triglyceride production. However, increased production was not always accompanied by increased triglyceride concentration in blood. During fasting, levels of insulin concentration in blood and lipoprotein lipase concentrations fell and triglyceride concentrations increased because of an impairment of removal (Streja et al. 1977). By contrast, high-carbohydrate feeding was accompanied by a sufficient increase in triglyceride removal so that no change in triglyceride concentration in blood occurred despite an increase in production (Steiner and Murase 1975). Thus, mild to moderate

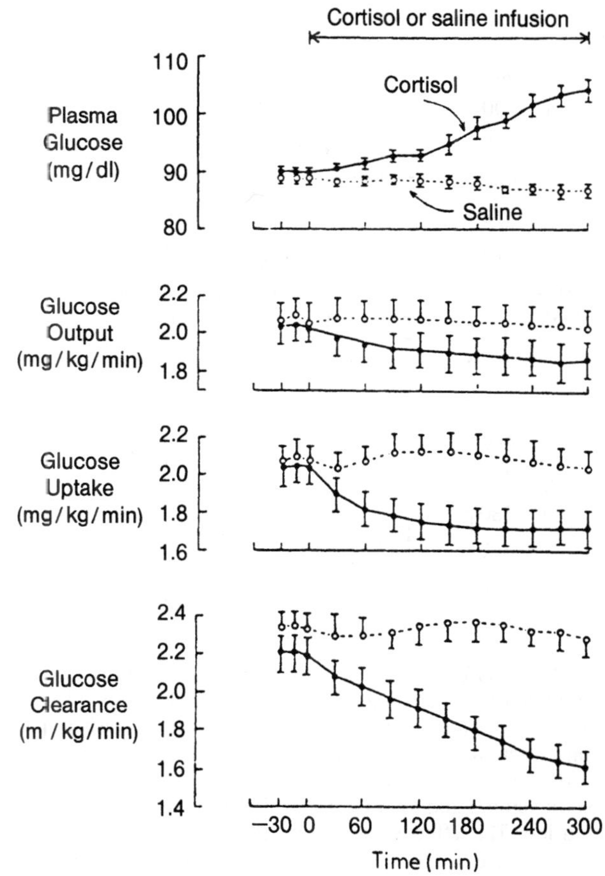

Fig. 3. The effect of cortisol infusion on concentrations of glucose in plasma and glucose kinetics in normal human subjects. *Abscissas* are time in minutes before and during intravenous infusion of cortisol or saline solution. *Ordinate* of the *top panel* is glucose concentration in plasma (mg/dl), of the *second panel* is glucose output (mg/kg/min), of the *third panel* is glucose uptake (mg/kg/min), and of the *bottom panel,* is glucose clearance (ml/kg/min). Note that plasma glucose gradually increased during cortisol infusion in spite of a gradual decline in glucose output. This increase reflected a marked reduction in glucose uptake and glucose clearance

changes in insulin concentration in blood were positively correlated with changes in rate of triglyceride production. Since the rates of triglyceride production and removal were both sensitive to changes in insulin levels, the effect of insulin resistance can be high levels of triglyceride concentration in blood. This resistance was reported to exist even in the absence of obesity (Steiner et al. 1980).

The turnover from triglyceride metabolism results in very low-density lipoprotein remnants (Reardon et al. 1978). These remnants are supposed to be atherogenic (Zilversmit 1979). If such is the case, the effect of high levels of insulin concentration in blood to increase turnover rates for triglycerides might be a possible mechanism that explains the role of insulin concentration in blood as a risk factor for coronary heart disease.

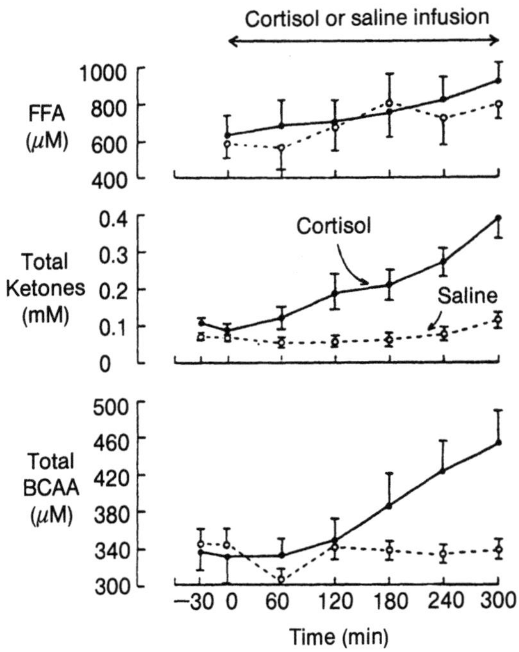

Fig. 4. The effect of cortisol infusion on concentrations of free fatty acids *(FFA)*, total ketones, and total branched chain amino acid *(BCAA)* in blood and plasma. *Abscissas* are the same as in Fig. 3. *Ordinate* of the *top panel* is FFA concentration in plasma (μ*M*), of the *second panel* is total ketone concentration in blood (m*M*), and of the *bottom panel*, is total BCAA concentration in plasma (μ*M*). Note that cortisol infusion had no significant effect on FFA concentration, whereas total blood ketones and total BCAA exhibited a greater rise during cortisol infusion than during saline infusion. This effect suggests that cortisol may have enhanced the release of FFA and simultaneously increased the hepatic conversion of FFA to ketones. Alternatively, cortisol may have inhibited the removal of ketones from blood

Metabolic Effects of Cortisol and Epinephrine

The influence of neuroendocrines on insulin sensitivity includes effects on glucose, ketones, free fatty acids, and amino acids in blood. Shamoon et al. (1980) infused cortisol intravenously during a 5-h period to raise plasma cortisol levels to high but physiologically acceptable levels. Normal adult men and women were studied after consuming a standard carbohydrate diet and fasting overnight before observations were made. The effect of cortisol infusion on plasma glucose and glucose kinetics in the normal human subjects is illustrated in Fig. 3. Infusion of cortisol increased levels of glucose in blood without influencing rates of glucose production. Removal of glucose from blood was reduced and this resulted in cortisol-induced hyperglycemia. These effects of cortisol on glucose metabolism occurred in the absence of significant changes in plasma insulin or glucagon concentration.

Concomitant effects on fatty acid and amino acid metabolism suggested that cortisol interfered with several cellular actions of insulin. No significant effect on free fatty acid concentrations in blood occurred, but total ketone concentrations rose during cortisol infusion (Fig. 4). These results suggest that cortisol enhanced the conversion of free fatty acids to ketones or inhibited mechanisms acting to remove ketones from blood. The rise in branched chain amino acid concentration in blood during cortisol infusion was consistent with a reduction in insulin sensitivity. These results suggest that cortisol interfered with several cellular actions of insulin.

Similar studies of epinephrine have also been performed. Soman et al. (1980) studied the effects of epinephrine on glucose and lipid metabolism. Epinephrine was infused intravenously into normal young men and women during a 4-h period. The authors reported an increase in glucose concentrations in blood of 45% above initial values, and an increase in free fatty acid concentrations in blood of 120% above initial values. These values returned to basal levels within 90 min. No significant effect on concentrations of insulin or glucagon in blood was observed. Rate of removal for glucose from blood decreased by 25% and remained suppressed throughout the 4-h period of observations. The authors concluded that epinephrine had a persistent effect in decreasing the removal of glucose from blood but only transiently increased the output of glucose and free fatty acids. Although no direct measurements of insulin activity were made, the results of these experiments are compatible with an interference by epinephrine in the influence of insulin on metabolic processes associated with glucose and lipid metabolism.

Behavioral Influences on Cortisol and Epinephrine

Psychological factors have been shown to influence secretion of cortisol and epinephrine. One characteristic of situations provoking increased secretion of cortisol is the novelty of an experimental situation. Davis et al. (1981) tested normal young men under a graded exercise tolerance test procedure. One group of 12 subjects was experienced with the incremental work test and another group of 7 subjects was inexperienced. The maximal capacities for work and the maximum heart rates of subjects in both groups were commensurate with the level of physical conditioning and age for each group, and no significant differences were noted between groups. High concentrations of lactate in blood were recorded in both groups, and no significant differences were determined between groups. Serum cortisol concentrations in blood rose during exercise in both groups, but the cortisol concentrations in blood after exercise were significantly greater in the inexperienced subjects (Fig. 5). Serum cortisol increased by 59% in the experienced subjects and by 138% in the inexperienced subjects. The authors concluded that novelty was the major determinant of the increased cortisol response in the inexperienced subjects compared to experienced subjects. Furthermore, this cortisol response bore little relationship to maximal oxygen uptake, heart rate, or venous lactate concentrations in blood. Apparently, the magnitude of response observed in cortisol concentrations was influenced more by psychological factors than the physiological effects of exercise.

Another characteristic of situations provoking increased secretion of cortisol is mental task demand, which elicits efforts to cope with those demands. Brandenberger et al. (1980) measured catecholamine and cortisol concentrations in blood of normal healthy male college students while they performed a short-term memory task under quiet or noisy conditions. As shown in Fig. 6, performing the task led to significant increases in cortisol concentration in blood. In a control session, there

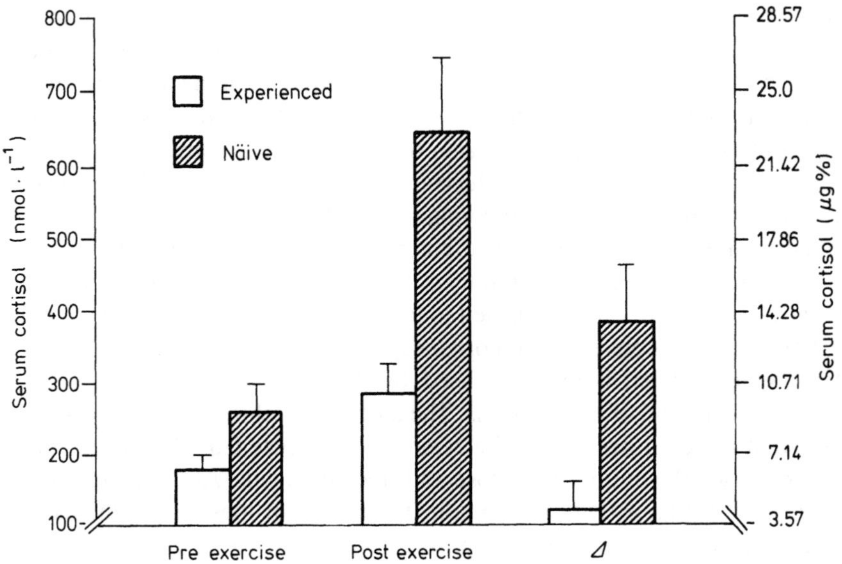

Fig. 5. Concentration of cortisol in serum before and after exercise on a bicycle ergometer in experienced and naive subjects. *Ordinate* on the *left* is concentration of cortisol in serum expressed as nmol/liter, and that on the *right* is concentration of cortisol expressed as μg/%. Note that the rise in concentration of cortisol after exercise was much greater in naive subjects than in experienced subjects

was a gradual decline in cortisol concentration in blood until about 12.00 noon, when a steep increase occurred after a meal. During the mental task performed either in quiet or in noise, the morning decline was interrupted. The difference in cortisol concentrations in blood between the three sessions was statistically significant. Varying the order of sessions revealed that carrying out the mental task for the first time in quiet produced a high cortisol concentration in blood with little additional effect when the second task session was carried out in noise.

Similarily, there were significant increases in epinephrine and norepinephrine concentrations in blood. Exposure to noise had little effect on the concentrations of epinephrine and norepinephrine in blood. In addition, a significant correlation was found between individual plasma cortisol increments and error-rates assessed from an accuracy of recall variable. As shown in Fig. 7, the relation between individual errors and cortisol concentrations in blood could be demonstrated. Although a relation between errors and cortisol concentrations in blood persisted in the second session, the increments in cortisol concentration were greatest during the first experimental session. The authors interpreted these results as providing evidence for a relationship between catecholamine secretion and attentional demand with an additional relationship between concentrations of cortisol in blood with successful coping under the demands of the mental task.

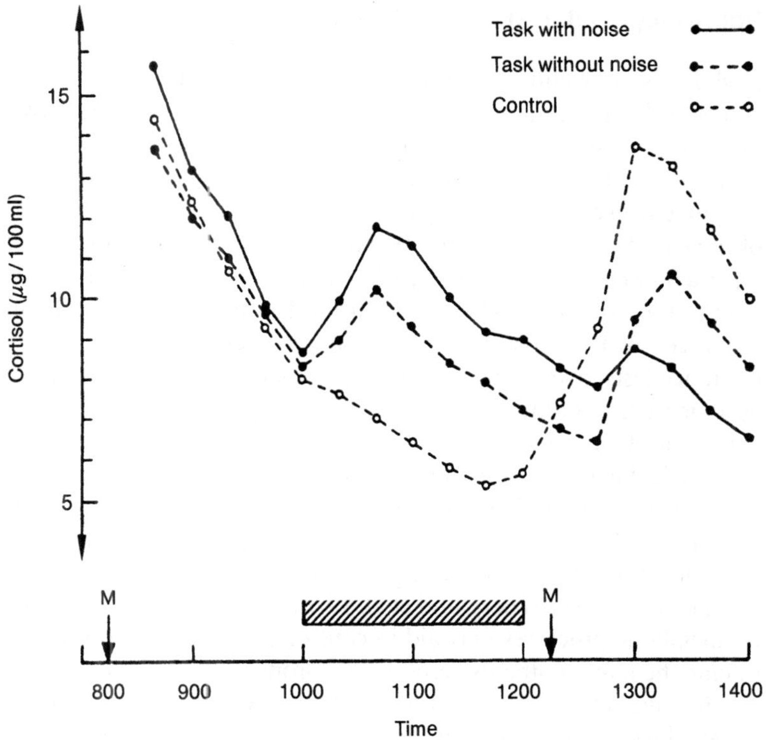

Fig. 6. Mean concentration of cortisol in plasma before, during, and after a short-term memory task under quiet and noisy conditions. *Abscissa* is clock time, and *M* represents meals taken at 8.00 a.m. and approximately 12.15 p.m. *Ordinate* is cortisol concentration in blood (μg/100 ml). Note the progressive morning decline in all sessions before 10.00 a.m. During the task performed either in quiet or noise, the morning decline was interrupted by a brief elevation that was most pronounced in subjects performing the memory task under noisy conditions

Fig. 7. Relation between errors and omissions during task performance and increases in concentration of cortisol in plasma. *Abscissa* is number of errors and omission committed by each individual expressed as a percentage of all responses. *Ordinate* is change in concentration of cortisol during task performance. The *filled circles* represent results obtained during each subject's first experimental session, and the *open circles* represent results obtained during each subject's second experimental session. Note that task-related errors and omissions were correlated with increases in individual maximum concentrations of cortisol in plasma. A significant reduction in the slope for data pertaining to the second session was found whether the task was performed in noise or in quiet

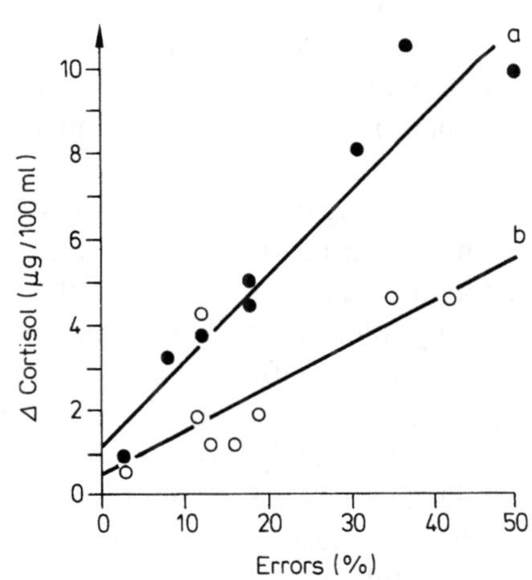

Improving Insulin Action on Metabolic Processes

High levels of insulin concentration in blood, either during fasting or during an oral glucose tolerance test, indicate reduced insulin sensitivity. Any therapeutic measure directed towards insulin-resistant conditions may be assessed from measurements of insulin concentration in blood in relation to glucose concentrations. A decreased insulin/glucose ratio following a therapeutic measure is interpreted as an indicator of increased insulin sensitivity. When glucose concentrations in blood during fasting are between 100 and 140 mg/dl, or glucose concentrations during glucose tolerance testing rise to levels between 120 and 180 mg/dl, glucose tolerance is said to be impaired (WHO Expert Committee on Diabetes Mellitus 1980). Although glucose tolerance tests give little insight to physiological mechanisms, they have been used as a measure of improvement following therapeutic measures designed to improve carbohydrate metabolism.

Physical inactivity and obesity both impair glucose tolerance and insulin sensitivity. In addition, individuals with arterial hypertension have been reported to be more often obese with impaired glucose tolerance and to have higher levels of insulin concentration in blood during fasting than individuals with normal levels of arterial blood pressure (Berglund et al. 1976). Consequently, improving insulin action on metabolic processes may aid in control of arterial blood pressure as well as reducing the risk for atherosclerosis and coronary heart disease.

Berglund et al. (1976) reported studies of body fat, body cell mass, fasting blood sugar, glucose tolerance, and insulin concentrations in blood for 106 hypertensive males aged 47-54 years. Similar studies were performed in a control group of 41 normotensive men 50 years in age. The hypertensive subjects were more often obese, more often had impaired glucose tolerance, and had higher levels of insulin concentration in blood. Differences between the groups remained when the hypertensive subjects were matched for percentage body fat with the normotensive controls. In addition, there was a weak, but significant, positive linear correlation between systolic blood pressure and levels of glucose concentration in blood 1 h after oral glucose loading when the two groups of men were combined (Campbell et al. 1975). The presence of high levels of insulin concentration in blood and decreased glucose tolerance in association with high levels of arterial blood pressure suggests that neuroendocrine function might influence blood pressure control as well as glucose metabolism.

Increasing physical activity and reducing body weight are therapeutic measures commonly used to improve glucose tolerance in obese individuals with non-insulin-dependent diabetes mellitus. Although diet and exercise are commonly prescribed, the physiological mechanisms involved in improving glucose tolerance are not well understood. Confusion arises because confounding factors such as endogenous insulin production, insulin sensitivity, relative body weight, and level of physical fitness are frequently unspecified.

Dietary changes which result in body weight reduction have been reported to improve glucose tolerance in middle-aged men. Lindgarde et al. (1982) performed glucose tolerance tests in 14 subjects before and 6 months after dietary changes involving substitution of complex carbohydrates for simple carbohydrates, reduced intake of saturated fat, substitution of polyunsaturated for saturated fat, and moder-

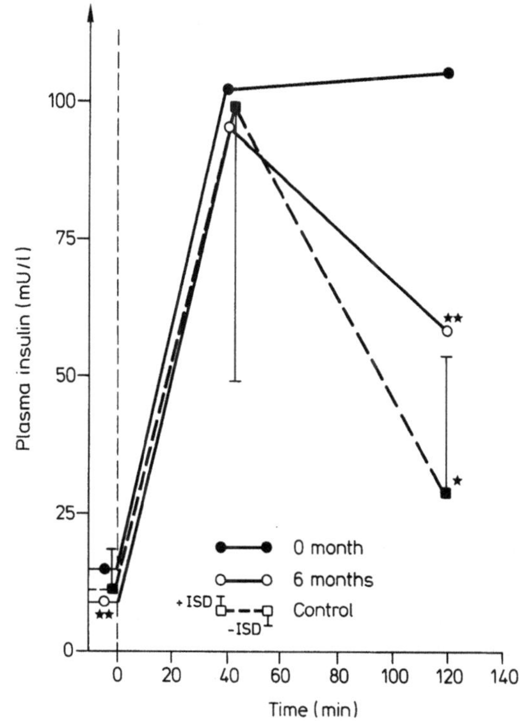

Fig. 8. Concentration of insulin in plasma at rest and during oral glucose tolerance test before and after 6 months of dietary changes and reductions in body weight for experimental subjects and concentration at rest and during oral glucose tolerance tests for control subjects. Note that dietary changes and reductions in body weight were associated with lower mean values for insulin concentrations in blood before and 120 min after the oral glucose tolerance test

ate caloric restriction. Body weight was reduced by 6.4 kg, physical work capacity was unchanged, and fasting levels of glucose and insulin concentration in blood were lowered. As shown in Fig. 8, levels of insulin concentration in blood during an oral glucose tolerance test were reduced towards normal values. The lack of any change in physical work capacity indicated that no changes in patterns of exercise or measures of physical fitness occurred during the study.

Regular exercise, which has a physical conditioning effect, does increase glucose tolerance and increase insulin sensitivity in obese subjects even without change in body weight or percentage body fat. Bjorntorp et al. (1977) reported results of studies with four men and four women who were severely obese. Before training, the obese subjects had decreased glucose tolerance, high levels of insulin concentration in blood, and elevated free fatty acid concentrations in blood. Exercise training consisted of 1-h sessions conducted three times each week for 6 weeks. Maximal oxygen consumption increased from 2.76 to 3.28 liters/min. Body weight, percentage body fat, and glucose tolerance were not changed. However, levels of insulin concentration in blood decreased, indicating increased insulin sensitivity. In addition, urinary cortisol output was decreased after physical conditioning in the obese subjects. These results suggest that physical conditioning may influence insulin sensitivity through a decrease in cortisol secretion.

Results of these clinical studies indicate that insulin sensitivity can be improved by changes in physical activity and diet. Although physical conditioning improves glucose tolerance and increases insulin sensitivity, the combination of regular exercise with weight reduction and restriction of fat in the diet has the most likelihood of reducing the risk for atherosclerosis and coronary heart disease.

Summary

The neuroendocrine mechanisms contributing to atherosclerosis apparently confound the association of genetic factors and traditional risk factors with development of atherosclerosis and coronary heart disease. High levels of insulin concentration in blood in proportion to glucose concentration indicate increased risk for atherosclerosis, and high levels of cortisol concentration in blood reduce insulin sensitivity. High circulating levels of insulin concentration may promote atherogenesis by direct effects on vascular smooth muscle proliferation and indirect effects through elevating circulating levels of triglyceride concentration and low-density lipoprotein concentration in blood. Evaluating the link between behavioral factors and atherogenesis, which may include alterations of insulin sensitivity, might be aided by measurements of hemoglobin A1c, measurements of insulin receptor concentration and affinity in red blood cells and monocytes, and the measurement of insulin/glucose ratios in blood (Koenig and Cerami 1980).

Behavioral influences which elicit strong neuroendocrine responses have also been identified. Tasks which elicit intense efforts to cope enhance secretion of cortisol and catecholamines. However, the situations which produce enduring neuroendocrine responses under normal daily conditions have not been identified.

Improving insulin sensitivity as a therapeutic approach to atherosclerosis would involve both physiological and behavioral measures. Physiological measures would include physical conditioning, control of body weight, and reducing dietary intake of saturated fat. Behavioral measures might include cognitive restructuring, relaxation training, increasing competence in performing daily tasks, and conditioning physiological responses to provocative situations.

References

Alford FP, Martin FL, Pearson MJ (1971) The significance and interpretation of mildly abnormal oral glucose tolerance. Diabetologia 7: 173-180

Armstrong DB, Dublin LI, Wheatley GM, Marks HH (1951) Obesity and the relation to health and disease. JAMA 147: 1007-1014

Bar RS, Gordon P, Roth J, Kahn CR, DeMeyts P (1976) Fluctuations in the affinity and concentration of insulin receptors on circulating monocytes of obese patients. J Clin Invest 58: 1123-1135

Bar RS, Harrison LC, Muggeo M (1979) Regulation of insulin receptors in normal and abnormal physiology in humans. Adv Intern Med 24: 23-52

Beck Neilson H, DePirro R, Pederson O (1980) Prednisone increases the number of insulin receptors on monocytes from normal subjects. J Clin Endocrinol Metab 50: 1-4

Berglund G, Larsson B, Andersson O, Larsson O, Svardsudd K, Bjorntorp P, Wilhelmsen L (1976) Body composition and glucose metabolism in hypertensive middle-aged males. Acta Med Scand 200: 163-169

Bjorntorp P, Holm G, Jacobsson B, Schiller-de-Jounge K, Lundberg P, Sjostrom L, Smith U, Sullivan L (1977) Physical training in human hyperplastic obesity. IV. Effects on the hormonal status. Metabolism 26: 319-328

Brandenberger G, Follenius M, Wittersheim G, Salame P (1980) Plasma catecholamines and pituitary adrenal hormones related to mental task demand under quiet and noise conditions. Biol Psychol 10: 239-244

Campbell IT, Jarrett RJ, Keen H (1975) Diurnal and seasonal variation in oral glucose tolerance: studies in the Antarctic. Diabetologia 11: 139

Chait A, Bierman EL, Albers JJ (1978) Regulatory role of insulin in the degradation of low density lipoprotein by cultured human skin fibroblasts. Biochim Biophys Acta 529: 292-299

Cherrington AD, Williams PE, Harris MS (1978) Relationship between the plasma glucose levels and glucose uptake in the conscious dog. Metabolism 27: 787-791

Christiansen I, Deckert T, Kjerulf K, Mitgaard K, Worning H (1968) Glucose tolerance, plasma lipids and serum insulin with ischaemic heart disease. Acta Med Scand 184: 283-287

Czech MP (1981) Insulin action. Am J Med 70: 142-150

Davis HA, Gass GC, Bassett JR (1981) Serum cortisol response to incremental work in experienced and naive subjects. Psychosom Med 43: 127-132

Dawber TR, Moore FE, Mann GV (1957) Coronary heart disease in the Framingham Study. Am J Public Health 47 [Suppl]: 4-24

DeFronzo RA, Tobin JD, Andres R (1979) Glucose clamp technique: method for quantifying insulin secretion and resistance. Am J Physiol 237: E214-E223

Ducimetiere P, Eschwege E, Papoz L, Richard JL, Claude JR, Rosselin G (1980) Relationship of plasma insulin levels to the incidence of myocardial infarction and coronary heart disease mortality in a middle-aged population. Diabetologia 19: 205-210

Eigler N, Sacca L, Sherwin RS (1979) Synergistic interactions of physiologic increments of glucagon, epinephrine, and cortisol in the dog. Clin Invest 63: 114-123

Epstein FH (1967a) Some uses of prospective observations in the Tecumseh Community Health Study. Proc R Soc Med 60: 56-61

Epstein FM (1967b) Hyperglycaemia - a risk factor in coronary heart disease. Circulation 36: 609-619

Fantus IG, Ryan J, Hizaka N, Gorden P (1981) The effect of glucocorticoids on the insulin receptor: an *in vivo* and *in vitro* study. J Clin Endocrinol Metab 52: 959-960

Flier JS (1983) Insulin receptors and insulin resistance. Annu Rev Med 34: 145-160

Fredrickson DS, Goldstein JL, Brown MS (1978) The familial hyperlipoproteinemias. In: Stanbury JB, Wyngaarden JB, Fredrickson DS (eds) The metabolic basis of inherited disease. McGraw-Hill, New York, pp 604-655

Garcia MJ, NcNamara PM, Gordon T, Kannel WB (1974) Morbidity and mortality in diabetics in the Framingham population - sixteen year follow-up study. Diabetes 23: 105-111

Gavin JR III, Roth J, Neville DM Jr, DeMeyts P, Buell DN (1974) Insulin-dependent regulation of insulin receptor concentrations: a direct demonstration in cell culture. Proc Natl Acad Sci USA 71: 84-88

Gertler MM, Leetma HE, Saluste E, Rosenberger JL, Guthrie RG (1972) Ischemic heart disease - insulin, carbohydrate and lipid interelationships. Circulation 46: 103-111

Gordon T, Castelli WP, Hjortland MC, Kannell WB, Dawber TR (1977) High density lipoprotein as a protective factor against coronary heart disease: the Framington Study. Am J Med 62: 707-714

Harrison L, Flier JS (1980) Secondary Diabetes. Raven, New York, pp 269-286

Himsworth HP, Kerr RB (1939) Insulin-sensitive and insulin-insensitive types of diabetes mellitus. Clin Sci 4: 119-152

Jarvelainen H, Halme T, Ronnema T (1982) Effects of cortisol on the proliferation and protein synthesis of human aortic smooth muscles cells in culture. Acta Med Scand [Suppl] 660: 114-122

Jenkins CD, Rosenman RH, Zyanski SJ (1974) Prediction of clinical coronary heart disease by a test for the coronary-prone behavior pattern. N Engl J Med 290: 1271-1275

Kashyap L, Magill F, Rojes L, Hoffman MM (1970) Insulin and nonesterified fatty acid metabolism in asymptomatic diabetics and atherosclerotic subjects. Can Med Assoc J 102: 1165-1169

Keen H, Rose G, Pyke DA, Boyns D, Clouverakis C, Mistry S (1965) Blood sugar and arterial disease. Lancet 2: 505-508

Koenig RJ, Cerami A (1980) Hemoglobin A(Ic) and diabetes mellitus. Annu Rev Med 31: 129-134
Kolterman OG, Insel J, Saekow M, Olefsky JM (1980) Mechanisms of insulin resistance in human obesity. J Clin Invest 65: 1273-1284
Lindgarde F, Erikkson KF, Lithell H, Saltin B (1982) Coupling between dietary changes, reduced body weight, muscle fibre size and improved glucose tolerance in middle-aged men with impaired glucose tolerance. Acta Med Scand 212: 99-106
Logan RL, Thomson M, Riemersma RA, Oliver MF, Olsson AG, Rossner S, Callmer E, Walldius G, Kaijser L, Carlson LA, Lockerbie L, Lutz W (1978) Risk factors for ischaemic heart-disease in normal men aged 40 (Edinburgh-Stockholm). Lancet 1: 949-955
Malherbe C, DeGasparo M, Berthet P, DeHertogh R, Hoett JJ (1970) The pattern of plasma insulin response to glucose in patients with a previous myocardial infarction - the respective effects of age and disease. Eur J Clin Invest 1: 265-270
Merimee TJ, Pulkkinen AJ, Loften S (1976) Increased insulin binding by lymphocyte receptors induced by β-OH butyrate. J Clin Endocrinol Metab 43: 1190-1192
Muggeo M, Bar RS, Roth J (1977) Change in affinity of insulin receptors following oral glucose in normal adults. J Clin Endocrinol Metab 44: 1206-1209
Nikkila EA, Miettinen AA, Vesenne MR, Pelkonen R (1965) Plasma insulin in coronary heart disease. Lancet 2: 508-511
Olefsky JM (1976) Decreased insulin binding to adipocytes and circulating monocytes from obese subjects. J Clin Invest 57: 1165-1172
Ostrander LD, Francis R, Hayner NS, Kjelsberg MO, Epstein FH (1965) The relationship of cardiovascular disease to hyperglycemia. Ann Intern Med 62: 1188-1198
Pyorola K (1979) Relationship of glucose tolerance and plasma insulin to the incidence of coronary heart disease: results from two population studies in Finland. Diabetes Care 2: 131-141
Reardon MF, Fidge NH, Nestel PJ (1978) Catabolism of very low density lipoprotein B apoprotein in man. J Clin Invest 61: 850-860
Ross R, Glomset JA (1973) Arteriosclerosis and the arterial smooth muscle cell. Science 180: 1332-1339
Ross R, Glomset J, Kariya B, Harker L (1974) A platelet-dependent serum factor that stimulates the proliferation of arterial smooth muscle cells *in vitro*. Proc Natl Acad Sci USA 71: 1207-1210
Roth J (1973) Peptide hormone binding to receptors: a review of direct studies *in vitro*. Metabolism 22: 1059-1073
Roth J, Kahn CR, Lesniak MA, Gorden R, DeMeyers P, Megyesi K, Neville DM Jr, Gavin JR III, Soll AH, Freychet P, Goldfine ID, Bar RS, Archer JA (1975) Receptors for insulin, NSILA-s, and growth hormone: applications to diseases states in man. Recent Prog Horm Res 31: 95-139
Santen RJ, Willis PW, Fajans SS (1972) Atherosclerosis in diabetes mellitus. Arch Intern Med 130: 833-843
Shamoon H, Soman V, Sherwin R (1980) The influence of acute physiological increments of cortisol on fuel metabolism and insulin binding to monocytes in normal humans. J Clin Endocrinol Metab 50: 495-500
Soman V, Shamoon H, Sherwin R (1980) Effects of physiological infusion of epinephrine in normal humans: relationship between the metabolic response and β-adrenergic binding. J Clin Endocrinol Metab 50: 294-297
Stamler J, Epstein FH (1972) Coronary heart disease: risk factors as guides to preventive action. Prev Med 1: 27-48
Steiner G, Murase T (1975) Triglyceride turnover: a comparison of simultaneous determinations using the radioglyceride and lipolytic rate procedures. Fed Proc 34: 2258-2262
Steiner G, Vranic M (1982) Hyperinsulinemia and hypertriglyeridemia, a vicious cycle with atherogenic potential. Int J Obes 6: 117-124
Steiner G, Morita S, Vranic M (1980) Resistance to insulin but not to glucagon in lean human hypertriglyceridemics. Diabetes 29: 899-905
Stout RW (1977a) The relationship of abnormal circulating insulin levels to atherosclerosis. Atherosclerosis 27: 1-13
Stout RW (1977b) The effect of insulin and glucose on sterol synthesis in cultured rat arterial smooth muscle cells. Atherosclerosis 27: 271-278
Stout RW (1981) The role of insulin in atherosclerosis in diabetics and nondiabetics. Diabetes 30: 54-57

Stout RW (1982) Hyperinsulinaemia as an independent risk factor for atherosclerosis. Int J Obes 1: 111-115

Stout RW, Bierman EL, Ross R (1975) Effect of insulin on the proliferation of cultured primate arterial smooth muscle cells. Circ Res 36: 319-327

Streja DA, Marliss EB, Steiner G (1977) The effects of prolonged fasting on plasma triglyceride kinetics in man. Metabolism 26: 505-516

Taggart H, Stout RW (1980) Control of DNA synthesis in cultured vascular endothelial and smooth muscle cells - response to serum, platelet-deficient serum, lipid-free serum, insulin and oestrogens. Atherosclerosis 37: 549-557

Thomopoulos P, Kosmakos FC, Pastan I, Lovelace E (1977) Cyclic AMP increases the concentration of insulin receptors in cultured fibroblasts and lymphocytes. Biochem Biophys Res Commun 75: 246-252

Tzagournis M, Chiles R, Ryan JM, Skillman TG (1968) Interrelationships of hyperinsulinism and hypertriglyeridemia in young patients in coronary heart disease. Circulation 38: 1156-1163

West KM (1978) Specific morbid effects (complications): atherosclerosis and related disorders. In: West KM (ed) Epidemiology of Diabetes and Its Vascular Lesions. Elsevier, New York, pp 353-402

WHO Expert Committee on Diabetes Mellitus (1980) Second report. Technical report series 646. World Health Organization, Geneva

Yasuda K, Kitabchi AE (1980) Decreased insulin binding of human erythrocytes after dexamethasone or prednisone ingestion. Diabetes 29: 811-814

Zilversmit DB (1979) Atherogenesis: a postprandial phenomenon. Circulation 60: 473-485

Some Working Hypotheses on the Significance of Behaviorally Evoked Cardiovascular Reactivity to Pathophysiology

P. A. Obrist, K. C. Light, A. Sherwood, M. T. Allen,[1] A. W. Langer,[2] and J. P. Koepke[3]

Introduction

A guiding hypothesis inherent in research on the role of behavioral influences in the etiology of cardiovascular pathophysiology is that repeated occurrences of environmentally induced myocardial, vascular, and blood pressure (BP) reactivity is the means by which life's events are translated into the disease process (Folkow 1982). While this assumption appears to have a certain face validity, there is evidence to indicate that reactivity *per se* does not have invariable pathophysiological consequences, since there are circumstances where reactivity serves a necessary adaptive function. For example, pressor responses facilitate tissue perfusion when one exercises (Obrist 1981) or changes state from sleep to awake (Floras et al. 1978). On other occasions, reactivity may reflect nothing more than a momentary disruption in the efficiency with which the individual adjusts cardiovascularly to the ever-changing events in the interaction of the organism and its environment (Obrist et al. 1970; Obrist 1984). The most definitive evidence implicating this interaction, and hence reactivity, in the development of cardiovascular disease, is from animal models (Lawler et al. 1981; Anderson et al. 1983; Kaplan et al. 1983; Manuck et al. 1983). But caution must be exerted in generalizing from such data, since we are not certain how much one can liken these models to the human condition. This paper is intended first to briefly overview some of the evidence which places some reservations on this hypothesis, and secondly to propose some specific hypotheses that attempt to provide a perspective of how we might better decipher when reactivity has the pathophysiological consequences we seek to ascertain. This discussion is most relevant to the hypertensive process but is also applicable to coronary heart disease, to the extent that hypertension is instrumental in the development of atherosclerosis.

First, it is necessary to emphasize that we are dealing with working hypotheses which are amenable to evaluation even in the human organism. While using humans places restraints on our methodology, generally restricting the assessment of visceral processes to the use of noninvasive procedures, this does not indicate that we should not use such a methodology. It does require a degree of caution and awareness of the error of measurement in the technology, and sometimes the resolve to settle for part truths.

1 University of North Carolina at Chapel Hill, North Carolina, USA
2 Department of Psychology, University of Syracuse, Syracuse, New York, USA
3 Department of Physiology, University of Iowa, Iowa City, Iowa, USA
(Correspondence should be addressed to Paul A. Obrist, Medical Research Building A. 218-H, Medical School, University of North Carolina at Chapel Hill, Chapel Hill 27514, North Carolina, USA)

Biological and Psychological Factors
in Cardiovascular Disease
Ed. by T. H. Schmidt, T. M. Dembroski, and G. Blümchen

Also, it has become apparent that those of us with our roots in behavioral science have commonly failed to understand the critical role the cardiovascular system plays in maintaining homeostatic processes. But those of us whose roots are in cardiovascular physiology and medicine have all too often ignored the continuous interaction of the organism with the world around it (Obrist 1981). Yet, how do we decipher this environment-organism interaction and its cardiovascular consequences?

Many of us have been raised on the notion that the sympathetic innervation of the cardiovascular system can appreciably modify its activity, particularly in emergencies such as Cannon's flight-fight syndrome. But this is only a starting point, and its functional significance and pathophysiological consequences have not proven obvious. We propose to start even more basically and attempt first to decipher the extent to which cardiovascular adjustments in the behaving individual represent an efficient and effective adjustment with regard to metabolic homeostasis. This is well documented when a physical demand is placed on the individual, as with exercise (Obrist 1981), where increased cardiac output (CO), blood flow in the active muscles, and BP can be enormous, although such adjustments are not considered to have pathophysiological consequences. However, these are not the usual circumstances encountered in the cariovascular psychophysiology laboratory, or, for that matter, under most conditions of real life when no great metabolic expenditure is required. Yet, the cardiovascular system is not insensitive to these other events and can evidence appreciable changes without obvious metabolic requirements. For example, it is now documented by the use of indwelling catheters that the BP is quite variable, even in normotensive individuals, over a wide variety of daily nonphysical activities, with the BP values reaching hypertensive levels in most (Bevan et al. 1969; Littler et al. 1975; Mancia and Zanchetti 1983). We have observed a similar degree of variability in young adult humans to a variety of laboratory situations as evaluated by myocardial as well as BP reactivity (Pollak and Obrist 1983). As Julius (1977) has pointed out with regard to borderline hypertensives, it is unlikely that the variability of the BP is a forerunner of hypertension in more than a minority of individuals. Almost any novel event can momentarily alter the BP (e.g., phasic anticipatory effects, Obrist et al. 1974). But since we do not all become hypertensive, the reactivity of the BP per se carries unknown significance. There are probably individuals and occasions where episodic elevations of the BP serve no other function than to sustain blood flow, such as when we arise from sleep (Littler et al. 1975; Floras et al. 1978). Blood pressure fluctuations may also reflect nothing more than "noise" in the system, whereby the interaction of its determinants; e.g., the cardiac output (CO) and vascular resistance, do not quite adjust in some sort of efficient synchrony, but where the consequences are minimal.

Focus of Investigation into BP Regulation

There is a strategy which might facilitate the resolution of these uncertainties. Essential hypertension has been viewed as a disorder of BP regulation involving an elevation of peripheral resistance in the presence of a normal CO (Freis 1960; Folkow 1982). There is also some consensus that the etiological process may involve any number of interacting influences which may be initiated by a variety of events whose significance is no longer obvious once hypertension is established, such as an initial elevated CO observed in some borderline hypertensives (Folkow 1982; Lund-Johansen 1983). Our task is to decipher when the control of the BP is faulty, such that there develops vascular consequences which sustain an elevated BP. In the light of the complexity of BP control it is reasonable for any given investigative effort to focus on only some ways in which disregulation might occur, knowing full well that one is dealing with only part of the scenario. This is no easy chore, since one can never be certain whether any disregulation is acute and short lived, or one involving more permanent disruption of regulation. Only long-term prospective studies can definitively resolve this issue, which may become deserving as we decipher mechanisms of BP control. Nonetheless, there are some leads from which two aspects of our research were derived. However, it should be borne in mind that we are working with young adult humans, who at this point in their life infrequently evidence elevated casual or resting BP; if they do, it is episodic, commonly only occurring when they are first exposed to the laboratory procedures (Obrist 1981; Obrist and Light 1984). This population is used on the assumption that any disregulation in BP control has as yet minimally influenced those processes which would act to sustain the BP at more elevated levels and thus cloud the etiological picture. It is immaterial, in one sense, whether the BP control mechanisms we hope to decipher should prove relevant to the etiological process. It is more important that we clarify BP control in the healthy behaving organism, believing that only such fundamental understanding, will point to the ways disregulation might occur. How can we understand disregulation if we do not understand regulation?

The two aspects of BP control we are focusing on concern myocardial and renal influences. This focus was suggested by clinical observations in individuals showing a marginally elevated BP, where there is evidence that an elevated CO mediated by increased beta-adrenergic drive is seen in a certain percentage of such individuals (Frohlich 1977; Lund-Johansen 1983). Second, there is evidence that the hypertensive process is either the result of or aggravated by the inability of the kidneys to maintain sodium balance efficiently (Doyle et al. 1980; Guyton 1980). In either case the potential for disregulation is appreciable because if either the myocardium or kidney adjust such that the heart is pumping too much blood or the kidney retaining excessive amounts of sodium relative to metabolic requirements, the consequences have been speculated to increase the peripheral resistance in various ways (Obrist 1981; Light and Obrist 1985). Our focus is on establishing whether laboratory-controlled stressors can modify myocardial and renal events in this manner. This may appear to some as proving the obvious, but a survey of relevant literature indicates little concern with neurohumoral control of myocardial and renal functioning in consciously behaving normotensive young adult humans. The survey revealed that a great deal had been left to assumption, and there were striking inconsistencies in the literature or very incomplete evidence (Obrist 1976, 1981; Obrist et al. 1974).

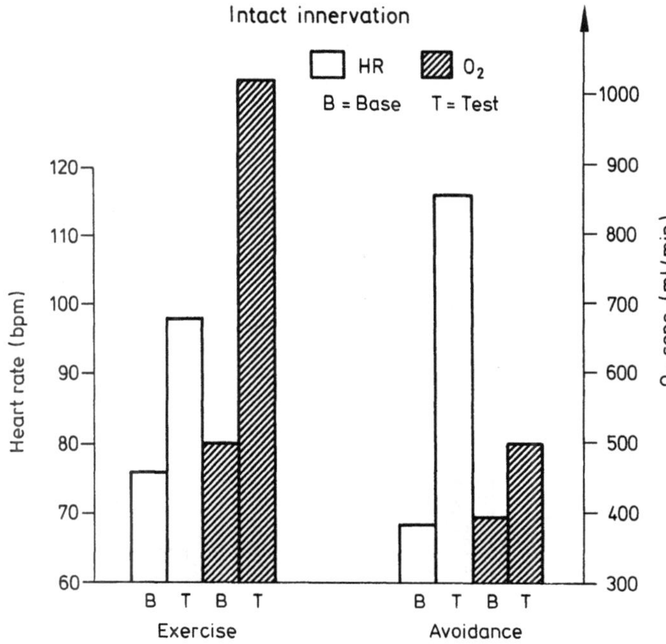

Fig. 1. Mean HR *(open bars)* and O_2 consumption *(checkered bars)* during baseline *(B)*, isotonic exercise *(T)*, and shock avoidance *(T)* in one reactive subject with the cardiac innervations intact. After Langer et al. 1984b)

Influence of Myocardial Adjustment on BP Regulation

First, consider the myocardial adjustments. Behavioral events seem to involve various degrees of engagement of the cardiac innervations. For example, during classic aversive conditioning phasic decreases in heart rate (HR), resulting from increased vagal excitation, mask sympathetic acceleratory effects, whereas phasic increases in HR are primarily due to a loss of vagal tone (Obrist et al. 1965). However, reasonably unequivocal sympathetic influences became obvious once individuals were placed in situations where they had to cope actively, and when attention was focused on the more reactive subjects (Obrist et al. 1974, 1978, 1979; Light and Obrist 1980, 1983; Obrist 1981; Light 1984; Obrist and Light 1984). They were seen not only in regard to HR but also in several indirect indices of myocardial contractility, as attested to by the effects of pharmacological antagonists such as beta-adrenergic blockade. Even then how can such myocardial be implicated in BP disregulation? First, the SBP tends to covary directly with the myocardial events (Obrist et al. 1978; Obrist 1981; Light 1984). However, such a relationship is at best suggestive. Second, and more importantly, recent data indicate that these myocardial events occur in the absence of any appreciable change in metabolic requirements as assessed by oxygen (O_2) consumption (Langer et al. 1985a). That is to say, they are metabolically excessive or inappropriate. This was seen with regard to HR (Langer et al. 1986), as well as the CO when the latter was evaluated by aortic blood flow in dogs (Langer et al. 1979) and impedance cardiography in humans (unpublished data; see also Lan-

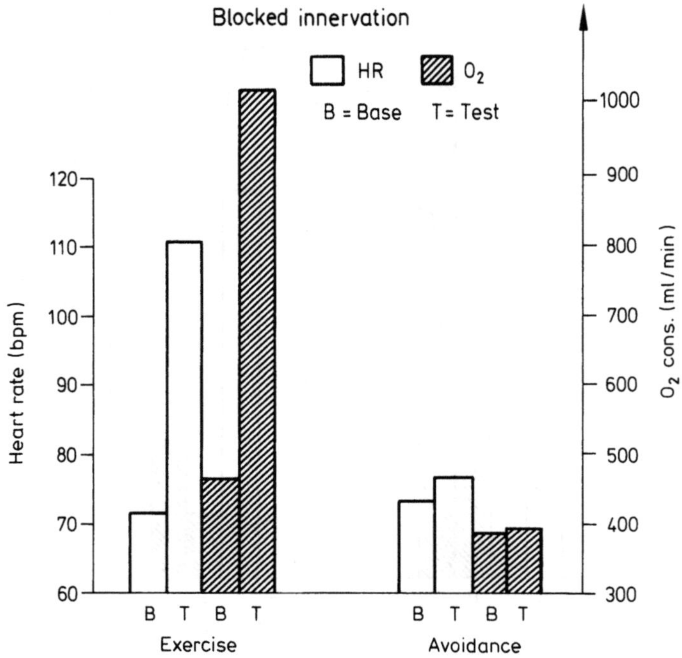

Fig. 2. Mean HR *(open bars)* and O_2 consumption *(checkered bars)* during baseline *(B)* isotonic exercise *(T)* and shock avoidance *(T)* in one subject with the adrenergic cardiac innervations blocked. (After Langer et al. 1984b)

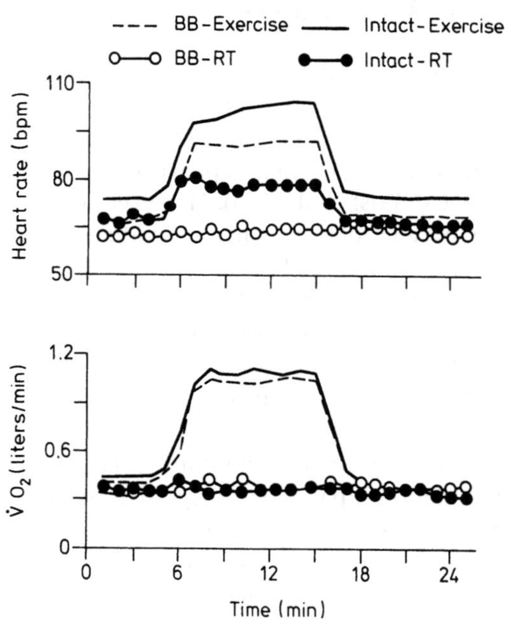

Fig. 3. HR and O_2 consumption during exercise and a shock avoidance task. Both tasks have a 10-min duration commencing at minute 6. *(BB,* beta blockade; *RT,* shock avoidance reaction time task. (After Langer et al. 1984b)

ger et al. 1985b). Such effects are most obvious in the more reactive individuals and are not seen once the myocardial adrenergic innervations are blocked pharmacologically.

These data are illustrated for HR and O_2 consumption for individual human subjects in Fig. 1 and 2 and are summarized for all subjects in Fig. 3. Figure 1 is derived from a reactive subject with an intact innervation and illustrates levels of HR and O_2 consumption during baseline and to both a mild level of isotonic exercise and shock avoidance. These data make the point that exercise evokes appreciable increases in O_2 consumption and HR, while the behavioral challenge (shock avoidance) evokes a smaller change in O_2 consumption, but an even greater increase in HR, thus exemplifying what is meant by a metabolically inappropriate adjustment associated with the behavioral stressor. Figure 2 illustrates in one individual the effects of beta-adrenergic blockade on HR and O_2 consumption during isotonic exercise and shock avoidance. During exercise a similar increase in HR and O_2 consumption is seen as with an intact innervation; however, with the adrenergic innervations now blocked, there is no longer any increase in HR.

Figure 3 summarizes the HR and O_2 consumption changes for all subjects during moderate levels of exercise, and illustrates the shock avoidance task by dividing it into two subgroups, one with an intact and another with a blocked beta-adrenergic innervation. During avoidance there is little change in O_2 consumption under either condition, but HR accelerates only with an intact innervation. With exercise, comparable increases in HR and O_2 consumption are observed with or without an intact sympathetic innervation. There are baseline differences in HR, with pharmacological blockade decreasing baseline. Nonetheless, the synergistic loss of vagal tone during exercise appears to compensate for any loss of sympathetic excitation with regard to change in HR from baseline to exercise.

Cardiac output has now been evaluated in humans in relation to O_2 consumption and HR. These data are still being evaluated, but the results so far quantified are consistent with that obtained in dogs, in which CO was measured invasively, and in humans, in whom only HR was evaluated. This study with humans also evaluated O_2 consumption and cardiovascular changes during the cold pressor test because preceding studies indicated that inescapable pain as encountered with this laboratory challenge evokes lesser beta-adrenergic effects than shock avoidance. This in turn is relevant to the issue of whether situations providing an individual with a means to cope actively with the behavioral challenges (shock avoidance) evokes a greater disruption of BP control than situations where the individual cannot control or actively cope with the challenge (cold pressor; Obrist 1981). Data so far evaluated indicate that these stressors evoked small changes in O_2 consumption relative to exercise. Yet, the avoidance task evoked a substantial increase in both CO and HR. While the cold pressor evoked an increase in HR, the change in CO was minimal.

Figure 4 illustrates the relationship between CO and O_2 consumption in one pilot subject. A linear regression line was first computed to depict the relationship between CO and O_2 consumption derived from three levels of isotonic exercise and rest, all evaluated in the sitting position. This serves as a reference for assessing the metabolic justification of CO modifications during the behavioral stressors. Then the points are presented (30-s averages) depicting the CO found during semire-

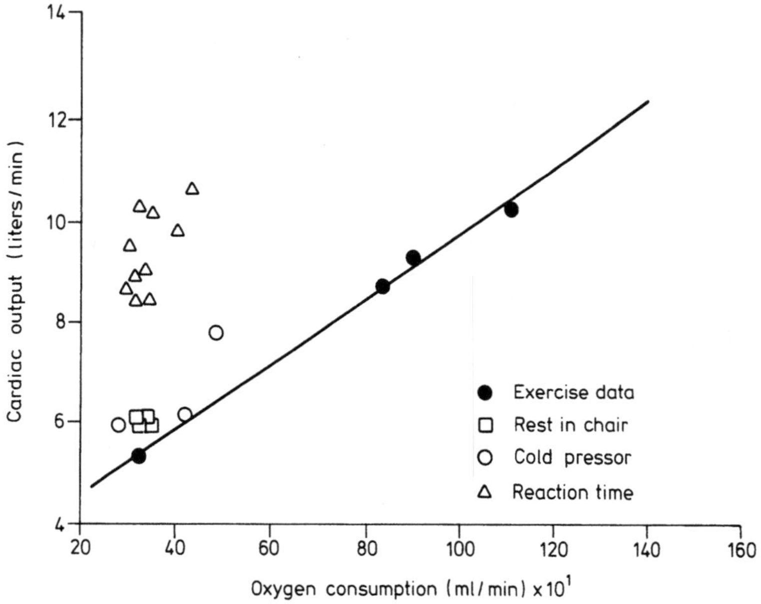

Fig. 4. The relationship between CO and O_2 consumption in one subject during exercise, cold pressor, and shock avoidance. Note O_2 consumption is expressed in units of ml/min × 10^1. Therefore, multiply all values by 10 to achieve actual O_2 consumption

Table 1. Mean CO and O_2 consumption in humans during four baselines, the cold pressor, shock avoidance, and three levels of exercise ($n = 24$)

	CO (liters/min)	O_2 consumption (ml/min)
Rest 1	5.6	248
Cold pressor (min 1-2)	5.6	312
Rest	5.4	255
Avoidance	6.7	303
Rest 3	5.4	264
Rest 4	5.4	260
Exercise		
25 w	7.2	671
50 w	8.8	973
75 w	10.3	1231

clined rest (chair rest), the cold pressor test, and a shock avoidance task, and with respect to O_2 consumption. The CO values during rest and the cold pressor test evidence minimal deviation from the regression line, while those during shock avoidance show a much more pronounced deviation. Thus, CO during avoidance is more or less comparable to that observed during exercise; yet O_2 consumption is similar to that at rest, illustrating in another way what is meant by a metabolically inappropriate cardiovascular adjustment.

Recent data on a group of 24 subjects are summarized in Table 1. Shock avoidance evokes an increase in CO almost comparable to the lowest level of exercise. O_2 consumption increases slightly during avoidance, but it is appreciably less than that seen during the lowest level of exercise. This disproportionate increase in CO relative to O_2 consumption during shock avoidance is most pronounced with the reactive subjects. In the eight more reactive subjects, as defined by the CO difference between baseline (Rest 4, Table 1) and shock avoidance, the increase in CO exceeded that seen during the lowest level of exercise (8.5 vs. 8.2 liters/min); yet O_2 consumption during avoidance was approximately half as great (333 vs. 683 ml/min). The less reactive subjects evidence very comparable and small increases in CO and O_2 consumption during shock avoidance. Thus, while the data averaged over all subjects provides evidence of a disproportionate increase in CO relative to O_2 consumption during avoidance (when compared to exercise), this metabolically inappropriate increase in CO is only pronounced in the more reactive individuals, and not seen during the cold pressor test, regardless of the reactivity dimension.

This evidence of an inappropriately elevated CO relative to O_2 consumption is suggestive of tissue overperfusion, particularly in the more reactive individuals. In conjunction with an elevated BP, conditions are provided which could have both immediate and long-term consequences with respect to vascular events, resulting eventually in an elevated vascular resistance characteristic of established hypertension. There are probably a number of mechanisms which could be involved in such vascular consequences, including functional autoregulation to excessive flow and pressure (Guyton 1980; Folkow 1982), as well as structural smooth muscle hypertrophy (Folkow 1982), and arteriolar rarefaction (Hutchins et al. 1982). However, discussion of these intrinsic mechanisms is beyond the scope of this chapter. It should suffice to emphasize that there are at our disposal guidelines for future inquiry as to the role these stress-induced myocardial events play in the intrinsic control of vascular resistance.

Influence of Renal Functioning on BP Regulation

Our recent work with renal functioning complement these results and points to still another means through which BP control could become disregulated. The data to be cited is primarily from a conscious dog preparation, but there is some human data as well. Renal functioning has not drawn much attention in the behaving individual, and where it has, the focus has been on such events as renal blood flow, events which do not provide a direct assessment of sodium (Na) balance (Grignolo et al. 1982). A necessary first step was to demonstrate whether behavioral challenges could alter Na balance, as assessed by Na excretion rates, and then affect the neurohumoral control of such events as well as their relationship, if any, to myocardial events and BP. To date, the data from dogs indicate that Na excretion rates are blunted by the laboratory stressors, and the mechanism involves primarily tubular reabsorption mediated by neurogenic rather than humoral influences (Grignolo et al. 1982; Koepke et al. 1983; Koepke and Obrist 1985. Furthermore, the magnitude of the decrease in Na excretion covaries inversely with HR and systolic blood pressure (SBP) changes. In other words, Na excretion decreases most in those dogs who

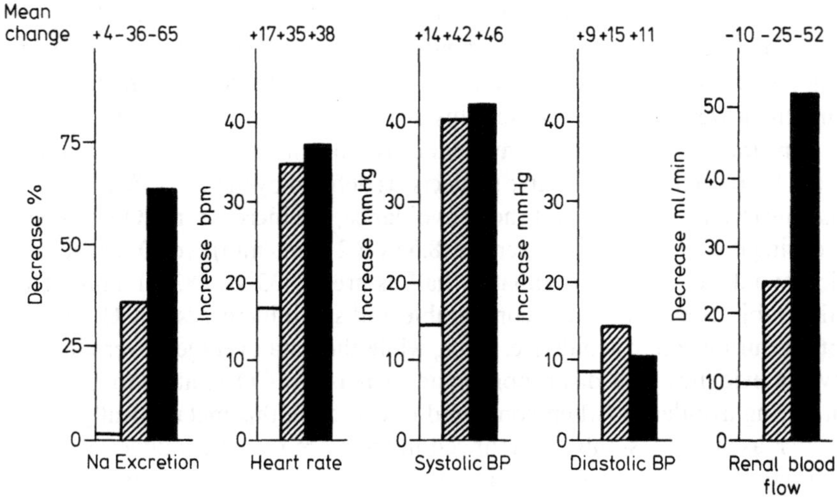

Fig. 5. Average HR, SBP and DBP and RBF changes in dogs ($n=30$) during shock avoidance as a function of the magnitude of Na excretion rate changes. (After Koepke 1982; Koepke et al. 1983)

Table 2. Mean HR and BP, and Na excretion changes during behavioral challenges in humans broken down by HR reactivity and the presence or absence of risk for hypertension based on parental history of hypertension after Light et al. 1983)

Group	HR (bpm)	BP (mmHg)		Change in excretion (%)	
		SBP	DBP	Na	Fluid
Low-risk					
Low HR reactors ($n=6$)	74±3	143±5	91±3	+ 6± 2	− 9±13
High HR reactors ($n=5$)	87±6	159±5	93±2	+12± 5	− 5±15
High-risk					
Low HR reactors ($n=6$)	69±3	142±4	87±2	+ 4± 6	+ 4± 6
High HR reactors ($n=7$)	88±4	159±7	93±3	−27±10	−35±11

exhibit the greatest increase in HR and SBP. The relationship between Na excretion rates and cardiovascular reactivity is summarized in Fig. 5. These data were derived from 30 dogs divided into three equal-size subgroups, ordered by the magnitude of the change in Na excretion during avoidance, i.e., the subgroups depict in the following order those dogs showing no change, intermediate change, and the most decreases in Na excretion, respectively. Appreciable decreases in Na excretion were associated with larger increases in HR and SBP, and greater decreases in renal blood flow (RBF). The relationship between changes in Na excretion rates and these three aspects of cardiovascular function is further indicated by significant correlations between Na excretion and HR ($r=-0.37$), SBP ($r=-0.58$) and RBF ($r=+0.48$). While these relationships between Na excretion, HR, SBP, and RBF are not satisfactorily clarified, the degree of covariation suggests a common mediating mechanism.

In humans, comparable blunting of Na excretion is seen, and it, too, relates to HR and SBP reactivity. However, it is only pronounced in individuals who evidence both HR and SBP reactivity and whom have either a parental history of hypertension and/or are individuals who have evidenced a marginally elevated SBP. This relationship is illustrated in Table 2, where the average HR, SBP, diastolic blood pressure (DBP), and change in Na excretion rates are depicted during challenging, nonaversive laboratory procedures. Four subgroups are shown. First, they were divided into those individuals without (i.e., 10 risk) and those with (i.e., hi risk) a parental history of hypertension (the latter also includes one individual with an elevated casual SBP). Each group was further dichtomized into those showing the highest and lowest HR during the hour-long laboratory challenge. As is apparent from Table 2, neither high levels of HR or SBP nor the presence of a higher risk of hypertension alone are associated with a decrease in Na excretion, but in combination an appreciable decrease is evident (Light et al. 1983).

Discussion and Summary

How do these stress-evoked myocardial and renal events become involved in BP disregulation and the hypertensive process? We do not know with any degree of certainty. They clearly indicate a disruption of metabolic efficiency in that they reflect excessive responses. An increase in the CO is a necessary event when one exercises, and in certain individuals these behavioral stressors elevate the CO to levels comparable to that seen at modest levels of exercise. However, there is no metabolic necessity for such an adjustment. The kidney's handling of Na bears similarities to the CO in that, as we must maintain a given CO in accordance with a given metabolic load, the kidney must retain most of the Na it filters, otherwise the osmolarity of the blood would be compromised. However, these behavioral stressors further augment Na retention without any metabolic necessity, such as Na loss associated with sweating or gastrointestinal disorders, or when one becomes overhydrated, when Na retention would act to maintain plasma osmolarity. Our observations indicate that these myocardial and renal adjustments covary during active coping tasks, suggesting that the exaggeration of normal functioning of two vital organs involved in the control of BP could interact or complement each other. The consequences in the behaving organism remain unknown, but at least when cardiovascular reactivity and the renal handling of Na are evaluated in this context a case can be made that we are dealing with events with a potential to disrupt BP control through their eventual influence on vascular resistance.

In summary, the goal of the research cited is rather straightforward, but the exact path and methodologies are not. Take for example, the exercise-like cardiovascular adjustment observed during active coping tasks [which also includes increased striate muscle blood flow (Brod 1963) and SBP (Sherwood et al. 1986)]. Most aspects of it do not appear to have pathophysiological consequences when one exercises. One principle difference is that peripheral resistance decreases more during exercise (Langer et al. 1979), probably because of the intrinsically mediated vasodilation in the active muscles. The net result is a lower mean BP during exercise. Does this mean that the higher mean BP encountered during the nonmetabolically demanding coping task triggers, over time, more sustained increases in vascular resistance? This would be suggested by the potential for the autoregulation of peripheral blood flow and its long-term consequences. The influence on vascular resistance of

Na retention, in conjunction with these other potentially relevant autoregulatory mechanisms could summate in some fashion (Light and Obrist 1985). The point is that we must decipher the means by which vascular resistance becomes elevated over time. The myocardial and renal effects, and evolving hypothesis outlined, provide a starting point, as well as a means to evaluate the organism-environmental interaction. Finally, since hypertension has been implicated as a risk factor in coronary heart disease, the elucidation of these behaviorally associated mechanisms of BP control seems quite important for determining when elevations of the BP facilitate atherogenesis. To underscore the point, the pronounced myocardial, renal, and BP effects observed during exercise are not considered to carry a risk; thus why should they carry a risk in the stressed but nonexercising organism? The elucidation of BP control should facilitate answers to this question.

Acknowledgment. This research was supported by grants from the National Institutes of Health: HL 18976 to Paul A. Obrist, and RCDA HL 01096 and Research Grant HL 30903 to Kathleen C. Light.

References

Anderson DE, Kearns WD, Better WE (1983) Progressive hypertension in dogs by avoidance conditioning and saline infusion. Hypertension 5: 286-291

Bevan AT, Honour AJ, Stott FH (1969) Direct arterial pressure recording in unresticted man. Clin Sci 36: 329-344

Brod J (1963) Hemodynamic basis of actute pressor reactions and hypertension. Br Heart J 25: 227-245

Doyle AE, Mendelsohn FAO, Morgan TO (1980) Pharmacological and therapeutic aspects of hypertension vol 2. CRC, Boca Raton, Florida, pp 86-96

Floras JS, Jones JV, Johnson JA, Brooks DE, Hassan MO, Sleight P (1978) Arousal and circadian rhythm and blood pressure. Clin Sci Mol Med 55: 395s-397s

Folkow B (1982) Physiological aspects of primary hypertension. Physiol Rev 62: 347-504

Freis ED (1960) Hemodynamics of hypertension. Physiol Rev 40: 27-53

Frohlich ED (1977) Hemodynamics of hypertension. In: Genest J, Koiw E, Kuchel O (eds) Hypertension: physiopathology and treatment. McGraw-Hill, New York, pp 15-49

Grignolo A, Koepke JP, Obrist PA (1982) Renal function and cardiovascular dynamics during treadmill exercise and shock avoidance in dogs. Am J Physiol 242: R 482-R 490

Guyton AC (1980) Arterial blood pressure and hypertension. Saunders, Philadelphia

Hutchins PM, Dusseau JW, Marr MC, Greene AW (1982) The role of arteriolar structural changes in hypertension. In: Henrich H (ed) Microvascular aspects of spontaneous hypertension. Huber, Bern, pp 41-53

Julius S (1977) Borderline hypertension: epidemiologic and clinical implications. In: Genest J, Koiw E, and Kuchel O (eds) Hypertension: physiopathology and treatment. McGraw-Hill, New York, pp 630-640

Kaplan JR, Manuck SB, Clarkson TB, Lusso FM, Taub DM, Miller EW (1983) Social stress and atherosclerosis in normocholesterolemic monkeys. Science 220: 733-735

Koepke JP (1982) Neurohumoral mechanisms of the decreased excretion of sodium and water resulting from behavioral stress in conscious dogs. Ph. D. dissertation, University of North Carolina, Chapel Hill

Koepke JP, Obrist PA (1983) Angiotensin II in the renal excretory response to behavioral stress in conscious dogs. Am J Physiol 245: R 259-R 264

Koepke JP, Light KC, Obrist PA (1983) Neural control of renal excretory function during behavioral stress in conscious dogs. Am J Physiol 245: R 251-R 258

Langer AW, Obrist PA, McCubbin JA (1979) Hemodynamic and metabolic adjustments during exercise and shock avoidance in dogs. Am J Physiol 5: H 225-H 230

Langer AW, Hutcheson JS, Charlton JD, McCubbin JA, Obrist PA, Stoney CM (1985a) On-line minicomputerized measurement of respiratory gas exchange during exercise. Psychophysiology 22: 50-58

Langer AW, McCubbin JA, Stoney CM, Hutcheson JS, Charlton JD, Obrist PA (1985b) Cardiopulmonary adjustments during exercise and an aversive reaction time task: effects of beta-adrenoceptor blockade. Psychophysiology 22: 59-68

Langer AW, Stoney CM, Obrist PA, Sutterer JR (1986) The integration and differentiation of cardiovascular and metabolic responses to stress. In: Grossman P, Janssen K, Vaitl D (eds) Cardiovascular-somatic-respiratory interactions in psychophysiology. (NATO Advanced Study Institute). Plenum, New York, pp 59-68

Lawler JE, Barker GF, Hubbard JW, Schaub RG (1981) Effects of stress on blood pressure and cardiac pathology in rats with borderline hypertension. Hypertension 3: 496-505

Light KC (1984) Cardiovascular and renal responses to competitive mental challenges. In: Orlebeke JF, Mulder G, van Doornen LJP (eds) Cardiovascular psychophysiology: theory and methods. Proceedings of the 1983 international conference, Noordwijkerhout, The Netherlands. Plenum, New York

Light KC, Obrist PA (1980) Cardiovascular response to stress: effects of opportunity to avoid, shock experience and performance feedback. Psychophysiology 17: 243-252

Light KC, Obrist PA (1983) Task difficulty, heart rate reactivity and cardiovascular response to an appetitive reaction time task. Psychophysiology 20: 39-115

Light KC and Obrist PA (1985) Renal and cardiovascular effects of psychological stress and sodium intake. In: Katkin ES and Manuck SB (eds) Advances in Behavioral Medicine. Jai, London, pp 89-114

Light KC, Koepke JP, Obrist PA, Willis PW (1983) Psychological stress induces sodium and fluid retention in men at high risk for hypertension. Science 219: 429-431

Littler WA, Honour AJ, Carter RD, Sleight P (1975) Sleep and blood pressure. Br Med J 3: 346-348

Lund-Johansen P (1983) Hemodynamic alterations in early essential hypertension: recent advances. In: Gross F, Strasser T (eds) Mild hypertension: recent advances. Raven, New York, pp 237-249

Mancia G, Zanchetti H (1983) Blood pressure variability and the assessment of BP: Implications for epidemiological research and for treatment. In: Gross F, Strasser T (eds) Mild hypertension: recent advances. Raven, New York, 251-262

Manuck SB, Kaplan JR, Clarkson TB (1983) Behaviorally induced heart rate reactivity and atherosclerosis in Cynomolgus monkeys. Psychosom Med 45: 95-108

Obrist PA (1976) The cardiovascular-behavioral interaction - as it appears today. Psychophysiology 13: 85-107

Obrist PA (1981) Cardiovascular psychophysiology: a perspective. Plenum, New York, p 237

Obrist PA (1984) General overview of the area of cardiovascular psychophysiology in relation to stress and disorders. In: Orlebeke JF, Mulder G, van Doornen LJP (eds) Cardiovascular psychophysiology: theory and methods. Plenum, New York

Obrist PA, Light KC (1984) Active-passive coping and cardiovascular reactivity: interaction with individual differences and types of baseline. In: Baum A, Gordon W, Herd JA (eds) Proceedings of the Academy of Behavioral Medicine Research 1981-82. Academic, New York

Obrist PA, Wood DM, Perez-Reyes M (1965) Heart rate during conditioning in humans: effects of UCS intensity, vagal blockade, and adrenergic block of vasomotor activity. J Exp Psychol 70: 32-42

Obrist PA, Webb RA, Sutterer JR, Howard JL (1970) The cardiac-somatic relationship: some reformulations. Psychophysiology 6: 569-587

Obrist PA, Lawler JE, Howard JO, Smithson KW, Martin PL, Manning J (1974) Sympathetic influences on the heart in humans: effects on contractility and heart rate of acute stress. Psychophysiology 11: 405-427

Obrist PA, Gaebelein CJ, Shanks-Teller E, Langer AW, Grignolo A, Light KC, McCubbin JA (1978) The relationship between heart rate, coratid dP/dt, and blood pressure in humans as a function of the type of stress. Psychophysiology 15: 102-115

Obrist PA, Light KC, McCubbin JA, Hoffer JL (1979) Pulse transit time: relationship to blood pressure and myocardial performance. Psychophysiology 16: 292-301

Pollak MH, Obrist PA (1983) Pulse transit time and ECG Q-wave to pulse wave interval as indices of beat-by-beat blood pressure changes. Psychophysiology 20: 21-28

Sherwood A, Allen MT, Obrist PA, Langer AW (1986) Evaluation of beta-adrenergic influences on cardiovascular and metabolic adjustments to physical and psychological stress. Psychophysiology 23: 89-104

Behavioral Aspects of Cardiovascular Reactivity in Essential Hypertension

M. FREDRIKSON[1]

Ischemic heart disease, myocardial infarction and angina pectoris, are major causes of chronic disease and premature death in most western societies (Alderman 1980). A high arterial blood pressure (BP) increases the risk for development of such cardiovascular-related diseases. Hypertension (HT) affects 10%-20% of the general population (Hypertension Detection and Follow-up Program Cooperative Group). Only 5% of all cases are secondary to organic or endocrine diseases, whereas the remaining 95%, called primary or essential HT, are of unknown origin (Berglund et al. 1976). Page (cf. 1977) put forward a mosaic theory of HT, stating that the disease is multifactorially determined. Some etiological factors that have been studied to a great extent are genetic predisposition (Ayman 1934), excessive salt intake (Dahl 1977), disturbances of the autonomic nervous system (Louis et al. 1973) or the renin-angiotensin-aldosterone system (Laragh et al. 1976), increased reactivity of the arterial vascular smooth muscle (Page 1977), involvement of the kidney (Guyton et al. 1974), the role of personality traits (Harrell 1980) and "stress" (Shapiro et al. 1979). Most students of HT (cf. Pickering 1961; Page 1977; Folkow 1982) agree that the disease is multifactorially determined and that the central nervous system, the autonomic nervous system, the cardiovascular system, and the hormonal system interact in initiating and maintaining essential hypertension. Also, it is generally agreed upon that genetic factors operate, and claims have been made that genetic influences account for anywhere between 30% and 70% of the BP variance (Pickering 1961). Consequently, between 70% and 30% of the variance may be caused by environmental and behavioral factors.

Essential Hypertension, Life-style and the Defense Reaction

Some (see Weiner 1977 for a review) view HT mainly as a psychosomatic disease and suggest that psychosocial or emotional factors are pathophysiologically important in initiating or aggravating the disease. It has been debated whether personality traits (see Harrel 1980 for a review) and life-style (see Shapiro et al. 1979 for a review) affect arterial BP. Some epidemiological studies and experimental models of hypertension have supported the notion that certain circumstances in life affect long-term regulation of BP. For example, hypertension is more prevalent among those having "stressful" occupations compared with less taxing jobs, (Cobb and Rose 1973), and is also more common among men experiencing a discrepancy between job responsibility and level of education than among those experiencing con-

1 Medical Psychology I, Punkthuset, Karolinska Hospital, P.O. Box 60500, S-10401 Stockholm, Sweden

Biological and Psychological Factors in Cardiovascular Disease
Ed. by T.H. Schmidt, T.M. Dembroski, and G. Blümchen

gruence (Theorell and Lind 1973). However, some studies have failed to establish a relationship between "life-stress" and BP (cf. Rahe et al. 1976). Such conflicting evidence may be due to the varying nature of "life-stress" or to different human styles of coping. For example, some transitions in life, such as getting employed, require behavioral activity, whereas others, such as losing a loved one, require passive adaptation. Also, there are probably individual differences in coping styles, the same event being coped with differently by different individuals. After reviewing the epidemiological literature on hypertension, Guttmam and Benson (1971) concluded that life-styles, including frequent behavioral adjustments, are associated with elevated levels of arterial BP.

In animal models of HT, it has been shown that repeated experimental elicitation of the defense reaction, directly through hypothalamic stimulation (Folkow 1982), or indirectly through overcrowding (Henry and Stephens 1977), may lead to the development of sustained HT. In the spontaneously hypertensive rat (SHR), transient pressor episodes elicited as part of the defense reaction are mediated primarily by an increased cardiac output, but translate into sustained high BP mediated by an increased peripheral resistance, resulting from structural vascular hypertrophy (Folkow 1982). This course of development seems to mirror the development of HT in man. Lund-Johansen (1967, 1977) followed borderline hypertensive patients longitudinally and observed that, initially, arterial BP was maintained by an increased cardiac output. Ten years later, BP was unchanged, while cardiac output had declined to a normal level and vascular resistance had increased to a high level. Consequently, the time course of cardiovascular hemodynamics in humans resembles that seen in the SHR during repeated elicitation of the defense reaction.

It is well known that acute emotional reactions and other physiological events may be accompanied by a temporary, and sometimes large increase in arterial BP. The question then arises whether the wear and tear of acute pressor episodes may accumulate and mediate the hypertensive effect of life transitions and coping styles. Therefore, one could ask whether HT patients, compared with normotensive (NT) subjects, show excessive BP reactivity, and if transient pressor episodes to behavioral events predict or eventually cause sustained high BP in genetically susceptible humans. In addition, the question has been raised whether BP reactivity to stimulation is part of a general defense response within the sympathetic nervous system (SNS) or instead is localized only within the cardiovascular system. Furthermore, the question remains whether BP reactivity is determined mainly by endogenous factors and is similar within a single individual in all types of situations, or is exogenous and unique for each situation.

Early studies indicated that HT patients compared with NT controls showed excessive BP reactivity to several different tasks, including the cold pressor test (Hines and Brown 1936), "stressful" interviews (Wolf et al. 1955), and memory tests (Jost et al. 1952). These results implied an endogenous factor as the cause for HT, and claims were made that hyperreactivity predicts development of high BP (Hines and Brown 1936). However, some studies failed to demonstrate reactivity differences between HT and NT (Pickering and Kissing 1935), and contradicted the view that hyperreactivity predicts subsequent hypertension (Harlan et al. 1964). Even though the reactivity concept is central in several theories on the etiology of human HT (Obrist 1981; Steptoe 1981; Folkow 1982; Surwit et al. 1982; v. Eiff 1984) and in animal models of HT (Folkow 1982), the experimental evidence linking human essential HT to early exaggerated BP reactivity is conflicting.

Cardiovascular Reactivity in Retrospect

Ever since a 1932 study by Hines and Brown, a number of studies have included comparisons of BP reactivity in HT and NT to various standardized laboratory manoeuvers, such as the cold pressor test, mental arithmetic, intelligence tests, color word tests, visual puzzles, sensory-motor tasks, interviews with an emotional content, and other social encounters. Table 1 summarizes 66 studies published between 1932 and 1985 on cardiovascular reactivity to behavioral/psychological tasks, but excludes all physiological or pharmacological manipulations (exercise tests, orthostatic tests, infusion studies, etc.). In 36 of 74 laboratory tasks (49%) a reliable systolic hyperresponse was found in HT; 44 of 93 tasks (47%) provoked a greater diastolic change or mean BP in HT than NT. If analyses are restricted to papers presenting statistically significant findings, 25 of 56 tasks (45%) were found to elicit systolic hyperreactivity in HT, and 29 of 70 (41%) tasks were accompanied by greater diastolic reactivity in HT patients than NT controls. Some papers have reported reactions as percent changes, and others as absolute changes. Percent change is chosen since the vasculature in HT shows an increased wall to lumen ratio, and, for geometrical reasons, will respond with a greater increase in arterial pressure to a given vasoconstrictor impulse than any vessel with a decreased ratio. By computing percent change, this factor is controlled for. Five of 16 tasks (31%) elicited a greater percent systolic blood pressure (SBP) change in HT than NT and six of 15 (40%) elicited a greater diastolic blood pressure (DBP) change. Only in three studies did NT show greater systolic or diastolic responses than (Weiner et al. 1962; Sullivan et al. 1981; Linden and Feurstein 1983). During 8 of 51 tasks (16%) heart rate (HR) reactivity was greater in HT than NT, but lower during 6 tasks (12%).

In summary, BP hyperreactivity among HT patients, compared with NT controls, is commonly, but not consistently, observed. Reactivity differences seem to be more readily observed with certain tasks than with others. Studies using sensory-motor manipulations, like motor tracing tasks, sorting of steel balls during noise, and reaction-time tasks have all reported greater BP reactivity in HT than NT. Studies using the cold pressor test have generally (see Table 1) reported only few reactivity differences between HT and NT. Conflicting results could reflect variations in study design, study populations, sampling procedures, drug treatment, or simply indicate that some HT subgroups are hyperreactive, whereas others are not. Furthermore, most studies were performed without any "blinding" procedures, and several did not even include adequate statistical comparisons. In addition, most studies have used a restricted number of tasks, predominantly discomforting stimuli or tasks that require cognitive elaboration. These tasks are associated with the defense reaction, and were called sensory-rejection tasks by the Laceys (Lacey and Lacey 1974). Little use has been made of "sensory-intake" tasks associated with vigilance behavior and outerdirected attention.

Table 1. Summary of studies on cardiovascular reactivity to behavioral challenge in essential hypertension published since 1932[a]

Reference	Groups and initial SBP/DBP or MBP (HR)			Age	Behavioral task/s Δ SBP/DBP or MBP (HR)		Study conclusion SBP/DBP or MBP	HR
					Cold pressor			
Hines and Brown (1932)	11 HT (retinal changes)	150/?	(?)	26–64	38.4/32.5	(?)		
	7 HT (labile, no retinal changes)	122/?	(?)	26–64	32.0/21.0	(?)		
	8 HT (potential)	?/?	(?)	19–44	30.1/21.1	(?)		
	40 NT	103/?	(?)	17–50	8.9/ 7.5	(?)		
					+/+		+/+	?
					Cold pressor			
Briggs and Oerting (1933)	46 HT	?/?	(?)	20–89	15.0/7.1	(?)		
	60 NT	?/?	(?)	20–79	9.9/9.9	(?)		
					+/=		+/=	?
					Cold pressor			
Hines and Brown (1933)	49 HT (retinal changes)	150/?	(?)	24–64	36.7/24.8	(?)		
	21 HT (no retinal changes)	150/?	(?)	24–64	37.2/25.0	(?)		
	18 NT (hyperreactors 16+mmHg)	122/?	(?)	17–40	29.3/23.8	(?)		
	69 NT (normoreactors 0–15 mmHg)	103/?	(?)	15–55	8.6/ 8.1	(?)		
					+/+		+/+	?
					Cold pressor			
Pickering and Kissin (1935)	12 HT	218/126	(?)	54	21/13	(?)		
	7 NT (cardiac enlargement)	120/78	(?)	33	8/ 6	(?)		
	9 NT	130/76	(?)	53	22/11	(?)		
					=/=		=/=	?
					Cold pressor			
Hines and Brown (1936)	66 HT (retinal changes)	?/114	(?)	25–62	47.2/34.3	(?)		
	127 HT (no retinal changes)	?/114	(?)	24–64	34.4/25.4	(?)		
	90 NT (hyperreactors, 22+mmHg SBP or DBP)	?/77	(?)	4–75	29.4/24.5	(?)		
	288 NT (normoreactors, 0–22 mmHg SBP or DBP)	?/66	(?)	4–86	11.4/10.6	(?)		
					⊕/⊕		⊕/⊕	?
					Cold pressor + arm arterial occlusion			
Alam and Smirk (1938)	9 HT	?/?	(?)	?	48/26	(?)		
	5 HT (renal origin)	?/?	(?)	?	21/10	(?)		
	14 NT	?/?	(?)	?	33/20	(?)		
					⊕/⊕		⊕/⊕	?
					Cold pressor			
Ayman and Goldshine (1938)	88 HT	?/?	(?)	50 24–68	33.5/19.0	(?)		
	10 NT (hyperreactors, 22+mmHg) SBP or DBP)	?/?	(?)		33.0/17.8	(?)		
	38 NT (normoreactors, 0–22 mmHg SBP or DBP)		(?)	50 14–76	10.5/ 9.0	(?)		
					+/+		+/+	?
					Cold pressor			
Miller and Brugger (1939)	52 HT	209/113	(?)	54	35/22	(?)		
	11 nephritis (with or without HT)	163/94	(?)	36	17/13	(?)		
	16 NT (normoreactors)	123/77	(?)	28	14/12	(?)		
	10 NT (hyperreactors)	129/80	(?)	27	37/25	(?)		
					⊕/⊖	(?)	⊕/⊖	?

Table 1 (continued)

Reference	Groups and initial SBP/DBP or MBP (HR)			Age	Behavioral task/s Δ SBP/DBP or MBP (HR)			Study conclusion SBP/DBP or MBP	HR
					Interview				
Wolf et al. (1948)	21 HT	?/?	(?)	?	No group data presented				
	16 NT	?/?	(?)	?					
					Sensory stimulation	Emotional questions	Digit span test with success		
Jost et al. (1952)	12 HT	?/?	(?)	(89)	HT 4.5 (-7)	9.5 (-5)	7 (1)		
	47 NT	?/?	(?)	(82)	NT 1.5 (-1)	3 (2)	3 (8)		
					+ -	+ -	+ -		
					Digit span test with failure				
					HT 2 (3)			+	–
					NT -0.5 (9.5)			+	–
					+ –			+	–
								+	–
					Interview				
Wolf et al. (1955)	62 HT	132	(?)	42	18 (?)				
	29 NT	91	(?)	34	10 (?)				
					⊕			⊕	?
					Psychodrama				
Kalis et al. (1957)	14 HT	172/107	(90)	?	17/8 (8)				
	22 NT	119/ 73	(81)	?	3/1 (2)				
					⊕/⊕ ⊕			⊕/⊕	⊕
					Cold pressor	Fear situation			
Schachter (1957)	18 HT	166/107	(?)	42	26.2/? (?)	?/16.8 (?)			
	15 HT (potential)	133/76	(?)	41	12.1/? (?)	?/16.3 (?)			
	15 NT	114/70	(?)	38	13.3/? (?)	?/ 7.5 (?)			
					⊕/⊖	⊖/⊕			
					Anger situation				
					26.1/? (?)				
					21.6/? (?)				
					14.5/? (?)				
					⊕/⊖			⊕/⊖	?
								⊖/⊕	?
								⊕/⊖	?
					Interview				
van der Valk (1957)	15 HT (benign or malignant)	?/?		?	No group data presented				
	3 NT (healthy)	?/?		?					
	11 NT (patients)	?/?		?					
					Mental arithmetic				
Brod et al. (1959)	10 HT,	178/112	(?)	37	39/23 (?)				
	8 NT,	129/ 77	(?)	37	26/16 (?)				
					⊖/⊖			⊖/⊖	?
					Cold pressor				
Boyer et al. (1960)	21 HT	177/94	(99)	45	33.1/20.1 (6.2)				
	20 NT	107/60	(77)	25	35.6/24.5 (4.8)				
					⊖/ ⊖ ⊖			⊖/⊖	⊖
					Cold pressor				
Remington et al. (1960)	9 HT (established)	191/121	(85)	43	31/28 (−13)				
	10 HT (labile)	135/84	(85)	32	31/21 (−11)				
	10 NT	107/63	(74)	32	19/23 (−13)				
					=/= =			=/=	=

Table 1 (continued)

Reference	Groups and initial SBP/DBP or MBP (HR)			Age	Behavioral task/s Δ SBP/DBP or MBP (HR)		Study conclusion SBP/DBP or MBP	HR
Engel and Bickford (1961)	20 HT	140-220/ 90-140	(?)	35	Horn, Mental arithmetic, Proverbs, Cold pressor, Static exercise			
	20 NT	?/?	(?)	34	Reactivity data not presented: 15 of 20 HT had their greatest reaction in BP compared with 5 of 20 HT. Intraclass correlations were higher in HT than NT			
					Saline-infusion	Repeated saline-infusion due to subjects mistake		
Shapiro (1961)	50 HT	172/103	(?)	51	31/13 (8)	27/13 (12)		
	36 NT	110/67	(?)	<51	15/10 (9)	?/? (?)		
					+/+ =	+/+ =		
					Cold pressor	Colour word test		
					36/27 (12)	21/6 (11)		
					17/21 (13)	12/6 (12)		
					+/+ =	+/+ =	++/++	= =
							++/++	= =
						Thematic Apprehension Test		
Weiner et al. (1962)	31 HT	?/?	(?)	41		10.7 (6.5)		
	41 NT	?/?	(?)	28	13 Young adults	14.0 (16.2)		
					13 Depressed ulcers-patients	6.4 (4.9)		
					15 Nondepressed ulcers-patients	8.9 (8.4)		
						⊖ ⊖	⊖	⊖
					Saline-infusion	Cold pressor		
Shapiro et al. (1963)	35 HT	127	(?)	47	19.3 (14.3)	30.1 (9.6)		
	33 NT	87	(?)	37	9.4 (10.1)	19.6 (10.0)		
					⊕ ⊕	⊕ ⊖		
					Colour word test			
					15.0 (10.0)		⊕⊕	⊕⊖
					8.1 (8.3)		⊕	⊖
					⊕ ⊖			
					Cold pressor			
Greene et al. (1965)	8 HT	172/102	(79)	44	31.8/17.5 (14.1)			
	10 NT	122/73	(72)	35	23.0/20.0 (12.3)			
					⊖/⊖ ⊖		⊖/⊖	⊖
					Cold pressor (before atropinization)	(after atropinization)		
Cuddy et al. (1966)	16 HT (labile)	135/85	(82)	40	10/8 (2)	21/22 (4)		
	13 NT	120/74	(84)	39	12/10 (1)	12/6 (1)		
					⊖/⊖ ⊖	⊕/⊕ ⊖	⊖/⊖	⊖
McKegney and Williams (1967)	13 HT	?/?	(?)	51	Word association test	Personal discussion		
	10 NT	?/?	(?)	41	Thematic Apprehension Test No data relevant for HT vs. NT comparisons presented Authors concluded that HT showed DBP hyperresponsivity to personal discussion only			
							?/⊕	?
							=/=	?
							=/=	?
					Ravens progressive matrices			
Nestel (1969)	20 BHT	147/95	(?)	35	35/25 (?)			
	18 NT	117/75	(?)	31	12/11 (?)			
					⊕/⊕		⊕/⊕	?

Table 1 (continued)

Reference	Groups and initial SBP/DBP or MBP (HR)			Age	Behavioral task/s Δ SBP/DBP or MBP (HR)			Study conclusion SBP/DBP or MBP	HR
					Sorting of steel balls during noise and light distraction				
Lorimer et al. (1971)	7 HT(M)	160/103	(?)	43	27.7/14.1 (?)				
	7 NT(M)	113/79	(?)	34	12.9/10.1 (?)				
					⊕/⊖				
	8 HT (F)	168/102	(?)	49	29.0/17.5 (?)				
	8 NT (F)	113/79	(?)	47	16.5/ 9.6 (?)				
					⊕/⊕			⊕/⊕	?
					Movie depicting "good" doctor	Movie depicting "bad" doctor	Interview		
Sapira et al. (1971)	19 HT	?/?	(?)	?	2 (2)	2 (1.6)	9.5 (7.9)		
	15 NT	?/?	(?)	?	0.1 (0.1)	−0.5 (−0.7)	0.5 (3)		
					⊕ ⊖	⊕ ⊕	⊕ ⊕		
								⊕⊕	⊕⊖
								⊕	⊕
					Mental arithmetic				
Bauman et al. (1973)	30 HT	135/81	(88)	15-20	10/7 (16)				
	20 NT	112/72	(73)	15-20	8/4 (10)			⊖/⊖	⊖
					⊖/⊖ ⊖				
					Ravens progressive matrices				
Esler and Nestel (1973)	10 HT (8 sustained)	144/100	(?)	?	16/2 (?)				
	6 NT	108/66	(?)	?	10/8 (?)				
					⊖/ ⊖			⊖/⊖	?
					Sentence information	Slide-presentation			
Hodapp et al. (1975)	11 HT (WHO II)	161/85	(85)	21-51	14/6 (13)	10/8 (5)			
	9 HT (WHO I)	130/110	(76)	21-51	12/2 (12)	8/4 (2)			
	31 NT	120/80	(72)	20-45	12/4 (13)	2/2 (1)			
					⊖/ ⊖ ⊖	⊕/⊕ ⊖		⊕/⊕	⊖
								⊖/⊖	⊖
					Mental arithmetic				
Richter-Heinrich et al. (1975)	90 HT	143/88	(?)	?	12/12 (?)				
	75 NT	122/76	(?)	?	8/6 (?)				
					+/+			+/+	?
					Mental arithmetic				
Nyberg (1976)	12 HT(M)	143/92	(79)	47	13/10 (10)				
	10 NT(M)	125/80	(66)	31	10/9 (12)				
					+/+ =				
	5 HT(F)	149/93	(78)	49	14/13 (7)				
	9 NT(F)	108/72	(72)	30	3/5 (8)				
					+/+ =			+/+	=
					Mental arithmetic				
Nyberg et al. (1977)	18 HT	155/94	(89)	47	8/5 (4.5)				
	6 NT	131/86	(67)	33	6/4 (15)				
					=/= =			=/=	=
					Cold pressor				
Voudoukis (1978)	31 HT(W)	M ?/?	(?)	?	29/23 (?)				
	42 NT(W)	M ?/?	(?)	?	24/20 (?)				
					⊖/ ⊖				
	26 HT(W)	F ?/?	(?)	?	28/33 (?)				
	48 NT(W)	F ?/?	(?)	?	33/22 (?)				
					⊖/ ⊖				
	23 HT(B)	M ?/?	(?)	?	31/22 (?)				
	20 NT(B)	M ?/?	(?)	?	24/22 (?)				
					⊖/ ⊖				
	28 HT(B)	F ?/?	(?)	?	31/24 (?)				
	34 NT(B)	F ?/?	(?)	?	32/22 (?)				
					⊖/ ⊖			⊖/ ⊖	?

Table 1 (continued)

Reference	Groups and initial SBP/DBP or MBP (HR)			Age	Behavioral task/s Δ SBP/DBP or MBP (HR)	Study conclusion SBP/DBP or MBP	HR
					Mental arithmetic		
Brod et al. (1979)	12 HT	185/111	(66)		33/22 15		
	19 HT (renal)	170/101	(68)		21/18 16		
	9 NT	126/76	(57)		12/12 16		
				$\bar{x}$=36	⊕/⊖ ⊖	⊕/⊖	⊖
					Mental arithmetic		
Falkner et al. (1979)	17 BHT	123/75	(88)	16	12.6/16.2 (16.2)		
	33 (positive FH)	112/71	(83)	15	8.5/11.3 (11.3)		
	25 NT (negative FH)	107/71	(79)	15	5.9/ 3.5 (7.2)		
					⊕/⊕ ⊕	⊕/⊕	⊕
					Colour word test		
Hjemdahl and Eliasson (1979)	7 HT	126/86	(72)	35	35/23% (20)		
	7 NT	107/74	(75)	35	21/14% (13.3)		
					⊖/ ⊖ ?	⊖/⊖	?
					Mental arithmetic during noise distraction		
Schulte and Neus (1979)	20 HT (WHO II)	142/91	(65)	45	26.8/13.5 (11)		
	12 HT (WHO I)	133/83	(73)	41	17.4/9.3 (12)		
	18 BHT	126/80	(75)	44	21.4/13.0 (14)		
	16 NT	117/75	(73)	41	14. /10.8 (16)		
					⊕/⊖ ⊖	⊕/⊖	⊖
					Sensory-motor tracing task		
von Scheuck et al. (1979)	32 HT (sustained)	148/?	(?)	26	13/? (9)		
	30 HT (labile)	133/?	(?)	25	3/? (7)		
	55 NT	120/?	(?)	18-30	6/? (5)		
	24 NT (hypotensives)	112/?	(?)	25	1/? (3)		
					⊕/⊕	⊕/⊕	?
					Auditory letter identification; Mental arithmetic		
Fredrikson et al. (1980)	14 HT	?/?	(?)	44	6/4 (?); 13/9 (?)		
	14 NT	?/?	(?)	44	3/2 (?); 6/6 (?)		
					⊖/⊖; ⊕/⊖	⊖/⊖	?
						⊕/⊖	?
					Cold pressor; Film; Shock avoidance		
Light and Obrist[a] (1980)	29 BHT (labile)	135/79	(74)	18-29	18/10 (15); 8/8 (1); 24/4 (20)		
	31 NT	125/72	(72)		14/11 (12); 6/8 (1); 19/5 (17)	+/+	=
					⊕/⊕ ⊖; ⊕/⊕ ⊖; ⊕/⊕ ⊖	+/+	=
						+/+	=
					Cold pressor		
Murakami et al. (1980)	19 HT (young labile)	81	(?)	29	24.9 (?)		
	15 HT (old labile)	113	(?)	49	28.1 (?)		
	25 HT (fixed)	123	(?)	52	24.7 (?)		
	17 NT	81	(?)	35	21.0 (?)		
					⊖	⊖	?
					Mental arithmetic (Peak value)		
Ambrosini et al. (1981)	14 HT	?/96	(?)	47	?/20 (?)		
	47 BHT	?/74	(?)	24	?/15 (?)		
	11 NT (positive FH)	?/70	(?)	22	?/10 (?)		
	8 NT	?/66	(?)	23	?/7 (?)		
					⊕/⊕	⊕/⊕	?

Table 1 (continued)

Reference	Groups and initial SBP/DBP or MBP (HR)			Age	Behavioral task/s Δ SBP/DBP or MBP (HR)	Study conclusion SBP/DBP or MBP	HR
					Ravens progressive matrices: Peak value; Mean value		
Hollenberg et al. (1981)	15 HT	98	(?)	40	8 (?); 0 (?)		
	8 NT (positive FH)	88	(?)	39	3 (?); 0 (?)		
	16 NT	81	(?)	39	0.5 (?); 0 (?)		
					⊕; ⊖	⊖	?
					Social conversation		
Lynch et al. (1981)	30 HT	149/85	(79)	55	7.1/10.4 (5.2)		
	15 NT	124/72	(73)	43	7.7/ 9.5 (6.3)		
					⊖/⊖ ⊖	⊖/⊖	⊖
					Mental arithmetic during noise distraction		
Schulte et al. (1981)	48 HT	132/82	(74)	44	24.6/13.1 19.3		
	48 NT	110/69	(70)	44	16.6/10.1 14.9		
					⊕/⊕ ⊖	⊕/⊕	⊖
					Mental arithmetic		
Sullivan et al. (1981)	15 HT	150/104	(?)	37	1/4% (16%)		
	13 NT	108/74	(?)	36	10/7% (8%)		
					⊖/⊖ ⊖	⊖/⊖	⊖
					Mental arithmetic		
Anderson et al. (1982)	10 HT	88	(?)	45	?/5 (?)		
	10 NT	72	(?)	37	?/7 (?)		
					/ =	?/ =	?
					Mental arithmetic		
Bahlmann et al. (1982)	12 HT	135	(?)	?	43.3 (?)		
	6 NT	91	(?)	?	21.0 (?)		
					⊕	⊕	?
					Auditory letter identification; Mental arithmetic[b]		
Fredrikson et al. (1982)	14 HT	152/99	(71)	42	6.6/2.2 (1); 13.6/9.4 (13)		
	14 NT	119/76	(66)	44	3.3/1.4 (0); 8.8/5.9 (11.5)		
					⊖/⊖ ⊖; ⊕/⊖ ⊖	⊕/⊖	⊖
						⊖/⊖	⊖
					Interview; Slide of parent/partner		
Groen et al. (1982)	11 HT	195/112	(78)	27-45	23/7 (3); 9/3 (−2)		
	11 NT	131/78	(70)	18-56	18/8 (3); 5/0 (−4)		
					⊖/⊖ ⊖; ⊖/⊖ ⊖	⊖/⊖	⊖
						⊖/⊖	⊖
					Mental arithmetic; Interview; 85 dB white noise		
Jern (1982)	24 BHT	131/70	(73)	?	21.6/23.9 (14); 14.9/14.1 (?); 3.0/2.2 (?)		
	11 NT	117/66	(72)	?	16.4/14.9 (11); 9.7/10.4 (?); 1.5/1 (?)		
					⊖/⊕ ⊖; ⊖/⊖; ⊖/⊖		
					Videodisplayed med. information; Anxiety situation	⊖/⊕	⊖
					5.2/3 (?); 7.5/5.2 (?)	⊖/⊖	?
					3.7/3 (?); 4.4/1.5 (?)	⊖/⊖	?
					⊖/⊖; ⊖/⊖	⊖/⊖	?
						⊖/⊖	?
					Roleplay with negative and positive emotional content		
Keane et al. (1982)	12 HT	151/83	(75)	47	16.3/6.2 (5.5)		
	12 NT (patients)	130/72	(74)	47	11.8/8.5 (6.3)		
	(12 NT (nonpatients)	128/69	(76)	47	14.1/8.5 (6.5)		
					⊖/ ⊖ ⊖	⊖/ ⊖	⊖

Table 1 (continued)

Reference	Groups and initial SBP/DBP or MBP (HR)	Age	Behavioral task/s Δ SBP/DBP or MBP (HR)			Study conclusion SBP/DBP or MBP	HR
			Colour word test				
Prikryl et al. (1982)	17 HT 145/94 (86)	25	6 /10.5 (4)				
	17 NT 123/77 (80)	22	10.5/ 6 (10)				
			=/= =			=/=	=
			Anxiety-provoking interview				
Svensson and Theorell (1982)	19 HT 141/85 (?)	18	6.4/6.0 (?)				
	15 NT 123/72 (?)	18	6.4/3.9 (?)				
	12 NT 110/64 (?)	18	2.9/5.2 (?)				
	(hypotensives)		⊖/ ⊖			⊖/ ⊖	⊖
			Cold pressor				
Bühler et al. (1983)	18 HT 117 (71)	30-65	29.6 13.8				
	15 NT 81 (53)	31-62	20.7 10.6				
			+ ?			+	?
			Cold pressor	Mental arithmetic			
Drummond (1983)	18 HT 129/88 (77)	25	12.2/12.9 (4.7)	13.9/9.7 (14.2)			
	18 NT 110/73 (70)	25	10.1/13.0 (7.3)	9.9/5.5 (13.7)			
			⊖/⊖ ⊖	⊖/⊕ ⊖		⊖/⊕	⊖
						⊖/⊖	⊖
			Color word test	Cold pressor			
Eliasson et al. (1983)	33 HT 155/103 (77)	40	33/30% (31)	36/35% (14)			
	16 BHT 141/92 (75)	36	37/40% (33)	30/42% (15)			
	17 NT 120/80 (72)	38	35/30% (25)	34/39% (13)			
			⊖/⊕ ⊖	⊖/⊖ ⊖		⊖/⊕	⊖
						⊖/⊖	⊖
			Cold pressor				
Frisk-Holmberg et al. (1983)	17 HT 156/105 (78)	43	18 (?)				
	17 NT 124/83 (68)	46	17 (?)				
			⊖			⊖	?
			Mental arithmetic during noise distraction				
Schulte and Neus (1983)	10 HT 140/86	33	24.9/16.9 (31%)				
	10 BHT 124/77	32	18.9/12.2 (25%)				
	10 NT 114/73	32	12.1/18.1 (19%)				
			⊕/⊕ ⊕			⊕/⊕	⊕
			Color word test	Distressing movie	Video-game		
Steptoe et al. (1983)	12 HT 147/95 (mild)	42	22/10 (11)	7/4 (1)	23/17 (6)		
	12 HT 147/90 (transient)	41	14/11 (18)	3/1 (2)	5/3 (7)		
	12 NT 131/84	43	18/7 (11)	5/3 (1)	13/7 (3)		
			⊕/⊕ ⊕	⊖/⊖ ?	⊕/⊕ ?	⊕/⊕	⊕
						⊕/⊕	?
						⊖/⊖	?
			Roleplay (low distress)	Roleplay (high distress)			
Linden and Feurstein (1983)	9 HT 151/95 (untreated)	41	18/9 (5)	19/3 (3)			
	9 HT 139/83 (drugtreated)	52	18/4 (3)	19/12 (3)			
	20 NT 130/75	43	10/6 (6)	13/10 (8)			
			⊕/⊕ ⊖	⊕/⊖ ⊖		⊕/⊕	⊖
						⊕/⊖	⊖
			Attentional demands	Mental arithmetic	Cold pressor		
Fredrikson et al. (1984)	14 HT 154/103 (74)	47	3/4 (1)	12/7 (6)	9/11 (2)		
	14 NT 124/76 (65)	40	2/1 (3)	9/6 (13)	9/13 (3)		
			⊖/⊖ ⊖	⊖/⊖ ⊖	⊖/⊖ ⊖	⊖/⊖	⊖
						⊖/⊖	⊖
						⊖/⊖	⊖
			Mental arithmetic + noise				
Schulte et al. (1984)	38 HT ?/? (?)		24/11 (?)				
	13 NT ?/? (?)		14/12 (?)				
		$\bar{x}$=39	⊕/⊖			⊕/⊖	?

Table 1 (continued)

Reference	Groups and initial SBP/DBP or MBP (HR)			Age	Behavioral task/s Δ SBP/DBP or MBP (HR)		Study conclusion SBP/DBP or MBP	HR
Fredrikson et al. (1985)	22 HT	(158/100)	(?)	46	Attentional demands, Mental arithmetic, Cold pressor, Isometric muscle work			
	22 NT	(?/?)	(?)	42	Reactivity data not presented: 9 of 22 HT had their greatest response in BP compared with 5 of 22 NT. Intraclass correlations were higher in HT than NT			
					Aversive reaction-time task			
Fredrikson and Engel (1985)	12 HT	104	(84)	53	14.6/7.7	(6)		
	12 BHT	100	(79)	41	8.3/7.5	(9)		
	12 NT	88	(64)	42	6.3/5.3	(4)		
					⊕/⊕	⊜	⊕/⊕	⊜

[a] Significant differences refer to BP levels and not reactivity (change)
[b] HT more reactive during first minute only.

Abbreviations: B, blacks; BHT, borderline hypertensives; DBP, diastolic blood pressure; F, females; FH, family history of hypertension; HR, heart rate; HT, essential hypertensives; M, males; MBP, mean blood pressure; NT, normotensives; SBP, systolic blood pressure; W, whites; WHO I, grade 1 according to the World Health Organisation classification scheme on the extent of organ damage; WHO II, grade 2; $\bar{x}$, mean value; ?, data not reported; +, HT more reactive than NT - no statistical test included; ⊕, HT more reactive than NT - statistical tests included; =, HT and NT equally reactive - no statistical tests included; ⊜, HT and NT equally reactive - statistical tests included; −, HT less reactive than NT - no statistical tests included; ⊖, HT less reactive than NT - statistical tests included.

Essential Hypertension, Laboratory Manoeuvers and the Defense Reaction

Fredrikson et al. (1982, 1985a) studied mild HT (⩾160/95 mmHg) and age- and sex-matched NT subjects recruited from the same population during one intake and one rejection task. None of the participants had any prior history of cardiovascular complications or of antihypertensive medication. Both Fredrikson et al. (1982) and Fredrikson et al. (1985a) subjected patients to a sensory-intake task consisting of auditory letter identification, and to a sensory-rejection task, involving mental arithmetic. Fredrikson et al. (1985a) also included the cold pressor test and isometric muscle exercise. We were primarily interested in analyzing (1) to what extent BP reactivity is part of generalized SNS activation, or is specific to the cardiovascular system; and (2) to what extent cardiovascular responses are intrinsic and similar in all situations, or extrinsic and unique for each situation. In both studies we recorded the following: SBP and DBP, hand and forearm blood flow, hand and forearm vascular resistance and HR. Skin conductance activity, which is closely related to SNS activity measured directly by microneurography (Lidberg and Wallin 1981), was recorded as an index of noncardiovascular SNS activation. Fredrikson et al. (1985a) also added urinary catecholamines as an additional SNS index. The rejection task (mental arithmetic) elicited a more widespread sympathetic-like response than the intake task (auditory letter identification; Figs. 1a, b).

There were only a few indications that the reaction patterns were different in HT and NT. During the first minute of the rejection task SBP reactivity was greater in

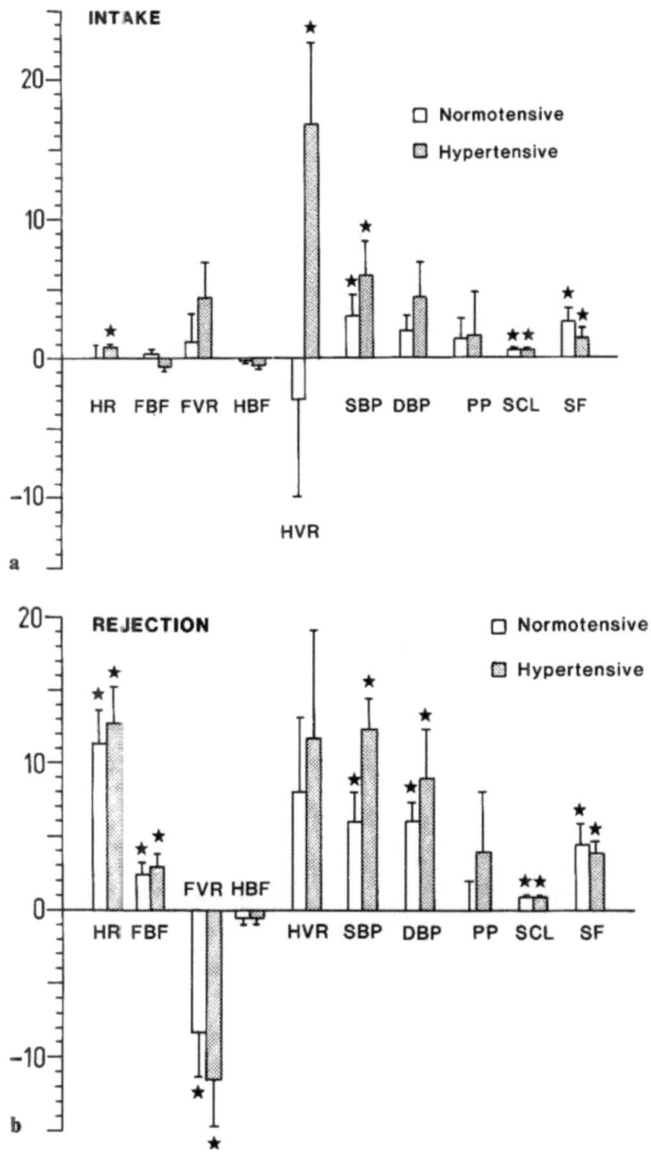

Fig. 1a, b. Physiological responses of hypertensives *(shaded bars)* and normotensives *(blank bars)* to the intake (**a**) and during the rejection task (**b**). Responses are shown in absolute values as follows: heart rate *(HR)* in bpm; forearm blood flow *(FBF)* and hand blood flow *(HBF)* in ml/100 ml tissue per min; forearm vascular resistance *(FVR)* and hand vascular resistance *(HVR)* in arbitrary units; systolic and diastolic blood pressures *(SBP* and *DBP)* and pulse pressure *(PP)* in mmHg; skin conductance level *(SCL)* in μmho; skin conductance fluctuations *(SF)* in frequency/min. Significant responses are indicated by *asterisks*. A *P*-level of 0.05 is adopted. (Fredrikson et al. 1982)

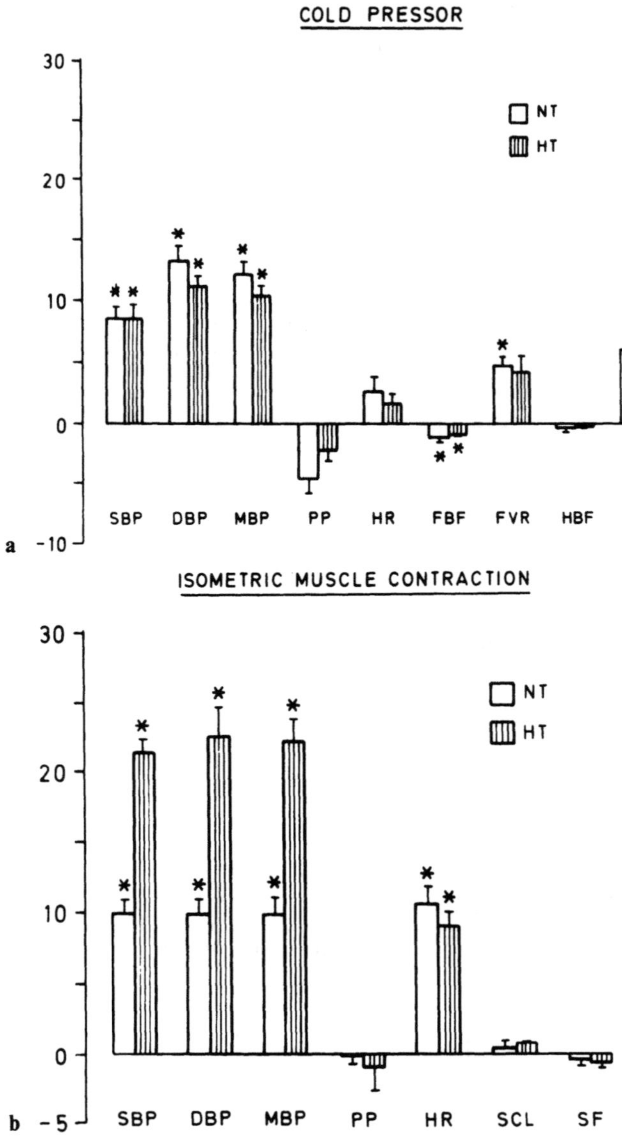

Fig. 2a, b. Mean (SEM) of physiological responses of hypertensives *(shaded bars)* and normotensives *(blank bars)* during the cold pressor test (**a**) and isometric exercise (**b**). Responses are shown in absolute values as follows: systolic and diastolic blood pressures *(SBP* and *DBP)*, mean blood pressure *(MBP)*, and pulse pressure *(PP)* in mmHg; heart rate *(HR)* in bpm; forearm blood flow *(FBF)* and hand blood flow *(HBF)* in ml/100 ml tissue per min; forearm vascular resistance *(FVR)* and hand vascular resistance *(HVR)* in arbitrary units; skin conductance level *(SCL)* in μmho; skin conductance level *(SCL)* in μmho; skin conductance fluctuations *(SF)* in frequency/min. An *asterisk* indicates a significant response. (Fredrikson et al. 1985a)

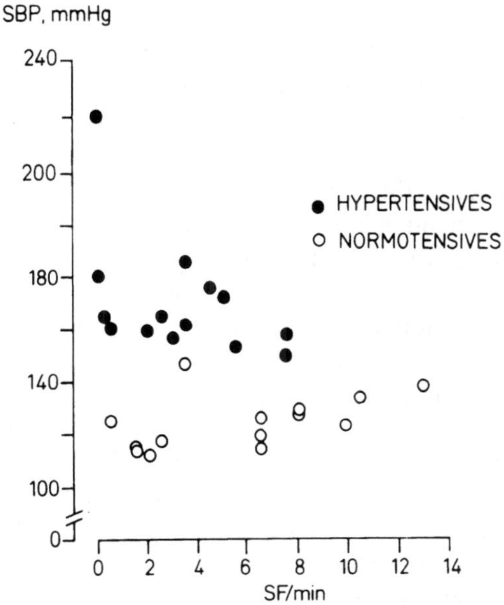

Fig. 3. A scatter plot of spontaneous fluctuations *(SF)* in skin conductance and systolic blood pressure *(SBP)* for hypertensive ($r = -0.48$; $P < 0.07$) and normotensive groups ($r = +0.48$; $P < 0.07$) during mental arithmetic. (After Fredrikson et al. 1982)

HT than NT. The sensory-intake task (Fig. 1 a) and the cold pressor task (Fig. 2 a) elicited similar BP responses in both groups. During isometric muscle contraction (Fig. 2 b), HT showed a greater increase in both SBP and DBP. Reactivity differences in BP during mental arithmetic and isometric muscle contraction were not paralleled by differences in skin conductance level or skin conductance fluctuations, which were similar in both groups during both tasks. Also, catecholamine excretion rates were similar in HT and NT. Thus, no support was obtained for any theory linking BP hyperreactivity to generalized SNS activation. In contrast, during mental arithmetic, SBP and skin conductance fluctuations were negatively correlated in HT, but positively correlated in NT (Fig. 3).

Generalized Sympathetic Arousal or Cardiospecific Activation?

In Fredrikson et al. (1985 a), the absence of a catecholamine difference between HT and NT might be age-specific. Goldstein (1983) reviewed reports on catecholamine excretion rate in HT and concluded that elevated plasma catecholamines characterized only a subgroup of HT, namely young borderline hypertensive (BHT) men. In our work the sample age averaged 46 years, which may account for the lack of a difference in catecholamine activity. Consistent with previous reports, no support was obtained for any general increase in skin conductance activity in HT compared with NT. Even though HT showed greater BP reactivity, Jost et al. (1952), Schachter (1957), and Steptoe et al. (1983) failed to observe differences between HT and NT in skin conductance activity. Jern (1982) observed greater electrodermal activation in NT than in BHT subjects during mental arithmetic. In addition, direct recordings of

SNS activity done via microneurography indicate that skin sympathetic activity is not different in HT and NT (Wallin et al. 1973). Thus, it seems unlikely that BP hyperreactivity in HT patients is part of generalized SNS activation.

Increased electrodermal activation and decreased cardiovascular activity is associated with good performance in tasks requiring vigilance behavior (cf. Lacey and Lacey 1974). This might be called "a state of sensory intake", where a great amount of attention is allocated to the environment, as opposed to a "state of sensory rejection," with less attention allocated to the environment. Fredrikson et al. (1982) observed decreased electrodermal activation together with increased cardiovascular activation in HT (see Fig. 5), and suggested that these data may indicate "a state of sensory rejection" in HT patients. This interpretation is consistent with data presented by Shapiro and co-workers showing impaired cognitive and perceptual abilities in HT compared with NT (Shapiro et al. 1982; Miller et al. 1984). Also, it has been shown that BP elevations reduce the effects of painful stimulation, since rats having intact baroreceptors tolerate more painful electrical stimulation than do rats with denervated receptors (Dworkin et al. 1979). Cognitive and perceptual abilities improve when BP decreases (Miller et al. 1984), indicating that BP may modulate sensory afferent activity.

Prognostic Value of Transient BP Changes

Fredrikson et al. (1985 a) observed that reactivity to one task was not predictive of reactivity to any other task, since BP reactivity across tasks was uncorrelated both in HT and NT. Thus, generalizing from one task to another might not be possible. Similar findings have been reported in NT subjects and in subjects having a family aggregation of high BP (see Krantz and Manuck 1985, for a review). Also, 17 studies summarized in Table 1 included several tasks, but only in 5 of these was hyperreactivity consistently observed across tasks. Thus, in 12 studies BP reactivity observed in one task did not generalize to other tasks. These findings may be of importance, since in some studies BP reactivity to the cold pressor test have failed to predict subsequent development of high BP or even BP levels (Harlan et al. 1964) and indicated that basal BP is a better predictor. Some data suggest that the predictive power of BP responsivity may increase with longer follow-up times. Wood et al. (1984) reported that early hyperreactivity to the cold pressor test was related to future hypertension 45 years later, whereas studies that have failed to establish a connection (cf. Harlan et al. 1964; Eich and Jacobsen 1967) have typically used shorter follow-up times.

However, if reactivity is not a unitary but a multifaceted phenomenon, it is not possible to conclude whether reactivity to the cold pressor test is of limited value in BP predictions, or whether the reactivity concept *per se* is ambiguous. Some studies indicate that beta-adrenergically mediated differences in BP reactivity may serve as a better vehicle in predicting BP development than those that are mediated alfa-adrenergically. The cold pressor test increases BP mainly due to alfa-adrenoceptor-mediated vasoconstriction (Bühler et al. 1983), whereas mental arithmetic raises it mainly as the result of beta-adrenergic activation (Schulte and Neus 1983). Cardiovascular reactivity among NT subjects is greater in situations stimulating beta-adrenoceptors compared with changes mainly determined by alfa-adrenoceptor activity (Obrist et al. 1978; Light 1981). Also, NT subjects with HT parents compared with NT subjects with NT parents commonly show greater BP hyperreactivity to tasks involving beta-adrenergic (Falkner et al. 1979; Hastrup et al. 1982), but seldom to tasks eliciting alfa-adrenergic activation (Feldt et al. 1942). In addition, Falkner et al. (1981) in a prospective study of adolescents, found BP development to be related to differences in beta-adrenoceptor-mediated BP reactivity. However, in the Falkner et al. (1981) study, it is not possible to evaluate the relative contribution of hyperreactivity independent of family history, since subjects who developed sustained HT manifested both characteristics. Thus, the speculation that beta-adrenergically-mediated differences in BP reactivity, but not differences mediated alfa-adrenergically, predicts development of sustained essential hypertension must await confirmation or refutation, since no prospective studies have included such a comparison. It has also been suggested that patterning of BP responses, rather than their response-magnitude or situational determinants, may have prognostic value. Eliot et al. (1982) suggested that BP elevations resulting from increased cardiac output, or from increased peripheral resistance, or both, all have differential prognostic value. The evaluation of this suggestion is also hampered by the lack of data. Cardiovascular hyperreactivity in an early phase of HT development may be directly involved in the causation of HT or may merely reflect another side of a single pathophysiological process simultaneously causing hyperreactivity and sustained HT (Manuck et al. 1985). The mechanism by which a hyperkinetic circulatory state may (or may not) transform to a normokinetic high vascular resistance state remains a controversy. It has been suggested that autoregulation with increased vascular resistance and normalization of cardiac output occurs because the perfusion is in excess of the metabolic needs (Cowely 1980). Julius claims that metabolic demands are increased in BHT and that the impetus for autoregulation is lacking, and then argues in favor of decreased cardiac responsivity in HT (cf. Julius et al. 1985). Folkow (1982) states that increased cardiac output resulting from genetic or behavioral factors causes structural changes in the arterioles, thereby directly raising vascular resistance.

However, even though the mechanisms of transition are controversial and the importance of cardiovascular reactivity is debated, it may be valuable to monitor transitory BP changes since these may relate to end-organ damage. Devereux et al. (1983) studied target organ damage in hypertension. They correlated measures of left ventricular hypertrophy with BP recorded under basal conditions and at work in borderline HT patients and in NT controls. Cardiac hypertrophy was more closely related to BP during "stressful" conditions at work than to basal pressure. Similar findings were reported by Sokolow et al. (1966). Thus, BP reactivity to behavioral challenge may be a valuable predictor of left ventricular hypertrophy.

Task-specific or Nonspecific Activation?

Fredrikson et al. (1982, 1985a) did not address the question of group selection directly, but it is worth noting that reactivity differences were sparse when both HT and NT subjects were recruited from the same general population. This suggests that self-referred HT groups might show comparatively greater reactivity than randomly recruited groups, or that NT controls consisting of laboratory and hospital staff may be less reactive than the general population (Steptoe 1984). Jern et al. (see Jern 1982) compared a population sample of mild HT patients with an outpatient group and found lower levels of anxiety and psychic symptoms in the population than in the clinic sample. Since Whitehead et al. (1977) observed that anxiety is positively correlated with SBP, it is likely that the use of clinic groups overestimates reactivity differences among HT and NT subjects. Also, a nonfamiliar laboratory environment probably produces greater nonspecific activation in patients than in laboratory staff traditionally used as NT controls (cf. Shapiro et al. 1963; Groen et al. 1982). However, even though these factors may exaggerate differences among HT and NT subjects, reactivity differences are not produced by preselection or nonspecific activation only. Steptoe et al. (1983) eliminated the effect of preselection by recruiting subjects via a mass screening program. They studied three groups of subjects, one with mild HT, one with transient HT, and NT controls. These were subjected to a color word test and a video game. Even though subjects were ignorant of their actual BP, greater reactivity was observed among HT than NT subjects. Reactivity differences also tend to vary with behavioral demands, a fact hard to account for by concepts like preselection of subjects or nonspecific activation.

Vigilance, Behavior, and Reactivity

Some of the discrepant results obtained in laboratory studies on BP reactivity in essential HT might be due to the fact that such differences are more easily observed during tasks requiring active coping on behalf of an individual than during tasks with no performance demands (Obrist 1981; Fredrikson et al. 1982, 1985a; Drummond 1983; Steptoe et al. 1983). Tasks requiring avoidance behavior produce cardiovascular activation, which seem to be part of general SNS activation. It would be expected then, that reactivity differences in SNS activation between HT and NT would be more easily obtained in tasks demanding active coping than nondemanding tasks (Obrist et al. 1978; Light 1981). Also, increased SNS reactivity might be most easily observed in BHT, since autonomic factors operate primarily in this phase of disease development (Julius and Schork 1971). Thus, in an attempt to optimize conditions for observing excessive SNS reactivity in essential HT, Fredrikson and Engel (1985) studied cardiovascular and noncardiovascular SNS responses during a task requiring vigilance behavior (and activity) in patients with BHT or sustained HT, and compared those with NT controls.

Twelve patients in each group were subjected to a signaled reaction time task which consisted of a 35-s pre-period that ended with a noxious 110 dB white noise, the delivery of which was contingent upon poor performance. Thus, the noxious sound could be avoided by performing at high speed, whereas it was sounded if

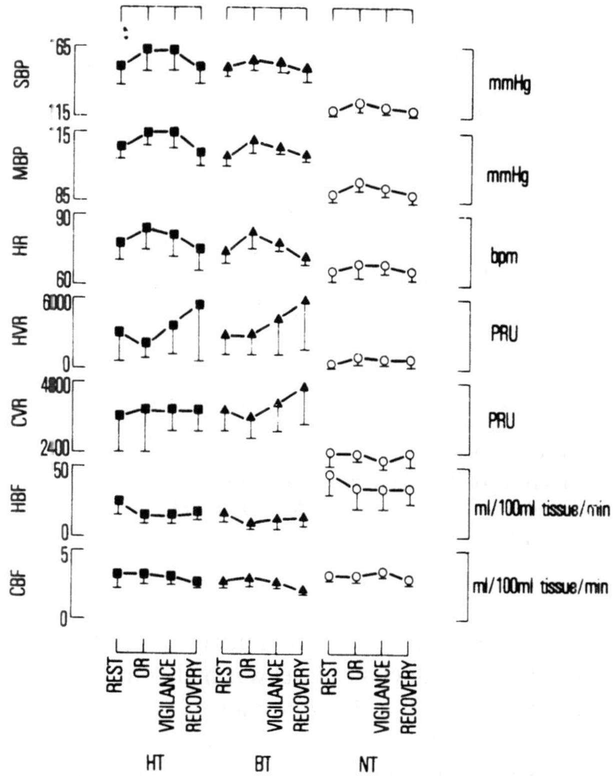

Fig. 4. Means and half standard deviations of systolic and mean blood pressures *(SBP* and *MBP)*, heart rate *(HR)*, hand and calf vascular resistances *(HVR* and *CVR)*, hand and calf blood flows *(HBF* and *CBF)* recorded from patients with essential hypertension *(HT)*, borderline hypertension *(BT)* and normotensive controls *(NT)* before, during and after a reaction time task. *REST* and *RECOVERY* are the means of 5 measurements taken 10 min before and after the task. *OR* includes responses from tone-presentation 1 and *VIGILANCE* the mean of tone-presentations 2–16. (Fredrikson and Engel 1985)

reaction times were slow. The experiment consisted of 16 repeated presentations, and during all pre-periods SBP and DBP, hand and calf blood flow, and HR were recorded. Skin conductance level, fluctuations and responses were recorded as non-cardiovascular SNS responses. The following questions were asked:

1. Do HT and BHT show pressor hyperreactivity during the reaction- time-contingent noise avoidance task?
2. Is pressor hyperreactivity during such a task specific to the cardiovascular system or part of generalized SNS-activation?

Reaction time performance was similar in all groups, meaning that they all had the same number of aversive tones delivered to them. The two HT groups showed greater pressor reactivity and increased vascular resistance compared with the NT controls (Fig. 4). Differences were most evident for SBP and for the established HT group. HR and SBP changes were positively correlated in BHT only ($r = 0.61$), indicating that BP changes were mainly determined by increased cardiac output in this

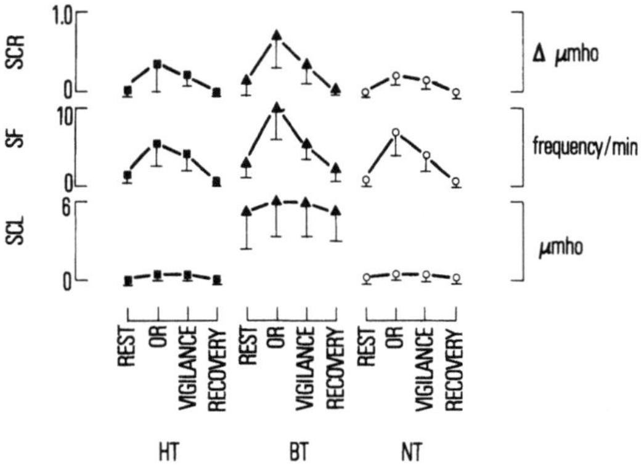

Fig. 5. Means and half standard deviations of skin conductance responses *(SCR)*, skin conductance fluctuations *(SF)* and skin conductance level *(SCL)* recorded from patients with essential hypertension *(HT)*, borderline hypertension *(BT)* and normotensive controls *(NT)* before, during, and after a reaction-time task. *REST* and *RECOVERY* are means of 5 measurements taken 10 min before and after the task. *OR* includes responses from tone-presentation 1 and *VIGILANCE* the mean of tone-presentation 2-16. (Fredrikson and Engel, 1985)

group. Consistent with the notion of a generally increased SNS activation in BHT, resting skin conductance level was higher in BHT patients than in any other group. However, this resting difference was not reflected in reactivity, since Fredrikson and Engel (1985) observed no reactivity differences between groups in any skin conductance variable (Fig. 5). BP changes were positively correlated with electrodermal activity in all groups, but more so in NT than HT. Since BP effects were not paralleled by or correlated with electrodermal effects, no support was found for the all-or-none notion of reactivity, but data supported the specificity notion. The fact that differences were observed in skin conductance activity at rest, but not for reactivity, points to the importance of distinguishing between measures of sympathetic tone at rest and sympathetic reactivity, since the two probably reflect different aspects of any pathophysiological process.

Vigilance, Sensitization, and Habituation

Besides reactivity effects, the study design of Fredrikson and Engel (1985) permitted evaluation of sensitization and habituation effects. A response is sensitized if it is augmented by successive stimulus presentations, and habituation occurs if responses decrease with repeated presentations. To study if reactions were more easily sensitized in HT patients than in NT subjects, we analyzed reactions to tones immediately following response failures, and thus delivery of the 110 dB white noise. Reactions to those tone presentations were substracted from responses recorded to tones immediately preceding failure trials. Any habituation mechanism would yield smaller responses on a later failure trial compared with a preceding success trial. SBP was sensitized more easily in patients with sustained HT than in BHT patients or NT controls (Fig. 6). No sensitization differences between HT, BHT, or NT in skin conductance were observed.

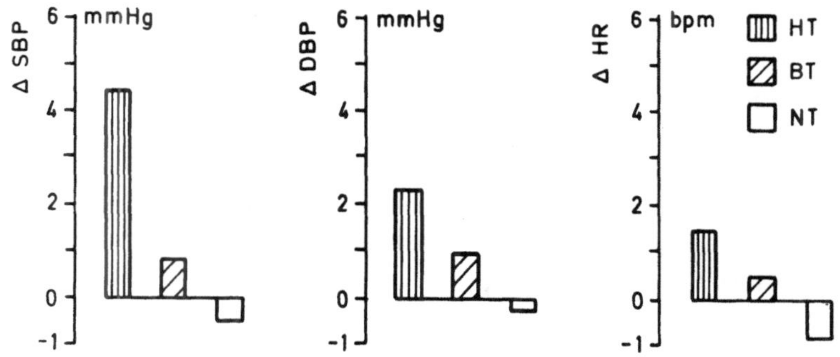

Fig. 6. Differences between average reactivity in systolic blood pressure *(SBP)* recorded from tone-presentations preceding and after response failures in patients with essential hypertension *(HT)*, borderline hypertension *(BT)* and normotensive controls *(NT)*. (After Fredrikson and Engel, 1985)

Fredrikson and Engel (1985) concluded: (1) that pressor hyperreactivity in HT and BHT was not part of generalized SNS activation, and (2) that HT and BHT showed similar response patterns, supporting the view that differences between HT and BHT are quantitative rather than qualitative.

Developmental Stages of Hypertension and Reactivity: a Summary

The series of studies conducted by Fredrikson and co-workers indicate:

1. That pressor hyperreactivity in HT is commonly but not consistently observed
2. That hyperreactivity in HT is specific to the cardiovascular system and not part of generalized SNS activation
3. That there is little intercorrelation of cardiovascular reactivity to different stimuli or tasks
4. That differences in BP reactivity among HT and NT may be more easily observed during mentally taxing or "active" conditions compared with less taxing or "passive" conditions; thus BP reactivity is not only constitutionally, but also situationally determined
5. That reactivity differences between BHT and HT are quantitative rather than qualitative

These conclusions regarding HT are consistent with the results obtained when BHT has been studied. Eliasson et al. (1983) and Steptoe et al. (1983) compared BHT and NT in situations demanding "active" (Stroop color word test) or "passive" coping (movie or cold pressor test) and observed differences in BP reactivity between BHT and NT only in situations characterized by active "coping efforts." Neither plasma catecholamines (Eliasson et al. 1983) or skin conductance activity (Steptoe et al. 1983), both of which are noncardiovascular SNS measures differed between BHT and NT.

In conclusion, data indicate that patients with sustained HT or BHT, and subjects having a family history of high BP commonly show pressor hyperreactivity to situations requiring active coping. In HT and BHT, BP hyperreactivity seems to be specific to the cardiovascular system rather than due to generalized SNS activation. In BHT, most studies have reported cardiospecific activation during behavioral activation (cf. Schachter 1957; Jern 1982; Eliasson et al. 1983; Steptoe 1983; Fredrikson and Engel 1985). However, some have obtained data indicating that BP hyperreactivity correlates with other signs of SNS activation (Nestel 1969; Falkner et al. 1979). In subjects with a family history of cardiovascular disease, data on the generality vs. specificity issue are not consistent. Some studies have reported greater noncardiovascular SNS reactivity to behavioral challenge, as reflected by plasma catecholamines (Falkner et al. 1979), plasma renin activity (Hollenberg et al. 1981), skin conductance activity (Collins et al. 1981), and greater sodium retention, possibly as a result of SNS influences on the kidney (Light et al. 1983). However, some studies have reported that differences in reactivity are localized within the cardiovascular system (Lawler and Allen 1981; Newlin and Levensson 1982).

Since environments that provoke active behavioral adjustments are associated with increased BP reactivity in epidemiological studies (Guttman and Benson 1971), it is tempting to speculate that observed individual differences in transient BP responses to behavioral demands (at various developmental stages of HT) may predict subsequent development of high BP. Some support for the notion that transient BP changes produced experimentally predict casual levels occurring during daily life was provided by Steptoe et al. (1983). They found that BP reactivity during "active" but not "passive" coping correlated positively with self monitored BP over a 14-day period. However, Steptoe et al. (1983) did not examine the correlation between self-monitored BP and BP levels recorded in the laboratory, leaving the possibility that estimates of responsivity do not add to the predictive power of casual levels recorded in the clinic. Studies listed in Table 1 indicate that HT patients are as likely to show systolic as diastolic hyperreactivity. Systolic hyperreactivity among HT patients was observed in 49% of the studies and diastolic hyperreactivity in 47% of the studies. Investigators who have found diastolic but not systolic hyperreactivity generally have used subjects with less severe HT (BHT) (cf. Jern 1982; Drummond 1983; Eliason et al. 1983). Diastolic hyperreactivity among BHT subjects is in line with reports indicating a vascular abnormality with decreased vasodilator capacity seen in patients with essential HT, as well as in subjects having an increased hereditary risk for development of HT. This risk is possibly due to derangement of dilatory beta-adrenoceptors in patients with essential HT (Bühler et al. 1980) and to structural abnormalities in subjects with a positive family history of HT (Takeshita et al. 1982). In most studies, cardiovascular hyperreactivity has been stimulus specific and not obtained in all tasks. This indicates that BP hyperreactivity is not completely intrinsic, but modified by behavioral demands. However, patterning of several physiological responses seems less dependent on extrinsic factors in HT than in NT.

Essential Hypertension and Individual Response Specificity

Responses may be elicited by stimuli or emitted by individuals. In psychophysiology the former has been termed "stimulus-response specificity" and the latter "individual-response specificity", defined as "a consistent hierarchy of responses to a set

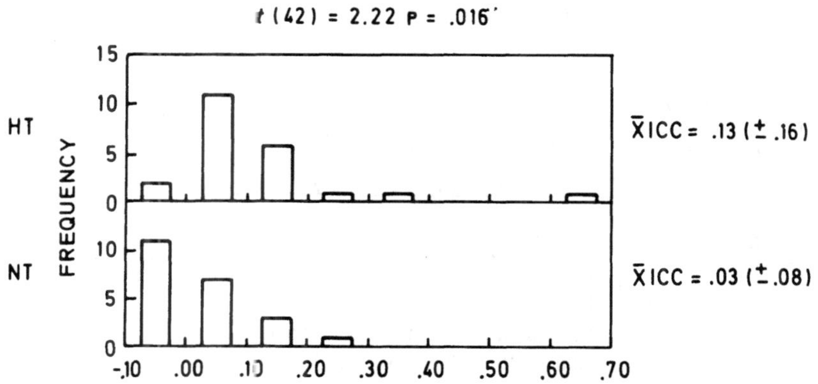

Fig. 7. Distribution of intraclass correlations *(ICC)*, mean correlations and *t*-test comparing hypertensive patients *(HT)* and normotensive controls *(NT)*, with blood pressure responses included. (After Fredrikson et al. 1985)

of stimuli" (Engel 1983). The first demonstration that the patterning of responses is less dependent on stimuli, but more closely tied to individuals in HT than NT was provided by Engel and Bickford (1961). They subjected female HT patients and NT controls to five laboratory "stressors": mental arithmetic, noise, a memory task, cold pressor test, and isometric work, while recordings were made of SBP and DBP, HR, respiration rate, skin conductance activity, and finger toe, and face temperature. To enable comparisons between groups and response systems all responses were standardized. In 15 of 20 female patients, BP was the greatest response irrespective of the task, whereas this was true in only 5 of 20 NT controls. Also, the numerical estimate of individual response specificity - the intraclass correlation coefficient - was higher in HT than NT. This general finding was replicated and extended by Fredrikson et al. (1985b). We subjected male HT patients and matched NT controls to four stimuli: letter identification, mental arithmetic, cold pressor, and isometric exercise, and recorded SBP and DBP, HR, respiration, forearm and hand blood flow, and skin conductance level and fluctuations. Replicating Engel and Bickford (1961), results showed that male HT patients had more consistent reactions than controls, evidenced by higher intraclass correlations (Fig. 7). HT patients showed their maximum responses in BP, whereas NT controls showed variable maximum responses. Individual response specificity was greater among HT patients than NT controls, both during anticipation of tasks and during actual stimulation, pointing to the possibility that HT subjects both prepare for and react to behavioral demands in a less flexible manner than do NT subjects.

In Engel and Bickford (1961), the greater BP reactivity observed in HT might have produced higher intraclass correlations in HT than NT. Consequently, Fredrikson et al. (1985b) excluded BP responses in the computation of intraclass correlations. When this was done, HT still showed greater individual response specificity, indicating a more consistent ordering of responses (other than BP) in HT than in NT (Fig. 8).

To further address the question whether intraclass correlations are independent of reactivity, beta-adrenoceptor antagonistis were administrated to a subgroup of

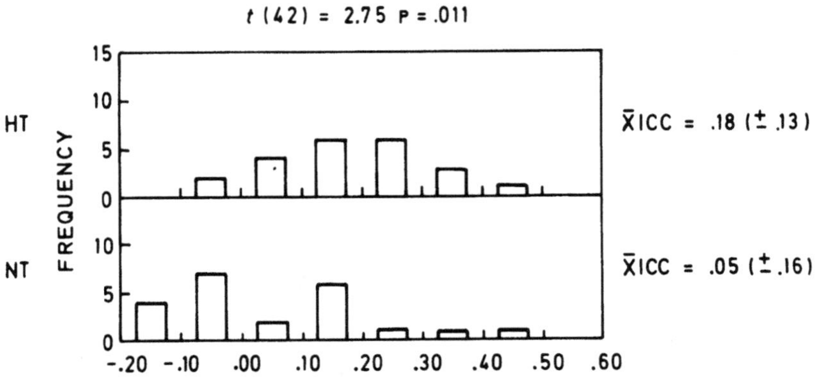

Fig. 8. Distribution of intraclass correlations *(ICC)*, mean correlations and *t*-test comparing hypertensive patients *(HT)* and normotensive controls *(NT)*, with blood pressure responses excluded. (After Fredrikson et al. 1985)

HT patients. Beta-adrenoceptor blockade attenuated SBP and HR reactivity, but failed to affect individual response specificity. The mean magnitude of the intraclass correlation coefficients were almost identical, and the correlation between the intraclass correlation coefficients obtained with and without drug treatment tended to be positive. Blood pressure was the most reactive and heart rate the least reactive system, whether patients were given blocking agents or not. Thus, neither the amount of consistency nor pattern end-points was affected by the attenuated reactivity. The greater consistency in HT is thus probably independent of BP reactivity. This indicates that individual patterns of autonomic activation are less flexible and less dependent on extrinsic factors in HT than NT.

Individual Response Specificity in Prospect

The theoretical significance of the concept of individual response specificity has been recognized (e.g., Engel and Bickford 1961; Foerster et al. 1983). In order to establish its clinical relevance, future studies must evaluate whether consistency is secondary or primary to HT. An important longitudinal issue is to determine if consistency changes as HT progresses. Also, since NT offspring of TH parents show enhanced cardiovascular reactivity (e.g., Falkner et al. 1979; Hastrup et al. 1982; Manuck and Proietti 1982) and data indicate that this hyperreactivity emerges across different behavioral tasks (Jorgenson and Houston 1981), it seems worthwhile to determine if these offspring also evidence greater individual response specificity, and, if so, whether that could be used as a marker for the development of HT or any other cardiovascular disease.

Acknowledgements. This research has been supported by grants from the National Defense Institute, Sweden, the National Institutes of Health, USA, and the Bergvalls Foundation, Sweden. The author was partially supported by a grant from the Swedish Work Environment Fund during preparation of this paper.

References

Alam M, Smirk FH (1938) Blood pressure raising reflexes in health, essential hypertension, and renal hypertension. Clin Sci 3: 259-266

Alderman MH (1980) The epidemiology of hypertension: etiology, natural history and the impact of therapy. Cardiovasc Rev Reports 1: 509-519

Ambrosini E, Costa FV, Montebugnoli C, Borghi C, Magnani B (1981) Intralymphocytic sodium concentration as an index of response to stress and excercise in young subjects with borderline hypertension. Clin Sci 61: 25s-27s

Anderson CD, Stoyva JM, Vaughn LJ (1982) A test of delayed recovery following stressful stimulation in four psychosomatic disorders. J Psychosom Res 26: 571-577

Ayman D (1934) Heredity in arteriolar (essential) hypertension: a clinical study of the blood pressure response of 1524 members of 277 families. Arch Int Med 53: 792-802

Ayman D, Goldshine AD (1938) Cold as a standard stimulus of blood pressure: a study of normal and hypertensive subjects. N Engl J Med 219: 650-655

Bahlman J, Brod J, Hubrich W, Pretscher P (1980) Beeinflussung der hämodynamischen Stressreaktion bei Hypertonikern durch eine kombinierte alfa- und beta-Blockade mit Labetalol. Dtsch Med Wochenschr 105: 1414-1418

Bahlman J, Brod J, Cachovan M (1982) Stress-induced changes of the venous circulation. Contrib Nephrol 30: 43-48

Baumann R, Ziprian H, Gödicke W, Hartrodt W, Naumann E, Läuter J (1973) The influence of acute psychic stress situations on biochemical and vegetative parameters of essential hypertensives at the early stage of the disease. Psychother Psychosom 22: 133-140

Berglund G, Andersson O, Wilhelmson L (1976) Prevalence of primary and secondary hypertension. Studies in a random population sample. Br Med J 2: 554-556

Boyer JT, Fraser JRE, Doyle AE (1960) The haemodynamic effects of cold immersion. Clin Sci 19: 539-550

Briggs JF, Oerting H (1933) Vasomotor response of normal and hypertensive individuals to thermal stimulus (cold). Minn Med 16: 481-486

Brod J, Fencl V, Hejl Z, Jirka J (1959) Circulatory changes underlying blood pressure elevation during acute emotional stress (mental arithmetic) in normotensive and hypertensive subjects. Clin Sci 18: 269-279

Brod J, Cachovan M, Bahlmann J, Bauer GE, Celsen B, Sippel R, Hundeshagen H, Feldmann U, Rienhoff O (1979) Haemodynamic changes during acute emotional stress in man with special reference to the capacitance vessels. Klin Wochenschr 57: 555-565

Bühler FR, Kiowski W, van Brummeln P, Amann FW, Bertel O, Landmann R, Ltold BE, Bolli P (1980) Plasma catecholamines and cardiac, renal and peripheral vascular adrenoceptor-mediated responses in different age groups of normal and hypertensive subjects. Clin Exp Hypertens 2: 409-426

Bühler FR, Bolli P, Hulthén UL, Amann FW, Kiowski W (1983) Alpha-adrenoceptors, adrenaline, and exaggerated vasoconstrictor response to stress in essential hypertension. Chest [Suppl] 83: 304-306

Cobb S, Rose RM (1973) Hypertension, peptic ulcer, and diabetes in air traffic controllers. JAMA 224: 489-492

Collins FH, Baer PE, Bourianoff GG (1981) Orienting behavior of children with hypertensive fathers. Psychophysiology 18: 181 (abstract)

Cowely AW Jr (1980) The concept of autoregulation of total blood flow and its role in hypertension. Am J Med 68: 906-916

Cuddy RP, Smulyan H, Keighley JF, Markuson CR, Eich RH (1966) Hemodynamic and catecholamine changes during a standard cold pressor test. Am Heart J 71: 446-454

Dahl CK (1977) Salt intake and hypertension. In: Genest J, Koiw E, Kuchel O (eds) Hypertension: physiopathology and treatment. McGraw Hill, New York

Devereux RB, Pickering TG, Harshfield GA, Kleinert HD, Denby L, Clark L, Pregibon D, Jason M, Kleiner B, Borer JS, Laragh JH (1983) Left ventricular hypertrophy in patients with hypertension: importance of blood pressure response to regularly recurring stress. Circulation 68: 470-476

Drummond PD (1983) Cardiovascular reactivity in mild hypertension. J Psychosom Res 4: 291-297

Dworkin BR, Filewich RJ, Miller NE, Craigwyle N, Pickering T (1979) Baroreceptor activation reduces reactivity to noxious stimulation: implications for hypertension. Science 205: 1299-1301
Eich RH, Jacobsen EC (1967) Vascular reactivity in medical students followed for ten years. J Chronic Dis 20: 583-592
Eliasson K, Hjemdahl P, Kahan T (1983) Circulatory and sympatho-adrenal responses to stress in borderline and established hypertension. J Hypertens 1: 131-139
Eliot RS, Buell JC, Dembroski TM (1982) Bio-behavioral perspectives on coronary heart disease, hypertension and sudden cardiac death. Acta Med Scand [Suppl] 606: 203-219
Engel BT (1983) Assessment and alteration of physiological reactivity. In: Dembroski TM, Schmidt TH, Blumchen G (eds) Biobehavioral bases of coronary heart disease. Karger, Basel
Engel BT, Bickford AF (1961) Response-specificity: stimulus-response and individual-response specificity in essential hypertensives. Arch Gen Psychiatry 5: 82-93
Esler MO, Nestel PJ (1973) Renin and sympathetic nervous system responsiveness to adrenergic stimuli in essential hypertension. Am J Cardiol 32: 643-649
Falkner B, Onesti G, Angelakos ET, Fernandes M, Langman C (1979) Cardiovascular response to mental stress in normal adolescents with hypertensive parents: hemodynamics and mental stress in adolescents. Hypertension 1: 23-30
Falkner B, Kushner H, Onesti G, Angelakos ET (1981) Cardiovascular characteristics in adolescents who develop essential hypertension. Hypertension 3: 521-527
Feldt RH, Weinstrand DEW, Milwaukee WS (1942) The cold-pressor test in subjects with normal blood pressure: report of observations on 350 subjects with special reference to the family history. Am Heart J 23: 766-771
Foerster F, Schneider HJ, Walschburger P (1983) The differentiation of individual-specific, stimulus-specific and motivation-specific response patterns in activation processes: an inquiry investigating their stability and possible importance in psychophysiology. Biol Psychol 17: 1-26
Folkow BS (1982) Physiological aspects of primary hypertension. Physiol Rev 62: 347-504
Fredrikson M, Engel BT (1985) Cardiovascular and electrodermal adjustments during a vigilance task in patients with borderline and established hypertension. J Psychosom 29: 235-246
Fredrikson M, Dimberg U, Frisk-Holmberg M (1980) Arterial blood pressure and electrodermal activity in hypertensive and normotensive subjects during inner and outer-directed attention. Acta Med Scand [Suppl] 645: 73-76
Fredrikson M, Dimberg U, Frisk-Holmberg M, Ström G (1982) Haemodynamic and electrodermal correlates of psychogenic stimuli in hypertensive and normotensive subjects. Biol Psychol 15: 63-73
Fredrikson M, Dimberg U, Frisk-Holmberg M, Ström G (1985 a) Arterial blood pressure and general sympathetic activation in essential hypertension during stimulation. Acta Med Scand 217: 309-317
Fredrikson M, Danielsson T, Engel BT, Frisk-Holmberg M, Ström G, Sundin Ö (1985 b) Autonomic nervous system function and essential hypertension: individual response specificity with and without beta adrenergic blockade. Psychophysiology 22: 167-174
Frisk-Holmberg M, Essén B, Fredrikson M, Ström G, Wibell L (1983) Muscle fibre composition in relation to blood pressure response to isometric exercise in normotensive and hypertensive subjects. Acta Med Scand 213: 21-26
Goldstein DS (1983) Plasma catecholamines and essential hypertension: an analytical review. Hypertension 5: 86-99
Greene NA, Boltax AJ, Lustig GA, Rogow E (1965) Circulatory dynamics during the cold pressor test. Am J Cardiol 16: 54-60
Groen JJ, Hansen B, Herrmann JM, Schäfer H, Schmidt T, Selbmann KH, v Uexüll Th, Weckman P (1982) Effects of experimental emotional stress and physical exercise on the circulation in hypertensive patients and control subjects. J Psychosom Res 26: 141-154
Guttman MC, Benson H (1971) Interaction of environmental factors and systematic arterial blood pressure. Medicine (Baltimore) 50: 543-553
Guyton A, Coleman TG, Cowley AW Jr, Manning RD Jr, Norman RA Jr, Ferguson JD (1974) A systems analysis approach to understanding longe-range arterial blood pressure control in hypertension. Circ Res 35: 159-176
Harlan WR Jr, Osborne RK, Graybiel A (1964) Prognostic value of the cold pressor test and the basal blood pressure: based on an eighteen year follow-up study. Am J Cardiol 13: 683-687

Harrel JP (1980) Psychological factors and hypertension. A status report. Psychol Bull 87: 482-501
Hastrup J, Light KC, Obrist PA (1982) Parental hypertension and cardiovascular response to stress in healthy young adults. Psychophysiology 19: 615-623
Henry JP, Stephans PM (1977) Stress, health and the social environment. A sociobiological approach to medicine. Springer, Berlin Heidelberg New York
Hines EA, Brown GE (1932) A standard stimulus for measuring vasomotor reactions: Its application in the study of hypertension. Proc Staff Meetings Mayo Clinic 7: 332-335
Hines EA, Brown GE (1933) A standard test for measuring the variability of blood pressure: its significance as an index of prehypertensive state. Ann Intern Med 7: 209-217
Hines EA, Brown GE (1936) The cold pressor test for measuring the reactibility of the blood pressure: data concerning 571 normal and hypertensive subjects. Am Heart J 11: 1-9
Hjemdahl P, Eliasson K (1979) Sympatho-adrenal and cardiovascular response to mental stress and orthostatic provocation in latent hypertension. Clin Sci 57: 189s-191s
Hodapp V, Weyer G, Becker J (1975) Situational stereotypy in essential hypertension patients. J Psychosom Res 19: 113-121
Hollenberg NK, Williams GH, Adams DF (1981) Essential hypertension: abnormal renal vascular and endocrine responses to a mild psychological stimulus. Hypertension 3: 11-17
Hypertension Detection and Follow-up Program Cooperative Group (1979) Five year findings of the hypertension detection and follow-up program. JAMA 2562-2577
Jern S (1982) Psychological and hemodynamic factors in borderline hypertension. Acta Med Scand [Suppl] 662: 1-54
Jern S, Hansson L, Sivertsson R (1985) Psychological differences between borderline hypertensives from a population sample and an outpatient hypertension clinic. (to be published)
Jorgensen RS, Houston BK (1981) Family history of hypertension, gender, and cardiovascular reactivity and stereotypy during stress. J Behav Med 4: 175-189
Jost H, Ruilman CJ, Hill TS, Gulo MJ (1952) Studies in hypertension II: central and autonomic nervous system reactions of hypertensive individuals to simple physical and psychologic stress situations. J Nerv Mental Dis 115: 152-162
Julius S, Schork MA (1971) Borderline hypertension - a critical review. J Chronic Dis 23: 723-759
Julius S, Schneider R, Egan B (1985) Suppressed anger in hypertension: facts and problems. In: Chesney M, Goldston S, Rosenman R (eds) Anger, hostility and behavioral medicine. Hemisphere, New York (to be published)
Kalis BL, Harris RE, Sokolow M, Carpenter LG (1957) Response to psychological stress in patients with essential hypertension. Am Heart J 53: 572-578
Keane TM, Martin JE, Berler ES, Wooten LS, Fleece EL, Williams G (1982) Are hypertensives less assertive? A controlled evaluation. J Consul Clin Psychol 50: 499-508
Krantz DS, Manuc SB (1985) Measures of acute physiologic reactivity to behavioral stimuli: assessment and critique. Psychol Bull (to be published)
Lacey J, Lacey BC (1974) Studies on heart rate and other bodily processes in sensorimotor behavior. In: Obrist PA, Black AH, Brener J, Di Cara LV (eds) Cardiovascular psychophysiology. Aldine, Chicago, pp 538-564
Laragh JH, Bear L, Brunner HR, Bühler FR, Sealy JE, Vaughn E (1976) The renin-angiotension-aldosteron system in pathogenesis and management of hypertensive vascular disease. In: Laragh JH (ed) Hypertension manual. New York Medical Books, New York, pp 313-320
Lawler KA, Allen MT (1981) Risk factors for hypertension in children: their relationship to psychophysiological measures. J Psychosom Res 23: 199-204
Lidberg L, Wallin BG (1981) Sympathetic skin nerve discharges in relation to amplitude of skin resistance responses. Psychophysiology 18: 268-271
Light KC (1981) Cardiovascular responses to effortful active coping: implications for the role of stress in hypertension development. Psychophysiology 19: 216-226
Light KC and Obrist PA (1980) Cardiovascular reactivity to behavioral stress in young males with and without marginally elevated causal systolic pressures. Hypertension 2: 802-808
Light K, Koepke JP, Obrist PA, Willis PW (1983) Psychological stress induces sodium and fluid retention in men at high risk for hypertension. Science 220: 429-431
Linden W, Feurstein M (1983) Essential hypertension and social coping behavior: experimental findings. J Human Stress 9: 22-31
Lorimer AR, Macfarlane PW, Provan G, Duffy T, Lawrie TDV (1971) Blood pressure and catechol-

amine responses to "stress" in normotensive and hypertensive subjects. Cardiovasc Res 5: 169-173
Louis WJ, Doyles AE, Anavcher S (1973) Plasma norepinephrine levels in essential hypertension. N Engl J Med 288: 599-605
Lund-Johansen P (1967) Hemodynamics in early essential hypertension. Acta Med Scand [Suppl] 482: 18
Lund-Johansen P (1977) Central hemodynamics in essential hypertension. Acta Med Scand [Suppl] 606: 35-42
Lynch JJ, Long JM, Thomas SA, Malinow KL, Katcher AH (1981) The effects of talking on the blood pressure of hypertensive and normotensive individuals. Psychosom Med 43: 25-33
Manuck SB, Proietti JM (1982) Parental hypertension and cardiovascular response to cognitive and isometric challenge. Psychophysiology 19: 481-489
Manuck SB, Morrison RL, Bellack AS (1985) Behavioral factors in hypertension: cardiovascular responsivity, anger, and social competence. In: Chesney M, Goldston S, Rosenman R (eds) Anger, hostility and behavioral medicine. Hemisphere, New York (to be published)
McKegney FP, Williams RB (1967) Psychological aspects of hypertension: II. The differential influence of interview variables on blood pressure. Am J Psychiatry 123: 1539-1545
Miller JH and Brugger M (1939) The cold pressor reaction in normal subjects and in patients with primary (essential) and secondary (renal) hypertension. Am Heart J 18: 329-333
Miller RE, Shapiro AP, King HE, Ginchereau EG, Hosutt JA (1984) Effect of antihypertensive treatment on the behavioral consequences of elevated blood pressure. Hypertension 6: 202-208
Murakami E, Hiwada K, Kokubu T (1980) Pathophysiological characteristics of labile hypertensive patients determined by the cold pressor test. Jpn Circ J 44: 438-442
Nestel PJ (1969) Blood-pressure and catecholamine excretion after mental stress in labile hypertension. Lancet I: 692-695
Newlin DB, Levenson RW (1982) Cardiovascular response of individuals with Type A behavior pattern and parental coronary heart disease. J Psychosom Res 26: 393-402
Nyberg G (1976) Blood pressure and heart rate response to isometric exercise and mental arithmetic in normotensive and hypertensive subjects. Clin Sci Mol Med 51: 681s-685s
Nyberg G, Graham RM, Stokes GS (1977) The effect of mental arithmetic in normotensive and hypertensive subjects and its modification by beta-adrenergic receptor blockade. Br J Clin Pharmacol 4: 469-474
Obrist PA (1981) Cardiovascular psychophysiology. Plenum, New York
Obrist PA, Gaebelein CJ, Teller ES, Langer AW, Grignolo A, Light K, McCubbin JA (1978) The relationship among heart rate, carotid dP/dt and blood pressure in humans as a function of the type of stress. Psychophysiology 15: 102-115
Page IH (1977) Some regulatory mechanisms of renovascular and essential arterial hypertension. In: Genest J, Koiw E, Kuchel O (eds) Hypertension: physiopathology and treatment. McGraw Hill, New York, pp 576-587
Pickering GW (1961) The nature of essential hypertension. Churchill, London
Pickering GW, Kissin M (1935) The effects of adrenaline and of cold on the blood pressure in human hypertension. Clin Sci 2: 201-207
Prikryl P, Rysanek K, Kuetnansky R, Kunovska V, Rechtorikova O, Dohnalova I (1982) Sympathethic activity in labile essential hypertension in young men. Part I: plasma catecholamines after orthostatic and emotional stress test. Act Nerv Super 24: 29-30
Rahe RH, Arajärvi H, Arajärvi S, Punsar S, Karvonen MJ (1976) Recent life change and coronary heart disease in east versus west Finland. J Psychosom 20: 431-437
Remington RD, Lambarth B, Moser M, Hoobler SN (1960) Circulatory reactions of normotensive and hypertensive subjects and of children of normal hypertensive parents. Am Heart J 59: 58-70
Richter-Heinrich E, Knust U, Miller W, Schmidt KH, Sprung H (1975) Psychophysiological investigations in essential hypertensives. J Psychosom Res 19: 251-258
Sapira JD, Scheib ET, Moriarty R, Shapiro AP (1971) Differences in perception between hypertensive and normotensive populations. Psychosom Med 33: 239-250
Schachter J (1957) Pain, fear, and anger in hypertensives and normotensives. Psychosom Med 19: 17-29

Schmeider R, Neus H, Schulte W (1982) Zur Beziehung zwischen Blutdruckvariabilität und Blutdruckrealitivität bei essentieller Hypertonie. Med Welt 33: 70/939-71/940
Schulte W, Neus H (1979) Bedeutung von Stressreaktionen in der Hypertoniediagnostik. Herz Kreislauf 11: 541-546
Schulte W, Neus H (1983) Hemodynamics during emotional stress in borderline and mild hypertension. Eur Heart J 4: 803-809
Schulte W, Neus H, v Eiff AW (1981) Blutdruckreaktivität unter emotionalem Stress bei unkomplizierten Formen des Hochdrucks. Klin Wochenschr 59: 1243-1249
Schulte W, Neus H, Thönes M, v Eiff AW (1984) Basal blood pressure variability and reactivity of blood pressure to emotional stress in essential hypertension. Basic Res Cardiol 79: 9-16
Shapiro AP (1961) An experimental study of comparative responses of blood pressure to different noxious stimuli. J Chronic Dis 13: 293-311
Shapiro AP, Moutsos SE, Krifcher E (1963) Patterns of pressor response to noxious stimuli in normal, hypertensive and diabetic subjects. J Clin Invest 42: 1890-1898
Shapiro AP, Benson H, Chobanian AV, Herd AJ, Julius S, Kaplan N, Lazarus RS, Ostfeld AM, Syme SL (1979) The role of stress in hypertension. J Human Stress 5: 7-26
Shapiro AP, Miller RE, King HE, Ginchereau EH, Fitzgibbon K (1982) Behavioral consequences of mild hypertension. Hypertension 4: 355-360
Sokolow M, Werdegar D, Kain HK, Hinman AT (1966) Relationship between level of blood pressure measured casually and by portable recorders and severity of complications in essential hypertension. Circulation 34: 279
Steptoe A (1981) Psychological factors in cardiovascular disorders. Academic, London
Steptoe A (1984) Psychophysiological processes in disease. In: Steptoe A, Mathews A (eds) Health care and human behaviour. Academic, London
Steptoe A, Melville DR, Ross A (1983) Behavioral response demands, cardiovascular reactivity and essential hypertension. Psychosom Med 45: 33-48
Sullivan P, Schoeutgen S, DeQuattro V, Procci W, Levine D, Van der Meulen J, Bornheimer J (1981) Anxiety, anger, and neurogenic tone at rest and in stress in patients with primary hypertension. Hypertension [Suppl II] 3: 119-123
Surwit RS, Williams RB, Shapiro D (1982) Behavioral approaches to cardiovascular disease. Academic, New York
Svensson JCh, Theorell T (1982) Cardiovascular effects of anxiety induced by interviewing young hypertensive male subjects. J Psychosom Res 26: 359-370
Takeshita A, Imaizumi T, Ashihara T, Yamamoto K, Hoka S, Nakamura M (1982) Limited maximal vasodilator capacity of forearm resistance vessels in normotensive young men with a familial predisposition to hypertension. Circ Res 50: 671-677
Theorell T, Lind E (1973) Systolic blood pressure, serum cholesterol, and smoking in relation to sociological factors and myocardial infarction. J Psychosom Res 17: 327-332
van der Valk JM (1957) Blood pressure changes under emotional influences in patients with hypertension and control subjects. J Psychosom Res 2: 134-146
von Eiff AW (1984) Pathophysiologie und Ätiologie der essentiellen Hypertonie. Münchener Medizinische Wochenschrift, 1984, 126, 165-170
von Scheuck K, Pietruschka WD, Schreiniche G, Gruber G, Huber B (1979) Differenzierung jugendlicher essentieller arterieller Hypertoniker durch psychophysiologische Untersuchungen und ihr Vergleich zum Verhalten physiologischer Parameter bei physischer Belastung. Deutsche Gesundheitswesen 34: 547-552
Voudoukis IJ (1978) Cold pressor test and hypertension. Angiology 29: 429-439
Wallin BG, Delius W, Hagbarth K-E (1973) Comparison of sympathetic nerve activity in normotensive and hypertensive subjects. Circ Res 333: 9-21
Weiner H (1977) Psychobiology and human disease. Elesevier, New York
Weiner H, Singer MT, Reiser MF (1962) Cardiovascular responses and their psychological correlates I: a study in healthy young adults and patients with peptic ulcer and hypertension. Psychosom Med 24: 477-497
Whitehead WE, Blackwell B, DeSilva H, Robinson A (1977) Anxiety and anger in hypertension. J Psychosom Res 21: 383-389
Wolf S, Pfeiffer JB, Ripley HS, Winter OS, Wolff HG (1948) Hypertension as a reaction pattern to

stress; summary of experimental data on variations in blood pressure and renal blood flow. Ann Intern Med 29: 1056-1076
Wolf S, Cardon PV, Shepard EM, Wollf HG (1955) Life stress and essential hypertension. Williams and Wilkins Baltimore
Wood DL, Sheps SG, Elveback LR, Schringer A (1984) Cold pressor test as a predictor of hypertension. Hypertension 6: 301-306

The Prognostic Significance of Exercise Induced Hypertension in Heart Infarction Patients

A.-T. TAMMEN, G. BIERCK, T. FENTROP, and G. BLÜMCHEN[1]

To determine the prognostic and clinical significance of exercise-induced hypertension (ExHPT) in heart infarction (HI) patients, blood pressure (BP) and course of disease in 83 HI patients with ExHPT were compared with those in a control (CT) group of 54 HI patients without ExHPT. After 7-8 years, 60 patients from the ExHPT-group and 30 patients from the CT group were reevaluated.

Patients and Methods

Exercise-induced hypertension (ExHPT) is defined as increases in BP over 200/100 mmHg at an ergometry exercise level of 100 w (Wink 1965; Franz 1982). Because under ergometer conditions, diastolic values are not always clearly determinable, the systolic BP value is considered to be the deciding factor. Initial study of the patients was made 8 months on an average after the infarction, while the patients were undergoing subsequent treatment. The reevaluation was done using ambulatory methods. The average age (49 vs. 46.4 years), sex (59 men and 1 woman vs. 30 men), as well as type of infarction (34 posterior HI, 23 anterior HI and 3 intramural HI vs. 17 posterior and 13 anterior wall HI), and average body weight were not significantly different between the reevaluated ExHPT patients and the CT group.

Amnestic hypertension, as well as antihypertensive therapy, was ruled out for every patient. The bicycle-ergometer test was performed with the patient in a supine position with the upper body slightly raised. Each exercise step of 40 or 20 w lasted for 4-min. BP was measured using a commercial measuring device containing a mercury column and standard cuff, as recommended by the WHO. Measurements were taken just before the start of the ergometer test and immediately after the end of each exercise step, until 5 min after the end of the exercise. Electrocardiogram (ECG) and pulse rate measurements were recorded regularly. The breakdown of the ergometer test followed the generally accepted guideline rules. None of the patients in the initial study suffered from angina pectoris under normal conditions. In the follow-up study, a careful anamnesis, a clinical examination, and an echocardiogram were performed. In addition to the ergometer test, BP was also measured at least three times at rest in a sitting position. The statistical evaluation was done by using the *t* test (paired and unpaired) and the chi-square test for a four-strip board.

1 Klinik Roderbirken der LVA Rheinprovinz, 5653 Leichlingen/Rhld. 1, Federal Republic of Germany

Biological and Psychological Factors
in Cardiovascular Disease
Ed. by T. H. Schmidt, T. M. Dembroski, and G. Blümchen

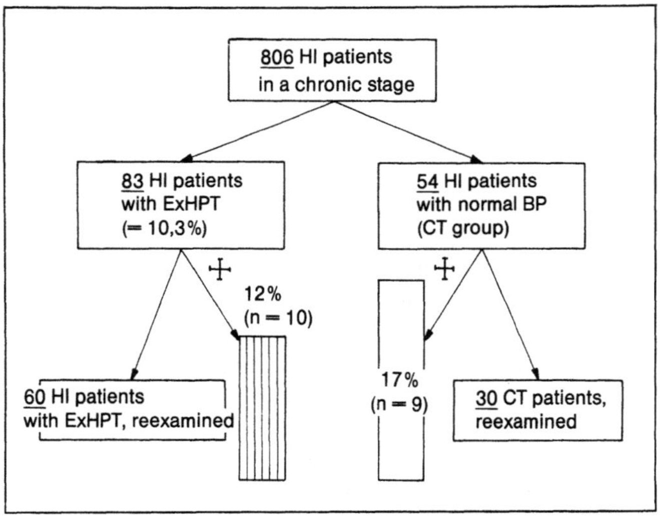

Fig. 1. Survey of the groups of patients investigated and of the mortality rates of the ExHT patients and CT groups

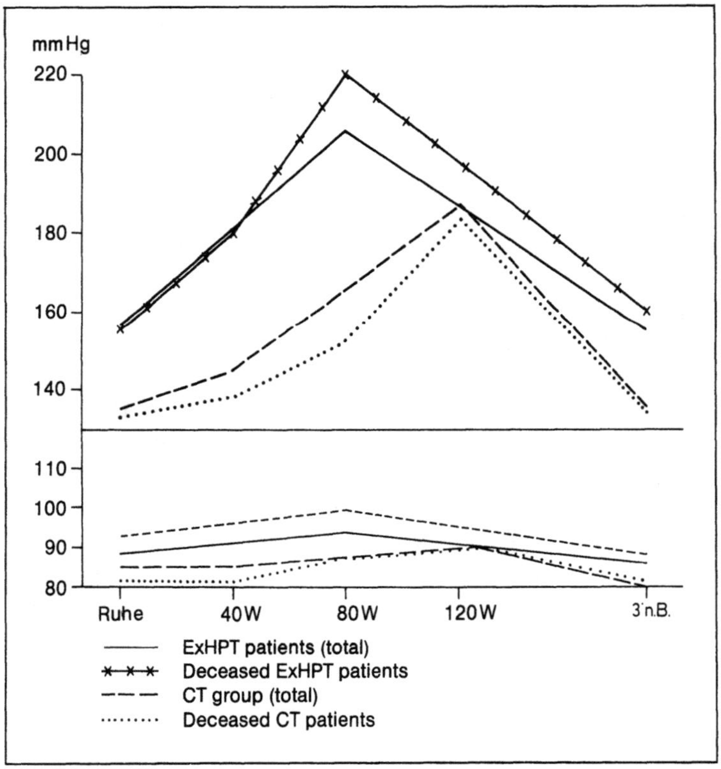

Fig. 2. Comparison of the ExBP reaction of the ExHT patients, CT group, and deceased patients from both collectives

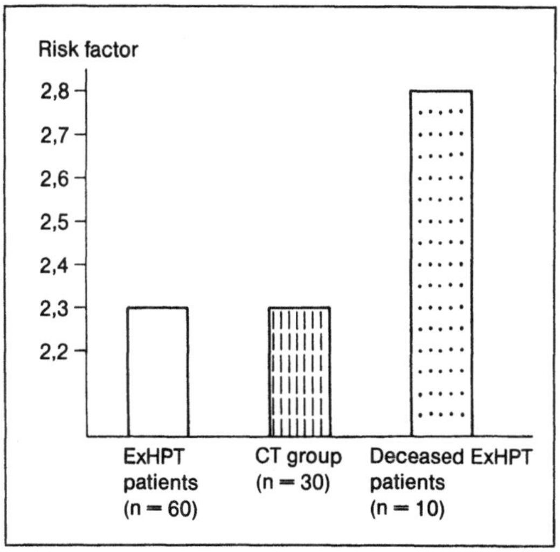

Fig. 3. Average number of risk factors per patient: A comparison of the total collective with the deceased ExHT patients. ("Risk-factor" valued as: cigarettes >10/day; serum cholesterol >260 mg/dl; serum triglycerides >200 mg/dl; uric acid >8 mg/dl, diabetes)

Results

The 83 ExHPT patients were recruited from a total of 806 HI patients. Thus, the frequency of exercise hypertension in our infarction patients amounted to 10.3%. At the time of the follow-up study, 7-8 years later, 10 (12%) of the 83 HI patients with ExHPT and 9 of the 54 HI patients from the CT group (17%) had died (Fig. 1).

The exercise-induced blood pressure (ExBP) of *the deceased ExHPT patients* was significantly higher than the average BP of the other ExHPT patients (16/4 mmHg at the 80-w level; Fig. 2).

However, it must be said that the number of anterior wall infarction patients (8 out of 10), as well as the incidence of additional cardiovascular risk factors (2.8 in comparison to 2.3) of the deceased ExHPT patients was also clearly higher than average (Fig. 3). Therefore, the strikingly high ExBP was not the only determining factor responsible for the premature death of this group. Additionally, coronary morphology was unknown.

Clear BP differences between the ExHPT patients and the CT group were already apparent at rest. In the initial study, *BP at rest,* measured during the intake examination, averaged 147/90 mmHg in the ExHPT patients, compared with an average of 132/89 mmHg in the CT group. Before the beginning of ergometry, BP values at rest averaged 154/88 and 136/85 mmHg, respectively (Fig. 4).

During hospitalization, 53 of the 60 ExHPT patients (88%), but only 8 of the 30 CT patients (27%), had BP values between 140/90 mmHg and 160/95 mmHg. This demonstrates that nearly all patients with ExHPT suffered from so-called borderline hypertension.

The follow-up study, 7-8 years later, showed the following results with regard to *BP development* (Tammen et al. 1984; Tables 1, 2, 3): A total of 37 patients (62% - Group I) from the ExHPT group and 7 patients (23%) from the CT group had developed manifest hypertension. A total of 7 former ExHPT patients (11% - Group 3) and 16 patients from the control group (56%) showed normal BP values at

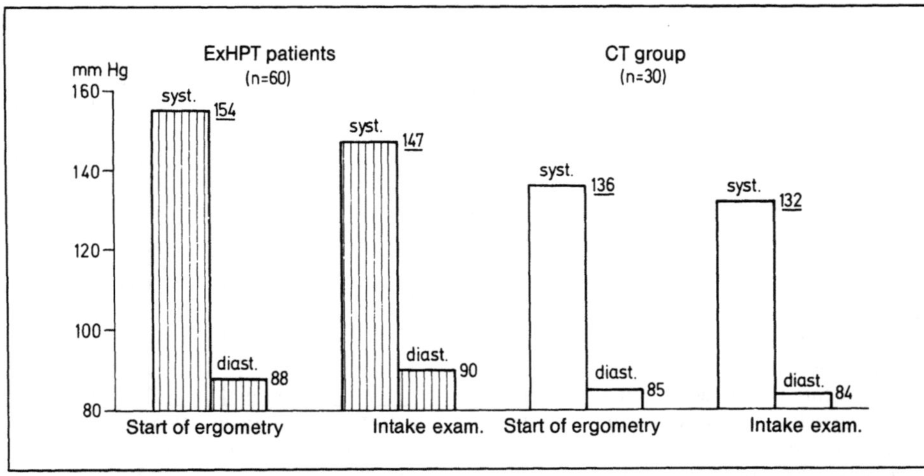

Fig. 4. Average BP at the intake examination of the ExHT patients and the CT group during their first medical check-up and at the beginning of the bicycle ergometer test

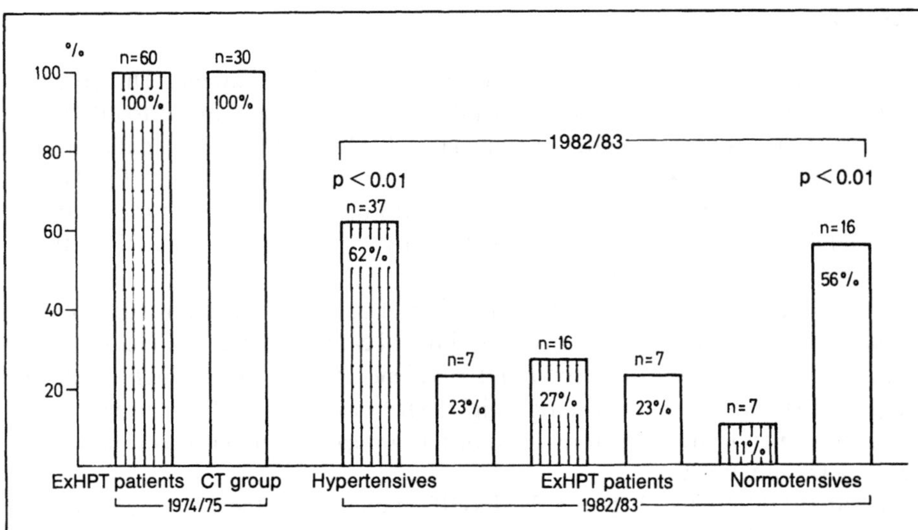

Fig. 5. Development of BP between 1974/75 and 1982/83 in the ExHT patients and in the CT group

rest and during exercise. Sixteen ExHPT patients (Group 2) showed no substantial change in their BP. Furthermore, they had borderline BP values at rest with an overshooting increase during exercise. Seven patients from the CT group (23%) reacted with newly discovered hypertension during exercise (Fig. 5). The follow-up study also shows a significantly greater *increase in average BP at rest* in the CT group in comparison with the ExHPT patients (25/14 vs. 13/10 mmHg; Fig. 6). Especially impressive was the massive BP increase of the patients developing hypertension within the CT group as compared with the patients developing hypertension in the

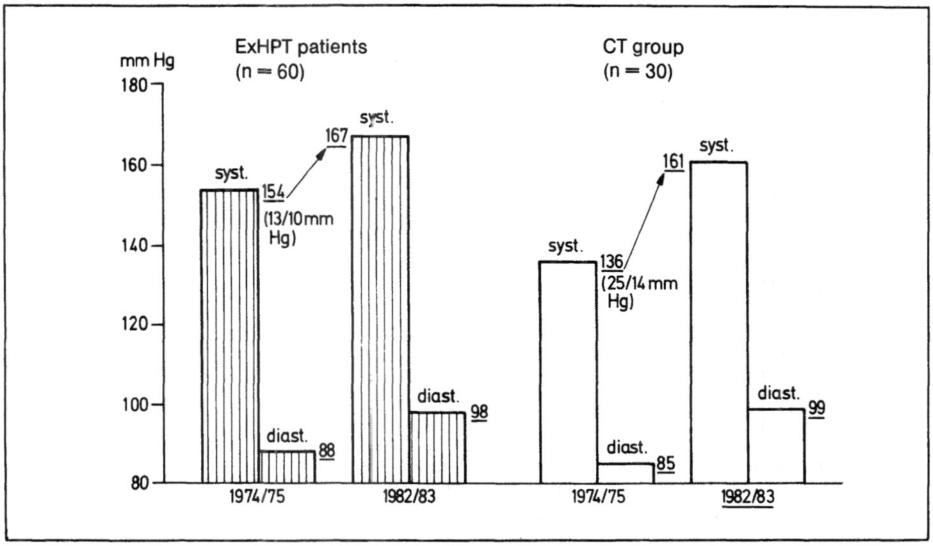

Fig. 6. Average increase in BP at rest (before the beginning of the ergometer test) from 1974/75 to 1982/83 in ExHT patients and CT group

ExHPT group. These patients with manifest hypertension in the CT group ($n = 7$) had developed an increase in BP of 50/28 mmHg in contrast to 26/13 mmHg for the manifest hypertension patients in the ExHPT group ($n = 37$). *BP during exercise* also showed a greater increase in the CT group than in the ExHPT patients. At the 80 w level, the BP increase in the CT group amounted to 28/20 mmHg, in contrast to a diastolic BP increase of only 10 mmHg in the ExHPT patients. Consequently, a rather small BP increase caused manifest hypertension in ⅔ of the ExHPT patients because of their rather high initial level of BP at the first examination.

At the time of the follow-up study, 22 (59%) of the ExHPT patients who had developed manifest hypertension were receiving *antihypertensive medication:* 13 patients received beta-blockers and 9 patients received diuretics. A significant difference in their antihypertensive effect on exercise hypertension was not found.

The clinical course of disease showed significant differences between the CT group and the ExHPT patients. Within the ExHPT group, differences between the patients who developed hypertension and those who did not were also noted. A total of 43% of the ExHPT patients, in comparison with 10% of the CT group, had developed *cardiovascular complications* (reinfarction, apoplectic insult, manifest heart insufficiency) or a progression of angina pectoris symptoms of at least one stage, according to NYHA. An increase of angina pectoris symptoms was largely responsible for these events. A deteriorating clinical course was observed most clearly in those ExHPT patients who had developed manifest hypertension (Fig. 7).

The *ergometric endurance* of the ExHPT patients was, from the beginning, on the average 22% lower than the endurance of the control group. At the time of the follow-up study, the ergometric endurance of the control group decreased to 17%, whereas it decreased to 29% in those ExHPT patients who had developed manifest hypertension (Fig. 8).

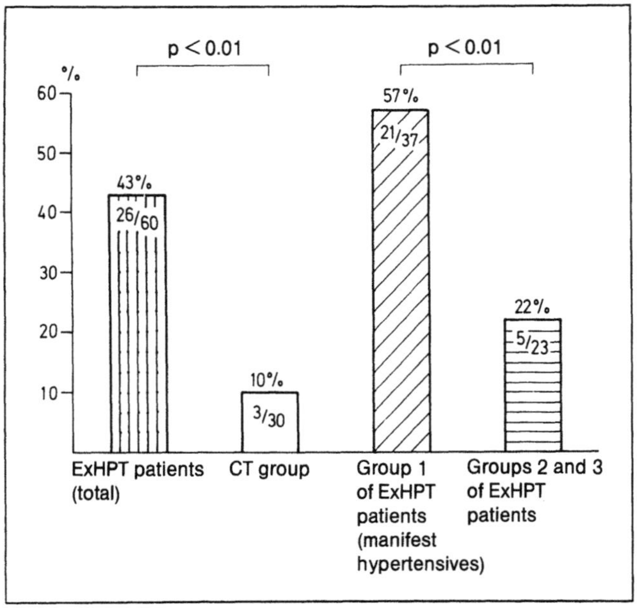

Fig. 7. Comparison of the clinical course from 1974/75 to 1982/83 in the total collective of the ExHT patients, CT group, and single groups of the ExHT collective. (For explanation, see text)

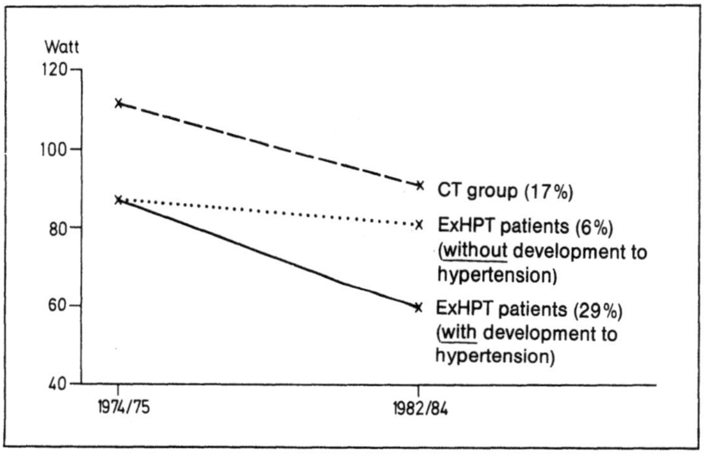

Fig. 8. Average decrease in ergometer capacity between 1974/75 and 1982/83

According to the Broca index, at the time of the initial study, the average *overweight* measurement of the patients in the ExHPT group and the CT group patients was 6 kg. At the time of the follow-up study, both groups had gained 2 kg and 4 kg, respectively; however, there was a slightly above average increase in the patients developing hypertension from both collectives (Fig. 9).

The *echocardiographic examination* showed that in 22 of the 60 ExHPT patients (37%), the end diastolic diameter of the left ventricle had dilated to at least 58 mm,

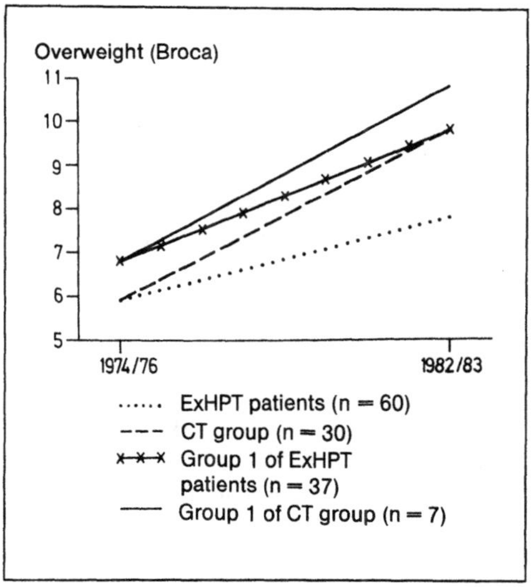

Fig. 9. Comparison of body weight between the total collective of ExHT patients, CT group, and those groups who developed hypertension

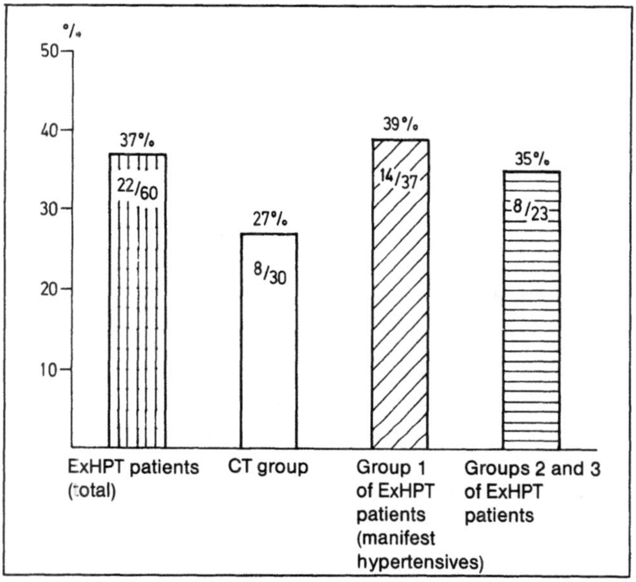

Fig. 10. Comparison of the echocardiographic end-diastolic diameter (> 58 mm) in the total collective of ExHPT patients and CT group, as well as in group 1 of the ExHPT patients and groups 2 and 3

indicating a reduced function of the left ventricle. This was the case in 8 out of 30 patients in the CT group (27%). A significant difference between patients with and patients without developing hypertension could not be established (Fig. 10). A septum hypertrophy of at least 13 mm was found in ten patients with manifest hypertension from the ExHPT group, but not in any patient from the CT group. A positive Sokolow index was found in four hypertension patients from the ExHPT collective.

Discussion

Methodological problems cannot be disregarded in the evaluation of the results of our study. The study-design was not prospective, the BP measurements were not standardized, and BP values of outpatients had to be compared with those of inpatients. Furthermore, possible influences of medicinal changes during the interim period, as well as the time factor of 7-8 years must be considered. However, in spite of these methodological problems, we think that the present results demonstrate a remarkable prognostic significance of the ExBP for the development of manifest hypertension. This phenomenon had already been demonstrated in a similar way for people without coronary heart disease, but borderline hypertension at rest (Franz 1981; Amecke and Rost 1983).

In our myocardial infarction patients, ExHPT was combined with borderline hypertension at rest in nearly 90% of the cases. There seems to be no fundamental difference in the prognostic value of the ExHPT reaction between people without coronary heart disease and those in a chronic myocardial infarction stage.

The overshooting BP reaction during exercise may "only" represent, in some of our patients, the revelation of a hypertensive BP state which already existed before the infarction event. In this case, the ergometer test could be seen as a provocation test that reveals a hypertensive BP state which had been hidden by the infarction event and the special circumstances of its treatment.

Because coronary status and ventricle function - the most important determinating factors of the prognosis of our HI patients - were unknown, it is not possible to draw conclusions about the mortality and the rank of ExHPT as a possible cardiovascular risk factor.

The mortality of only 12% 7 years after the myocardial infarction event is a strong argument against the importance of ExHPT as a cardiovascular risk factor, because the average mortality after this time amounts to 25%-30% (Proudfit 1978). Moreover, it must be considered that our ExHPT group was a positive selection of myocardial infarction patients because of their good ergometric endurance. Nevertheless, the clearly deteriorating clinical course, especially the serious progression of angina pectoris, may indicate the significance of the development of manifest hypertension for the further prognosis of the coronary heart disease. Therefore, in our opinion, an antihypertensive therapy with beta-blockers should be considered early for infarction patients with ExHPT, because, for a variety of reasons, they seem to improve the prognosis in secondary prophylaxis after infarction (Norwegian Multicenter Study Group 1981).

The outstanding increase of BP at rest in the CT group, which was almost double the average BP increase of the ExHPT patients and caused manifest hypertension in one-quarter of the CT group patients, is a rather surprising result of our study. At present we are not prepared to advance reasons for the high BP increase in normotensive infarction patients. Perhaps some of these patients also had latent hypertension before the infarction event, but the "provocation test bicycle-ergometer" did not, in their case, provoke ExHPT.

Summary

Comparison of BP and course of disease in 83 HI patients with and 54 without ExHPT yielded the following results after 7-8 years:

The death rate, 12% or 17%, respectively, was not significantly different; however, the course of disease in the ExHPT patients was more severe. A total of 62% of the ExHPT patients and 23% of the CT group developed manifest hypertension at rest. The average BP increase at rest and at exercise was clearly higher in the CT group than in the ExHPT group.

Acknowledgments. The authors are grateful to the Verein für Gefäßerkrankungen e.V., Engelskirchen and to the Landesversicherungsanstalt Rheinprovinz, Düsseldorf.

References

Amecke F, Rost R (1983) The prognostic significance of an overshooting exercise blood pressure as an indicator for subsequent manifestation of hypertension. Sportwissenschaftlicher Verlag, Tübingen

Franz IW (1981) Belastungsblutdruck bei Hochdruckkranken. Springer, Berlin Heidelberg New York

Franz IW (1982) Ergometrie bei Hochdruckkranken. Springer, Berlin Heidelberg New York

Norwegian Multicenter Study Group (1981) Timolol-induced reduction in mortality and reinfarction in patients surviving acute myocardial infarction. N Engl J Med 304: 801

Proudfit WL (1978) Minor prognostic associations. Cleve Clin Q 45: 141

Tammen AT, Bierck G, Fentrop T, Blümchen G (1984) Prognostische Bedeutung des Belastungsblutdrucks bei Herzinfarktpatienten. In: Anlauf M, Bock KD (eds) Blutdruck unter körperlicher Belastung. Dr. Steinkopf Verlag, Darmstadt

Wink K (1965) Statistische Untersuchungen über den arteriellen Blutdruck unter Ruhe- und Belastungsbedingungen und Versuch einer Normenbildung. Inaugural Dissertation, Freiburg

IV. Animal Models

Atherosclerosis, Social Dominance and Cardiovascular Reactivity

S. B. Manuck,[1] J. R. Kaplan, and T. B. Clarkson[2]

Introduction

Animal models play an important role in the study of atherogenesis because, under suitable dietary conditions, many species develop atherosclerotic lesions more rapidly than do human beings. In addition, use of animals permits experimental manipulation of pertinent environmental variables, as well as a more precise quantification of lesion characteristics (e.g., size, composition) than is feasible in clinical studies of human subjects. Moreover, among vertebrate species the nonhuman primates - in particular, Old World monkeys - have attracted the greatest interest of atherosclerosis researchers. Old World primates do not develop extensive atherosclerosis in their natural environments, yet all are susceptible to diet-induced hyperlipoproteinemia and the resulting patterns of atherosclerosis are similar, in many species, to those seen in human beings. Of the Old World monkeys, the macaques, especially rhesus and cynomolgus monkeys, are considered to be exceptionally useful models. This is due not only to the fact that the characteristics of lesions seen in these species closely resemble important features of human atherosclerosis, but also to pragmatic considerations such as the macaque's convenient size, commercial availability, and acceptance of experimental diets (Kaplan et al. 1985).

In addition, nonhuman primates provide a good model for the study of psychosocial influences on atherogenesis. The behavioral repertoires of primates are remarkably complex, with relationships among individuals defined by elaborated patterns of agonistic and affiliative interaction. The organization of most primate social groups is characterized, too, by a matrix of relational bonds (e.g., male-female, mother-infant, matrifocal subunits) and by interindividual hierarchies of social dominance (Lancaster 1975). Thus, many of the prominent dimensions of primate behavior - affiliation, social status, competition, aggression - reflect significant aspects of human social behavior as well. That certain of these behaviors (e.g., competitiveness, aggression) are also thought to promote atherogenesis in man - and others (e.g., affiliation) to have a protective influence on lesion development - further underscores the appropriateness of nonhuman primates in studies of experimentally induced atherosclerosis.

The purpose of this paper is to describe recent research, conducted at the Arteriosclerosis Research Center of Bowman Gray School of Medicine, Wake Forest University, investigating behavioral influences on coronary artery atherogenesis in

1 Department of Psychology, Clinical Psychology Center, 604 Engineering Hall, 4015 O'Hara Street, Pittsburgh, PA 15260, USA

2 Arteriosclerosis Research Center, Bowman Gray School of Medicine, Wake Forest University, Winston-Salem, NC 27109, USA

Biological and Psychological Factors
in Cardiovascular Disease
Ed. by T. H. Schmidt, T. M. Dembroski, and G. Blümchen

male cynomolgus macaques *(Macaca fascicularis)*. First, we review the results of two experiments that examine effects of psychosocial variables (viz., environmental stress, social status) on lesion development (Kaplan et al. 1982, 1983). The findings of both studies demonstrate that disruption of ordinary social relationships potentiates atherogenesis, especially among monkeys of high social rank (i.e., in dominant animals). We next describe related psychophysiological observations which demonstrate that monkeys that had shown the largest heart rate responsivity to a common laboratory challenge also had significantly increased atherosclerosis when compared to animals exhibiting a less pronounced cardiac response to stress (Manuck et al. 1983). The latter finding offers preliminary support to speculation that acute psychophysiological reactivity mediates associations between behavioral factors and atherogenesis. Yet, interestingly, social dominance - the behavioral characteristic related most appreciably to atherosclerosis in our initial work - did not covary significantly with animals' heart rate reactions to our standard laboratory stressor. Observations described in the latter section of this paper, however, document that in disrupted social environments the heart rates of dominant animals do fluctuate greatly, but as a function of naturally occurring changes in physical proximity and affiliative contact with other monkeys. Together, these results suggest: (1) that psychosocial variables contribute significantly to coronary artery atherogenesis in this animal model; and (2) that some monkeys may be susceptible to development of atherosclerosis because of a generalized cardiac hyperresponsivity to behavioral stimuli, while others may have an increased risk which is associated with autonomic responses to the behavioral demands of retaining dominant social status in an unstable, or stressful, environment.

Experiment I

The 30 animals employed in this experiment were all adult, male cynomolgus monkeys, imported from Malaysia and the Philippine Islands. The chief advantage of the cynomolgus macaque as a model of atherosclerosis is its high susceptibility, given a moderate hyperlipoproteinemia, to development of fatty streaks, and the rapid progression of these initial lesions to the formation of fibrous plaques (Kramsch and Hollander 1968; Armstrong and Megan 1975; Malinow et al. 1976; Wagner et al. 1978). Additionally, atherosclerotic lesions induced in these animals by the feeding of dietary cholesterol often show necrosis, mineralization, and the pooling of fat droplets or crystalline lipid (Armstrong et al. 1980; Clarkson 1980). Cynomolgus macaques experience myocardial infarction as well, with an incidence similar to that seen in man (Bond et al. 1980). Also, as in human beings, coronary artery atherosclerosis in male cynomolgus monkeys is more extensive than that observed among females (Rudel and Pitts 1978; Hamm et al. 1983).

Animals were assigned to one of two experimental conditions. These were designated the "stable" and "unstable" social conditions, and each consisted of three, five-member social groups. All groups were housed in identical pens and were fed a moderately atherogenic diet for 22 months. This diet derived 43% of calories from fat and had a cholesterol concentration of 0.34 mg/kcal; the latter is equivalent to a daily consumption, in man, of approximately 680 mg cholesterol.

Our psychosocial stressor involved the periodic reorganization of group memberships in the unstable social condition. Animals assigned to the three unstable groups were redistributed on a regular basis and in a manner ensuring that each monkey would be housed with either three of four new animals on every reorganization. The actual redistribution of monkeys took place once every 12 weeks during the first year of the study, and once every 4 weeks thereafter. We hypothesized that reorganization of group memberships would constitute a potent social stressor in this experiment, based on previous reports by other investigators describing the reactions of members of macaque social groups to the sudden introduction of unfamiliar monkeys (Bernstein et al. 1974). The appearance of strangers is experienced as a threat to existing relationships among monkeys and leads to intensification of agonistic encounters (including an increased frequency of overt aggression) as animals seek to reestablish generalized hierarchical associations and affiliative coalitions. Moreover, in order to promote further competition and social uncertainty among the monkeys in this investigation, an estrogen-primed, ovariectomized female was added to the unstable groups for half of each 4-week period occurring during the final 10 months of the study.

In contrast to the unstable condition, animals assigned to the stable (or unstressed) social condition lived in groups of fixed memberships throughout the experiment. Hence, "stable" animals were neither redistributed nor exposed to unfamiliar monkeys after placement into their initial social groupings. Also, unlike the unstable condition, females were never introduced into the stable social groups as a stimulus for heightened intragroup competition.

Over the course of the study, repeated measurements were made of a number of pertinent physiological variables, including total serum cholesterol (TSC) and high-density lipoprotein cholesterol (HDLC) concentrations, systolic and diastolic blood pressure (SBP, DBP), ponderosity, and fasting glucose concentration. Behavioral observations were also recorded routinely, using a focal sampling technique (Altmann 1974). Frequencies of aggressive, submissive, and affiliative acts were assessed in each monkey, based on approximately 50 h of behavioral monitoring per animal.

We also evaluated the relative rank, or social status, of the individual monkeys. Macaque social groups are characterized by linear dominance hierarchies, in which the rank of each animal is determined by its ability to defeat other group members in fights (Kawai 1958; Sade 1967; Bernstein 1970). Thus, our measurement of social status was derived from the observed outcomes of each monkey's aggressive interactions with other members of the same social group. In this experiment, the social status of individual animals showed considerable stability over time, and, in the unstable condition, across successive group reorganizations. In obtaining an overall descriptor of each animal's status, monkeys ranked first or second in their respective groups during a majority of the social evaluations conducted across the study (i.e., monkeys of consistently high rank) were identified as "dominant" monkeys for the experiment; the remaining, lesser ranked animals were designated "subordinates."

At necropsy, the animals' coronary arteries were perfused at a pressure of 100 mmHg. Five tissue blocks were cut perpendicularly to the long axis of each of three arteries, the left anterior descending, left circumflex, and right coronary ar-

Table 1. Mean coronary artery intimal area measurements (± SEM) among dominant and subordinate monkeys in the stable and unstable social conditions (Kaplan et al. 1982; Reprinted by permission of the American Heart Association, Incorporated)

Social condition	Social status	
	Dominant	Subordinate
Stable	0.32 mm^2 (±0.13)	0.45 mm^2 (±0.12)
Unstable	0.74 mm^2 (±0.12)	0.38 mm^2 (±0.10)

teries. Sections cut from each block were stained with either hematoxylin and eosin or Verhoeff Van Gieson stains. The Verhoeff Van Gieson-stained sections were then projected, and the area occupied by intima and/or intimal lesion (i.e., the area between the internal elastic lamina and lumen of the artery) was measured with the aid of a Zeiss image analyzer. Our principal pathological measurement in this study was the mean intimal area of 15 arterial sections, expressed in mm^2. A second index of atherosclerosis, lumen stenosis, was calculated as the ratio of intimal area to total area within the internal elastic lamina.

Early mortality claimed two animals before completion of the experiment, leaving 28 monkeys on which all data were available for analysis. Six of these monkeys were dominant animals and nine were subordinates from the unstable social condition; in the stable condition, seven monkeys were dominant and six were subordinate.

Effects of social condition (i.e., stable, unstable) and social status (i.e., dominant, subordinate) on the two measures of atherosclerosis described above were examined by analysis of variance. Listed in Table 1 are the mean intimal area (± SEM) and mean lumen stenosis (± SEM) of each of the four groups of animals. Note that on both dependent measures, the coronary artery atherosclerosis of dominant monkeys from the unstable social condition greatly exceeded that seen in the three remaining groups. This effect was reflected in a significant $\text{Conditions}_{\text{stable, unstable}}$ by $\text{Social Status}_{\text{dominant, subordinate}}$ interaction term on each of the two dependent measures (intimal area: $P=0.034$; lumen stenosis: $P=0.003$).[3] Subsequent comparisons revealed that dominant animals housed in unstable groups had more atherosclerosis than their dominant counterparts from the stable social condition; "unstable" dominants were also more severely affected than similarly housed (i.e., unstable) subordinate animals. It should be noted that neither analysis showed overall effects of Conditions (unstable vs. stable) or Social Status (dominant vs. subordinate) when these variables were considered alone. Hence, disruption of social group memberships in this investigation led to increased coronary artery atherosclerosis, but only among those animals that successfully maintained positions of social dominance over the course of the study.

Shown in Fig. 1 are photomicrographs of a section of left circumflex coronary artery from a respresentative monkey in each of the four experimental groups. The arterial sections depicted in the figure also approximate, in extent of atherosclero-

3 The analysis of intimal area measurements was performed after an initial data transformation of the form $X' = \sqrt{X} + \sqrt{X+1}$, as recommended by Sokol and Rohlf (1981) and Freeman and Tukey (1950).

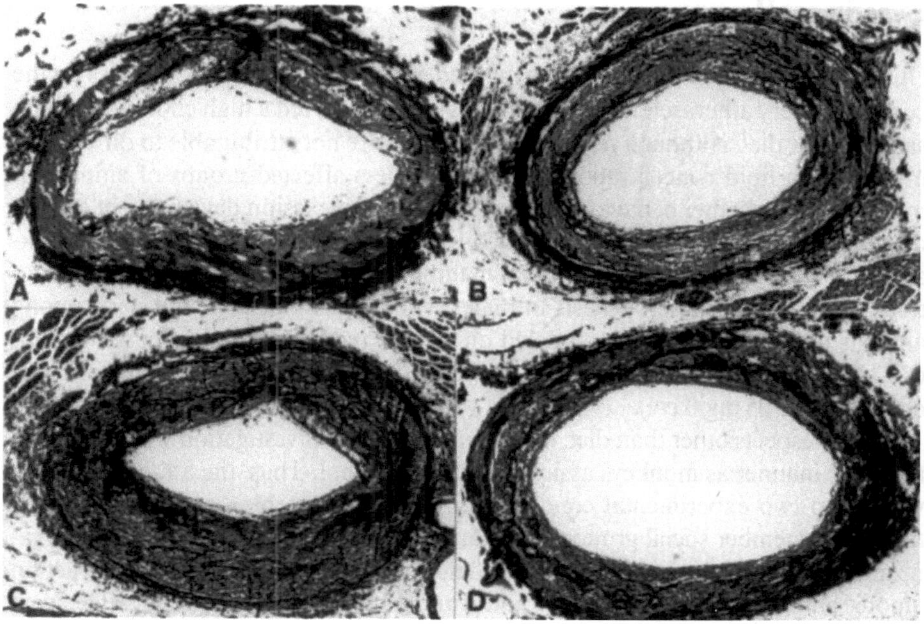

Fig. 1 A–D. Photomicrographs of sections of left circumflex coronary arteries representing the mean intimal area measured in the socially stable dominant (**A**), stable subordinate (**B**), unstable dominant (**C**), and unstable subordinate (**D**) groups. All photomicrographs are of paraffin sections stained by the Verhoeff Van Geison method X 40. (Kaplan et al. 1982; Reprinted by permission of the American Heart Association, Incorporated)

sis, the average intimal area of the group to which each animal belonged. The lesions seen in this experiment contained numerous foam cells, extracellular lipid, increased amounts of collagen and elastin, and, occasionally, mineralization. Medial changes were similar to those found in macaques fed equivalent diets and intergroup differences here appeared to reflect differences in lesion size, rather than composition.

Finally, the increased coronary artery atherosclerosis of dominant monkeys from the unstable condition could not be attributed to corresponding elevations in serum lipids, blood pressure, ponderosity, or fasting glucose concentration. Indeed, only TSC and HDLC concentrations were associated significantly with atherosclerosis; statistical adjustment for the influences of these variables (by analysis of covariance) did not weaken the interaction observed between experimental conditions and social status (intimal area: $P=0.038$; lumen stenosis: $P=0.004$). On the other hand, behavioral observations did reveal a number of differences among the four groups. In the unstable condition, for instance, dominant monkeys tended to engage in more overt aggression (e.g., biting, hitting), and subordinates exhibited more extreme forms of submission (e.g., cowering, fleeing), by comparison with their status-matched counterparts from the stable social condition. Beyond the accentuation of agonistic encounters, ordinary affiliative behaviors, such as grooming and passive body contact, were also disrupted among animals subjected to periodic social group reorganization.

Experiment II

Our first investigation documented a marked effect of psychosocial variables on the coronary artery atherosclerosis of cynomolgus monkeys fed a high cholesterol/high saturated fat diet. Although results of this study were not attributable to differences in the serum lipid concentrations of more and less affected groups of animals, it may be asked whether behavioral factors can potentiate lesion development even in normolipoproteinemic monkeys. Hence, in a second experiment, we again examined the effects of our psychosocial manipulation - recurrent group reorganization - on coronary atherogenesis in male, cynomolgus monkeys, but here among animals fed a "prudent" diet modeled on current recommendations of the American Heart Association. This diet was low in saturated fat and contained almost no cholesterol (0.05 mg/kcal).

In all respects other than diet, the 30 animals in this investigation were treated in the same manner as monkeys assigned to Experiment I. Thus, the animals were divided into two experimental conditions (i.e. stable, unstable), each consisting of three, five-member social groups. As in our first experiment, the deliberate reorganization of group memberships disrupted normal patterns of behavioral interaction among animals housed in the unstable condition. Such effects were reflected in higher rates of contact aggression, displays of more extreme forms of submission, and engagement in significantly less passive affiliation (body contact) among animals housed in the unstable (or stressed) social condition. One other effect of the psychosocial manipulation in this investigation (which was not observed in Experiment I) was that status relationships of several of the "unstable" animals tended to fluctuate over the course of the study, thus hampering identification of comparably-defined groups of dominant and subordinate monkeys from the stable and unstable conditions. For this reason, our primary analysis of the data in this experiment was based on an overall comparison of atherosclerosis in the two experimental conditions, collapsing across levels of social status.

The relative protection conferred by consumption of a "prudent", or low cholesterol, diet is suggested by the limited extent of coronary atherosclerosis seen in this study; in fact, the lesions observed here averaged less than a twentieth of the size of intimal area measurements recorded in Experiment I. Yet, despite the restricted range of intimal lesions produced under the "low cholesterol/low saturated fat" diet, monkeys from the unstable social condition had significantly more atherosclerosis than their unstressed counterparts (median IA = 0.021 and 0.004 mm^2, respectively; $P < 0.002$). A related measurement, intimal thickness (the maximum distance [in millimeters] observed at any one point between the internal elastic lamina and lumen of the artery), was also significantly greater among animals housed in the unstable social groups (median intimal thickness: $\bar{X}_{unstable} = 0.042$ mm; $\bar{X}_{stable} = 0.022$ mm; $P < 0.022$). With respect to lesion characteristics, 11 of 15 "unstable" monkeys had a least one coronary artery in which fatty streaks had progressed to small plaques, with evidence of smooth muscle cell proliferation; lesions of similar severity were found in only 4 of 14 animals from the stable social condition ($P < 0.05$). Moreover, as in Experiment I, effects of our behavioral manipulation on coronary artery atherosclerosis were not attributable to corresponding group differences in TSC or HDLC concentrations, systolic or diastolic blood pressures, ponderosity, or fasting glucose concentration.

Finally, it should be noted that even though dominance relationships were more variable here than in our first experiment, two animals from the unstable condition did occupy dominant social positions throughout the investigation. Also, consistent with the results of Experiment I, these few habitually dominant monkeys had the greatest coronary artery atherosclerosis of all animals in the study ($P < 0.05$). Hence, results of our second experiment suggest that repeated disruption of social group memberships exerts an atherogenic influence even on presumably well-protected (i.e., normolipoproteinemic, normotensive) animals, and that this influence may be especially pronounced among monkeys of high social rank.

Behaviorally-induced Heart Rate Reactivity and Atherosclerosis

It is noteworthy that behavioral influences on atherogenesis in the preceding studies were not related to the concomitant effects of other variables commonly associated with atherosclerosis, such as blood pressure and serum lipid concentrations. This is consistent also with epidemiological studies of the behavioral precursors of coronary heart disease (CHD) in man. In the well-known Western Collaborative Group Study, for instance, the Type A (or coronary-prone) behavior pattern was found to predict clinical CHD even after statistical adjustment for effects of other major risk factors, including serum cholesterol, blood pressure, smoking and age (Review Panel 1981; Matthews et al. 1985).

The apparently independent contribution of behavioral factors to CHD in human beings has generated, in turn, considerable speculation concerning the potential role of autonomic and neuroendocrine activity in the development of atherosclerosis and its clinical sequelae (Manuck and Krantz 1984). Two observations, in particular, have attracted the interest of scientists in this area: (1) that individuals vary greatly in the magnitude of their acute physiological responses to behavioral challenge (Krantz and Manuck 1984); and (2) that persons thought to possess a behavioral predisposition to CHD (i.e., Type A individuals) often show excessive cardiovascular and neuroendocrine (e.g., catecholamine) responses to challenging laboratory tasks and stressors (Wright et al. 1985). Extrapolating from these findings, several investigators have proposed that recurrent episodes of acute psychophysiological reactivity may promote atherogenesis in susceptible individuals, either through hemodynamic disturbances associated with abrupt rises in heart rate and blood pressure (e.g., turbulence, sheer stress) (Williams 1978; Manuck et al. 1983; Clarkson 1984) or through an increased release of neuroendocrine hormones, such as the catecholamines and cortisol (Henry 1983; Herd 1983; Schneiderman 1983). It is suggested, too, that the latter substances may be directly toxic to the artery wall and also influence related pathogenic processes, such as platelet aggregation (Schneiderman 1983).

Unfortunately, there is yet little evidence that the physiological mechanisms mentioned above do account for the increased CHD incidence attributable to behavioral factors like Type A (Manuck and Krantz 1984). On the other hand, data derived from animal models lend plausibility to the notion that enhanced psychophysiological reactivity may contribute to the development of coronary artery atherosclerosis. We believe that such evidence favors especially the proposal that arterial damage arises from acute hemodynamic disturbances accompanying the organism's sympathetic nervous system responses to stress. In the following paragraphs, we will elaborate on this hypothesis and describe initial data bearing on the relationship between cardiovascular response to stress and atherosclerosis.

First, it should be noted that there now exists considerable agreement that the initiating event in atherogenesis involves some form of insult or injury to the arterial endothelium. In addition, it is currently thought that when the endothelium is injured, cells that die are pushed out into the circulation through the replication of adjoining cells. Termed "nondenuding desquamation," this process prevents development of a denuded or endothelium-free surface at the site of injury. In contrast to the normal endothelium, however, replicating endothelium exhibits an increased permeability to low-density lipoproteins, thus permitting infiltration of plasma lipids into the intima of the artery. Moreover, newly generated endothelial cells promote proliferation of the smooth muscle cells that lie beneath, along with associated disturbances in the lipid metabolism of those cells (Clarkson 1984; Ross 1981; Schwartz et al. 1981).

Although the exact manner in which endothelial injury occurs is unclear, there is some evidence that hemodynamic forces play a significant role. In one recent experiment, for example, Hirsch et al. (1984) subjected laboratory rats to physical restraint, a manipulation that produced marked rises in both heart rate and blood pressure. These animals, and unstressed controls, were infused with radioactive thymidine, a label that is taken up preferentially by the nuclei of actively replicating cells. Autoradiographic examination of the aortic intimas of these animals showed endothelial cell replication rates of the stressed rats to be 500% higher than among control animals. In addition, Hirsch et al. (1984) explored the role of sympathetic influences on stress-induced endothelial cell removal and replacement by administering propranolol to groups of stressed rats during the period of restraint. Blocked animals showed no significant rise in heart rate and blood pressure under stress, nor were their endothelial cell replication rates greater than among autonomically intact, unstressed controls. Hence, beta-adrenergic blockade attenuated the hemodynamic response to physical restraint and protected the artery against endothelial injury.

Beere et al (1984) propose further that *elevated heart rate* represents an important predisposing hemodynamic factor in atherogenesis, especially at arterial sites subject to abrupt changes in the direction and strength of pulsatile blood flow (i. e., carotid bifurcation, proximal coronary arteries). In examining the influence of relative differences in heart rate on development of coronary artery atherosclerosis, Beere et al. (1984) lowered the heart rates of a small group of cynomolgus monkeys by surgical ablation of the sinoatrial node. Both these animals and sham-operated controls were then placed on an atherogenic diet for 6 months. Monkeys having the lower postoperative heart rates developed less than half the coronary atherosclerosis of animals with more elevated heart rates. "High" and "low" heart rate groups did not differ, however, in SBP or DBP, serum cholesterol, triglycerides, or body weight. Hence, the investigators conclude that an increased heart rate alone promotes atherogenesis in the coronary arteries; they also suggest that protracted elevations in heart rate caused by behavioral perturbations may account for epidemiological associations between psychosocial variables and development of CHD in human beings.

Because of the growing interest in cardiovascular response to stress and the apparently exaggerated hemodynamic reactions of Type A persons to common laboratory challenges, we sought to "model" individual differences in behaviorally induced heart rate reactivity among the animals assigned to our first experiment (Manuck et al. 1983). Our primary objective here was to determine whether monkeys (like human beings) vary in their cardiac responsivity to a behavioral stressor, and, if so, whether such variability is related to severity of atherosclerosis and/or behavioral characteristics of the animals. We selected heart rate as a parameter of interest, in part, because of the availability of commercial ECG radiotelemetry devices, which permit physiological monitoring in a social environment and without undue disturbance of the animals. As the data of Beere et al. (1984) suggest, however, heart rate may also have special relevance for the understanding of atherogenesis and, to the extent heart rate is influenced by psychosocial factors, in the mediation of behavior-atherosclerosis relationships.

As noted, heart rate response to a behavioral stressor was evaluated in the study animals from Experiment I. Actually, these recordings were made on only a single occasion and at a point near the completion of the overall study. Since these data were thus collected shortly before the animals were sacrificed, the findings reported below are basically retrospective.

Measurements were obtained under both resting and stressed conditions on days following the attachment of portable ECG telemetry units. Baseline heart rates were recorded during an interval of relative quiet, when no human beings were present or visible to the monkeys. Stress-period heart rate measurements were obtained on a subsequent day and involved a standard challenge, during which the experimenter displayed prominantly and threateningly before the target animals a large "monkey glove." This procedure was conducted in a stylized manner reminiscent of encounters commonly preceding the capture and physical handling of animals. Baseline heart rates in these animals averaged 128 bpm, but rose quite dramatically, to a mean of 219 bpm, during the stress manipulation. That the marked heart rate acceleration observed between baseline and stress conditions was due primarily to the "threatening" qualities of the experimenter's display, rather than to his presence alone, is suggested by heart rate recordings obtained on a third occasion, in which the experimenter merely paraded, without glove, before the animals. With the experimenter present, but without threat, the mean heart rate of all monkeys was 144 bpm, reflecting only a modest elevation over baseline.

Although heart rate increased by an average of 91 bpm between the baseline and stress periods, responses of individual monkeys ranged from +34 to +123 bpm. Similarly, six monkeys exhibited heart rate elevations less than 50% above baseline, while stress-period heart rates of seven animals increased over baseline measurements by more than 100%. Thus, our experimental challenge involving the threatened capture and physical handling of animals elicited a substantial mean heart rate acceleration, although among the monkeys tested there existed a considerable range of individual differences. Data we have collected subsequently on several other groups of cynomolgus monkeys indicate that these differences reflect stable individual characteristics (i.e., are reproducible on retesting) and generalize to other conditions of measurement.

In regard to atherosclerosis, our primary analyses involved comparisons of animals representing clearly differentiated groups of high and low heart rate reactive monkeys. These two groups consisted of animals falling within the upper and lower 30%, respectively, of the overall distribution of heart rate reactions. Although the baseline heart rates of high and low reactors were quite similar ($\bar{X}=126$ and 123 bpm, respectively), stress-period heart rates differed between the two groups by more than 35 bpm ($\bar{X}=236$ and 199 bpm, respectively). Most importantly, examination of the intimal area measurements of high and low reactors revealed that high heart rate reactive animals had about twice the coronary artery atherosclerosis of their low reactive counterparts. This difference in extent of atherosclerosis between high and low heart rate reactors was statistically significant ($P<0.05$), both on an overall "coronary index" and on analysis of intimal lesions in the individual coronary arteries.[4]

High and low heart rate reactive animals did not differ, however, in their SBP or DBP, body weights, or serum lipid concentrations. Although HDLC comprised a slightly smaller proportion of the total cholesterol of high, compared with low, heart rate reactors, this difference only approached significance ($P=0.10$). Among the behavioral variables examined, indices of aggression (recorded over the 22 months of the study) did differentiate high and low heart rate reactors; moreover, this relationship was especially pronounced when direct acts of contact aggression (e.g., biting, hitting) were considered apart from more ritualized, or noncontact, aggression. Interestingly, social status per se was not related significantly to animals' heart rate reactivity, nor were dominant monkeys from the unstable social condition - the most severely affected group of animals in Experiment I - disproportionately represented among our high heart rate reactors. Hence, the distribution of individual differences in heart rate response to a fear-eliciting laboratory challenge, while itself related to lesion development and to animals' overt aggressiveness, did not "explain" the principal psychosocial effect in this experiment, namely, the interactive influence of social status and environmental stress on coronary artery atherosclerosis.

At first glance, it is perplexing that our index of heart rate reactivity was associated with aggression, but not with dominance, since social dominance (as described previously) derives from an animal's ability to defeat other group members in fights. Actually, high social status and the propensity to engage in aggressive behavior (i.e., aggressiveness) are imperfectly correlated attributes in many nonhuman primates. One monkey may initiate few fights, for example, yet win nearly all

4 It does not appear that differences in the stress-related heart rates of high and low reactive monkeys are themselves a consequence of the different amounts of atherosclerosis observed in the two groups of animals. In recordings made an other groups of male cynomolgus monkeys, for example, we have found no differences in the stressed heart rates of animals fed atherogenic and prudent diets; these are groups which also differ greatly in extent of atherosclerosis, but due only to dietary manipulation. In addition, we have noted recently that distributions of individual differences in heart rate response to our laboratory challenge are also remarkably stable over time, even though the animals observed are fed an atherogenic diet and, therefore, are developing progressively more atherosclerosis across successive testing intervals.

of the contests in which it is involved; such an animal is clearly dominant, but not particularly aggressive. Conversely, another monkey may provoke a great many fights, yet habitually lose to the majority of its partners; this individual is subordinate, albeit highly aggressive. In accord with these observations, we noted only a moderate relationship in Experiment I between animals' rates of contact aggression and the distribution of social ranks ($r = 0.47$). In contrast, frequencies of submissive gesturing (which refers to highly ritualized behaviors used by an animal to signal defeat in a fight) were related quite strongly to social dominance. Among the animals in Experiment I, this inverse association was reflected in a Spearman coefficient of -0.91. Thus, highly aggressive monkeys were not necessarily socially dominant animals, nor was social status associated appreciably with the instigation of fights or the severity of aggressive behaviors. Instead, socially dominant monkeys tended to be those animals which, aggressive or not, were least likely to submit when engaged in fights with other group members.

These considerations help to explain how individual differences in heart rate response to our laboratory challenge - threat of capture - might be correlated with rates of contact aggression, yet not with social dominance. Our psychophysiological observations also provide initial support for the hypothesis that a cardiovascular hyperreactivity under stress may be implicated in atherogenesis. The fact that heart rate responses here covaried with the aggressiveness of our experimental animals is consistent, too, with the findings of epidemiological and laboratory studies of man. In human subjects, for example, aggressiveness or high "potential for hostility" is also related significantly to the magnitude of individuals' heart rate and pressor responses to experimental stressors (Dembroski et al. 1978; Van Egeren 1979; Manuck et al. 1985). Moreover, these same behavioral characteristics have emerged recently as independent predictors of CHD events and as correlates of angiographically documented coronary artery atherosclerosis (Williams et al. 1980; Barefoot et al. 1983; Shehelle et al. 1983).

Psychophysiology of Naturally-occuring Social Behavior

It is still unclear why dominant animals from the unstable social condition developed more extensive atherosclerosis than similarly housed (i.e., unstable) subordinate monkeys or animals assigned to stable social groups. We believe, however, that the particular behavioral challenges experienced by dominant monkeys when faced with abrupt changes in the composition of their customary social groups also elicited very pronounced autonomic and neuroendocrine responses, which in turn promoted atherogenesis. In this regard, it is worth recalling the proposal by Beere et al. (1984) that protracted elevations in heart rate predispose to development of coronary artery atherosclerosis. In a behavioral context, such elevations might be achieved in a variety of ways. First, certain individuals may possess an intrinsic cardiac hyperresponsivity, which finds expression in the form of large heart rate reactions to any of a number of different behavioral stimuli. Compared to our low heart rate reactive monkeys, for instance, animals identified in the preceding section as high reactors showed large heart rate responses both to our deliberate laboratory challenge (threatened capture) *and* to the more benign manipulation in which the experimenter merely appeared in the area where monkeys were housed. Other animals, however, may have a less generalized propensity to respond to behavioral stimuli with large heart rate reactions, yet still exhibit marked rises in heart rate if exposed to particularly salient or provocative environmental challenges. In Experiment I, for instance, it is conceivable that recurrent redistribution of animals in the unstable condition posed an especially severe threat to socially dominant monkeys, since the status of these animals was more often and more aggressively contested than that of dominant animals in the stable condition. Thus, "unstable" dominant monkeys may have experienced frequent and pronounced disruptions of heart rate and other hemodynamic parameters in this experiment - reactions that may have arisen from the specific behavioral demands of achieving or retaining social preeminence in an unstable social environment.

Unfortunately, testing the hypothesis that dominant animals exhibit an enhanced physiological responsivity when faced with abrupt changes in the composition of their customary social groups presents significant methodological difficulties. Since the heightened reactivity of such monkeys is dependent on the social context in which the animals are housed, standardized, non-social laboratory challenges (e.g., our "threat of capture" manipulation) will necessarily prove ineffective as eliciting stimuli. More appropriate are observations reflecting the physiological correlates of naturally arising social behaviors, especially those occurring while the members of newly formed groups of monkeys are first establishing hierarchical and affiliative associations. Although we did not collect data of this type in our first two experiments, we are currently conducting an investigation which does focus, in part, on the psychophysiology of macaque social behavior during periods of group reorganization. Pathological results from this study are not yet available; however, our preliminary observations shed some light on the physiological concomitants of behavioral states associated with dominant and subordinate social status, as seen in an unstable environment.

The experimental animals in this investigation are, again, 30 adult male, cynomolgus monkeys. Here, though, all animals are housed in periodically reorganized social groups (i.e., there is no stable social condition). The actual heart rate observations to be described below were obtained by radiotelemetry on the first 4 days following the placement of animals into their initial five-member groups. In order to achieve simultaneous heart rate and behavioral monitoring of these monkeys, telemetered ECGs were preserved on a strip chart recorder during intervals in which animals' social behaviors were observed. Since the ECG recorder advances at a constant speed and the exact timing of each behavioral event is known (i.e., stored in memory on our behavioral monitoring device), it is possible to attach heart rate measurements to the specific behaviors that they accompanied. Finally, the social status of each animal was also established, based on the outcomes of fights occurring among group members during 4 weeks of behavioral observation.

Our initial analyses of these data involve comparisons of the heart rates of dominant and subordinate animals, as recorded during behavioral states that are presumed to differ in their social "meaning." However, we have not focused on heart rate as a correlate of one category for behavior, aggression, despite the importance of agonistic encounters in the determination of social status. Partly, this is due to the fact that the motivational interpretation of aggression-related heart rate measure-

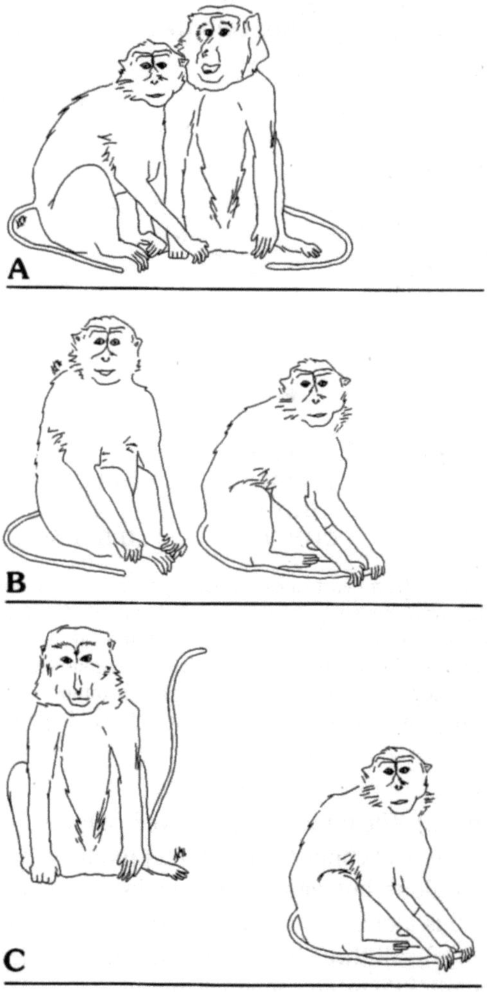

Fig. 2 A–C. Stylized drawings depicting monkeys in three different behavioral states passive body contact (**A**); close proximity (**B**); and alone at a distance (**C**)

ments is frequently confounded by cardiovascular adjustments associated with somatic components of the aggressive act itself, as in lunging, charging, or hitting. We have also noted very little difference in the heart rates of aggressing and submitting animals in recordings obtained *during* the course of ongoing fights. As importantly, the fighting that occurs among socially housed groups of macaques is of brief duration (i.e., seconds, rather than minutes), and aggressive behavior, overall, accounts for only a small proportion of the activities of such animals (typically less than 3%). Consequently, it does not seem to us plausible that pathogenic processes related to atherosclerosis – at least those mediated by hemodynamic forces – are influenced appreciably by the cardiovascular concomitants of aggressive acts *per se*.

What we have explored, on the other hand, are the heart rates of our experimental animals during three other behavioral states which, taken together, absorb up to 80% of the daytime activities of monkeys living under these laboratory conditions

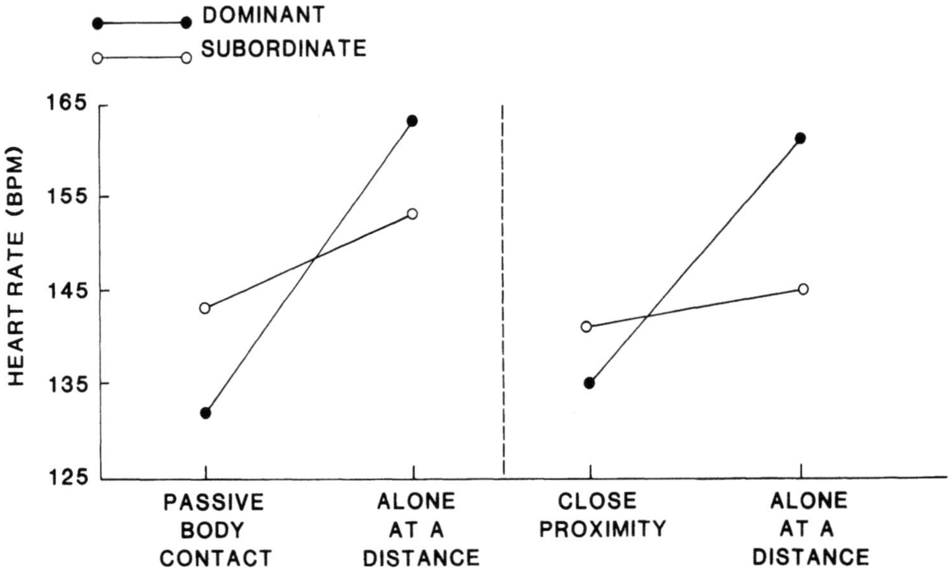

Fig. 3. Mean heart rates (in beats per minute) of dominant and subordinate animals, as recorded during occurrences of different behavioral states. Illustrated in the *left panel* are heart rates observed during "passive body contact" and "alone at a distance". In the *right panel* are heart rates recorded when animals were in "close proximity" and "alone at a distance." Note that the heart rates depicted in each panel reflect matched samples, in which the two behavioral states contrasted were both exhibited by the same animal within a single 10-min sampling interval

(Fig. 2). The three states involve instances in which (1) an animal is sitting passively, in physical contact with another monkey (passive body contact); (2) a monkey is sitting alone, but within touching distance of another (close proximity); and (3) an animal is alone and not within touching distance of another monkey (alone at a distance). All three conditions can be considered "quiescent," in the sense that they entail little or no somatic activity.

It should be noted that the actual heart rate measurements selected for analysis involved matched samples, in which two of the three behavioral states were exhibited by the same monkey within a single 10 min sampling interval. Each heart rate sample was 1 min in duration and was separated by temporal "buffers" from preceding and subsequent behaviors.

Unfortunately, even though each of the experimental monkeys might be found in all three behavioral states many times during the day, the co-occurrence of two of these states in a given 10-min period was a relatively rare event. As a result, only a portion of the animals observed actually contributed data suitable for analysis. Nevertheless, we have discovered a few consistent relationships between behavioral states and heart rate. In particular, heart rate measurements recorded while animals were in "close proximity" or in "passive body contact" with another monkey were significantly lower than when the same animals were sitting "alone at a distance." These heart rate differences were also quite appreciable, averaging between 15 and 20 bpm. However, the magnitude of the relationships observed varied substantially between monkeys, and, as depicted in Fig. 3, much of this variability could be accounted for by differences in animals' social status. Perhaps most striking are the exceptionally high heart rates that dominant monkeys exhibited when remaining "alone at a distance" (i.e., >160 bpm). These values were, respectively, 31 and 25 bpm higher than heart rate measurements recorded from the same animals during "passive body contact" and "close proximity" to other monkeys. In contrast, corresponding differences among subordinate animals, albeit in the same direction, averaged less than 10 bpm.

Thus, compared with their subordinate counterparts, dominant monkeys show greater fluctuations in heart rate, as a function of varying proximity and physical contact (affiliation) with other animals, at least during the initial formation of new social groupings. This interaction between social status and the behavioral states of the animal is attributable, in the main, to the greatly elevated heart rates that dominant monkeys exhibit when *not* engaged in active social interactions (i.e., sitting beyond touching distance of others and not communicating to other animals through vocalizations, or changes in posture or facial expression). While it is not entirely clear why this heart rate-behavior association should be most pronounced among dominant monkeys, we have noted that the majority of agonistic interactions taking place during social group reorganizations also follow periods in which fight participants are sitting at a relative distance from other animals. During the week that these heart rate data were collected, for instance, 29% of all instances in which animals were observed to be "alone at a distance" were terminated by fighting; in contrast, periods of "passive body contact" and "close proximity" to other animals were followed by fighting in only 12% of instances.

Taken together these considerations provide a possible explanation for the interactive effects of social status and environmental stress on atherogenesis in our earlier experimental work. Since it is the dominant animal's status which is in jeopardy when group composition is altered (subordinate status being retained by default), it is the dominant monkey that must be most attentive to any movements, gestures or facial expressions conveying the agonistic intentions of potential competitors. In turn, it is reasonable to suspect that such vigilance will be especially pronounced during those intervals most likely to precede aggressive interactions, such as periods when the animal is "alone at a distance." The fact that monkeys may spend 40%-60% of the day in this behavioral state suggests that associated elevations in heart rate, as seen among dominant animals, may also persist over substantial periods of time. Hence, we hypothesize that when dominant monkeys are exposed to unfamiliar animals on repeated occasions and over many months or years, consequent increases in heart rate - possibly in conjunction with other hemodynamic and neuroendocrine disruptions - induce significant endothelial injury (e.g., in the manner described previously) and thereby potentiate the development of coronary artery atherosclerosis.

Acknowledgments. This research was partly supported by grants from the National Institutes of Health (HL 14164, HL 29028, HL 26562) and a grant from R. J. Reynolds Industries Inc.

References

Altmann J (1974) Observational study of behavior: sampling methods. Behaviour 48: 1-41

Armstrong ML, Megan MB (1975) Arterial fibrous proteins in cynomolgus monkeys after atherogenic and regression diets. Circ Res 36: 256-261

Armstrong ML, Trillo A, Prichard RW (1980) Naturally occurring and experimentally induced atherosclerosis in nonhuman primates. In: Kalter SS (ed) The use of nonhuman primates in cardiovascular diseases. University of Texas Press, Austin

Barefoot JJC, Dahlstrom WC, Williams RB (1983) Hostility, CHD incidence, and total mortality: a 25-year follow-up study of 255 physicians. Psychosom Med 45: 59-63

Beere PA, Glagov S, Zarins CK (1984) Retarding effect of lowered heart on coronary atherosclerosis. Science 226: 180-182

Bernstein IS (1970) Primate status hierarchies. In: Rosenblum LA (ed) Primate behavior: developments in field and laboratory research, vol I. Academic, New York

Bernstein IS, Gordon TP, Rose RM (1974) Aggression and social controls in rhesus monkey (Macaca mulatta) groups revealed in group formation studies. Folia primatol 21: 81-107

Bond MD, Bullock BC, Bellinger DA, Hamm TE (1980) Myocardial infarction in a large colony of nonhuman primates with coronary artery atherosclerosis. Am J Pathol 101: 675-692

Clarkson TB (1980) Symposium summary. In: Kalter SS (ed) The use of nonhuman primates in cardiovascular diseases. University of Texas Press, Austin

Clarkson TB (1984) Implications for atherogenesis. In: Stress, reactivity, and cardiovascular disease. NIH, Bethesda, (publication no 84-2698)

Dembroski TM, MacDougall JM, Shields JL, et al (1978) Components of the Type A coronary-prone behavior pattern and cardiovascular responses to psychomotor performance challenge. J Behav Med 1: 159-176

Freeman MF, Tukey JW (1950) Transformations related to the angular and the square root. Ann Math Stat 21: 607-611

Hamm TE, Kaplan JR, Clarkson TB, Bullock BC (1983) Effects of gender and social behavior on the development of coronary artery atherosclerosis on cynomolgus macaques. Atherosclerosis 48: 221-233

Henry JP (1983) Coronary heart disease and arousal of the adrenal cortical axis. In: Dembroski TM, Schmidt TH, Blümchen G (eds) Biobehavioral bases of coronary heart disease. Karger, Basel

Herd JA (1983) Physiological basis for behavioral influences in atherosclerosis. In: Dembroski TM, Schmidt TH, Blümchen G (eds) Biobehavioral bases of coronary heart disease. Karger, Basel

Hirsch EZ, Maksem JA, Gagen D (1984) Effects of stress and propranolol on the aortic intima of rats. Arteriosclerosis 4: 526 (abstract)

Kaplan JR, Manuck SB, Clarkson TB, Lusso FM, Taub DB (1982) Social status, environment, and atherosclerosis in cynomolgus monkeys. Arteriosclerosis 2: 359-368

Kaplan JR, Manuck SB, Clarkson TB, Lusso FM, Taub DB, Miller EW (1983) Social stress and atherosclerosis in normocholesterolemic monkeys. Science 220: 733-735

Kaplan JR, Manuck SB, Clarkson TB, Pritchard RW (1985) Animal models of behavioral influences on atherogenesis. In: Katkin ES, Manuck SB (eds) Advances in behavioral medicine, vol I. JAI, Greenwich (unpublished)

Kawai M (1958) On the rank system in a natural group of Japanese macaques. Primates 1: 84-98

Kramsch DM, Hollander W (1968) Occlusive atherosclerotic disease of the coronary arteries in monkeys *(Macaca irus)* induced by diet. Exp Mol Pathol 9: 1-22

Krantz DS, Manuck SB (1984) Acute psychophysiologic reactivity and risk of cardiovascular disease: a review and methodologic critique. Psych Bull 96: 435-464

Lancaster J (1975) Primate behavior and the emergence of human culture. Holt, Rinehart and Winston, New York

Malinow MR, McLaughlin P, Papworth L, Nato HK, Lewis L, McNully WP (1976) A model for therapeutic interventions on established coronary atherosclerosis in a nonhuman primate. Adv Exp Biol Med 67: 3-31

Manuck SB, Krantz DS (1984) Psychophysiologic reactivity in coronary heart disease. Behav Med Update 6: 11-15

Manuck SB, Kaplan JR, Clarkson TB (1983) Behaviorally-induced heart rate reactivity and atherosclerosis in cynomolgus monkeys. Psychosom Med 45: 95-108
Manuck SB, Proietti JM, Rader SJ, Polefrone JM (1985) Parental hypertension, affect and cardiovascular response to cognitive challenge. Psychosom Med 47: 189-200
Matthews KA, Jamison JW, Coddington EM (1985) Assessment of type A, anger and hostility: a review of measures through 1982. Proceedings of the NHLBI workshop. In: Measuring psychosocial variables in epidemiologic studies of cardiovascular disease. NIH, Bethesda (to be published)
Review Panel (1981) Coronary-prone behavior and coronary heart disease: a critical review. Circulation 19: 583
Ross R (1981) Atherosclerosis: a problem of the biology of arterial wall cells and their interactions with blood components. Arteriosclerosis 1: 293-311
Rudel LL, Pitts LL (1978) Male-female variability in the dietary cholesterol-induced hyperlipoproteinemia of cynomolgus monkeys (Macaca fascicularis). J Lipid Res 19: 992-998
Sade DS (1967) Determinants of dominance in a group of free ranging rhesus monkeys. In: Altman S (ed) Social communication among primates. University of Chicago Press, Chicago
Schneiderman N (1983) Behavior, autonomic function and animal models of cardiovascular pathology. In: Dembroski TM, Schmidt TH, Blümchen G (eds) Biobehavioral bases of coronary heart disease. Karger, Basel
Schwartz S, Gajdusek C, Shelden S (1981) Vascular wall growth control: the role of endothelium. Arteriosclerosis 1: 107-126
Shekelle RB, Gale M, Ostfeld AM, Paul O (1983) Hostility, risk of coronary heart disease, and mortality. Psychosom Med 45: 109-114
Sokol R, Rolhf FJ (1981) Biometry. Freeman, San Francisco
Van Egeren L (1979) Cardiovascular changes during social competition in a mixed-motive game. J Pers Soc Psychol 37: 858-864
Wagner WD, St Clair RW, Clarkson TB (1978) Angiochemical and tissue changes in Macaca fascicularis fed an atherogenic diet for three years. Exp Mol Pathol 28: 140-153
Williams RB (1978) Psychophysiological processes, the coronary-prone behavior pattern, and coronary heart disease. In: Dembroski TM, Weiss SM, Shields JL, Haynes SG, Feinleib M (eds) Coronary-prone behavior. Springer, Berlin Heidelberg New York
Williams RB, Haney T, Lee K, Yong Y, Blumenthal J, Whalen R (1980) Type A behavior, hostility and coronary atherosclerosis. Psychosom Med 42: 539-549
Wright RA, Contrada RJ, Glass DC (1985) Psychophysiologic correlates of Type A behavior. In: Katkin ES, Manuck SB (eds) Advances in behavioral medicine. JAI, Greenwich

Psychosocial Stress and Its Pathophysiological Effects in Tree Shrews *(Tupaia belangeri)*

D. VON HOLST[1]

Introduction

Every animal species has its own typical social structure, which can change predictably under the influence of certain factors (e.g. food availability, reproductive cycle, number of individuals) but which is, in general, constant. The form taken by the social structure is determined and also maintained by the continual contact between animals. Each individual in a society is thus a part of every other individual's environment and continually exerts an effect on them, both from a behavioural and physiological point of view. Changes in the social relationships between animals (e.g. because of an increase in animal numbers or a change in rank order) thus have an effect on the physiological state of the individuals either positively or negatively, depending on the situation. This paper will illustrate some of these effects in tree shrews, especially those related to behaviour and physical health as a result of confrontation.

Tree shrews *(Tupaia belangeri)* are diurnal mammals approximately the size of squirrels and are widely distributed throughout South East Asia. On the basis of a number of morphological and physiological parallels they were considered as primates until a few years ago. Today, however, they are accorded their own order, the Scandentia, since they obviously branched off from the other Eutherian mammals in the early Tertiary. They thus represent a recent model of the ancestors of all present-day placental mammals (Martin 1968; Starck 1978).

In the wild, tree shrews usually live as pairs in territories which are vigorously defended against strangers of the same sex (Kawamichi and Kawamichi 1979). In the laboratory, adult tree shrews, especially the males, also attack intruding (or introduced) individuals of their own sex immediately and usually defeat them within a few minutes. A short while after the fight, the winners show no further signs of arousal and pay virtually no attention to the defeated animals. The losers, in contrast, creep into any hiding place, which they only leave to eat and drink. During the following days, fights between the animals are very rare or non-existent. Nevertheless, the losers die within less than 20 days. Death is not a result of physical exertion during the fight; nor are wounds the cause of death, since, while fighting, the animals usually inflict only superficial scratches and bites on one another. Death is associated, rather, with the continual presence of the winner, as the following results show: If the animals are separated after the fight by a non-transparent partition, the losers recover from the fight just as fast as the winners and do not die prematurely, even when they are subjected to a fight on each day over a period of weeks. If, how-

1 Department of Animal Physiology, University of Bayreuth, Universitätstrasse 30, 8580 Bayreuth, Federal Republic of Germany

Biological and Psychological Factors
in Cardiovascular Disease
Ed. by T. H. Schmidt, T. M. Dembroski, and G. Blümchen

ever, the two animals are separated by a wire mesh partition so that the loser can no longer be attacked but can see the "threatening" winner continually, then it dies within a few days. Anthropomorphically, if can be said that the loser dies of constant "anxiety" (for details see von Holst 1972, 1977; von Holst et al. 1983).

The introduction of a rival into a male's cage presents a form of extreme stress for a territorial animal such as the tree shrew. To determine the physiological changes resulting from slighter stress, two strange male tree shrews were introduced into a cage unknown to both of them (cage size: 120 × 70 cm; height: 50 cm; the cage contained two separate feeding places, water bottles and sleeping boxes). In this situation, the animals did not start to fight immediately but first hesitantly explored and marked the cage. Fights, however, usually started after a short time, leading to a clear dominance relationship between the two within less than 4 days. The behaviour of all males was more or less comparable before the fights started, but this changed after the dominance relationship was established, depending on the rank of the animals.

Although both males lived together continuously in the relatively small cage, the winners more or less ignored the losers; attacks on the latter were rare or completely lacking. The losers, on the other hand, changed their behaviour drastically. On the basis of differences in their behaviour, two groups could be distinguished: submissive and subdominant animals. Submissive animals crept into a corner of the cage or into a sleeping box and only left this hiding place to drink or eat hastily. They even withstood the rare attacks of the winner without any attempts to defend themselves or to flee. They ceased grooming themselves and their coats rapidly looked rough and dirty, distinguishing them clearly from all the other animals. To the observer they gave an impression of apathy or depression. Subdominant animals, in contrast, showed a great increase in locomotor activity; they watched the movements of the dominant continually and attempted to avoid possible confrontations by giving way or fleeing. If a confrontation could not be avoided, they even defended themselves.

Finally, there were a few cases in which short fights took place daily between the two males; however, these did not lead to the establishment of a clear dominance relationship. The majority of the time was spent by both animals attempting to avoid any possible confrontation with the rival. Since these animals were found to show no difference in behaviour or physiology to the subdominant males when a definite dominant was present, they were included in the subdominant group.

Confrontation Study

The study was conducted with 104 male tree shrews that were held isolated for at least 6 months before the experiments began. Their average age was approximately 4 years (tree shrews can live up to 10 years in the laboratory); their average body weight was 210 ± 2 g (mean ± SE). All animals were kept under constant conditions (light : dark = 12 : 12 h; ambient temperature 25 ± 1 °C; relative air humidity approx. 55%), with food *(Altromin Tupaja Standard-Diät)* and water ad lib. A total of 20 animals were used as controls. Of the 84 animals which were used in confrontations with other males, 28 became dominant, 36 subdominant and 20 submissive. Together with 17 control animals, 6 dominants, 19 subdominants and 10 submissive animals were sacrificed about 10 days after the start of the experiment to determine the weight and morphology of certain organs.

In addition, the activities of the adrenal medullary enzymes tyrosine hydroxylase (TH) and phenylethanolamine *N*-methyltransferase (PNMT) from the right adrenal glands (according to Witte and Matthaei 1980) together with the norepinephrine content of the left adrenals were determined[2], to obtain an indication of the sympathetic nervous system activity (Thoenen et al. 1969). The remaining animals were kept for up to 23 days in the experiment. With the exception of those sacrificed for the study, all dominant animals survived the experiment. In contrast, two subdominants died after 3 weeks and all submissives died within 2 weeks.

Before the start of the experiments and then at intervals of 2–5 days, the majority of the animals (together with 14 isolated controls) had blood samples taken to determine various parameters. Here, only the concentrations of the hormones cortisol, corticosterone and testosterone will be reported on, these all being determined by means of highly specific radioimmunoassays. All blood samples were taken at 8.00 a. m., i. e. 2 h before the light/activity phase of the animals, and all animals were also sacrificed at this time. In 14 other tree shrews the heart rate was determined continually by means of transmitters implanted subcutaneously dorsally. The transmitters were developed by one of my collegues, Dr. W. Stöhr. They weighed (including battery) 1.5 g and remained functional for approx. 6 months (details: Stöhr 1982).

Physiological Effects

Body Weight

The average weight of dominant males at the start of the experiment showed no difference to that of the controls and prospective losers. During the first few days of the confrontation, the dominants lost weight slightly; however, once the dominance relationship was established, their weight increased steadily, finally reaching an average value slightly above that at the start of the experiment. This increase is all the more surprising since the body weight of controls, which were kept isolated and undisturbed – apart from regular blood sampling – in their original cages, decreased gradually over the experimental period. Compared with dominants, subordinate animals showed a greater weight loss during the first 2 days after the start of the experiment (approximately 10%). While the body weight of subdominants after establishment of the dominance relationship remained at this level, the submissive animals continued to lose weight until death (Fig. 1).

Endocrine Changes in the Blood

Experimental groups (dominants, subdominants and submissives) showed no difference in their hormone concentrations at the start of the experiment from controls. The average value of hormone concentrations for all animals at the start of the experiment was therefore taken as a base or control value. As can be seen in Fig. 2,

2 These studies were conducted by my previous collegue Dr. E. Fuchs (present address: Deutsches Primatenzentrum, Göttingen).

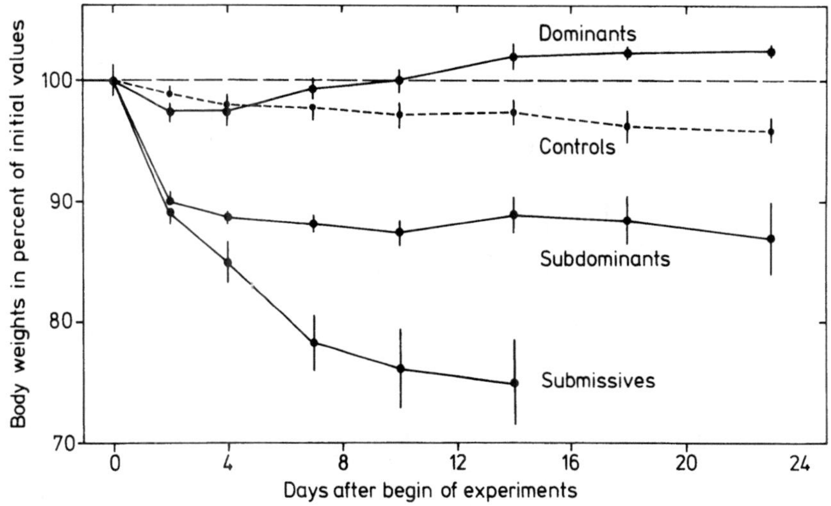

Fig. 1. Changes in body weight shown by the 84 experimental animals and 20 controls after the start of the experiment (see text for details)

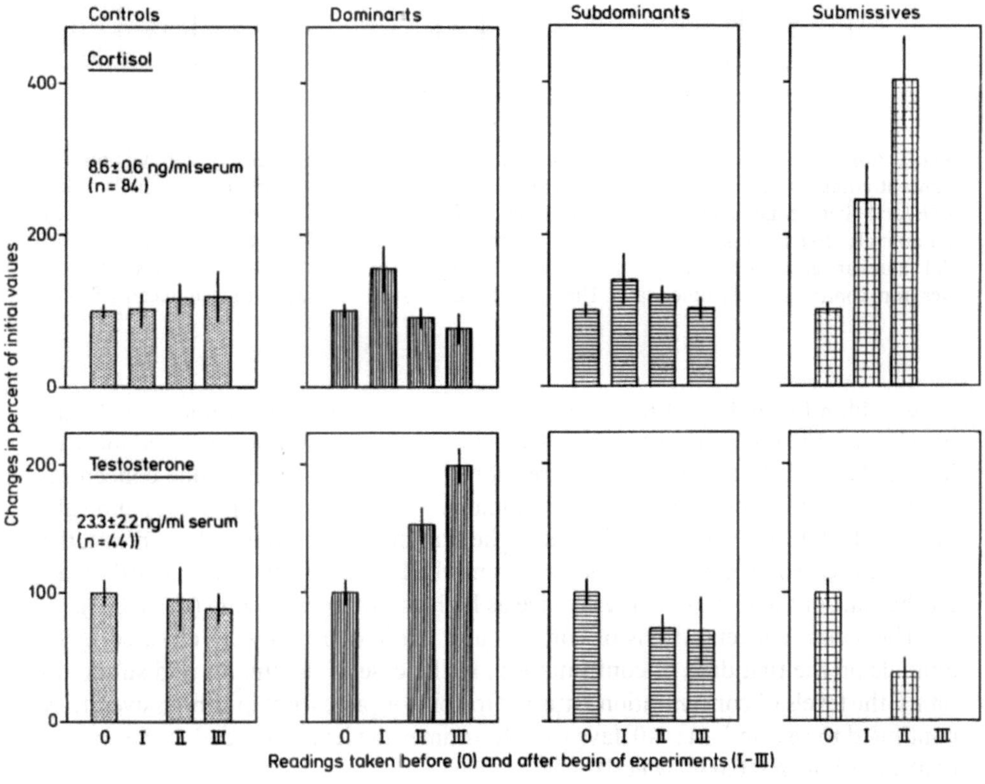

Fig. 2. Changes in the cortisol and testosterone concentrations of control and experimental animals during the experiment expressed as percentage of control value. The absolute control value is given (mean ± SE). The values before *(0)* and for the days 2 *(I)*, approx. 10 *(II)* and approx. 20 *(III)* after the start of the experiment are shown

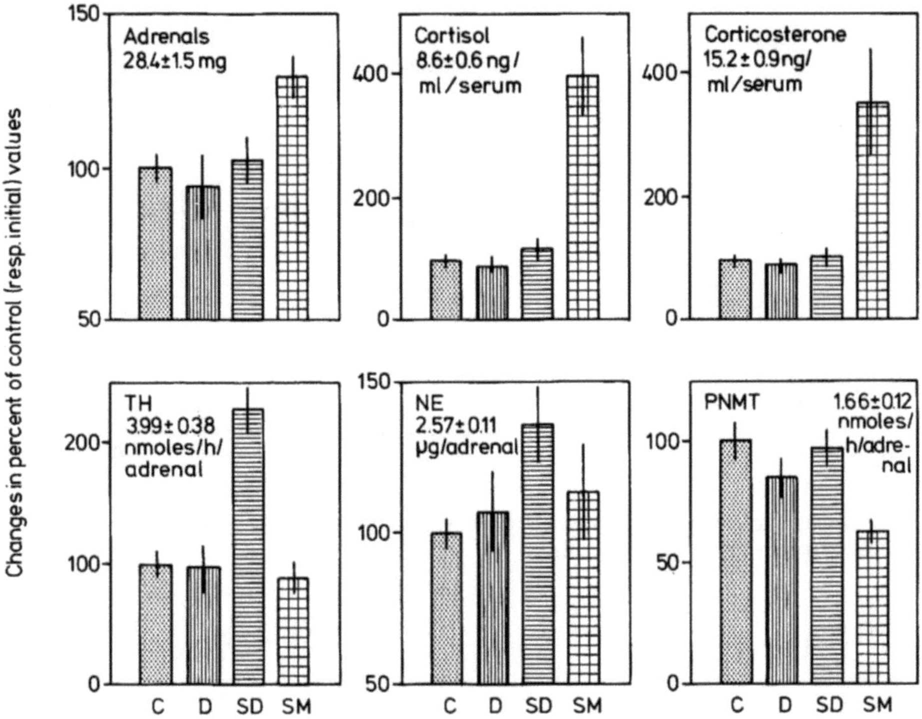

Fig. 3. Adrenal weights, serum hormone concentrations (cortisol, corticosterone), adrenal hormone concentrations (norepinephrine: *NE*), and activities of the adrenal enzymes tyrosine hydroxylase *(TH)* and phenylethanolamine *N*-methyltransferase *(PNMT)* of control animals *(C)* and experimental animals after 10 days of confrontation. (*D*, dominants; *SD*, subdominants; *SM*, submissives.) All values are given as percentages of the base values (glucocorticoids) or as percentages of the values from control animals (other data). The absolute base or control values are given (mean ± SE)

regular blood sampling of the control animals resulted in a slight and non-significant increase in their cortisol values, while the serum testosterone remained more or less unchanged. In the subordinate tree shrews, the serum testosterone concentrations decreased significantly (in subdominants by approx. 30% ($P < 0.05$) and submissives by 60% ($P < 0.001$) 10 days after the start of the experiment. In contrast, the serum testosterone of dominants showed a marked increase and at about 20 days after the start of the experiment was twice as high as the control value ($P < 0.001$).

The serum concentrations of cortisol (and corticosterone) were elevated in all animals on the first days of confrontation. In the case of dominants and subdominants, the levels of concentration returned to control values, but in submissives, they continued to rise and after 10 days were four times the level recorded at the start of confrontation ($P < 0.001$) (Fig. 2).

The same applies to the serum corticosterone values and adrenal weights of the three groups of animals (Fig. 3).

Parallel to this increased adrenocortical activity, the numbers of basophile and eosinophile leucocytes and of lymphocytes were reduced to about 30% of the con-

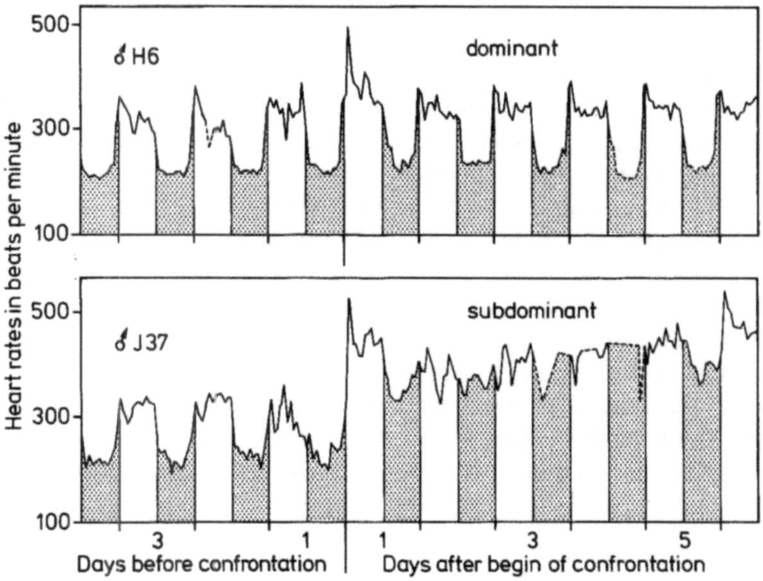

Fig. 4. Heart rates of two experimental animals before and after confrontation (see text for details). The dark phases (= sleeping periods) are *shaded*

trol levels ($P < 0.001$) in submissive animals only. This finding indicates a drastic reduction in immunological resistance and, in conjunction with the increased glucocorticoid values, a reduced wound-healing ability in the passive submissives. This was not the case for animals of the other two groups.

In contrast to this, the TH activity in the adrenals of submissive animals showed no difference to that of dominant tree shrews or control animals, while, in subdominants, it increased by more than 100% ($P < 0.001$) (Fig. 3).

The norepinephrine concentrations of the adrenals show comparable differences in the four groups. This finding points to a great increase in sympathetic nervous system activity in the behaviorally active subordinates while the TH and PNMT values of the passive subordinates (submissives) indicate rather a reduced sympathetic nervous system activity. This could possibly be associated with the 20% lower heart weight ($P < 0.01$) of submissives in comparison with all other groups.

Heart Rate Changes

The heart rates of 14 males were determined telemetrically over a period of months before and during the experiment (details: Stöhr 1986, see p. 491). Prior to the start of confrontation, all animals showed comparable day/night changes of their average heart rates, the day level lying about 50% above the night levels (Fig. 4). In all cases, confrontation led to a marked increase in heart rates, to levels that could reach 600 bpm over short periods of time. Once a dominance relationship was established, the heart rates of dominants ($n = 5$) returned to their initial levels. In subdominant tree shrews ($n = 6$), however, the day levels remained elevated to a greater or lesser extent, depending on the dominance relationships among the animals.

Even more drastically the heart rates of subdominants increased during the nights, thereby reaching values comparable with those during the day, thus eradicating the original day-night rhythm (see Fig. 4). This increase in heart rate was present in situations where a subdominant male lived together with an obvious dominant (as in Fig. 4) and also in cases where both animals were so-called subdominants with no clear dominance relationships between them.

This increase in heart rate, together with the other results mentioned above points to a constant high activation of the sympathetic-adrenomedullary system in subdominants - and this not only during the day when the dominant animal is present and an attack can take place at any time, but also during the night when both animals are completely quiet and sleeping (?) in their separate nest-boxes. To date, it has not been possible to determine the heart rates of submissives, since, in this group, the transmitters were regularly rejected after 1-2 days; however, we have the impression that in contrast to the active subdominants, submissives have a reduced heart rate and lowered blood pressure (recognisable during blood sampling).

Summary of Findings

These findings show the following: A social confrontation leading to a dominance relationship has, apparently, no negative effects on the dominant animal, even when it has to reassert its position through occasional fights; on the contrary, its gonadal activity and with this, its reproductive capacity is improved. Vanquished tree shrews, on the other hand, are typified by a lowered body weight, reduced gonadal activity and many other physiological changes which will not be dealt with in detail here. In general, the physiological changes are qualitatively the same in both groups of subordinate animals, differing only in degree. However, there is a clear qualitative difference between subdominants and submissives with respect to their adrenal functions. Subdominants (i.e. animals which adapt to the situation actively) show no change of adrenocortical function but an increase in sympathetic-adrenomedullary activity, which ultimately could lead to damage of the cardiovascular system and cardiac arrest (Beere et al. 1984). Submissives (i.e. animals which passively succumb to the situation) show no activation of their sympathetic-adrenomedullary system. In contrast, their adrenocortical activity is drastically increased, leading to a marked catabolism of muscular and fat tissues together with a reduction of wound-healing and immunological resistance.

These findings support the hypothesis advanced by Henry and Stephens (1977) that, in mammals, dependent on their "valuation" of the situation or dependent on their "behavioural strategy", the adrenal medullary or adrenal cortical systems can be activated independently of one another while, under generally unstable conditions, both systems are activated together (such as in all tree shrews during the first days of confrontation). Although the animals in the confrontation experiments could be easily separated as to status on the basis of their behaviour, observation before the experiments started gave no clue as to whether an animal would become dominant or subordinate after a confrontation, and, particularly, whether a subordinate would respond passively or actively to the situation (i.e. whether it would become submissive or subdominant). Also the base levels of all physiological parameters measured before confrontation showed no differences in the animals from the different groups and had therefore as little prognostic value as differences in body weight or how the fights were conducted.

Reaction Test

Since a confrontation causes ethological and physiological reactions within the individual, we started to study the physiological responses of tree shrews under control and chronic stress conditions to an acute standard stress (=reaction test). For this, the animals were brought in their sleeping boxes to a neighbouring laboratory at 8.00 a.m., and blood samples were taken 1, 5, 15 and 30 min after their room had first been entered. Blood was taken (250 μl per sample) from the tail vein. Between sampling the animals were returned to their sleeping boxes but remained for the entire period in the laboratory. Amongst others, the following blood parameters were determined: concentrations of epinephrine, norepinephrine, dopamine, cortisol, corticosterone and glucose; in addition, the heart rates of certain animals were continually monitored telemetrically.

Physiological Effects

The reaction test was an activating stressor for all the tree shrews. The heart rates of the animals were elevated for the entire experimental period and the levels of catecholamines, glucocorticoids and glucose in the blood showed great increases. Shortly after the reaction test, however, the heart rate and all other parameters returned to the control level; 2 days after the test at the latest no residual effects could be determined. Here, only the cortisol values will be dealt with.

On an average, the cortisol values of control animals increased within 30 min to approx. 60 ng/ml serum (203 experimental animals); however, there were great differences between individuals. For example, in male K 4, values of nearly 120 ng cortisol/ml serum were reached, whereas in male K 37 the cortisol concentration only rose to less than 40 ng/ml (Fig. 5). A repetition of the reaction test after 8 days resulted in almost identical (and individually different) values for all animals (see Fig. 5).

Although the starting values (1-min values) do not correlate significantly with one another, the 15- and 30-min values of different individuals were highly correlated (correlation coefficients of the 10 individuals in Fig. 5: $r \gg 0.90$; $P < 0.001$).

To date, up to 6 reaction tests with more than 50 control animals have been carried out over a period of more than 2 years. Again the maximal cortisol values differed from individual to individual between less than 30 ng/ml serum and more than 150 ng/ml serum, but were quite constant for each individual over the entire period of 2 years. In-vitro superfusion analyses of the adrenals from control animals showed a high correlation between the in-vitro cortisol production of the individuals after maximal stimulation of secretion through the addition of ACTH to the superfusions medium and the serum cortisol values obtained approximately 10 days before reaction tests ($r = 0.81$; $P < 0.001$) (Hutzelmeyer 1984). The individual differences of cortisol reaction values are therefore mainly due to corresponding differences in the adrenal capacity of the individuals to form and secrete corticoids after ACTH application.

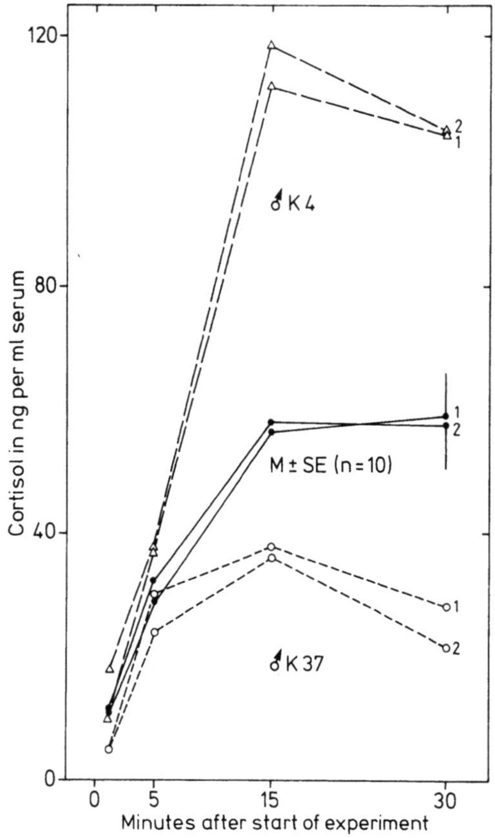

Fig. 5. Increase in cortisol concentrations in the serum of 10 experimental animals during two acute reaction tests *(1* and *2)* performed at an interval of 8 days. The average increase in cortisol levels for all animals (mean ± SE) and the individual values of the animals with the highest *(K 4)* and lowest *(K 37)* responses are given

Chronic stress always leads to an increase in cortisol reaction values. After transference of animals to a new cage, their values rose approximately 50% after only a single day but, at the latest, 8 days afterwards, the cortisol values had returned to their original low levels (six animals). Social confrontations had an even more marked effect: in both subdominant and submissive animals, the cortisol reaction values 10 days after the start of confrontation (the earliest measurements) were elevated by up to 100% (examples Fig. 6). The same was true of males (and females) which lived in partnership with a member of the opposite sex without real fights and dominance relationships but in continual social tension (see Fig. 6: non-harmonic pair). On the other hand, the opposite was found when males became dominant after confrontation with rivals: Their cortisol reaction values either sank if they had a high starting value or remained unchanged if the initial values were low (Fig. 7).

The same reduction in reaction values was found in males in three confrontation experiments which, owing to unknown reasons, did not result in agonistic interactions, the males responding to each other sexually (examples: Fig. 7). A harmonic

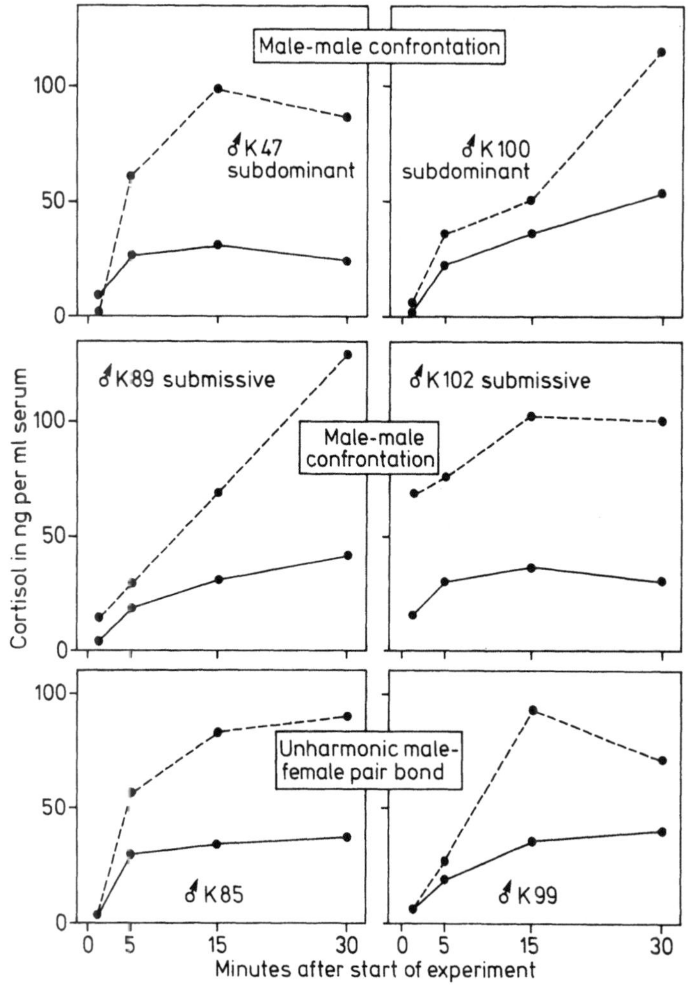

Fig. 6. Cortisol responses of males in the reaction test before *(solid lines)* and 10 days after *(broken lines)* the start of a constant stress

relationship between the individuals of mated pairs also led to a marked drop in the cortisol reaction values, resulting in extremely low levels (examples: Fig. 7). Parallel to this, the heart rates of individuals in harmonic pairs dropped during the day and especially at night by up to 20% and remained at these low levels, whereas the heart rates of individuals in non-harmonic pairs showed a marked increase (details: Stöhr, this volume).

Summary of Findings

Stresses of various types, such as the transference to a strange cage, acute fights with a rival, living together in a non-harmonic situation with a female conspecific or adopting the subordinate position in a confrontation experiment in male tree shrews, leads to an increase in their cortisol (and corticosterone) reaction values,

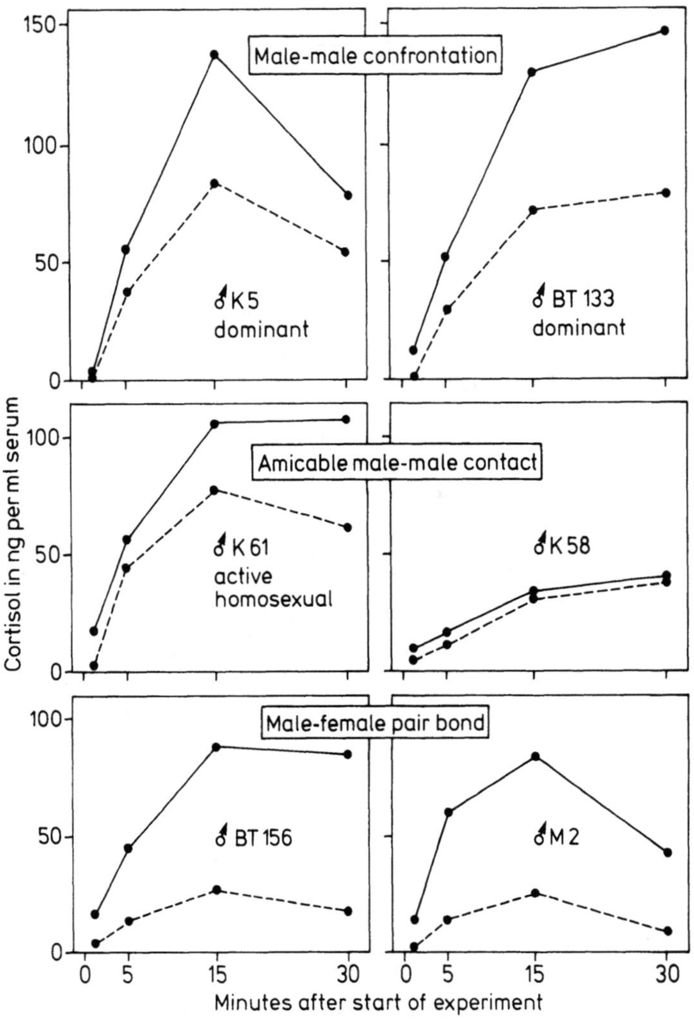

Fig. 7. Cortisol responses in the reaction test of males before *(solid lines)* and 10 days after the attainment of a dominant position or after 10 days of friendly contact with a conspecific *(broken lines)*

while a dominant position, friendly interaction with a conspecific of the same sex or life in a harmonic pair bond lowers the cortisol reaction values. The same could be true of other animal species. Thus, the corticosterone levels in the blood of subordinated mice in the "open field test" or after the injection of ACTH increase much more than in dominant animals (Ely and Henry 1978). The same is true in rhesus monkeys (Sassenrath 1970). Dominant squirrel monkeys respond to capture and anaesthetisation with a lesser increase in serum cortisol than subordinate individuals, despite their higher starting values (Coe et al 1979).

These findings indicate that a low cortisol response of a tree shrew in the reaction test could be an indicator that the animal lives in a situation which it can control, in which it receives social support from a conspecific or, anthromorphically, that the animal has high "self-confidence". A high cortisol response, on the other

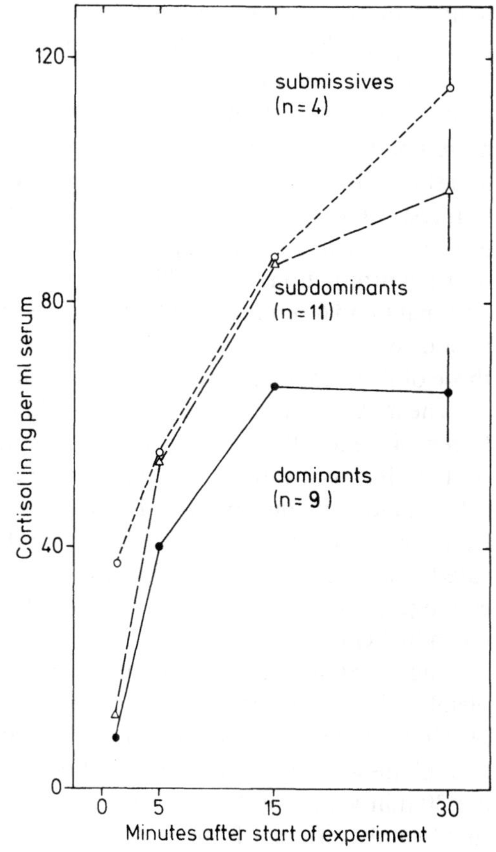

Fig. 8. Cortisol responses in the reaction test of males 10 days after the start of confrontation. The mean values and, in the case of the 30-min values, the SE, are given

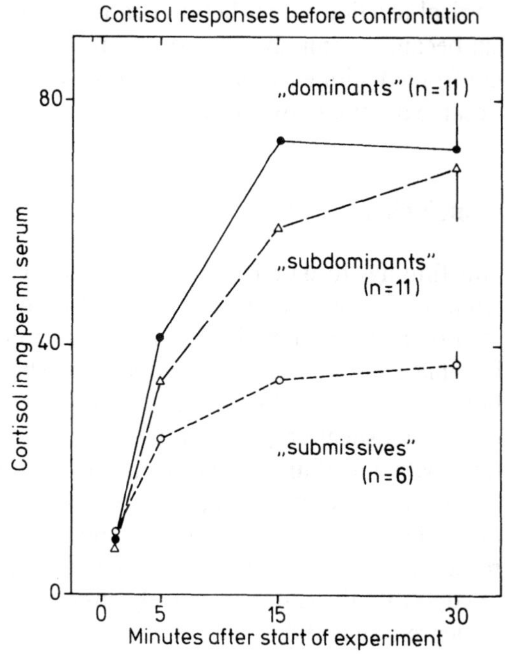

Fig. 9. Cortisol responses of the experimental groups shown in Fig. 8 before confrontation. The mean values and, in the case of the 30-min values, the SE, are given

hand, would be an indicator of loss of control, insecurity, subordination or, anthromorphically, "lack of self confidence".

Hence the question arises: Do these cortisol reaction test values of control animals allow a prediction as to their behaviour in the case of a confrontation? Put more simply, have these individual cortisol reactions a prognostic value? To date, 28 tree shrews have been studied, which, independent of their initial levels in the reaction test, were paired, as previously described, in the confrontation test. Reaction tests were made on all animals about 8 days before and then 10 days after the start of the confrontation. Of the 28 experimental animals, 11 became dominant, 11 subdominant und 6 submissive. Of the submissives, two animals died during the experiment, so that their reaction values at the end of the stress period, together with those of their dominant rivals, are not available.

The maximal starting values (=30-min reaction values) of all animals varied between 24.4 and 118.1 ng cortisol/ml serum (average approx. 60 ng/ml). As was expected, the basal values (=1-min values) of the dominants and the behaviourally active subdominants lay, after 10 days of confrontation, within the range of those from control animals, while the values for the passive submissives were clearly elevated. The cortisol reaction values (5 to 30-min values) of dominants lay in the lower range of starting values for all animals, while those of the subordinates were much higher (Fig. 8).

The reaction values of animals before confrontation, however, showed a completely different picture (Fig. 9). Prospective dominants and subdominants had approximately the same average cortisol reaction values, while those of the prospective submissives lay, on an average, about 50% below those of the other two groups; the 30-min values of "dominants" ($P<0.001$) and "subdominants" ($P<0.01$) are significantly different from those of "submissives". Comparison of the individual starting values also showed the same trend: Of the eight animals with the lowest cortisol reaction values before confrontation (between 24.4 and 42.3 ng/ml serum) six became submissive, one dominant and one subdominant, the latter two being confronted with each other. Again the male with the higher cortisol starting value became dominant over its rival.

Conclusion

Our findings to date can be interpreted in the following way: Physiological data from undisturbed animals (basal or 1-min values) and reaction values before the start of confrontation give us just as little information as to whether an animal will become a winner or a loser as does the behaviour of an animal before the fight. If, however, an animal loses a fight, its original cortisol response in the reaction test allows a statistical prognosis to be made regarding its behaviour in this situation: A male with a medium to high cortisol response in the reaction test (i.e., according to the previous interpretation, with less "self-confidence") would, after the subordination, attempt to cope with the situation actively. In contrast, a male with low cortisol reaction values (i.e. with a high level of "self-confidence") would make no attempt to cope with the situation actively after subordination but would become apathetic or depressive and die.

These findings, at present, are based on data from a small number of experimental animals which lived for months or years with no direct contact with conspecifics before confrontation. The conclusions are, therefore, despite their clarity, to be considered with caution. Moreover, a series of questions and contradictions have been raised which will be mentioned here only briefly: The attainment of a dominant position lowers the cortisol reaction values of male tree shrews; with this, theoretically, there should be an increasing danger of becoming a submissive after a fight. Basically, however, in tree shrews, as in other species, success in a fight increases the chances that the animal will win future fights (see "trained fighters") so that the decision - submissive or subdominant - would only occur rarely for successful dominants. However, the possibility that a dominant male, if he happens to be beaten in a fight, would become a submissive cannot be excluded. For certain species with a strict hierarchy the loss of an individual animal's dominant position usually does not result in its taking the second place in the rank order but in its relegation to the lowest position, where it often becomes apathetic and dies.

In addition to this, in our experiments to date, dominant tree shrews during confrontations have never reached the low cortisol reaction values typical of later submissives before the confrontation. Low values comparable with these have only been recorded for the individuals in harmonic pairs, but even these are, in general, very successful in fights, and it is not known whether they would react submissively once defeated.

The central question, however, is why the submissives described here have such extremely low cortisol reaction values before the start of the fight, i.e. why they have such a high "self confidence". Genetic influences do not appear here to be of any great importance, since even in the case of twins the whole range of possible reaction variations is present. However, it is possible that social influences during ontogeny can play a part. On the basis of many observations we have the impression that males which have had no negative social contact with parents or other conspecifics during ontogeny (either because of early separation from the parents or removal of the father) are the ones which "give up" most easily and quickly during a confrontation and become submissive. Whether these animals have especially low cortisol reaction values before the fight, however, is not known to date.

References

Beere PA, Glagov S, Zarins CK (1984) Retarding effect of lowered heart rate on coronary atherosclerosis. Science 226: 180–182

Coe CL, Mendoza SP, Levine S (1979) Social status constrains the stress response in the squirrel monkey. Physiol Behav 23: 633–638

Ely DL, Henry JP (1978) Neuroendocrine response pattern in dominant and subordinate mice. Horm Behav 10: 156–169

Henry JP, Stephens PM (1977) Stress, health, and the social environment. A sociobiologic approach to medicine. Springer, Berlin Heidelberg New York

Hutzelmeyer U (1984) Nebennierenrinden-Aktivität bei *Tupaia belangeri:* Beziehung zwischen in-vitro und in-vivo Daten. Thesis University of Bayreuth

Kawamichi T, Kawamichi M (1979) Spatial organization and territory of tree shrews *(Tupaia glis).* Anim Behav 27: 381–393

Martin RD (1968) Reproduction and ontogeny in tree shrews *(Tupaia belangeri)* with reference to their general behaviour and taxonomic relationships. Z Tierpsychol 25: 409-495, 505-532

Sassenrath EN (1970) Increased adrenal responsiveness related to social stress in rhesus-monkeys. Horm Behav 1: 283-298

Starck D (1978) Vergleichende Anatomie der Wirbeltiere auf evolutionsbiologischer Grundlage. Vol 1: Theoretische Grundlagen Stammesgeschichte und Systematik unter Berücksichtigung niederer Chordata. Springer, Berlin Heidelberg New York

Stöhr W (1982) Telemetrische Langzeituntersuchungen der Herzfrequenz von *Tupaia belangeri:* Basalwerte sowie phasische und tonische Reaktionen auf nichtsoziale und soziale Belastungen. Inaugural Dissertation, University of Bayreuth

Stöhr W (1986) Heart rate of tree shrews and its persistent modification by social contact. In: Schmidt TH, Dembroski TM, Blümchen G (eds) Biological and psychological factors in cardiovascular disease. Springer, Berlin Heidelberg New York, pp 491-499

Thoenen H, Mueller RA, Axelrod J (1969) Trans-synaptic induction of adrenal tyrosine hydroxylase. J Pharmacol Exp Ther 169: 249-254

von Holst D (1972) Renal failure as the cause of death in *Tupaia belangeri* exposed to persistent social stress. J Comp Physiol 78: 236-273

von Holst D (1977) Social stress in tree-shrews: problems, results, and goals. J Comp Physiol 120: 71-86

von Holst D, Fuchs E, Stöhr W (1983) Physiological changes in male *Tupaia belangeri* under different types of social stress. In: Dembroski TM, Schmidt TH, Blümchen G (eds) Biobehavioral bases of coronary heart disease. Karger, Basel, pp 382-390

Witte PU, Matthaei H (1980) Mikrochemische Methoden für neurobiologische Untersuchungen. Springer, Berlin Heidelberg New York

Heart Rate of Tree Shrews and Its Persistent Modification by Social Contact

W. STÖHR[1]

Introduction

The physiological state of an animal is influenced by a multitude of external factors. Physical factors like ambient temperature, for instance, have a profound effect on oxygen consumption and heart rate. Equally powerful are the effects of social environment upon the physiological state of an individual. Socially induced changes of the endocrine system are comparatively well documented both in field and laboratory studies, but few investigations deal with the effects of the social environment on other neurovegetative parameters like heart rate.

Squirrel monkeys show rank-dependent differences in heart rate during the formation of status orders (Candland et al. 1970). In groups of macaques and baboons heart rates of the individual members were found to be inversely correlated with their rank order (Cherkovich et al. 1973). These investigations, however, were based on sporadic radiotelemetric recordings covering only minutes or hours. It is therefore still an open question whether these heart rate changes are persistent or transient.

In tree shrews under social stress, von Holst (1969) found increased activation of the sympathetic nervous system that was maintained for weeks without any sign of habituation. To investigate this long-lasting effect of sociobehavioral interaction, we decided to record the heart rate of tree shrews *(Tupaia belangeri)* continuously over long periods of time and a wide range of social situations.

Methods

The detection of slow, incremental changes of heart rate, especially in small, highly active animals, requires a number of methodological prerequisites:

1. Measurements must be very precise and free of artifacts.
2. The measurement method must not have an effect on the animal whose heart rate is being measured. This excludes, for instance, the use of wire leads or external backpacks (Bohus 1974). We consider extremely miniaturized, implanted radiotransmitters the only feasible method to avoid such methodological side effects.
3. Before studying the effects of social interactions, the true baseline heart rate of each experimental animal must be known. This means recording heart rate continuously while the animal lives in a stable environment (especially one with a

1 Department of Animal Physiology, University of Bayreuth, Universitätstrasse 30, 8580 Bayreuth, Federal Republic of Germany

Biological and Psychological Factors
in Cardiovascular Disease
Ed. by T. H. Schmidt, T. M. Dembroski, and G. Blümchen

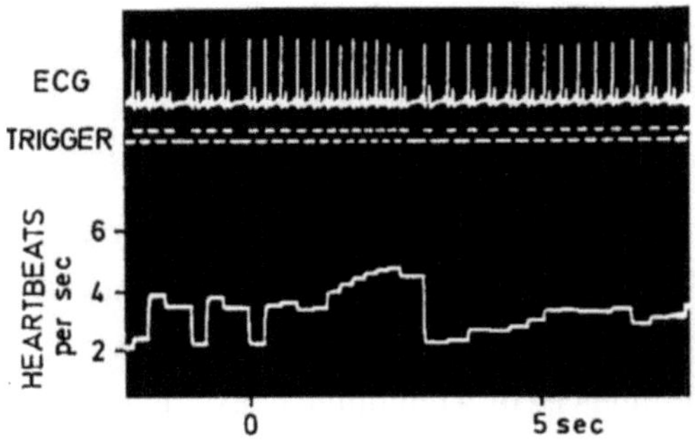

Fig. 1. Oscillogram of performance check: *Top*, ECG; *middle*, R-wave trigger with T-wave suppression; *bottom*, interbeat-intervals expressed in voltage steps = heart rate in beats per sec

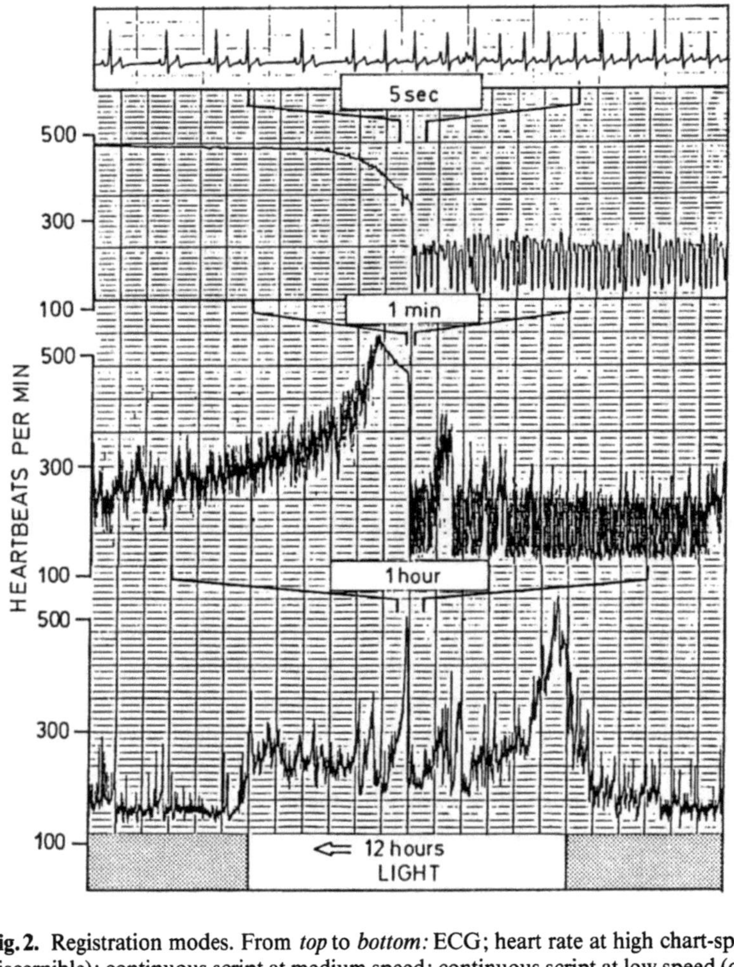

Fig. 2. Registration modes. From *top* to *bottom:* ECG; heart rate at high chart-speed (single beats discernible); continuous script at medium speed; continuous script at low speed (dampened for diurnal pattern recognition)

stable temperature), until all postoperative effects have disappeared and the animal has habituated to the experimental situation. This state is indicated by a low, stable mean heart rate and a stable diurnal pattern of heart rate.

As no suitable radio transmitters are commercially available, we developed a miniature transmitting system that is especially optimized for long-term recordings of heart rate in small animals. The transmitters measure 13 × 9 × 3.5 mm. Depending on the size of the battery used, their weight is between 0.9 and 1.5 g, and their corresponding lifetime between 2 and 6 months. The transmitters were subcutaneously implanted in the back of the animals with electrodes extending to the thoracic region (Stöhr 1982). The receiving system includes several stages of noise suppression and artifact distinction. Precise determination of heart rate is based on quartz-controlled measurement of interbeat-intervals. ECG, R-wave triggering, and heart rate can be displayed on an oscilloscope for continuous surveillance of proper performance (Fig. 1).

Four registration modes were employed (example: Fig. 2):
1. Frequent recordings of ECG on paperstrips
2. Heart rate recordings at fast chart-speed in acute tests
3. Continuous heart rate registration at medium chart-speed throughout the lifetime of the transmitter
4. Continuous registration of heart rate at very slow chart-speed to elucidate diurnal fluctuations

To date we have recorded heart rates from 19 tree shrews for more than 50000 h. The animals were kept single (unless mentioned otherwise), with food (Altromin Special Diet) and water ad lib; light: dark cycle was 12:12 h; ambient temperature was 25 ± 1 °C; and relative humidity was 55 ± 5%.

Results and Discussion

Following the implantation of the transmitter the high postoperative heart rate gradually declines to a steady baseline within a period of 1-6 weeks, depending on the animal's familiarity with the experimental situation (Fig. 3). Baseline heart rates found after this habituation period differ considerably from individual to individual (night means lay between 131 and 275 bpm; day means between 215 and 383 bpm), but they are very stable over a long time (see Fig. 3). These heart rates are low for animals of this size (ca. 200 g), since according to allometric equations their resting heart rate should be 335 bpm. We attribute the low values we found to our nonstressing transmitting method.

Each animal has an individual pattern of diurnal heart rate fluctuations, with mean day levels about 50% higher than mean night levels. While night heart rate is rather stable, day heart rate fluctuates between three periodically recurrent phases which are correlated with ongoing behaviour (Fig. 4). Very low heart rates are found at rest, medium heart rates at physical activity (running, jumping, climbing). The high peaks of heart rate coincide with the termination of resting periods, before the animal become active again. These phases are characterized by a very attentive be-

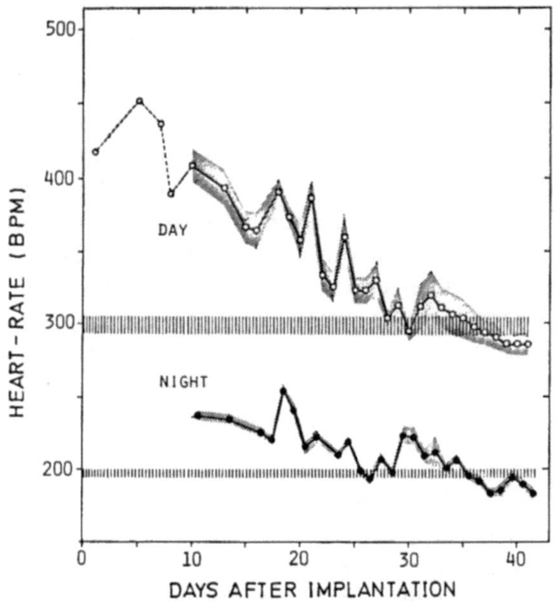

Fig. 3. Long habituation period. Heart rate (mean ± SE) during day (○) and night (●). Early data missing or incomplete because of registration problems. *Horizontal shadings* indicate mean heart rate (mean ± SE) between days 186 and 196 after implantation of transmitter

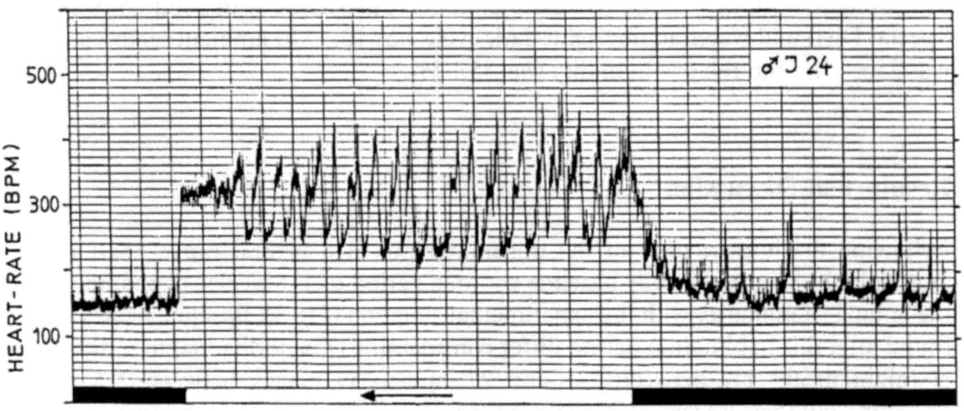

Fig. 4. Typical diurnal heart rate pattern of an undisturbed tree shrew (light : dark cycle = 12 : 12 h)

haviour. During the consecutive cage exploration and cage marking, heart rate gradually comes down to medium levels and the animal turns to miscellaneous activities. Thus, the whole range of physical activity can be performed at heart rates of 250–350 bpm, depending on the individual. Maximum heart rates of 500–650 bpm are only reached in emotionally arousing situations – regardless of physical activity.

Conspecific interaction drastically changes the individual heart rate pattern. Olfactory and acoustic signals from a female placed in an adjacent cage (no visual

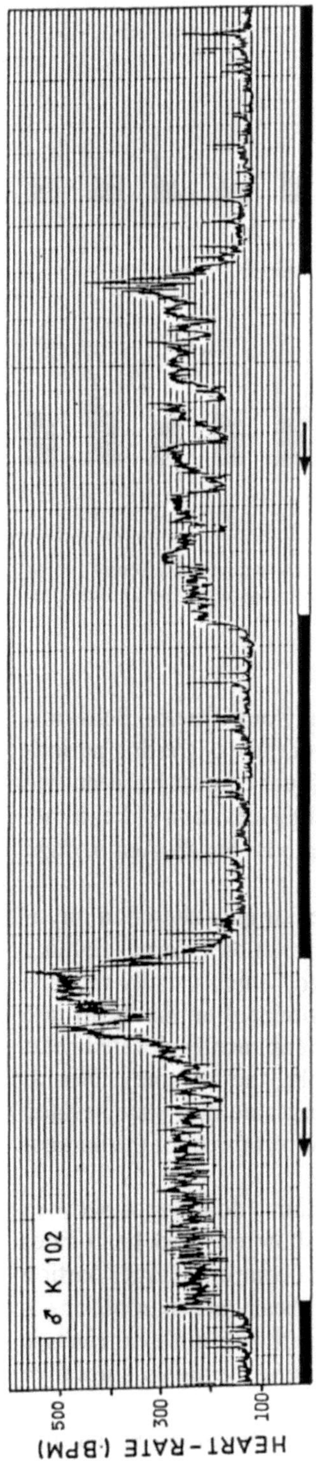

Fig. 5. Heart rate reaction of a male tree shrew to a female placed in the adjacent cage

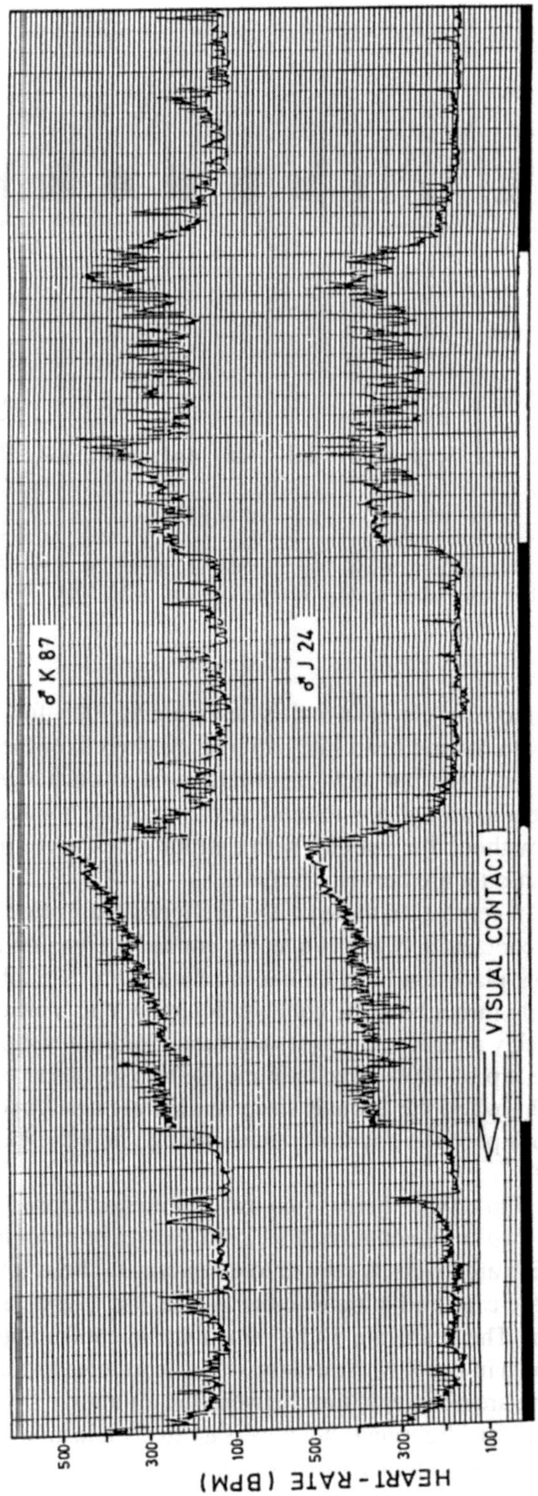

Fig. 6. Heart rate reaction of two male tree shrews upon visual contact

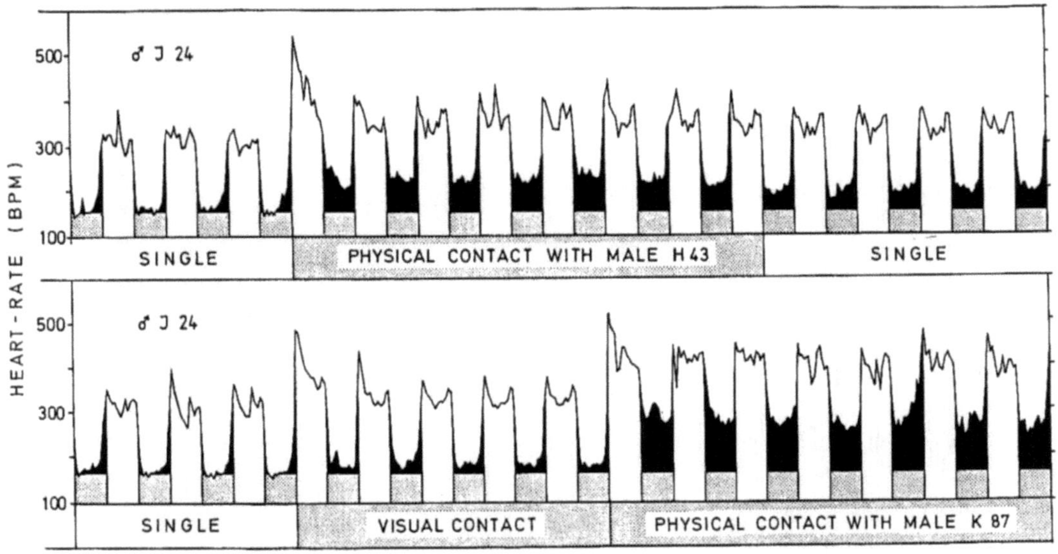

Fig. 7. Heart rate reaction of a male tree shrew in physical contacts with two different males. *Shaded areas*, dark cycle; *white areas*, light cycle. Night changes from prefight levels are emphasized in *black*

contact) can elevate a male's heart rate by 100% for several hours (Fig. 5). Behavioral patterns and heart rate patterns are altered for the rest of the day (resting periods are reduced), but night heart rate remains unchanged. Visual contact between two animals through a wire-mesh partition elicits a longer-lasting elevation of heart rate throughout the first day, with a striking lack of resting periods (Fig. 6). Again, night heart rates are hardly affected.

In contrast to these transient effects, heart rate can be lastingly altered in physical contacts between two males. Immediately upon confrontation vigorous fighting takes place until a dominance relationship is established, which usually remains stable throughout the cohabitation. While in a clearly dominant animal heart rate quickly returns to prefight values, subdominants show a permanently elevated heart rate, up to 100% over baseline values (see also von Holst, this volume). Even at night, when the animals sleep in separate nest-boxes, heart rate may stay elevated above previous day-time values, though here there is no direct threat of the antagonist.

If in a fight there is no clear "winner and loser," a relative dominance between the two opponents results. In this case, both animals show elevated heart rates which are inversely related to dominance: The animal that controls a larger portion of the cage and initiates more attacks has a less elevated heart rate than his opponent. The heart rate of the same male in confrontations with two different rivals is shown in Fig. 7. Most striking is the heart rate elevation during the nights, since then there are no interactions between the animals.

Actual fighting is not necessary to elicit lasting heart rate elevations. Social contact between females or ill-matched pairs of opposite sex causes remarkably high heart rate levels in both animals, though in these cases there is hardly any open ag-

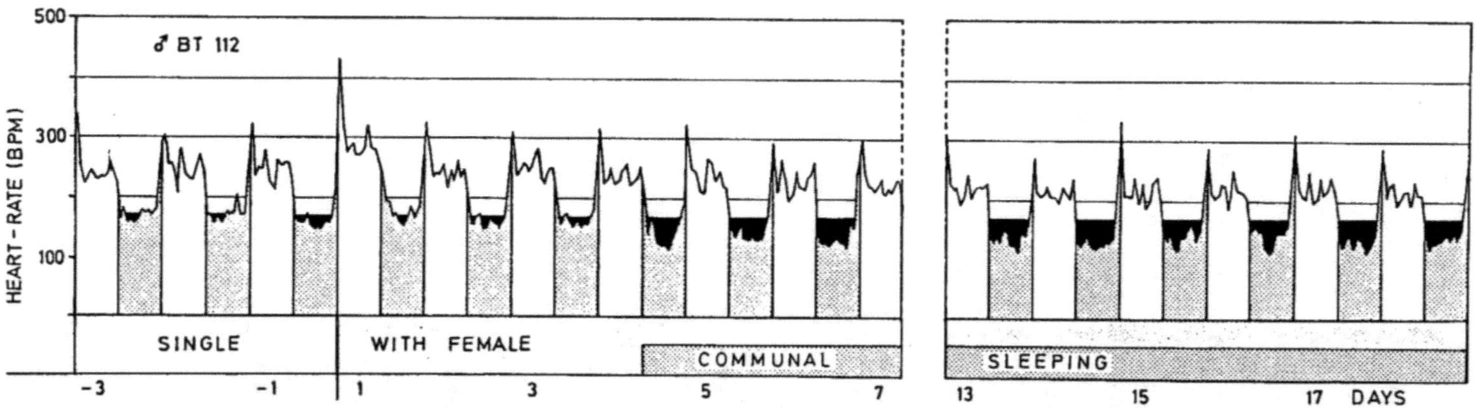

Fig. 8. Heart rate reaction of a male tree shrew to physical contact with a female. *Shaded areas,* dark cycle; *white areas,* light cycle. Night changes from precontact level are emphasized in *black*

gression but rather a sort of social tension. In any of these aversive contacts heart rate elevation becomes somewhat chronic, i.e., it does not return immediately to normal levels after complete separation of the animals. Original baseline values are only regained after weeks.

Tree shrews have strong individual preferences or aversions to partners of the opposite sex. The spontaneous accord of some couples could be described as "love at first sight." Mutual affection is indicated by mouth-licking, intensive mutual grooming, frequent communal resting (huddling), and sharing the same nest-box at night. To date, despite attempts with several experimental groupings, we have not been able to study heart rate in such a truly harmonic couple, since the outcome of arbitrary coupling is absolutely unpredictable. However, in the four couples that lived in moderate harmony after a few days of adjustment, heart rates in both animals were reduced by up to 20% below the baseline heart rates of the same animals living undisturbed and single (Fig. 8).

Heart rate elevations during the formation of a dominance order are not surprising, but to be expected in a situation of fighting and strong emotional engagement. Surprising to us, however, was the magnitude of elevation (up to 100%), its persistence (throughout the cohabitation and for weeks after), and its presence even during sleep. This means that an aversive social contact can double the total work load of a tree shrew's heart during both day and night for the duration of the contact, without any interval of rest and recovery.

High heart rate reacting macaques that were fed a moderately atherogenic diet developed significantly more atherosclerosis than low reactors. (Manuck et al. 1983). In contrast, reduced atherosclerosis was found in the same species when heart rate was reduced by ablation of the sinoatrial node (Beere et al. 1984). As in Manuck's study, there was no difference in serum cholesterol, body weight, and blood pressure as compared with the control group. This suggests that heart rate alone may contribute to the development or absence of atherosclerosis.

Conclusion

Our data show that heart rate in tree shrews is determined to a great extent by the social environment. Aversive social situations elevate heart rate, while positive social situations, such as the presence of a harmonic partner, lower heart rate persistently. On the basis of the data presented by Manuck and Beere et al., our results indicate that social influences may contribute to a large extent to the development as well as to the prevention of cardiovascular disease.

References

Beere PA, Glagov S, Zarins ChK (1984) Retarding effect of lowered heart rate on coronary atherosclerosis. Science 226: 180-182

Bohus B (1974) Telemetered heart rate responses of the rat during free and learned behavior. Biotelemetry 2: 193-201

Candland DK, Bryan DC, Nazar BL, Kopf KJ, Sendor M (1970) Squirrel monkey heart rate during formation of status orders. J Comp Physiol Psychol 3: 417-423

Cherkovich GM, Tatoyan SK (1973) Heart rate (radiotelemetrical registration) in macaques and baboons according to dominant - submissive rank in groups. Folia Primatol 20: 265-273
Manuck StB, Kaplan JR, Clarkson ThB (1983) Behaviorally induced heart rate reactivity and atherosclerosis in Cynomolgus monkeys. Psychosom Med 45, 2: 95-108
Stöhr W (1982) Telemetrische Langzeituntersuchungen der Herzfrequenz von *Tupaia belangeri:* Basalwerte sowie phasische und tonische Reaktionen auf nichtsoziale und soziale Belastungen. Inaugural Dissertation, University of Bayreuth
von Holst D (1969) Sozialer Streß bei Tupajas *(Tupaia belangeri).* Die Aktivierung des sympathischen Nervensystems und ihre Beziehung zu hormonal ausgelösten ethologischen und physiologischen Veränderungen. Z Vergl Physiol 63: 1-58
von Holst D (1986) Psychosocial stress and its pathophysiological effects in tree shrews *(Tupaia belangeri).* In: Schmidt TH, Dembroski TM, Blümchen G (eds) Biological and psychological factors in cardiovascular disease. Springer, Berlin Heidelberg New York, pp 476-490

Blood Pressure Regulation by Sodium Intake and Behavioral Stress

D. E. ANDERSON[1]

Introduction

Several studies have shown that acute pressor responses evoked by "mental stress" tend to be of greater magnitude in hypertensive patients and their offspring than in normotensive controls (Engel and Bickford 1962; Nestel 1969; Light and Obrist 1980; Eliasson et al. 1983). On the basis of these observations, it has sometimes been suggested that cardiovascular hyperreactivity is genetic in origin and that it precedes the development of chronic hypertension. One theory is that sympathetically mediated pressor responses to behavioral interactions lead to chronic elevation of total peripheral resistance and hypertension in individuals who exhibit this trait of cardiovascular hyperreactivity. Indirect support for this view can be found in studies of genetic hypertension in rodents. For example, spontaneously hypertensive rats (SHR) are "hyperreactive" to acute environmental stimulation and show attenuated development of high blood pressure if they are reared in protected environments (Lais et al. 1974) or if their sympathetic nervous system function is impaired (Folkow and Hallback 1977).

The evidence also suggests, however, that cardiovascular reactivity itself is subject to environmental influence and that its role in the pathogenesis of hypertension may depend on multiple environmental inputs. This view calls into question the usefulness of a general trait of cardiovascular hyperreactivity, but suggests that elucidation of the extrinsic factors which affect reactivity may lead to an understanding of long-term blood pressure regulation.

This chapter is based on the premise that the magnitude of cardiovascular response to environmental stimuli depends on the dietary intake of sodium and potassium. High sodium and/or low potassium intake typically have little direct effect on blood pressure in individuals with homeostatic physiologic function. However, high sodium intake potentiates the acute cardiovascular response to adrenergic stimulation and behavioral stress. It has also been found that specific behavioral stresses alter rates of excretion of ingested sodium and potassium. Thus, tonic psychobehavioral stress factors and dietary micronutrient intake jointly determine the cardiovascular response to acute stimulation. The potential relevance of these interactions to long-term control of arterial pressure is illustrated in a discussion of a model of progressive, 24-h hypertension in laboratory dogs that results from a combination of behavioral stress (producing sustained bradycardia) and high sodium intake, even though neither factor alone is sufficient to increase arterial pressure

1 Department of Psychiatry and Behavioral Medicine, University of South Florida College of Medicine, and J. A. Haley Veterans Administration Hospital, Tampa, FL 33612, USA

Biological and Psychological Factors
in Cardiovascular Disease
Ed. by T. H. Schmidt, T. M. Dembroski, and G. Blümchen

progressively. It has also been found that concurrent potassium intake mediates the combined effects of sodium intake and behavioral stress on arterial pressure. The interaction of such dietary micronutrients with specific neuroendocrine adaptations to recurrent stresses may play a significant role in the pathogenesis of hypertension (Folkow 1982).

Dietary Sodium and Potassium and Arterial Pressure

Epidemiologic studies have shown that hypertension tends to be more prevalent in cultures in which dietary sodium intake is high and lower in cultures in which sodium consumption is low (Freis 1976). Dietary sodium restriction can decrease blood pressure in hypertensive (e.g., Morgan et al. 1978; McGregor et al. 1982) and even normotensive individuals (Miller et al. 1983). Moreover, it has been shown recently that the decreases in blood pressure of hypertensive patients produced by sodium restriction are accompanied by decreases in intralymphocytic sodium levels (Ambrosioni et al. 1982) and that such patients exhibit decreased vascular responsiveness to mental arithmetic stress (Ambrosioni et al. 1982).

However, it cannot be inferred from these observations that high sodium intake alone reliably "causes" hypertension. Under normal conditions, relatively constant levels of total body sodium are maintained in the healthy individual despite wide fluctuations in dietary intake. The average daily sodium intake of United States citizens, based on analyses of 24-h urinary sodium excretion, ranges between 80 and 115 mEq/day (Dahl and Love 1957; Altman and Dittmer 1974); in comparison, some oceanic fish-eating societies consume several times as much (Yamori et al. 1981). Sodium balance is maintained by several interrelated physiologic mechanisms, including renal glomerular filtration, the renin-angiotensin-aldosterone system, arterial pressure, and the sympathetic nervous system. The concentration of sodium remains high in the extracellular fluid, but low inside the cell. The reverse is true for potassium.

The limits of the ability of the body to regulate sodium balance have been probed in dietary studies with normotensive human subjects. For example, one study showed that 10 days on a 400-mEq diet did not increase arterial pressure, though it did increase forearm vasodilation (Mark et al. 1975). More recently, it has been reported that a high sodium diet maintained for a whole year did not increase arterial pressure, though increases in stroke volume and cardiac output and decreased total peripheral resistance were maintained by this diet (Sullivan and Ratts 1983). Small but significant elevations in arterial pressure (7–15 mmHg systolic) were observed over a period of 6 days in subjects exposed to very high sodium diets (800–1500 mEq/day) (Murray et al. 1978; Luft et al. 1979). This increase was mediated by increases in stroke volume and cardiac output, while plasma renin activity and plasma aldosterone concentrations were decreased.

These observations of changes in hemodynamics resulting from high sodium intake appear to be relevant to the whole-body autoregulation theory of hypertension. Briefly, this theory states that hypertension involves a two-stage process: one in which cardiac output is elevated and excessive for metabolic need and a second in which total peripheral resistance increases reflexively to reduce local blood flows and maintain the hypertensive state even after cardiac output has returned to normal. It has been proposed (Obrist 1981) that beta-adrenergic influences on the heart associated with behavioral stress could engender this kind of process. Evidently, a high sodium diet by itself, which increases cardiac output, does not produce such whole-body autoregulation of blood pressure, at least over a 1-year interval.

The epidemiologic evidence suggests that potassium intake by humans may be inversely related to arterial pressure (Watson et al. 1980; Yamori et al. 1981). In addition, plasma potassium and total body potassium levels have also been found to be negatively correlated with blood pressure (Lever et al. 1981; Ueshima et al. 1981). Several recent studies have suggested that a marked reduction in the ratio of sodium to potassium intake decreases blood pressure in hypertensive patients (reviewed by Treasure and Ploth 1983). Thus, the evidence to be reviewed below should be looked at with the understanding that potassium intake can modulate these sodium-blood pressure relationships. Thus, the discussion is about sodium/potassium intake, rather than simply sodium intake.

Hyperreactivity to Dietary Sodium

Even though high sodium intake alone does not raise arterial pressure in most humans, there are those whose blood pressure does increase in response to this dietary stimulus. Sodium sensitivity is especially prevalent in the offspring of individuals who are hypertensive and in individuals with early or "borderline" hypertension. For example, Mark et al. (1975) reported that "borderline" hypertensives responded not only with forearm vasoconstriction, but also with increased blood pressure to the same diet that did not increase pressure in the normotensive control group. These effects were found to be accompanied by decreases in plasma catecholamines (Fujita et al. 1980). It was also found that individuals aged over 40 years and blacks tend to be relatively salt sensitive and excrete proportionally less sodium in response to a high salt diet (Luft et al. 1979).

It is clear that, by itself, cardiovascular responsiveness to sodium depends to some extent on genetic factors. Rats that become hypertensive in response to a high sodium diet have been bred (S strain), while others have been bred to be resistant to the hypertensinogenic effects of the same diet (R strain) (Dahl et al. 1962). Sodium hypertension in S rats results from increased total peripheral resistance, with part of the increase in total peripheral resistance being neural and part nonneural (Takeshita and Mark 1978; Falkner et al. 1981). The genetic factor apparently includes a blood-borne humoral factor, since cross-perfusion of salt-loaded S and R rats alters blood pressure of each in opposite directions. Rats with a genetic predisposition to become hypertensive in response to sodium intake also tend to be reactive to aversive stimulation. Dahl S rats, but not Dahl R rats, placed in a conditioning situation that involves "conflict" show progressively increased blood pressure over periods of weeks (reviewed by Friedman 1981).

Even though the SHR becomes hypertensive on a normal sodium diet, its hypertension is exacerbated if it is fed a high sodium diet (Aoki and Yamori 1972). Experiments with young SHRs have shown that both high sodium diet and behavioral stress (crowding) altered central nervous system catecholamines and aggravated the hypertension (Ely and Wiegand 1983). Sodium loading of SHRs was found to increase (a) the concentration of sodium in the extracellular fluid of these subjects and (b) the reactivity of vascular smooth muscle of SHRs in proportion to the increase in plasma sodium concentration (Dietz et al. 1982). When arteries of young SHRs were transplanted into control rats, the electrical potential of the arterial cell membrane came to resemble that of the host, and vice versa (Campbell et al. 1981). These effects were observed only in young SHRs, but not in adults with established hypertension. Again, these experiments indicate that the circulation of the SHR contains a substance that alters the electrical characteristics of the cell membrane and its permeability to sodium.

A recent study with human hypertensives examined the effects of sodium restriction on the blood pressure of normotensive subjects with and without a family history of hypertension (Skrabal et al. 1984). Two weeks of moderate sodium restriction resulted in a small but significant decrease in blood pressure in a subset of these subjects. Members of this group were 2.5 times as likely to have a positive family history of hypertension as members of the group that did not respond to sodium restriction. The responsive group was also found to have a higher initial blood pressure level and a lower concentration of salivary sodium. On the basis of these findings, it was speculated that the cause of the enhanced sodium sensitivity was increased activity of the sympathetic nervous system. Paradoxically, the cause of the enhanced sodium sensitivity might also involve the parasympathetic nervous system, even though the neurotransmitter acetylcholine induces acute relaxation of vascular smooth muscle. Recent studies by Numa and colleagues in Japan have shown that the binding of acetylcholine to its receptor causes a small change in the voltage of the cell membrane and an increase in the influx of sodium into the cell (Marx 1985). These effects can alter the cells' responses, such as the firing of neurons or the contraction of muscle cells.

Aspects of renal function of salt-sensitive individuals have also been shown to be quantitatively different from those of salt-insensitive controls. Hollenberg et al. (1981) showed that a nonverbal IQ test decreased renal blood flow and increased plasma renin activity, blood pressure, and heart rate to a greater degree in hypertensive subjects and in normotensive subjects with a family history of hypertension than in a control group of normotensive subjects with a negative family history of hypertension. In another study (Light et al. 1983), it was reported that performance of a competitive perceptual-motor task was associated with decreased urinary fluid volume and sodium excretion in saline-loaded young adults with hypertension or with a positive family history of hypertension, but not in a control group of normotensive subjects with a negative family history of hypertension. The magnitude of diuresis occurring under these conditions was negatively correlated with the magnitude of blood pressure and heart rate response to the task. Animal studies have also shown that acute pressor responses and suppression of renal excretory activity to an aversive stimulus were greater in genetically hypertensive rats than in genetically normotensive rats (Lundin and Thoren 1982). Thus, individuals who show increases in pressure to sodium intake may have a decreased ability to autoregulate body sodium levels.

Sodium Potentiation of Adrenergic Stimulation Effects

A high sodium diet can also affect neural structure and function in genetically normotensive animals. For example, although a high sodium intake decreased basal sympathetic nervous system activity (Dietz et al. 1978) and the turnover of norepinephrine in the central nervous system of rats (Tanaka et al. 1982), it was also found to increase the density of alpha receptors in the kidneys (Sanchez and Pettinger 1981) and especially in the kidneys of genetically hypertensive rats (Pettinger et al. 1982). These increases in alpha receptor density could enhance the response of vascular smooth muscle to sympathetic stimulation. The salt-induced decreases in resting levels of peripheral catecholamines might be due to the central nervous system changes, since interruption of the neural connections between the brain and periphery by drugs or surgery prevented peripheral, but not central catecholamine responses to salt feeding (Nakamura et al. 1971; van Ameringen et al. 1977). A high sodium diet has also been found to potentiate the pressor response to sympathetic nerve stimulation in Dahl S rats, while destruction of peripheral sympathetic nerves with 6-hydroxydopamine prevented the onset of hypertension (Ikeda et al. 1978). Moreover, the pressor response to hypertonic saline administered into the left lateral ventricle was greater in S rats than in salt-resistant (R) rats, even when all subjects were maintained on a low salt diet. It was suggested by these investigators that a high sodium diet may influence hypertension via heightened responsivity of the central nervous system to stimulation.

Other studies have shown that a high sodium diet increases the magnitude of the pressor response to intraventricular administrations of hypertonic saline or angiotensin II in normotensive rats (Reid and Laragh 1965; Campbell and Schmitz 1978). These effects were attenuated if the subjects were maintained on a high potassium diet (Goto et al. 1981). Increasing dietary sodium intake has also been shown to augment the effects of adrenergic stimulation on cardiovascular activity of dogs. For example, when the sodium diet of dogs was increased from 5 to 240 mEq/day, the magnitude of pressure elevation induced by intrarenal norepinephrine infusion increased by more than 100%, while the effective renal plasma flow and glomerular filtration rate decreased and renal vascular resistance increased progressively. Plasma renin activity was not increased under these conditions (Cowley and Lohmeier 1979). The latter studies indicate that the combined effects of sodium intake and sympathomimetic agents can be sustained over time.

Similar findings have been reported in studies with human subjects. For example, when normotensive human subjects received a diet with 800 mEq/day sodium for 5 days, the pressor response to the intra-arterial infusion of norepinephrine was enhanced, even though plasma norepinephrine levels preceding the infusion were decreased (Rankin et al. 1981; Falkner et al. 1981) monitored blood pressure and heart rate of two groups of teenage subjects during a 10-min mental arithmetic task before and after 2 weeks of a high sodium diet (oral supplement of 175 mEq/day). Those with a positive family history of hypertension showed a larger increase in blood pressure (but a smaller increase in heart rate) to the mental arithmetic after the salt loading period. The pressor response to the task was comparable before and after the salt loading period in the control group with no family history of hypertension. It has also been reported that the magnitude of pressor response to mental arithmetic performed by borderline hypertensive subjects was reduced after 6 weeks on a low salt diet (Ambrosioni et al. 1982). The diet did not reduce blood pressure at rest, but was associated with a decrease in intralymphocytic sodium levels, the magnitude of which was correlated in the individual subject with the reduction in pressor response to the arithmetic task. Another study showed that the magnitude of pressor response to norepinephrine infusion was larger in subjects who responded to 2 weeks of sodium restriction with a decrease in resting blood pressure than in another group of subjects for whom the sodium restriction did not change blood pressure (Skrabal et al. 1984).

Behavioral Conditioning, Sympathetic Activation and Renal Function

It is well established that renal sympathetic activity is importantly involved in several kinds of experimental hypertension (reviewed by Katholi 1983). Renal sympathetic activity (Okamoto et al. 1967) and renal norepinephrine turnover (Patel et al. 1981) are increased in SHRs compared with normotensive control rats. Renal denervation of young SHRs was found to increase sodium excretion and to delay the development of hypertension (Dietz et al. 1978; Liard 1979; Winternitz et al. 1980). However, attenuation of hypertension was not observed following renal denervation of mature SHRs with established hypertension, showing that the nervous system in this form of hypertension is pathogenetically involved in the development rather than the maintenance of high blood pressure. Renal sympathetic activity has also been found to be important in salt-deoxycorticosterone acetate hypertension (de Champlain et al. 1968; Katholi et al. 1980) and in one-kidney renal hypertension (Katholi et al. 1981).

Sustained hypertension can be produced in genetically normotensive but uninephrectomized dogs by continuous infusion of the sympathetic neurotransmitter norepinephrine (Katholi et al. 1977). This hypertension was accompanied by increases in renal vascular resistance and total peripheral resistance, together with decreases in cardiac output, variable changes in renal hemodynamics, and a positive sodium balance. By contrast, continuous electrical stimulation of the stellate ganglion of intact dogs was found to produce sustained hypertension which was associated with increases in cardiac output and no change in sodium balance (Liard et al. 1975). This hypertension was reversed by adrenergic blocking drugs.

Stress-Salt Hypertension

Studies of behavioral stress effects on chronically instrumented laboratory animals have focused on two specific patterns of hemodynamic response (Cohen and Obrist 1975; Brady and Harris 1976). One is the sympathetically mediated "defense" or "fight or flight" reaction, which involves an increase in cardiac output and arterial pressure, accompanied by vasodilation in skeletal muscle and little change in total peripheral resistance (Folkow and Neil 1971; Forsyth 1971). This response includes increased oxygen consumption and appears to facilitate an emergency behavioral response. The other is the more subtle, but no less important, "orienting," "sensory intake," or "vigilance" reaction. This parasympathetically mediated response includes decreases in heart rate and respiration. Further, blood vessels in skeletal muscle constrict, total peripheral resistance increases, and arterial pressure is maintained or actually increased (Sokolow 1963; Anderson and Tosheff 1973; Williams et al. 1975; Zanchetti et al. 1979). This pattern typically emerges under conditions of behavioral inhibition, apparently in the service of attention to the environment.

Both of these cardiovascular response patterns can be produced reliably in animals in the context of avoidance conditioning schedules. There are two kinds of avoidance conditioning: discriminated and free operant. In discriminated avoidance, a specific warning signal precedes each occurrence of an unconditional aversive stimulus (UAS), typically a brief electric shock or high-intensity auditory stimulus. In free-operant avoidance, no such warning signal is present, but a recycling timer runs continuously. Each time the subject makes a response, the timer is reset immediately. If the timer is permitted to complete its cycle (say, 20 s), a UAS is presented. Thus, the elapsed time since the last response or the last UAS are the only cues for the animal regarding the imminence of the next UAS. Free-operant avoidance conditioning produces a stable series of behavioral responses during each session which enables the animal to avoid virtually all UASs. The relative loss of potency of the UAS which would otherwise be associated with recurrent presentations is prevented by the rarity of its occurrence. Performance of free-operant avoidance behavior by dogs or monkeys reliably evokes a sustained "defense" reflex, with increases in cardiac output and arterial pressure, but not in total peripheral resistance (Forsyth 1971; Anderson and Tosheff 1973; Lawler et al. 1975). Regional blood flow changes include increases in blood flow in the heart, skeletal muscle, and liver and decreases in blood flow in the brain, skin, gastrointestinal system, spleen, pancreas, and, notably, the kidneys (Forsyth 1971).

Acute inhibition of renal excretion of water and sodium also occurs under these conditions, even in the absence of renal hemodynamic changes (Grignolo et al. 1982; Koepke et al. 1983). The renal excretory changes are not prevented by administration of the alpha-adrenergic blocking agent, phenoxybenzamine, perhaps because of compensatory increases in vasopressin produced by the drug (Koepke et al. 1982). Conditioned inhibition of renal excretory activity is prevented by beta-adrenergic blocking drugs, but only if they cross the blood-brain barrier (Koepke et al. 1983). In addition, avoidance conditioning procedures have been shown to produce increases in plasma renin activity in baboons (Blair et al. 1976).

It has also been found that, if a dog is confined in the experimental environment for a fixed period of time immediately preceding each avoidance session, blood pressure increases gradually, owing to a progressive rise in total peripheral resistance, while heart rate and cardiac output decrease (Anderson and Tosheff 1973; Lawler et al. 1975). The chronotropic effects are clearly due to increased parasympathetic nervous system activity, and it is thought that the increase in total peripheral resistance is due to an increase in alpha-adrenergic activity. This complex physiologic response may arise from the fact that the subject will receive the first UAS of the session if it does not maintain vigilant attention to the environment so as to initiate prompt avoidance responding after the onset of the session (typically signalled by a change in illumination in the experimental chamber).

Bradycardia and peripheral vasoconstriction in cats induced by confrontation with other animals has also been found to be associated with decreases in renal blood flow (Zanchetti et al. 1979). These effects are mediated by the renal sympathetic nerves, since renal denervation abolishes the response. It has also been shown that the peripheral vasoconstriction and bradycardia occurring during the "diving" reflex (Andersen 1966) is accompanied by a dramatic decrease in renal blood flow, glomerular filtration rate, and renal plasma flow (Murdaugh et al. 1961).

A few studies have shown that prolonged exposure to behavioral stress can result in sustained elevations in arterial pressure in chair-restrained primates with no genetic bias to hypertension. Herd et al. (1969) found that squirrel monkeys who were trained to work on escape-avoidance tasks two h/day maintained elevations in pressure between as well as during performance periods over several months. Similarly, Forsyth (1969) also reported that rhesus monkeys developed sustained hypertension after several months on avoidance schedules. These pioneering studies suggested that chronic hypertension might result from prolonged exposure to behavioral stresses in genetically normotensive animals, but replication and extension of such experiments is expensive of time, and others with similar procedures were unable to produce hypertension in baboons (Findley et al. 1971).

A clue regarding a procedure for developing behavioral hypertension more rapidly might be found in the observation that surgically produced reductions in renal excretory capacity resulted in hypertension in dogs within 10 days if they also received increased sodium in the form of intravenous saline infusion (Coleman and Guyton 1969). From these findings, it was hypothesized that a behavioral conditioning procedure that decreased renal excretion of sodium (and water) in combination with an increase in sodium intake would also produce a sustained hypertensive adaptation over a comparable period. In order to test this hypothesis, a system was constructed that enabled 24-h monitoring of cardiovascular activity in the semi-freeranging dog (Kearns et al. 1981). The dogs' body weight ranged from 13 to 22 kg. Each dog wore a vest which contained a pressure transducer, the cable of which ascended vertically through a hollow tether to a swivel, permitting the dog freedom of activity in the environment. The swivel was attached to a 60-cm-long boom, the other end of which was connected to the wall via a universal joint 2.13 m above floor level. The boom was counterbalanced so that there was minimal tension on the tether. A saline infusion line descended through the swivel and tether to the transducer, permitting administration of pharmacologic agents into and/or withdrawal of blood samples from an indwelling arterial catheter without disturbing the dog.

Arterial pressure and heart rate were monitored continuously for 24 h/day, 7 days/week. A computer system analyzed the data in terms of averages of systolic and diastolic arterial pressure and heart rate over successive 10-min and 60-min intervals. Typically, dogs were trained on the avoidance conditioning procedures prior to implantation of the catheter. The avoidance training period required daily sessions over periods of weeks to produce promptly initiated and stably maintained avoidance behavior. Following the acquisition of the avoidance performance, an arterial catheter was implanted into the aorta during aseptic surgery. During the subsequent experiments, the dog resided in the experimental chamber for 24 h/day. Patency of the catheter was ensured by a very slow (5 ml/h) but continuous infusion of lightly heparinized saline, powered by a peristaltic pump.

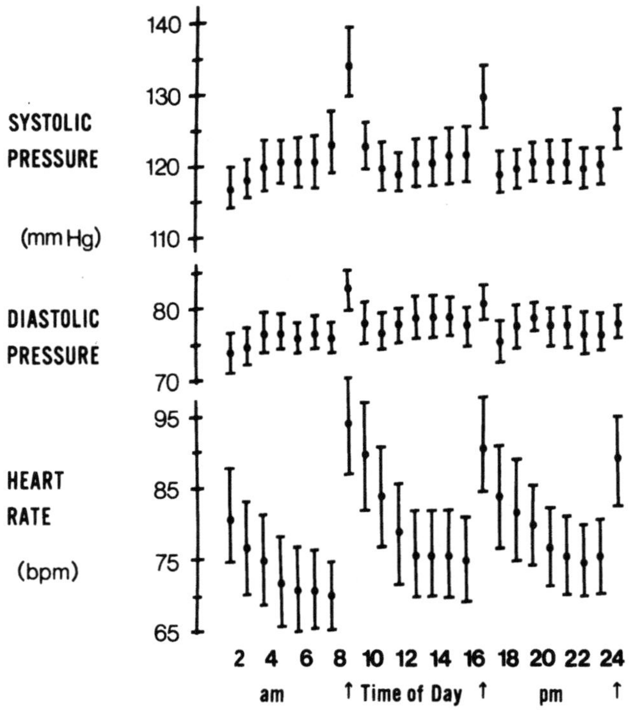

Fig. 1. Mean levels of systolic and diastolic pressures and heart rate during each hour of the day, averaged for a total of 80 days for eight dogs

Avoidance sessions were presented three times per day, at 12 midnight, 8 a.m., and 4 p.m. Each session was 30 min in duration and was signalled by the illumination of a light above the response key. Avoidance sessions were programed for at least 15 successive days, during which isotonic saline was infused continuously into the catheter at a constant rate of 50 ml/h. This procedure resulted in a 24-h intake of 185 mEq of sodium (less than 11 g), in addition to the 35–70 mEq ingested each day in food. Since the daily fluid intake from the infusion pump of 1340 ml exceeded amounts which would be consumed each day on an ad lib basis, no additional drinking water was provided.

The avoidance schedule produced a cyclic pattern of cardiovascular adaptation in each dog (Fig. 1). Both arterial pressure and heart rate were elevated during the hours in which the avoidance sessions occurred. However, heart rate levels declined progressively between sessions, while blood pressure remained stable or increased somewhat. These patterns indicate that total peripheral resistance increased and cardiac output decreased as the onset of the next avoidance session approached.

The administration of high levels of sodium in the form of saline in the context of this schedule of avoidance sessions resulted in a gradual increase in mean 24-h levels of arterial pressure over the 15-day periods (Fig. 2) (Anderson et al. 1983 a). The slope of the increase for the mean of the eight dogs was significant and relatively linear ($r=0.61$; $P<0.01$). Individual dogs varied considerably in the magnitude of hypertension achieved and in the rate at which blood pressure increased over

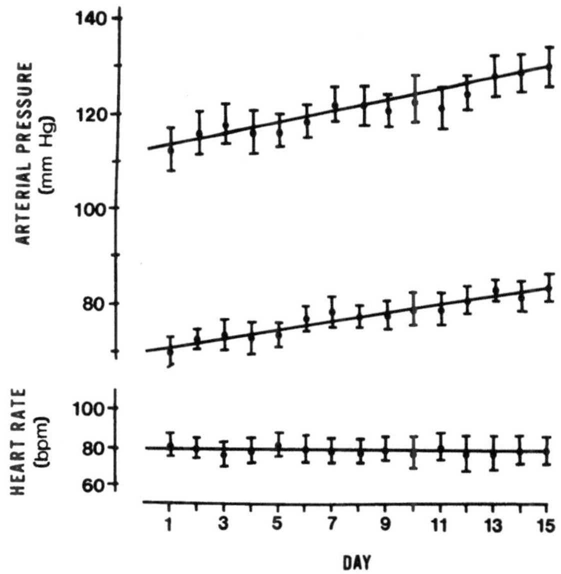

Fig. 2. Mean 24-h levels of systolic and diastolic pressures and heart rate for 15 successive days of avoidance sessions and saline infusion, averaged for eight dogs

time. One dog showed a rise in systolic pressure of 55 mmHg over this period, while another showed no significant change. It is not yet clear whether these differences reflect the effect of variations in genetic influence or procedural variations (e.g., differences in UAS intensity). Figure 2 also shows that 24-h heart rate levels did not increase. It is clear, therefore, that this progressive 24-h hypertension was not simply a sustained cardiovascular "defense" reflex to the avoidance contingencies.

The hypertension was reversible by termination of the avoidance schedules and saline infusion. The reversibility of the hypertension suggests that structural damage to the kidneys was not involved. Typically, continuation of the saline infusion following termination of the avoidance schedules resulted in a continuation of the hypertension, presumably due to conditioned effects of the behavioral procedures.

Progressive hypertension did not develop in dogs who were run on the avoidance schedule for 15 days in the absence of a high rate of saline infusion. Similarly, a high rate of saline infusion typically did not increase blood pressure in dogs that had not been trained on the avoidance task. Thus, the hypertension did not result from the additive effects of two separate factors, but developed because of synergistic interactions between behavioral procedures and high sodium intake. It should be emphasized that the bradycardia between sessions was an essential component for the hypertension to develop. Saline infusion of dogs maintaining 24-h tachycardia may not be as effective.

Development of experimental hypertension by removal of renal mass and salt loading was found to be accompanied by a significant increase in the retention of both water and sodium (Coleman and Guyton 1969). It was hypothesized, therefore, that hypertension in saline-loaded dogs on avoidance schedules also involved retention of both water and sodium. As an initial attempt to test this hypothesis, sodium and water balance were studied in dogs before and during the development of

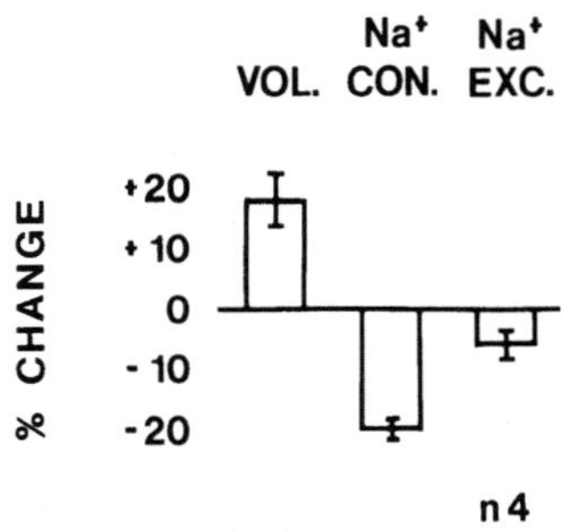

Fig. 3. Mean percentage difference in 24-h urine volume, sodium concentration, and sodium excretion between 14 days of baseline rest and 14 days of avoidance sessions, averaged for four saline-loaded dogs

avoidance-saline hypertension. For these experiments, 24-h urine volume was measured daily in dogs for 14 days of saline infusion only (baseline) followed by 14 days of a combination of saline infusion and avoidance schedules (conditioning).

Figure 3 shows the 24-h mean urine volume, urinary sodium concentration, and total urinary sodium excretion, averaged for four dogs under 14 days of each of these two conditions, baseline and conditioning. The data show that, contrary to expectations, urine volume was actually almost 20% greater during the 14-day conditioning period than during the 14-day baseline period, even though water intake was identical under both conditions. However, the concentration of sodium in the urine of each dog decreased to an even greater extent during the conditioning period, with the result that total daily sodium excretion decreased slightly during conditioned hypertension. Presuming that sodium balance was maintained during the 14-day baseline period of stable pressure, a progressively positive sodium balance (i.e., an increase in total body sodium) occurred during the conditioning period. Additional experiments will be necessary to quantitate this effect with confidence, but a 10% increase in total body sodium over the 15-day conditioning interval is a reasonable approximation. Thus, there was a marked divergence in the effects of the behavioral stress procedures on the excretion of water and sodium. The observation of a negative water balance and positive sodium balance in stress-salt hypertension suggests the possibility of an increase in total peripheral resistance resulting from an increase in intracellular sodium in vascular smooth muscle cells.

It has also been found that avoidance-saline hypertension can be reversed by increases in intake of potassium (Anderson et al. 1983b). When potassium chloride was gradually infused into the arterial circulation of dogs for 14 days at a rate of 100 mEq/24 h, arterial pressure of dogs made hypertensive by 14 days of avoidance-saline exposure decreased progressively. When the potassium infusion was discontinued, the pressure levels began to rise again. Potassium may operate at central, arterial, and/or renal levels to affect blood pressure. The experiments show clearly that sodium is not the only micronutrient that affects the blood pressure of dogs during exposure to behavioral stress, and they emphasize the ratio of sodium to potassium intake as an important variable. Recently, it has also been found that substitution of a low potassium dog chow for a normal potassium dog chow results in an enhancement of the hypertension, further underlining the importance of the ratio of sodium to potassium intake in the regulation of blood pressure in stressed animals. Studies are also needed to assess the potential role of other dietary micronutrients, such as calcium and magnesium.

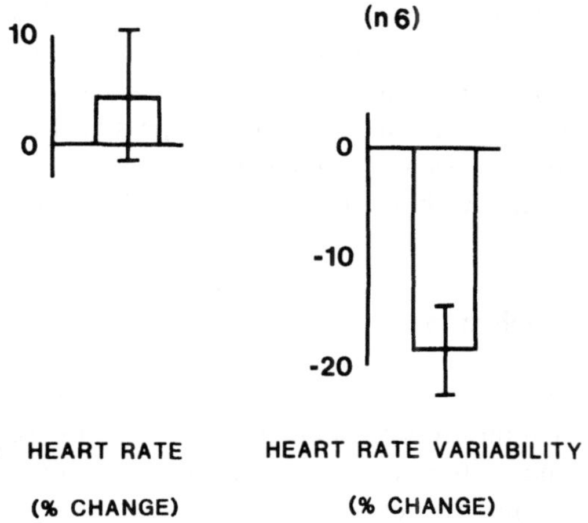

Fig. 4. Difference in mean and standard deviation of hourly heart rate within 24-h intervals between 7 days of baseline rest and 7 days of saline infusion, averaged for six dogs

Sodium Intake and Cardiac Variability

Blood pressure and heart rate of hypertensive and normotensive humans vary almost continuously during the 24-h day. Recently, Mancia et al. (1983) reported that the absolute variability of blood pressure of ambulatory human hypertensives (derived from direct and continuous recording) is greater than that observed in normotensive subjects. They also found, however, that variabilities in the heart rate of human hypertensives were not greater than those of normotensive controls. Some investigators (e.g., Julius et al. 1983) have even suggested that the responsiveness of the heart to sympathetic nervous system stimulation may be decreased in hypertensive patients.

Studies in our laboratory suggest that the infusion of isotonic saline at a rate of 1340 ml/24 h for 7 days is associated with no consistent change in 24-h mean heart rate of nonstressed dogs, but does result in a significant decrease in the variability of the heart rate, as assessed by the standard deviation of successive 1-h means within 24-h intervals. Figure 4 shows that the mean heart rate of six dogs averaged 75.5 bpm during 7 days of a low saline infusion rate (335 ml/24 h) and 78.6 during 7 days of the high rate of infusion, a nonsignificant group difference. The data also show, however, that the standard deviation of the hourly mean heart rate levels decreased by 18.5 ± 5.1% in response to the high rate of saline infusion ($t = 3.11$; $P < 0.025$). These effects were consistent in five of the six dogs, with the sixth showing no change. The standard deviations of mean blood pressure variability decreased under conditions of high salt intake in four of the six dogs, who also showed no significant change in 24-h pressure levels in response to saline infusion in the absence of avoidance sessions.

The variability of heart rate and blood pressure have also been examined in four other dogs who received the low rate of saline infusion for 7 days and the high rate of saline infusion for the following 7 days while they were on avoidance schedules. The mean systolic (19.5 mmHg) and diastolic (13.8 mmHg) pressures increased in response to the high saline infusion rate in these stressed dogs, and variability of blood pressure also increased by 59% (systolic) and 69% (diastolic). By contrast, mean heart rate levels did not change significantly under these conditions, and three of the four dogs showed a decrease in variability of heart rate. At the very least, these preliminary findings indicate that saline infusion has differential effects on the heart and blood vessels. It is possible that these differences are related to different densities of alpha- and beta-adrenergic receptors in heart and vascular tissue associated with the sodium-loading procedures.

Conclusion

It is apparent that sodium and potassium intake modulate the effects of acute behavioral stress on blood pressure. Progressive 24-h hypertension can be produced in genetically normotensive dogs by maintaining them for days or weeks on high-sodium-low-potassium intake under conditions of avoidance schedules that maintain bradycardia during the long intersession intervals. This form of experimental hypertension requires no surgical impairment of kidney function or administration of salt-retaining hormones. It is associated with an increase in total body sodium levels without an increase in total body water. The low 24-h heart rate levels and no increase in body water make it unlikely that the hypertension is due to increased cardiac output. Rather, it is more probable that it is due to increased total peripheral resistance.

One intriguing possibility is that neuroendocrine adaptations to the behavioral procedures alter permeability of the vascular smooth muscle cell membrane to sodium, thereby increasing vascular smooth muscle contraction to adrenergic input. Although it seems evident that the sympathetic nervous system is intimately involved in this process, the role of the parasympathetic nervous system should also not be overlooked. Altered ion transport across cell membrane is an important area of modern research on blood pressure control (Postnov and Orlov 1983), following earlier observations that sodium content of cells is increased in hypertension (Tobian and Binion 1952). It will be of interest to know whether specific behavioral procedures can alter sodium transport into the cells, and, if so, by what mechanism. Finally, it will be important to know whether prolonged exposure to these behavioral procedures under conditions of high-sodium-low-potassium intake results in structural adaptations of the peripheral vasculature and chronic hypertension (Folkow 1982). From such studies, rational interventions for prevention of hypertension in man may emerge.

Acknowledgments. The author wishes to thank William Kearns and Michael Sharinus for their technical assistance. This research was supported in part by grant HL 28462 from the National Heart, Lung, and Blood Institute.

References

Altman PL, Dittmer DS (1974) Handbook of biological data. Federation of American Societies of Experimental Biology. Bethesda, Md, p 1469

Ambrosioni E, Costa FV, Montebugnoli L, Borghi C, Magnani B (1981) Intralymphocytic sodium concentration as an index of response to stress and exercise in young subjects with borderline hypertension. Clin Sci 61 [Suppl 7]: 25s–27s

Ambrosioni E, Costa FV, Borghi MD, Montebugnoli L, Goirdani MF, Magnani B (1982) Effects of moderate salt restriction on intralymphocytic sodium and pressor response to stress in borderline hypertension. Hypertension 4: 789-794
Andersen HT (1966) Physiological adaptations in diving vertebrates. Physiol Rev 46: 212-243
Anderson DE, Tosheff JG (1973) Cardiac output and total peripheral resistance changes during preavoidance periods in the dog. J Appl Physiol 35: 650-654
Anderson DE, Kearns WD, Better WE (1983a) Progressive hypertension in dogs via avoidance conditioning and saline infusion. Hypertension 5: 286-291
Anderson DE, Kearns WD, Worden TJ (1983b) Potassium attenuates avoidance-saline hypertension in the dog. Hypertension 5: 414-421
Aoki K, Yamori Y (1972) Effects of high or low sodium intake in spontaneously hypertensive rats. Jpn Circ J 36: 539-545
Blair MF, Feigl EO, Smith OA (1976) Elevations in plasma renin activity during avoidance performance in baboons. Am J Physiol 231: 772-776
Brady JV, Harris AH (1976) The experimental production of altered physiological states. In: Honig W, Staddon J (eds) Handbook of operant behavior. Prentice Hall, New Jersey, p 596
Campbell WB, Schmitz JM (1978) Effects of alterations in dietary potassium on the pressor and steroidogenic effects of angiotensin II and III. Endocrinology 103: 2098
Campbell GR, Chamley J, Campbell J, Short N, Robinson RB, Hermsmyer K (1981) Effects of cross transplantation on normotensive and spontaneously hypertensive rat arterial muscle membrane. Hypertension 3: 534-543
Cohen DH, Obrist PA (1975) Interactions between behavior and the cardiovascular system. Circ Res 37: 693-706
Coleman TG, Guyton AC (1969) Hypertension caused by salt loading in the dog. III. Onset transients of cardiac output and other variables. Circ Res 25: 153-169
Cowley AW, Lohmeier TE (1979) Changes in renal vascular sensitivity and arterial pressure associated with sodium loading during long-term intrarenal norepinephrine infusion in dogs. Hypertension 1: 549-558
Dahl LK, Love RA (1957) Etiological role of sodium chloride intake in essential hypertension in humans. JAMA 164: 397-400
Dahl LK, Heine M, Tassarini L (1962) Role of genetic factors in susceptibility to experimental hypertension to chronic excess salt ingestion. Nature 194: 480-482
de Champlain J, Krakoff LR, Axelrod J (1968) Relationship between sodium intake and norepinephrine storage during the development of experimental hypertension. Circ Res 23: 479-491
Dietz R, Schomig A, Haebara H, Mann JFE, Rasher W, Luth JB, Grunberz N, Gross F (1978) Studies on the pathogenesis of spontaneous hypertension in the rat. Circ Res 43 [Suppl 1]: 98-106
Dietz R, Schomig A, Rascher W, Strasser R, Kubler W (1980) Enhanced sympathetic activity caused by salt loading in spontaneously hypertensive rats. Clin Sci 59: 171s-173s
Dietz R, Schomig A, Rascher W, Strasser R, Luth JB, Ganten U, Kubler W (1982) Contribution of the sympathetic nervous system to the hypertensive effect of a high sodium diet in stroke-prone spontaneously hypertensive rats. Hypertension 4: 773-781
Eliasson K, Hjendahl P, Kahan T (1983) Circulatory and sympatho-adrenal responses to stress in borderline and established hypertension. J Hypertension 1: 131-139
Ely DL, Wiegand J (1983) Stress and high sodium effects on blood pressure and brain catecholamines. Clin Exp Hypertens 9: 1559-1587
Engel BT, Bickford AF (1962) Response specificity. Arch Gen Psychiatry 5: 82-89
Falkner B, Onesti G, Angelakos E (1981) Effect of salt loading on the cardiovascular response to stress in adolescents. Hypertension 3 [Suppl 2]: 95-99
Findley JD, Brady JV, Robinson WW, Gilliam WJ (1971) Continuous cardiovascular monitoring during long-term behavioral monitoring in the baboon. Commun Behav Biol 6: 49-58
Folkow B (1982) Physiological aspects of primary hypertension. Physiol Rev 62: 347-504
Folkow B, Neil E (1971) Circulation. Oxford University Press, London
Folkow B, Hallback M (1977) Physiopathology of spontaneous hypertension in rats. In: Genest J, Koiw E, Kuchel O (eds) Hypertension. McGraw-Hill, New York, pp 507-528
Forsyth RP (1969) Blood pressure responses to long-term avoidance schedules in the rhesus monkey. Psychosom Med 31: 300-309

Forsyth RP (1971) Regional blood flow changes during 72-hour avoidance schedules in the monkey. Science 173: 546-548
Freis ED (1976) Salt, volume and the prevention of hypertension. Circulation 53: 589-595
Friedman R (1981) Experimental psychogenic hypertension. In: Wheatley D (ed) Stress and the heart. Raven, New York, pp 209-228
Fujita T, Henry WL, Bartter FC (1980) Factors influencing blood pressure in salt-sensitive patients with hypertension. Am J Med 69: 334-344
Goto A, Tobian L, Iwai J (1981) Potassium feeding reduces hyperactive central nervous system pressor responses in Dahl salt sensitive rats. Hypertension 3 [Suppl 1]: 128-134
Grignolo A, Koepke JP, Obrist PA (1982) Renal function, heart rate and blood pressure during exercise and avoidance in dogs. Am J Physiol 242: R482-R490
Herd JA, Morse WH, Kelleher RT, Jones LG (1969) Arterial hypertension in the squirrel monkey during behavioral experiments. Am J Physiol 217: 24-29
Hollenberg NK, Williams GH, Adams DF (1981) Essential hypertension: abnormal renal vascular and endocrine responses to a mild psychological stimulus. Hypertension 3: 11-17
Ikeda T, Tobian L, Iwai J, Gossen P (1978) Central nervous system pressor responses in rats susceptible and resistant to sodium chloride hypertension. Clin Sci 55: 225s-227s
Julius S, Weder AB, Egan BM (1983) Pathophysiology of early hypertension: implications for epidemiologic research. In: Gross F, Strasser T (eds) Mild hypertension: recent advances. Raven, New York, pp 219-235
Katholi RE (1983) Renal nerves in the pathogenesis of hypertension in experimental animals and humans. Am J Physiol 245: F1-F14
Katholi RE, Carey RM, Ayers CAR, Vaughan ED, Yancy MR (1977) Production of sustained hypertension by chronic intrarenal norepinephrine infusion in conscious dogs. Circ Res 40 [Suppl 1]: 118-125
Katholi RE, Naftilan AJ, Oparil S (1980) Importance of renal sympathetic tone in the development of DOCA-salt hypertension in the rat. Hypertension 2: 266-273
Katholi RE, Winternitz SR, Oparil S (1981) Role of the renal nerves in the pathogenesis of one-kidney renal hypertension in the rat. Hypertension 3: 404-409
Kearns WD, Better WE, Daley LA, Anderson DE (1981) A tether system for physiological studies in the dog. Behav Res Methods Instrumentation 13: 323-327
Koepke JP, Light KC, Obrist PA (1982) Alpha adrenoceptors in the renal excretory response to avoidance in conscious dogs. Fed Proc 41: 1105
Koepke JP, Grignolo A, Light KC, Obrist PA (1983) Central beta adrenoceptor medication in the antinatriuretic responses to behavioral stress in conscious dogs. J Pharmacol Exp Ther 227: 73-77
Lais LT, Bhatnagar RK, Brody MJ (1974) Inhibition by dark adaptation of the progress of hypertension in the spontaneously hypertensive rat (SHR). Circ Res 34 [Suppl 1]: 155
Lawler JE, Obrist PA, Lawler KA (1975) Cardiovascular function during preavoidance, avoidance and post-avoidance in dogs. Psychophysiology 12: 4-11
Lever AF, Beretta Piccoli C, Brown JJ, Davis DL, Fraser R, Robertson JS (1981) Sodium and potassium in essential hypertension. Br Med J 283: 463
Liard JF (1979) Renal denervation delays blood pressure increase in the spontaneously hypertensive rat. Experientia 33: 339-340
Liard JF, Tarazi RC, Ferrorio CM, Manner WM (1975) Hemodynamic and humoral characteristics of hypertension induced by prolonged stellate ganglion stimulation on conscious dogs. Circ Res 36: 455-464
Light K, Obrist PA (1980) Cardiovascular reactivity to behavioral stress in young males with and without marginally elevated casual systolic pressures. Comparison of clinic, home and laboratory measures. Hypertension 2: 802-808
Light KC, Koepke JP, Obrist PA, Grignolo A, Willis PW (1983) Psychological stress induces sodium and fluid retention in man at high risk for hypertension. Science 220: 429-431
Luft FC, Rankin LI, Bloch R, Weyman AE, Willis LR (1979) Cardiovascular and humoral responses to extremes of sodium intake in normal black and white men. Circulation 60: 697-706
Lundin S, Thoren P (1982) Renal function and sympathetic activity during mental stress in normotensive and spontaneously hypertensive rats. Acta Physiol Scand 115: 115-124
Mancia G, Ferrari A, Gregorini L, Parati G, Pomidossi G, Bertineri G, Grassi G, diRienzo M, Pe-

dotti A, Zanchetti A (1983) Blood pressure and heart rate variabilities in normotensive and hypertensive human beings. Circ Res 53: 96-104
Mark AL, Lawton WJ, Abboud FM, Fitz AE, Conner WE (1975) Effects of high and low sodium intake on arterial pressure and forearm vascular resistance in borderline hypertension. Circ Res 36, 37 [Suppl 1]: 1194-1198
Marx JL (1985) A potpourri of membrane receptors. Science 230: 649-651
McGregor GA, Best FE, Can JM, Markandic ND, Elder DM, Saganella SA, Squires M (1982) Double blind, randomized, crossover trial of moderate sodium restriction in essential hypertension. Lancet 1: 351-354
Miller JZ, Daugherty SA, Weinberger MH, Grim CE, Christian JC, Lang CL (1983) Blood pressure response to dietary sodium restriction in normotensive adults. Hypertension 5: 790-795
Morgan T, Gillies A, Adams W, Wilson N, Carney S (1978) Hypertension treated by salt restriction. Lancet 1: 227-230
Murdaugh HV, Schmidt-Neilsen JW, Wood JW, Mitchell WL (1961) Cessation of renal function during diving in the trained seal. J Cell Comp Physiol 58: 261-265
Murray RH, Luft CF, Bloch R, Weyman AE (1978) Blood pressure response to extremes of sodium intake in normal man. Proc Soc Exp Biol Med 159: 432-436
Nakamura K, Gerold M, Thoenen H (1971) Experimental hypertension of the rat: reciprocal changes of norepinephrine turnover in heart and brain stem. Naunyn Schmiedebergs Arch Pharmacol 268: 125-139
Nestel PJ (1969) Blood pressure and catecholamine excretion after mental stress in labile hypertension. Lancet 1: 692-694
Obrist PA (1981) Cardiovascular psychophysiology. Plenum, New York
Okamoto K, Nosako S, Yamori Y, Matsumoto M (1967) Participation of renal factors in the pathogenesis of hypertension in the spontaneously hypertensive rat. Jpn Heart J 8: 168-180
Patel KP, Kline RL, Mercer PF (1981) Noradrenergic mechanisms in the brain and peripheral organs of normotensive and spontaneously hypertensive rats at various ages. Hypertension 3: 682-690
Pettinger WA, Sanchez A, Saavedra J, Haywood JR, Gandler T, Rodes T (1982) Altered renal alpha$_2$-adrenergic receptor regulation in genetically hypertensive rats. Hypertension 4 [Suppl 2]: 188-192
Postnov YV, Orlov SN (1983) Alteration of cell membranes in primary hypertension. In: Genest J, Kuchel O, Hamet P, Cantin M (eds) Hypertension. McGraw-Hill, New York, pp 95-107
Rankin LI, Luft FC, Henry DP, Gibbs PS, Weinberger MH (1981) Sodium intake alters the effects of norepinephrine on blood pressure. Hypertension 3: 650-656
Reid WD, Laragh JH (1965) Sodium and potassium intake, blood pressure and pressor responses to angiotensin. Proc Soc Exp Biol Med 120: 65
Sanchez A, Pettinger WA (1981) Dietary sodium regulation of blood pressure and renal alpha$_1$ and -$_2$ receptors in WKY and SH rats. Life Sci 29: 2795-2802
Skrabal F, Herholz H, Neumayr M, Hanberger L, Ledochowski M, Sporer H, Hortnagl H, Schwarz S, Schonitzer D (1984) Salt sensitivity in humans is linked to enhanced sympathetic responsiveness and to proximal tubular reabsorption. Hypertension 6: 152-158
Sokolow EN (1963) Perception and the conditioned reflex. Pergamon, Oxford
Sullivan JM, Ratts TE (1983) Hemodynamic mechanisms of adaptation to chronic high sodium intake in normal humans. Hypertension 5: 814-820
Takeshita A, Mark AL (1978) Neurogenic contributions to hindquarters vasoconstriction during high sodium intake in Dahl strain of genetically hypertensive rat. Circ Res [Suppl 1] 43: 86-91
Tanaka T, Seki A, Fujii J (1982) Effect of high and low sodium intake on norepinephrine turnover in the cardiovascular tissues and brain stem of the rabbit. Hypertension 4: 294-298
Tobian L, Binion JT (1952) Tissue cations and water in arterial hypertension. Circulation 5: 754-758
Treasure J, Ploth D (1983) Role of dietary potassium in the treatment of hypertension. Hypertension 5: 864-872
Ueshima H, Tanigaki M, Iida M, Shimamoto T, Konishi M, Komachi Y (1981) Hypertension, salt and potassium. Lancet 1: 504
van Ameringen MR, de Champlain J, Imbeault S (1977) Participation of central noradrenergic neurons in experimental hypertension. Can J Physiol Pharmacol 55: 1246-1251

Watson RL, Langford HG, Abernethy J, Barnes TY, Watson MI (1980) Urinary electrolytes, body weight, and blood pressure: pooled cross-sectional results among four groups of adolescent females. Hypertension 2 [Suppl 1]: 193

Williams RB, Bittker TE, Buchsbaum MS, Wynne LC (1975) Cardiovascular and neurophysiologic correlates of sensory intake and rejection. I. Effects of cognitive tasks. Psychophysiology 12: 427-433

Winternitz S, Katholi RE, Oparil S (1980) Role of the renal sympathetic nerves in the development and maintenance of hypertension in the spontaneously hypertensive rat. J Clin Invest 66: 971-978

Yamori Y, Kihara M, Nara Y, Ohtaka M, Horie R, Tsunematsu T, Note S (1981) Hypertension and diet: multiple regression analysis in a Japanese farming community. Lancet 1: 1204

Zanchetti A, Stella A, Baccelli G, Mancia G (1979) Neural influences on kidney function in the pathogenesis of arterial hypertension. In: Onesti G, Klimt CR (eds) Hypertension: determinants, complications and intervention. Grune and Stratton, New York, pp 99-109

Individual Differences in Blood Pressure Reactivity and Behavior of Male Rats

J. M. Koolhaas, D. S. Fokkema, B. Bohus, and G. A. van Oortmerssen[1]

Introduction

One of the major concerns in research on the aetiology of coronary heart disease (CHD) and hypertension has been the question why some individuals suffer from these diseases while others are healthy, although exposed to seemingly identical external conditions. Since the early studies by Friedman and Roseman (1959), it has become increasingly clear that apart from environmental circumstances, personality factors are also important. In order to study the complex interplay between environmental variables and personality factors in the pathophysiology of the cardiovascular system, animal research is indispensable.

Many animal studies have been focused on the role of aversive environmental stimulation on the development of hypertension or CHD (see for a review Schneiderman 1983). Only studies on social stress, however, allow some possibility of studying the role of "personality factors." Von Holst et al. (1983), for example, found two distinct types of submissive male tree shrews. Submissive males that actively tried to escape from dominant males had longer survival times in a social stress situation than submissive animals that hardly responded to threats and attacks by the dominant ones. These findings suggest that individual differences may be important in stress susceptibility in relation to behavior. The importance of environmental factors was demonstrated by Raab and Oswald (1979). Subordinate male tree shrews that lived in the permanent visual presence of the dominant male, but were physically separated by a wire-mesh screen, died within a week. However, in a situation in which the dominant animal had free access to the subordinate one, but in which the latter could hide, mortality was much lower. The influence of social stress in cardiovascular pathophysiology has been studied mainly in complex colony situations. Dominant male mice had higher systolic blood pressures than the subordinate males living in the same colony (Henry and Stephens 1977; Ely 1981). In male cynomolgus monkeys, social dominance was associated with increased coronary artery atherosclerosis, but only in a situation with recurrent threat to the status of the dominant animal (Kaplan et al. 1982).

Although these experiments show that factors such as social status are important in the development of cardiovascular disease in animals, one may wonder to what extent individual difference characteristics predispose animals both behaviorally and physiologically to develop certain stress pathologies. The experiments by von Holst et al. (1983) indicate that such a behavioral and physiological differentiation between individuals might indeed be present.

1 Department of Animal Physiology, State University of Groningen, P.O. Box 14, 9750 AA Haren, The Netherlands

Biological and Psychological Factors
in Cardiovascular Disease
Ed. by T. H. Schmidt, T. M. Dembroski, and G. Blümchen

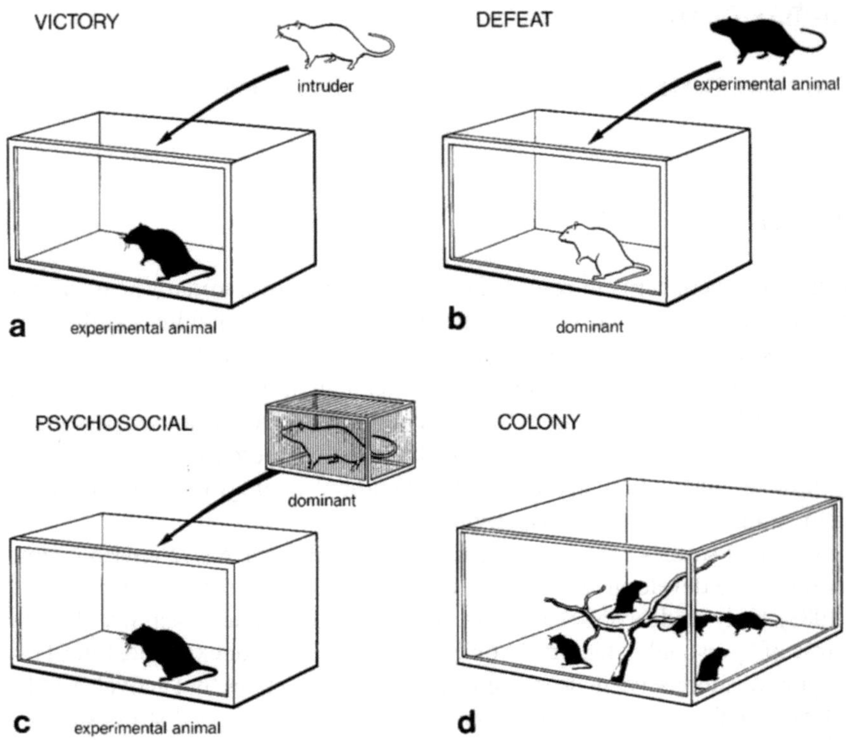

Fig. 1. Summary of the four social test situations

In this paper we shall attempt to identify factors in the social environment that may be important in the development of hypertension in male rats, with special emphasis on the individual differentiation in physiological and behavioral reaction patterns to these factors.

Methods

In order to study the physiological and behavioral effects of various social factors, it is important to have good experimental control over the social environment of the experimental animal. As has been described elsewhere (Koolhaas et al. 1980), this can be achieved reliably by using male Tryon Maze Dull S3 rats to establish a territory when housed in a fairly large cage (85 × 50 × 50 cm) together with a female. The following three situations were studied:

1. *Victory:* When the experimental animal is confronted with an unfamiliar male intruder in its home cage, it will attack the intruder. As a rule the experimental animal in its home cage will be the victor in this interaction (Fig. 1 a).
2. *Defeat:* The same experimental rat can also be used as an intruder in the home cage of a trained fighter. In a case like this, the experimental animal will almost certainly be defeated (Fig. 1 b).

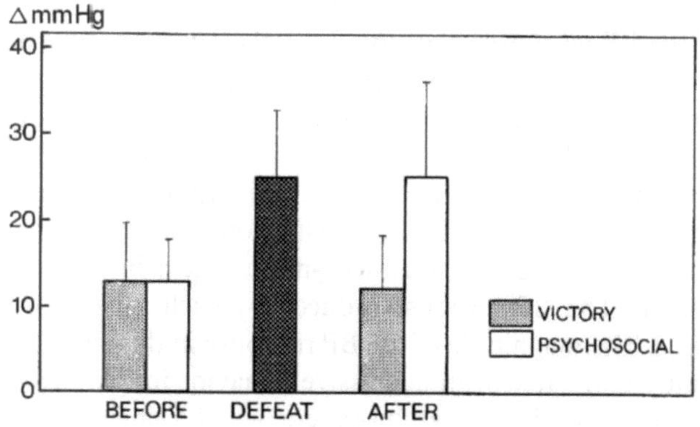

Fig. 2. Mean blood pressure responses in various social test situations. The response during victory and psychosocial stimulation is presented both before and after a single defeat experience

3. *Psychosocial stimulation:* In order to study the psychosocial components separately from the physical aspects of situations 1 and 2, the subordinate or dominant opponent was presented briefly, enclosed in a small wire-mesh cage (Fig. 1 c).

The effects of these three social situations on the behavior and physiology of the experimental animal was studied in 10-min tests. In order to investigate the predictive value of the findings based on short-term experiments for the development of hypertension in the long run, we studied male rats in a semi-natural colony situation. Before being housed in this colony each animal was characterized behaviorally in five victory tests. Each colony consisted of ten male rats and five females housed in an enriched environment of 2 × 3 metres, which contained sufficient food and water supply (Fig. 1 d).

Blood pressure (BP) recordings were made using chronic intra-arterial catheters. Blood samples (0.2 ml) for hormone assays were taken via chronic jugular vein cannulas. Using these chronic cannulation techniques, it is possible to study physiological and endocrinological processes in free-moving animals living in a variety of social situations (Koolhaas et al. 1983). However, the physiology of colony-housed animals was studied immediately after the 2-month period of colony housing.

Blood Pressure

All three social stimuli, i.e. victory, defeat and psychosocial, resulted in a rise in both systolic and diastolic BP. This BP response usually returned to baseline levels within a few minutes after the end of the stimulation. Figure 2 shows the average BP response in these three social situations. Although the BP response during defeat was significantly larger than during victory, the rather large standard deviations indicate a large variation in BP response between individual animals.

Usually there was a large variation between animals in the tendency to attack an intruder in the home territory. Some animals readily attacked, whereas others did not engage in any aggressive behaviour at all, or only after a long latency. It appeared that the duration of aggressive behaviour performed in the presence of an unfamiliar male conspecific (victory) was positively correlated with the magnitude of the BP response ($r=0.76$; $P<0.01$). The more time a male spent engaged in aggressive behavior during victory, the higher the BP response. This relationship may simply be a result of a difference in physical activity during the social interaction, but it may also reflect a difference between more and less aggressive animals in the "psychosocial appreciation" of the situation. A strong indication that such differences in appreciation indeed exist is found in the psychosocial test, in which an opponent enclosed in a small wire-mesh cage is briefly presented to the experimental animal. The BP response induced by such a psychosocial stimulus is shown in Fig. 2. The magnitude of the BP response in this situation before defeat was significantly correlated with aggressive behavior in the victory tests ($r=0.73$; $P<0.05$). Figure 2 also shows that the experience of a single defeat strongly enhanced this response. This conditioned BP response, i. e. the difference between pre- and post-defeat BP response, is again correlated with the duration of aggressive behavior in the victory test ($r=0.84$; $P<0.01$). Because the experimental animals performed little or no physical activity during these psychosocial tests, these results suggest differences between individual animals in the "appreciation" of a social situation. The aggressive animals seem to have a much more reactive blood pressure than the non-aggressive rats. Similar results were obtained by Manuck et al. (1983), who found that more aggressive monkeys relative to others showed a higher heart rate reactivity.

It is tempting to compare these results with the data on hostility scores and blood pressure reactivity in human Type A personalities. Type A individuals, especially those with high hostility, appeared to have a hyper-reactive BP response during the Type A interview and under appropriately challenging conditions (Dembroski et al. 1978).

The data just presented concern BP responses to social stimuli of relatively brief duration. It is important to consider the significance of these short-term changes to the basal BP during resting conditions in the long run. This issue has been approached by studying the relationship between the position of an animal in the social hierarchy of a rat colony and its basal BP under resting conditions. By means of regular behavioral observations, we measured the amount of victories and defeats each animal experienced during the 2-month period of existence in each colony. Before the animals were placed in the colony cage they were tested for their tendency to defend their home territory against unfamiliar male conspecifics in victory tests. It is not surprising that the aggressive animals in these tests were likely to take the higher positions in the social hierarchy of the colony ($r=0.54$; $P<0.01$; Fokkema 1984). However, only one of these animals became dominant in each colony. This dominant animal directed most of its aggressive behavior towards the other potentially dominant animals that were originally aggressive in their home cage. Hence, in the colony these latter animals displayed high levels of flight and submissive behaviors in response to approaches by the dominant animal. The originally non-aggressive animals received little attention from the dominant animal or other colony members and lived seemingly undisturbed.

Recordings of basal BP taken immediately after the 2-month period of colony life showed, in most colonies, a significant positive correlation with flight behavior. This means that, in particular, the potentially dominant males developed increased basal BP levels. About 60% of this group of males had BP levels that reached hypertensive values. It is important to realize that both the non-aggressive males and the dominant animal were usually normotensive. These findings suggest that the group of animals that had a high tendency to perform aggressive behavior in the home territory can be considered at risk for the development of hypertension. The individual differences in BP reactivity in the psychosocial test situation is consistent with this notion. It seems that the basal BP may become affected when animals from this high-risk group live in a social situation in which they are constantly psychosocially stimulated because of the continuous presence of the dominant animal.

Corticosteroids and Free Fatty Acids

A large body of literature provides evidence that the activity of the pituitary-adrenocortical system is related to social status. However, the exact relationship between the two is not clear. Several reports indicate that dominance status coincides with low basal corticoid levels in mice (Henry and Stephens 1977) and monkeys (Sapolsky 1982; Sassenrath 1973). Others, however, report high plasmacorticoid levels (Coe et al. 1979) or urinary corticoid levels (Leshner and Candland 1972) in dominant squirrel monkeys. A similar conflicting picture exists in studies on the pituitary-adrenocortical responsiveness during stress or in reaction to a standard dose of ACTH. A low responsiveness in dominant animals was found by Sassenrath (1973), Coe et al. (1979) and Henry and Stephens (1977), whereas Sapolsky (1982) reported high responsiveness of the adrenal cortex in dominant wild baboons. These data were all obtained after the animals had lived in a social group for a long period of time. Hence, the differences in results may be due to variations in the social environment at the time of sampling.

The main question, in the context of the present discussion, is to what extent the (re)activity of the pituitary-adrenocortical system may predict or determine subsequent status in social groups. Again two conflicting data sets can be found in the literature. Golub et al. (1979) concluded that low basal cortisol levels in weanling rhesus monkeys are good predictors of the development of dominance. On the other hand, Coe et al. (1979) did not find a relationship between basal corticoid levels in individually housed squirrel monkeys and subsequent status in social groups.

In our rat studies, we measured basal plasma corticosterone levels after 2 weeks of home cage housing (before any behavioral testing was done), after experience with five victory tests, and immediately after the 2-month period of colony housing. Corticosterone responses during psychosocial tests were determined before experience with territorial fights and after five victory tests. Neither the basal corticosterone level nor the response during the very first psychosocial test was significantly related to subsequent aggressive behavior during victory tests or to status in the colony (Table 1). However, after experience with five victory tests, the aggressive animals usually reacted with high corticosterone responses during a psychosocial test, whereas the non-aggressive animals had a low, or sometimes even a negative, response (Table 1). Immediately after colony housing we found a positive correlation between aggressive behavior and basal corticosterone levels in three out of four colonies, which reached significance in one colony. It seems, therefore, that the activity of the pituitary-adrenocortical axis in male rats can be considered as a reflection

Table 1. Relationship between home cage aggression and plasma corticosterone after various degrees of social experience (Spearman rank correlation coefficient)

	Basal corticosterone	Corticosterone
Naive males	NS	NS
Experience with five victories	NS	0.82
After 2 months of colony life	0.55–0.82	–

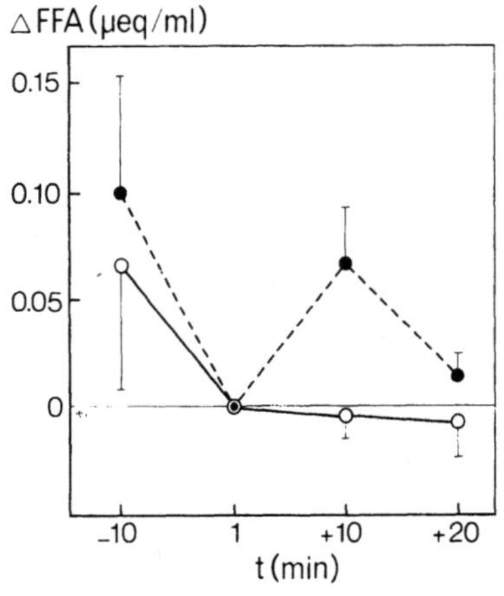

Fig. 3. Changes in plasma FFA concentration in response to psychosocial stimulation in naive animals. The *broken line* represents the subsequently aggressive animals; the *solid line* represents the non-aggressive males

rather than a predictor or determinant of the actual social status. Variables such as number of potentially dominant males, duration of colony housing, intensity of social interactions, species differences, etc. may account for the large variation of findings in the literature and our own results concerning corticoid levels and social status.

In contrast to the corticosteroids, we did find differences in plasma free fatty acid (FFA) concentrations that were related to subsequent aggressive behavior. During the very first psychosocial test in normally raised, but otherwise socially inexperienced rats, we observed high FFA responses in potentially aggressive animals, whereas the later non-aggressive males showed no rise in FFA (Fig. 3). Because the level of FFA is strongly dependent on the catecholamines, it is likely that these hormones differentiate in a similar way in relation to aggressive behavior.

Behavior

The data mentioned above show that (potentially) aggressive animals have a physiological reaction pattern that is different from that of the (potentially) non-aggressive animals, indicating an individual difference in the "appreciation" of the social situation. One may wonder what behavioral characteristics coincide with a particular pattern of physiology. Is there a more general behavioral variable that extends beyond the differentiation in aggressive behavior? In order to answer this question, we have studied the behavior of individual male rats in a variety of situations. In

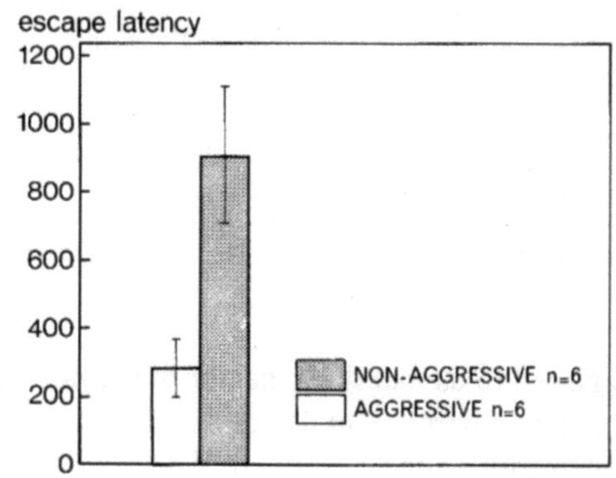

Fig. 4. Differences between aggressive and non-aggressive animals in escape latency (seconds) during confrontation with a dominant opponent (defeat)

these studies, special attention was paid to the relationship between the performance in these situations and the tendency to defend the home cage against unfamiliar male conspecifics.

As already mentioned, aggressive animals are likely to take higher positions in the social hierarchy of a colony. A detailed cluster analysis of the distribution of behavioral elements over the individual members of the colony revealed two major types of behavioral strategies. One type of strategy is characterized by the presence of threatening postures, approach and flight behavior. Animals that are characterized by this strategy will sometimes approach and threaten other animals and will flee immediately when approached or threatened by the dominant. This is in contrast to the second strategy, which is characterised by defensive behaviors and freezing. These animals do not take the initiative in a social interaction, but perform defensive behaviors or freezing in reaction to approach or threat by another animal.

The first strategy is mainly performed by the originally aggressive animals, whereas the latter strategy is related to those animals that performed little or no aggression in their home territory. This suggests that aggressive animals may be characterized by the fact that they actively determine their own social situation, whereas the non-aggressive animals are more passive. This idea of active versus passive behavioral strategies is confirmed by an analysis of behavior during defeat by a dominant animal. The flight or escape behavior during such a defeat appears to be highly correlated ($r=0.81$; $P<0.01$) with the tendency to perform aggressive behaviour in the home territory (Fig. 4). The aggressive animals readily escape from the dominant one, whereas the non-aggressive animals engage in freezing behavior instead.

Also, in non-social situations, the behavior of individuals differentiates in relation to the tendency to defend the home territory. Both aggressive and non-aggressive animals were tested in a problem solving task in a maze modelled after procedures used by Rabinovitch and Rosvold (1951). A food-deprived animal had to run for a startbox through a maze towards a goalbox in which it could obtain a small pellet of food. The configuration of the maze, and hence the route the animal had to follow to get to the goalbox changed, however, every three trials. In fact, the animal had to find its way in a continually changing environment. Table 2 shows that the non-aggressive animals made fewer errors than the aggressive animals. This result

Table 2. Relationship between home cage aggression and maze performance (Spearman rank correlation coefficient)

	Latency	Errors
A % aggressive behavior	NS	0.78
B % aggressive behavior	−0.64	−0.70

A, Rabinowitch % Rosvold maze; B, change in maze position of 90°.

suggested to us that the behavior of the non-aggressive animals may be more determined by environmental stimuli, whereas the behavior of the aggressive animals is more intrinsically determined. We tested this notion in an additional experiment in which a new series of animals were extensively trained to a standard of performance in one configuration of the maze. After reaching the set criterion, a minor change was introduced; that is, the maze was turned 90° with respect to the extra-maze cues. However, the maze itself remained unchanged. Table 2 shows that in this situation the performance of the aggressive animals was not affected, whereas the non-aggressive animals reacted with a longer latency and a higher number of errors. This experiment again shows that the behavior of the aggressive animals is much less under the control of external stimuli than the behavior of the non-aggressive animals. These latter animals readily notice a minor change in the environment, whereas the aggressive animals are unaffected by the external environment, once they are well trained. Taken together, these behavioral differences between individuals suggest that animals may differ more generally in the way in which they respond to a changing social or non-social environment. Although our evidence is still far from complete, we are working to test the hypothesis that the behavior of some animals (non-aggressive) is mainly determined by external stimuli, whereas other animals (aggressive) are characterized by a more intrinsic behavioral control. These latter animals seem to be able to develop routines that are, once into action, relatively insensitive to external stimuli.

Conclusion

The behavioral data indicate that animals differ individually on a scale from active to passive in responce to changing (social) situations. The reported results on BP responses, which can be considered as part of Cannon's fight/flight reaction, seem to be consistent with this view. The BP response is most prominent in the active animals during victory (fight) and is most strongly conditioned by defeat (flight) in these animals. Also, the high FFA responses in the active animals show that these animals readily prepare for physical activity.

Blood pressure recordings in animals living in a complex social structure showed a high incidence of hypertension in these active animals. It can be concluded, therefore, that in a normal population of male rats a high-risk group for the development of hypertension can be distinguished on the basis of behavioral and physiological parameters. However, apart from these "personality" factors, environmental factors do also play a role. Hypertension was only observed in the subtop of the colony and not in the top dominant animal, although both have the active behavioral strategy as a risk factor. It seems therefore, that a continuous lack of sufficient active control of the social environment is a necessary environmental condition in the development of hypertension.

One might predict that a dominant animal of a colony would develop hypertension provided that it lives together with a relatively large proportion of potentially dominant (active) animals. This might explain why Ely (1981) did find hypertension in the dominant males of mice colonies. In contrast to rats, dominant male mice tolerate little or no adult males in their vicinity. Similarly, Kaplan et al. (1982) found that social environmental conditions that provide recurrent threat to the status of the dominant animal are essential in the development of coronary artery atherosclerosis in monkeys.

The present model seems to us suitable for the study of the psychophysiology of hypertension and CHD. In the first place, because various cardiovascular parameters differ in relation to behavioral characteristics of individuals. Secondly, the model has some predictive value: On the basis of our results we can predict which combination of behavioral characteristics and environmental factors may affect basal BP.

A question that is open for further research is the origin of the individual differences. We are currently focusing on the relative contributions of genetic and ontogenetic factors in the development of behavioral differences and stress susceptibility using different strains of rats and mice.

Acknowledgment. This research was partly supported by a grant from the Dutch Heart Foundation to D.S. Fokkema.

References

Coe CL, Mendoza SP, Levine S (1979) Social status constrains the stress response in the squirrel monkey. Physiol Behav 23: 633–639

Dembroski TM, MacDougall JM, Shield JL, Petitto J, Lushene R (1978) Components of the type A coronary-prone behavior pattern and cardiovascular responses to psychomotor performance challenge. J Behav Med 1: 159–176

Ely DL (1981) Hypertension, social rank and aortic arteriosclerosis in CBA/J mice. Physiol Behav 26: 655–661

Fokkema DS (1985) Psychosocial stimuli and blood pressure in individual rats. In: Orlebeke JF, Mulder G, van Doornen LJP (eds) Psychophysiology of cardiovascular control. Methods, models and data. Plenum, New York 703–714

Friedman M, Rosenman RH (1959) Association of specific overt behavior pattern with blood and cardiovascular findings. JAMA 169: 1286–1296

Golub MS, Sassenrath EN, Goo GP (1979) Plasma cortisol levels and dominance in peer groups of rhesus monkey weanlings. Horm Behav 12: 50–59

Henry JP, Stephens PM (1977) Stress, health, and the social environment. Springer, Berlin Heidelberg New York

Kaplan JR, Manuck SB, Clarkson TB, Lusso FM, Taub DM (1982) Social status, environment and atherosclerosis in cynomolgus monkeys. Arteriosclerosis 2: 359–368

Koolhaas JM, Schuurman T, Wiepkema PR (1980) The organisation of intraspecific agonistic behaviour in the rat. Prog Neurobiol 15: 247–268

Koolhaas JM, Schuurman T, Fokkema DS (1983) Social behavior of rats as a model for the psychophysiology of hypertension. In: Dembroski TM, Schmidt TH, Blümchen G (eds) Biobehavioral bases of coronary heart disease. Karger, Basel, pp 391-400

Leshner AI, Candland DK (1972) Endocrine effects of grouping and dominance rank in squirrel monkeys. Physiol Behav 8: 441-445

Manuck SB, Kaplan JR, Clarkson TB (1983) Behaviorally induced heart rate reactivity and atherosclerosis in cynomolgus monkeys. Psychosom Med 45: 95-108

Raab A, Oswald R (1979) Coping with social conflict. Impact on the activity of tyrosine hydroxylase in the limbic system and in the adrenals. Physiol Behav 23: 837

Rabinovitch MS, Rosvold HE (1951) A closed-field intelligence test for rats. Can J Psychol 5: 122-128

Sapolsky RM (1982) The endocrine stress-response and social status in the wild baboon. Horm Behav 16: 279-292

Sassenrath EN (1973) Increased adrenal responsiveness related to social stress in rhesus monkeys. Horm Behav 1: 209-212

Schneiderman N (1983) Behavior, autonomic function and animal models of cardiovascular pathology. In: Dembroski TM, Schmidt TH, Blümchen G (eds) Biobehavioral bases of coronary heart disease. Karger, Basel, pp 304-351

von Holst D, Fuchs E, Stöhr W (1983) Physiological changes in male *Tupaia belangeri* under different types of social stress. In: Dembroski TM, Schmidt TH, Blümchen G (eds) Biobehavioral bases of coronary heart disease. Karger, Basel, pp 382-390

A Peculiar Breathing Pattern and Consequent Blood Pressure Oscillation During Social Stress

D. S. FOKKEMA and J. M. KOOLHAAS[1]

Introduction

The primary wave in blood pressure, which finds its origin in the cardiac pulse, is well known to vary in amplitude and frequency as a result of various environmental stimuli (Cacioppo and Petty 1982). Less attention has been given to the reactivity of the secondary blood pressure wave. Nor has its cause, the normal respiratory movement, been studied extensively in relation to environmental factors (Grossman 1983). Although its significance to other physiological responses has been well recognized, in experiments this has only infrequently been taken into consideration by controlling the respiratory rate (McCaul et al. 1979; Ahmed et al. 1982).

In some of the social and psychosocial situations used in the study of blood pressure in rats, as described in the previous paper, an interesting respiratory phenomenon has been observed. This breathing pattern and its effect on blood pressure will be described. During and after the social defeat experience of an experimental rat, and during the associated psychosocial stimulation that was part of the described experiments, a distinct and pronounced wave pattern was often observed in the continuous recordings of blood pressure. Systolic and diastolic blood pressure ran parallel to each other. Synchronous recording of blood pressure, intrathoracic pressure and diaphragm activity demonstrated that this blood pressure oscillation was associated with a specific respiratory pattern (Fokkema et al. 1986).

As a result of a social fight the blood pressure and the respiratory frequency increased. However, when the experimental rat changed its active "fighting back" strategy into passive "freezing" behavior, the respiratory rate dropped to below prefight level and the expiratory phase became very prolonged compared with inspiration. During expiration the intrathoracic pressure rose, often accompanied by ultrasonic vocalizations. This "pressure breathing" coincided with blood pressure oscillation. The blood pressure rose with the rising intrathoracic pressure and both pressures fell sharply again with the short inspiration (Fig. 1). The maximal amplitude of the blood pressure oscillation was 30 mmHg. The duration of the phenomenon ranged from several minutes, during the confrontation, to about an hour afterwards.

Blood pressure oscillation of such amplitude has rarely been described in conscious subjects. It reminded us of the alternating high and low blood pressure values demonstrated during yoga breathing exercises, as reported by Schmidt (1983). Also, in two of the three exercises described by Schmidt, a relative prolonging of the expiratory phase occurred by means of holding the breath, and breathing was ac-

1 Department of Animal Physiology, State University of Groningen, P.O. Box 14, 9750 AA Haven, The Netherlands

Biological and Psychological Factors
in Cardiovascular Disease
Ed. by T. H. Schmidt, T. M. Dembroski, and G. Blümchen

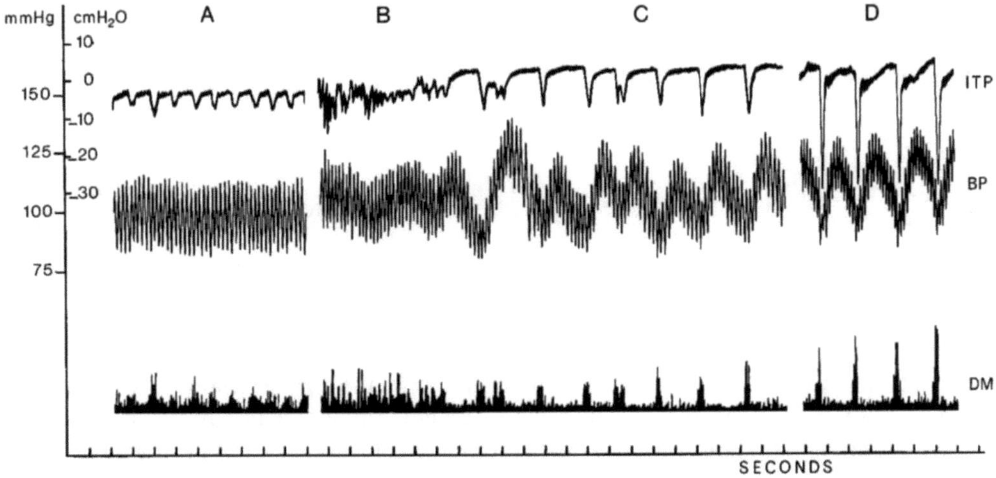

Fig. 1. Synchronous recording of intrathoracic pressure (*ITP*, cmH_2O) blood pressure (*BP*, mmHg) and diaphragm myography *(DM)* in an unrestrained rat. *A* during rest; *B* during a confrontation while the rat is panting; *C* after defeat during pressure breathing and oscillating blood pressure; *D* similar to *C*, but more pronounced after being attacked a second time

companied by a hissing sound. In addition, exaggerated heart rate variability occurred in phase with, but inversely related to the oscillating blood pressure. However, there is a fundamental difference between the breathing of a rat and yoga breathing. In the rat's pressure breathing the elevated intrathoracic pressure resulted in a rise in blood pressure, and thus may be considered as a series of Valsalva maneuvers. In contrast, the yoga breathing exercise caused a decrease in blood pressure during breath-holding, despite the elevated intrathoracic pressure. Although the stroke volume of the heart during expiration has been shown to be only one-third as large as the value during inspiration, the complete hemodynamic nature of this response is not yet understood (Schmidt 1983). It may be argued that, in rats, the possibly functional respiratory manipulation results in recurrent blood pressure elevations that eventually may be harmful to the vascular system. In contrast, the yoga breathing exercise may have overcome this problem by combining the same respiratory manipulation with an as yet unclarified technique to lower blood pressure.

It has been suggested that pressure breathing may be of value to attentional processes because of the enhancing influence of prolonged expiration on vagal activity (Fokkema et al. 1986). This is not in contradiction to the subjective feelings of being more aware and an expansion of conciousness that have been reported during yoga breathing exercises. Bohus (1985) reported that during "passive coping" in rats, vagal activation (decrease in heart rate) and sympathetic activation (rise in blood pressure) may occur concurrently, and that under these circumstances the high vagal activity may serve to temper the blood pressure elevations. Despite the reversed blood pressure oscillation with respect to respiration, the parallel of the prolonged expiration in both the rat's respiratory response to aversive social stimulation and the yoga breathing exercise leads to the suggestion that the latter may be an ingenious, cultural form of a natural response.

The description of yoga breathing mentions a return of the blood pressure to pre-exercise values after completion, and also that it has been recommended for people with high blood pressure (Schmidt 1983). Interestingly, in rats both a single or repeated defeat, accompanied by pressure breathing, results in a significant decrease in baseline blood pressure the following day (mean BP: 99→92 mmHg; $n = 10$; two-way ANOVA; $F1, 60 = 6.12$; $P < 0.025$) (Fokkema and Koolhaas 1985).

A study by McCaul et al. (1979) is one of the few that demonstrated an effect of respiration on mental processes and physiology. It was shown that a paced respiration rate at half the resting frequency using deeper breaths resulted in reduced physiological arousal measured as finger pulse volume and skin resistance. In addition there was a reduction in self-reported anxiety in shock-threatened experimental subjects practising such controlled breathing, compared with shock-threatened subjects without respiratory control or with a controlled higher rate. It remains an important question for further investigation to what extent and by which mechanisms such conscious or unconscious respiratory manipulations, as well as their acute effects on blood pressure, influence the state of mind and baseline blood pressure in the long term.

References

Ahmed AK, Harness JB, Mearns AJ (1982) Respiratory control of heart rate. Eur J Appl Physiol 50: 95-104

Bohus B (1985) Acute cardiac responses to emotional stressors in the rat: the involvement of neuroendocrine mechanisms. In: Orlebeke JF, Mulder G, van Doornen LJP (eds) Psychophysiology of cardiovascular control. Plenum, New York

Cacioppo J, Petty R (eds) (1982) Perspectives in cardiovascular psychophysiology. Guilford, New York

Fokkema DS, Koolhaas JM (1985) Acute and conditioned blood pressure changes in relation to social and psychosocial stimuli in rats. Physiol Behav 34: 33-38

Fokkema DS, Koolhaas JM, v d Meulen J, Schoemaker R (1986) Social stress induced pressure breathing and consequent blood pressure oscillation. Life Sci 38: 569-575

Grossman P (1983) Respiration and stress-related cardiovascular risk. Psychophysiology 20 (3): 284-300

McCaul K, Solomon S, Holmes D (1979) Effects of paced respiration on physiological and psychological responses to threat. J Pers Soc Psychol 37: 564-571

Schmidt TH (1983) Cardiovascular reactions and cardiovascular risk. In: Dembroski TM, Schmidt TH, Blümchen G (eds) Biobehavioral bases of coronary heart disease. Karger, Basel, pp 130-174

V. Prevention and Control

Prevention Paradox in Coronary Heart Disease

C. PATEL[1]

National crises or catastrophes not only arouse emotions but also lead to discoveries and innovations, usually because of astute observations and scientific enquiries made by a few individuals. The media and politics also play their part, and the entire process eventually ensures that further catastrophes are prevented, or at least their impact on society is softened. For example, the thalidomide tragedy affected 500 babies in the UK. The media sensationalized the reports, arousing public sympathy for the victims; this led to massive compensation from the drug company, in addition to the establishment, in 1964, of the Committee on Safety of Drugs. The loss of 4000 lives during the intense fog of London in December 1952 aroused public opinion and political debates which resulted in the Clean Air Act of 1956. Similar catastrophes - like infectious disease epidemics, road accidents, train or plane crashes, diseases resulting from industrial or occupational exposures - have led to the discovery of antibiotics, mass immunisation, numerous safety regulations, stronger legal action concerning drinking and driving, and compulsory seat belt wearing.

It seems ironical that over 200 000 lives in the UK (World Health Statistics Annual 1981), and many more thousands in other industrialized countries, continue to be lost every year - at least half of them prematurely - as a result of ischaemic and other hypertension-related cardiovascular diseases. Why does this not lead to a great public hue and cry and a flurry of scientific activity to combat this modern-day plague? One of the reasons put forward for this apparent failure is that we do not know what causes coronary heart disease (CHD) and without a knowledge of the exact aetiology, prevention is difficult.

The argument is only partly valid. Smoking and a high intake of saturated fat in the diet have long been implicated, but tobacco companies enjoy apparent immunity from law suits for the diseases caused by cigarette smoking and the Government, instead of prohibiting the companies from producing such lethal products, actually depend on them for a substantial revenue. Huge amounts of money are poured into dairy farming, which was an appropriate policy in the 1930s and 1940s, but now results in butter mountains and milk lakes and commercial exhortation of the public to consume amounts which are unhealthy. A competitive Type A behaviour is shown to be coronary prone, and yet society as a whole and corporations in particular continue to reward such behaviour, which can seem highly successful in the short term.

1 Department of Community Medicine, University College and Middlesex Hospital Medical School, 66-72 Gower Street, London WC1E 6EA, Great Britain

Biological and Psychological Factors
in Cardiovascular Disease
Ed. by T. H. Schmidt, T. M. Dembroski, and G. Blümchen

Why the Recent Decline in CHD in Mortality Some Countries?

A recent decline in CHD mortality in the USA, Australia and Canada by as much as 25% and to a lesser extent in Finland, the Netherlands and Switzerland, gives the impression that CHD is preventable. Unfortunately, we do not understand the exact cause of decline in these more fortunate countries. There have been changes in medical and surgical practices, in public health policies by governments and in the life-style of individuals. A conference organized by the National Institutes of Health in the USA to consider the causes of the decline agreed that the decline was real but could not pinpoint the causes with sufficient accuracy. It was suggested that all the above changes may have been responsible (Havlik and Feinleib 1979). The decline affected men and women, whites and blacks, young and old, with black women having the largest decline in mortality (28%) from CHD between 1968 and 1976.

Even though high serum cholesterol is associated with increased chances of having CHD, its aetiological role remains controversial. Japan is an outstanding exception to this diet-heart theory. Despite a greater than 200% increase in saturated fat consumption, the ischaemic heart disease mortality in Japan continues to decline, even though it had the lowest incidence to start with (Marmot et al. 1982). However, this relative immunity in the Japanese is not due to hereditary factors, as is shown by the increased incidence in those Japanese who move to Hawaii and California (Gordon 1957). In Switzerland, consumption of both saturated and polyunsaturated fats have increased, but CHD mortality decreased, while in Sweden the treatment of blood pressure is well advanced, smoking has decreased, saturated fat consumption has decreased, polyunsaturated fat consumption has increased, but heart disease rates in men have increased (Marmot et al. 1982; Alfredsson and Ahlbom 1983).

Trends in smoking habits fit the heart disease trend even less. The proportion of men who smoke has decreased, but the proportion of women smokers has increased; yet mortality has decreased more in women than in men (Havlik and Feinleib 1979). Reduction in smoking may have benfited British physicians (Doll and Peto 1976), but the general decline in smoking among men in the UK has not yet been equated by a decline in CHD mortality. Similarly, the rigorous approach to treating high blood pressure in the USA probably did not develop until the early 1970s; thus, even though it may be contributing to the continuing decline, it could not have initiated it.

Jogging is undoubtedly fashionable, but it is unlikely that it is predominantly the preoccupation of black women, who are the greatest beneficiaries of the CHD decline in the USA! The number of aortocoronary bypass operations has increased greatly in the USA but it could not account for more than a tiny fraction of the total decline. The importance of coronary care units can be played down by lack of positive proof from randomized controlled trials (Mather et al. 1971; Mather et al. 1976; Hill et al. 1976). Since a large proportion of patients with myocardial infarction die before reaching hospital, it is unlikely that coronary care units can improve overall CHD mortality by more than 4%-5% (Rose 1975).

Despite these anomalies, it is generally believed that scientific scepticism concerning the value of preventive efforts, together with public as well as professional apathy are largely responsible for the poor record in prevention of CHD deaths in the UK. Other possible reasons for the conflicting results mentioned above might be that the measures taken are too little and too late, and that many poorly understood risk factors like social, cultural, psychological and occupational factors have been ignored altogether in the preventive strategies.

Risk Factor Reduction as a Basis for Prevention

On the basis of strength of relationship, dose-response curve, temporal sequence, consistency of observation in different studies and independent predictive capacity, the major risk factors are male gender, hypertension, raised plasma cholesterol and cigarette smoking (Intersociety Commission for Heart Disease Resources 1970). Other factors are Type A behaviour pattern characterized by aggressive competitiveness, intense achievement striving, easily aroused hostility and extreme sense of time urgency (Friedman and Rosenman 1974), obesity, physical inactivity (Morris et al. 1980) and "stress", which encompasses several heterogenous factors. Occupational stress, for example, includes work overload, understimulation, piecework remuneration, role ambiguity, job conflict, job dissatisfaction or lack of fulfilment (Russek and Zohman 1958; Buell and Breslow 1960; Friedman and Hellerstein 1968; Sales and House 1971; Theorell and Floderus 1977). Similarly, psychosocial stress includes bereavement, anxiety or depression (Parkes et al. 1969; Cottington et al. 1980; Engel 1971; Connolly 1976), lack of self-esteem and control over one's life (Karasek 1979; Karasek et al. 1981). Difficulty in being assertive or expressing one's emotions have been reported to be associated with high blood pressure and increased incidence of hypertension (Harburg et al. 1979). Other risk factors considered to be important are belonging to low socioeconomic class (Marmot et al. 1978), lack of social support (Syme 1975; Marmot and Syme 1976), social and cultural mobility demanding excessive behavioural adjustments in life (Syme et al. 1964, 1965; Tyroler and Cassel 1964; Kaplan et al. 1971) and lack of resilience, which can buffer an impact of stressful life events on the health of an individual (Kobasa 1982).

In view of the association it would seem logical that reducing the above risk factors more comprehensively might reduce CHD mortality. The problem, however, becomes more complex when a decision has to be made as to who should receive such an intervention and how it should be made.

Mass Strategy or High-Risk Strategy?

The protagonists of mass strategy (Rose 1981) point out that the majority of deaths occur from the masses of people exposed to the mild and moderate ranges of risk factor levels. For example, in the London Whitehall Study (Reid et al. 1976; Rose et al. 1977) involving 20000 middle-aged male civil servants, it was shown that two-thirds of coronary mortality occurred in men with phase 4 diastolic blood pressure of less than 110 mmHg (approximately 105 mmHg if measured in Phase 5), while half the deaths occurred in men with diastolic BP of less than 100 mmHg (or approximately 95 mmHg if measured in phase 5). Even seemingly normal blood pressure was not without substantial risk. Thus, it would seem that to reduce CHD in a meaningful way we need to treat a large number of people with mildly elevated blood pressure (Rose 1981).

Similar logic would apply when it comes to reducing the level of plasma cholesterol. Illustrating the argument with the data from the Framingham Study, Rose (1981) pointed out that the risk indeed rises steeply with increasing cholesterol concentration, but the number of people affected by very high levels is fortunately low. Over a 10-year follow-up period, only 3 out of 34 excess deaths per 1000 occurred at concentrations of 310 mg/100 ml. (8 mmol/litre) or more, which would be considered abnormal and worthy of treatment by conventional clinical standards, although 90% of CHD deaths would arise from the masses of people exposed to a smaller relative risk.

Statistics can play a very confusing trick on our thinking for preventive strategy. It is important to understand very clearly the difference between relative risk and absolute risk. In younger people the rise in blood pressure would very steeply increase the *relative risk* of dying from complications compared with that in older people. This statement is hardly surprising since the average pressure and, hence, the average mortality are higher in the older generation, thus reducing the relative risk, which merely compares the risk of, say, higher systolic pressure with the average risk of dying in that age group.

On the other hand, if we consider the *absolute risk* or the actual number of people dying in different age groups as a result of risk factor elevation, the picture would be quite different. Since there are many more people with hypertension in the older age groups, the actual number of people who die from it are greater in the older age group. Thus, a policy of treating younger persons with moderately severe risk factor levels more energetically at the expense of older patients and those with mildly elevated risk factors is not likely to produce the largest benefit to the community, although it would confer larger benefit on the individual.

Viewing mass strategy in this manner, one could say that it does seem to make sense. Why are the protagonist of "high-risk" strategy (Oliver 1983) opposing this sensible approach? The argument is based on the generally poor results of several multiple risk factor intervention trials.

Multiple Risk Factor Intervention Trials

Because the results of single factor intervention studies were disappointing, it was thought that meaningful results might be achieved by reducing all major risk factors simultaneously. The North Karelia region of Finland, having the highest mortality from CHD in the world, started a risk factor intervention programme involving the entire community in 1972. At the end of 5 years, the predicted net CHD reduction based on risk factor changes was estimated to be 17% (Puska et al. 1979). However, the actual mortality, although lower in North Karelia, was not statistically significant (Salonen et al. 1979). It was argued that the district of Kuopio was not a good control because the CHD rate was naturally falling there, as it has been falling in the rest of Finland to a varying degree.

In the Multiple Risk Factor Intervention Trial (1982) in the USA, 366287 healthy volunteers were screened to identify 12866 high-risk men, who were randomly allocated to either special intervention (SI) group or usual care (UC) groups. The SI group had an active programme of counselling from physicians, nutritionists, psychologists and the media to reduce smoking, decrease saturated fat and increase polyunsaturated fat in the diet and control hypertension with drugs. The UC group was referred to the usual sources of care in the community. At the end of 7 years, CHD mortality was 7% lower, but the total mortality was 2% higher in the treatment group, neither of which was significant. Two explanations were offered:

1. Intervention was effective but could not be demonstrated in a short period of 7 years, especially since mortality in the control group happened to be particularly low.
2. The beneficial effects of reducing cigarette smoking and dietary changes were wiped out by the adverse effect of antihypertensive drugs in a subgroup of hypertensives with ECG abnormality at entry to the study.

The WHO Collaborative Group (1983) recently reported the results of its European trial in the prevention of coronary heart disease. In this study, 60881 men from the UK, Belgium, Italy and Poland participated. In the UK section, 18210 men aged between 40 and 59 years from 24 factories took part. The factories were arranged in pairs and randomly allocated. Intervention consisted of advice to stop smoking, reduce saturated fat in the diet, lose weight in the obese, take active exercise and control hypertension by drugs. The changes in risk factors were very modest. Predicted net reduction of CHD mortality from risk factor reduction was 4% overall and 11% in the high-risk group. The actual result in the intervention group showed 11% increase in total mortality (most of which was from CHD) and 4%–5% increase in coronary incidence, both of which were non-significant.

The Belgian section of the study comprised 19409 men. Similar intervention, although with more personal care, led to an estimated reduction in CHD mortality using multiple logistic function of 15.8% and an actual reduction in coronary mortality of 20.8% (non-significant). However, both total mortality (17.5%) and non-fatal myocardial infarction (26.1%) were significantly reduced. In Cracow (Poland) the predicted result from risk factor reduction was 4%, but the actual CHD mortality reduction was 20% (non-significant). In Italy, the estimated prediction was 14% reduction, but the actual reduction in CHD mortality was 28%. The study as a whole, however, did not show a significant difference in CHD mortality or in incidence between treatment and control groups.

Not all observations have been negative. In Oslo, Hjiermann and his colleagues (1983) screened 16202 men aged between 40 and 49 years and randomly allocated 1232 healthy normotensive (systolic BP below 150 mmHg) men with serum cholesterol between 7.5 and 9.8 mmol/litre (290–380 mg/dl) and cigarette smoking. The men in the intervention group were advised (in collaboration with their wives) to consume less calories, mainly by reducing sugar, alcohol and fat and increasing vegetable fibre. Antismoking advice was given individually to all the smokers in the intervention group. The net reduction in serum cholesterol and triglycerides were 13% and 20% respectively. Although the reduction in mean tobacco consumption was

45% greater in the intervention group, only 25% stopped smoking compared with 17% in the control group. Total coronary events were 3.1% in the intervention group compared with 5.7% in the control group, a statistically significant difference.

Nonetheless, the results of these studies taken overall are disappointing. In addition, several things are clear: (1) even though the traditional major risk factors are predictive of future CHD, there is no consistent relationship between reduction in risk factors and reduction in CHD mortality; (2) dietary advice does not result in an impressive reduction in serum cholesterol; (3) the results of advice to stop smoking are on the whole disappointing; and (4) mass medication may be hazardous. On the last point, however, both lobbies agree.

Mass Medication

The WHO-coordinated European trial of clofibrate (Committee of Principal Investigators 1978) was the largest primary prevention trial, in which 30000 apparently healthy men were screened and 10000 men in the high-risk group were randomly allocated to clofibrate or placebo groups. Although there was significantly less nonfatal myocardial infarction in the treated group (131 compared with 174), the total mortality was actually higher (162 compared with 127), mostly caused by diseases of the liver, gallbladder and intestines. This finding has an important implication in the strategy for prevention. Although clofibrate had been used in a substantial number of patients over a period of many years, there was no hint that it could kill. In the light of the results one may still say that benefit would outweigh the risk in cases of severe hypercholesterolaemia. However, treatment of a large number of people exposed to small relative risk poses a different dilemma.

Similarly, essential hypertension affects as many as a quarter of the population. There is no dispute that diastolic blood pressure of 105 mmHg or more should be treated with antihypertensive drugs, and there is evidence that lowering mild hypertension with diastolic blood pressure between 90 and 104 mmHg is likely to be beneficial (Hypertension Detection and Follow Up Program 1979; Management Committee 1980). Mild hypertension accounts for about 70% of all hypertensives. Many physicians are reluctant to treat hypertension. Up to half of the patients do not comply with their drugs regularly, and, of those who do, a large proportion report side effects.

Since the probability of complications in individual patients is no more than about 1% per annum, we face what has been described as the prevention paradox: "A measure that brings large benefits to the community, offers little to each participating individual" (Rose 1981). In other words, 99 out of 100 patients have to take antihypertensive drugs for a whole year with no apparent benefit. The results of the Medical Research Council's Mild to Moderate Hypertension (DBP 90-109 mmHg) Study (Medical Research Council 1977) have recently been published (Medical Research Council Working Party 1985).

A group of 17354 patients with mild hypertension were randomly allocated to antihypertensive drugs or placeboes similar in appearance. The drugs used were a diuretic (bendroflumethiazide) or a beta-blocker (propranolol). After 5 years of follow-up or 85572 patient years of observation, it was shown that treatment made no difference to the overall rates of coronary heart disease or mortality related to any other cause, but stroke rate was reduced on active treatment. However, subgroup analysis showed that both propranolol and bendrofluaridezide were effective in reducing strokes, but only in nonsmokers. In smokers, strokes were reduced on bendrofluaridezide but actually increased on propranolol. In conclusion, about 850 patients have to be treated for 1 year to prevent one stroke. Treatment did not appear to save lives and a substantial percentage of patients were subjected to chronic side effects, not all of which were minor.

Thiazide diuretics have been in use with a good safety record for many years. Although they were known to increase glucose intolerance and increase the possibility of developing gout, it took a massive trial to detect that about 20% of men report impotence on this treatment. Beta-blockers caused fewer side effects in men, but as many as 15% of the women experienced serious side effects. Altogether 15% of the patients had to be withdrawn from the trial because of side effects (Medical Research Council 1981). In addition to side effects, there are also metabolic consequences, such as elevation of cholesterol and triglycerides, which are likely to counteract the possible beneficial effects. In view of these findings, the question is being asked: Are there no other safe, effective and acceptable alternatives to life-long antihypertensive drugs?

Thus, it is clear that although a large number of CHD deaths occur in people exposed to small relative risk, a preventive strategy using pharmacological agents with a small inherent risk may outweigh the benefit when applied to large masses of people with mild to moderate range of risk factor levels. To that extent it makes sense to pursue a selective policy of pharmacological intervention confined to subjects exposed to relatively high risk.

Cost of Treatment

When planning preventive strategy, the aspect of cost benefit must also be taken into consideration. Development of high technology therapeutics including heart transplants and involved immunological intricacies make sensational news and interesting and intriguing reading. Science must continue to advance, but we should not fool ourselves into believing that these advances would make an impressive impact on the total burden of CHD mortality, and it is important to decide in advance how much of our resources we are prepared to spend on high technology developments and how much on real prevention. The type of preventive strategy we choose is also important.

Recently, results of a trial of cholestyramine were published in the USA (Lipid Research Clinics Trial Investigators 1984). Some 480000 men aged between 35 and 59 years were screened to identify 18000 men with cholesterol levels of 265 mg/dl or more. They were put on a cholesterol-reducing diet for 4 months. A total of 3806 men (0.8% of the original sample) whose cholesterol level was still 265 mg/dl or more at the end of 4 months were randomly allocated to treatment and control groups. The treatment group was given 24 G of cholesteryramine per day, while the control group was given an inactive silica mixture. Both the groups continued on a cholesterol-reducing diet.

At the end of 7 years, there were 155 fatal and non-fatal CHD events in the cholestyramine group compared with 187 in the control group - significant at 5% level, but only on a one-tailed *t* test. The total mortality was equal in both groups because of increased deaths from accidents and violence in the treated group. Even if we take this finding to be due to coincidence, the strategy does not make financial sense. Altogether 7% in the treatment group suffered heart attacks, compared with 8.6% in the control group; thus, a reduction of 1.6% was made over 7 years, or a 0.25% per year, or 1 in every 400 men year treated. This result is applicable to the high-risk group, which in the study comprised only 0.8% of the screened population.

Let us extrapolate the results in real terms to the population of the UK. Providing that the results are also applicable to women, approximately 192 000 men and women (0.8% of 24 million estimated in the age group) will qualify for treatment, thus reducing annual CHD events by 480 (not deaths). Compare that with our present figures of 200 000 deaths per year (World Health Statistics Annual 1981). When we consider the cost involved in screening the entire adult population, irrespective of the method of screening we adopt, and putting 192 000 individuals on cholestyramine at a total cost of £ 250 million per year in drugs bill, the return is so negligible that even the most affluent country is unlikely to be able to afford such a preventive strategy. It must also be remembered that in this study no less than 58% suffered side effects, mainly gastrointestinal, at least in the initial stages.

A Desirable Strategy

From the above discussion it is clear that a mass strategy of primary prevention is the only answer for a mass disease. Such a mass strategy should be effective like an immunisation procedure, safe like drinking purified water and cheap like wearing seat belts. Mass medication has no place in this strategy, although drugs must be used in selected high-risk patients where the non-drug approach is either ineffective or only partially effective.

Non-pharmacological Methods

In recent years there has been increasing interest in the development of the non-drug approach in the management of hypertension. The results are encouraging. The main areas of development are weight reduction, decreasing dietary sodium and/or increasing potassium intake, exercise and various form of psychological and the behavioural approach to stress management, including relaxation, meditation and biofeedback. The secret of success may lie in combining these approaches, but before that can happen each individual method is expected to prove its worth in properly controlled trials. This paper discusses the value of relaxation-based behavioural and psychological techniques in the treatment of hypertension and the possible prevention of CHD.

Relaxation Therapies

A variety of techniques like yoga (Datey et al. 1969; Patel 1973, 1975 a, 1975 b), biofeedback (Benson et al. 1971; Miller 1972; Elder et al. 1973; Blanchard et al. 1975; Elder and Eustis 1975; Kristt and Engel 1975; Walsh et al. 1977; Surwitt and Shapiro 1977; Richter-Heinrich et al. 1975), progressive muscle relaxation (Jacobson 1939; Brady et al. 1974; Kallinke et al. 1982), meditation and techniques derived from the principles of meditation (Benson et al. 1974 a; Blackwell et al. 1976; Stone and DeLeo 1976; Pollack et al. 1977), autogenic training (Luthe 1969; Klumbies and Eberhardt 1966), and hypnosis (Deabler et al. 1973; Friedman and Taub 1977) were reported to reduce blood pressure in hypertensive patients in preliminary studies. These studies lacked the clarity of methods used in drug evaluation trials but they showed at least that blood pressure may be lowered by behavioural methods and that most patients are willing to play an active role in the management of their own health in the short term. Even though it is not possible to carry out double-blind trials of behaviour therapy, carefully executed, randomised controlled trials, usually using a combination of some form of relaxation and stress management, have now shown that statistically significant and clinically meaningful reduction in BP ranging from 6 to 26 mmHg systolic and from 5 to 15 mmHg diastolic are possible (Patel and North 1975; Shoemaker and Tasto 1975; Taylor et al. 1977; Bali 1979; Brauer et al. 1979; Seer and Raeburn 1980; Richter-Heinrich et al. 1981; Patel et al. 1981; McGrady et al. 1981; Glasgow et al. 1982; Southam et al. 1982; Crowther 1983; Irvine 1983; Little et al. 1984; Waddon 1984). Some methods appear to be superior to others, although a large amount of variation in results has been explained by the height of the initial BP (Jacob et al. 1977).

Patel and North (1975), in a randomized controlled trial, reported a fall in mean BP from 168/100 to 141/84 mmHg in the behaviour modification group compared with a fall from 169/101 to 160/90 mmHg in the control group, who attended the same number of sessions, for the same length of time and had the same number of BP measurements. Both the groups were receiving antihypertensive medications which, nevertheless, were kept constant. Similar results have been reported by Patel et al. (1981) in another study in which 192 male and female employees of one industry aged between 35 and 64 years with two or more of the following risk factors – BP $\geq$140/90 mmHg, not on antihypertensive drugs, plasma cholesterol $\geq$ 6.3 mmol/litre and current smoking of $\geq$10 cigarettes/day – were identified through a screening programme and were randomly allocated to treatment and control groups. Both the groups were given health education leaflets advising them to stop smoking, to reduce animal fat in the diet and to remain under the supervision of their own physicians. The treatment group, in addition, had group sessions of 1 h once a week for 8 weeks in breathing exercise, deep muscle relaxation, meditation and stress management, with skin resistance biofeedback as an aid to learning relaxation. The patients were also asked to practise relaxation for 15–20 min twice a day as well as to relax briefly during everyday life situations such as while waiting at red traffic lights while driving, before picking up the telephone or every time they looked at their wrist watch. The results showed a fall in BP from 163/100 to 141/88 mmHg in the intervention group compared with a fall from 160/99 to 149/96 mmHg in the control group at the follow-up at 8 months.

A number of studies have now shown that relaxation can be combined with smaller doses of antihypertensive drugs than would be necessary in the control of essential hypertension (Datey et al. 1969; Patel 1973; Taylor et al. 1977; Brauer et al. 1979). Recently, Little et al. (1984) have reported that relaxation therapy can not only reduce pregnancy hypertension but also the frequency of hospital admission without compromising the fetal or maternal outcome.

Long-term Follow-up

Several studies have now reported reasonably long-term follow-ups. Patel et al. (1985) have recently reported a 4-year follow-up of the study reported earlier. Approximately 90% of the patients were followed up. Significantly greater reduction in both systolic and diastolic BP in the treated group was maintained in comparison with the control group, and this was true for the entire group as well as separately for those who were initially hypertensive (BP ≥140/90 mmHg) and normotensive (BP <140/90). Although the subjects were initially unmedicated, 18% of the treatment group and 20% of the control group were on antihypertensive medication at the 4-year follow-up. Despite the tendency for BP to rise somewhat during the 4 years, the differences between the groups were maintained. Body weight and alcohol consumption remained unchanged, while the reduction in animal fat was greater in the control group.

Morbidity data at the 4-year follow-up were rather intriguing. More people in the control group reported symptoms of angina, of having suffered other complications of hypertension or were on long-term medication. Such reports are, however, subject to bias. ECG changes, on the other hand, are more objective. Initial ECGs, however, were available in only 69 out of 86 of the treatment group and 57 out of 75 of the control group (unselected) and were blindly coded (Minnesota code). There were five new incidents of myocardial ischaemia in the control group compared with one in the treatment group. In addition, there was one fatal myocardial infarction in the control group. Fisher's exact test for these objective data was statistically significant ($P<0.05$). Caution is, however, necessary in interpreting the data in view of the small sample and incomplete follow-up.

Negative Results

There have been occasional reports where relaxation treatment has failed to produce a significant reduction in BP (Schwartz and Shapiro 1973; Surwit et al. 1978; Frankel et al. 1978; Christoph et al. 1978; Luborsky et al. 1982; Goldstein et al. 1982), but they usually omitted some essential components of the treatment, included inappropriate comparison groups or studied patients with rather low initial BP. For example, Luborsky et al. (1982) took 51 hypertensive patients, 20 of whom were on antihypertensive medication until 3 days before entering the trial. It is known that BP may not revert to its original level for months after drug withdrawal, which can confound the true effect of any treatment which follows.

Christoph et al. (1978) compared relaxation training with quiet reading in a single session and failed to detect any difference in BP between the groups. One session could hardly be called training in relaxation. Goldstein et al. (1982) found no difference in BP between relaxation and non-specific control groups. The patients had enlisted through a newspaper advert expecting to get biofeedback training, so it is possible that the relaxation group patients may have thought that they were controls. There was not much difference in the intervention and control procedures. Patients in both the groups rested in a comfortable chair, but the relaxation group was asked to count breaths. There was no home practice and the patients were not trained in stress management. With such diluted procedure and only nine patients in each group, it is quite possible not to detect a difference.

Is Reduction in BP by Behavioural Treatment Real?

It has been argued that observed reduction in BP may be due to subjective or objective bias or to the relaxation of the subjects at the time of measurement. Significant reductions were reported even when control group patients were seen as many times as treatment group patients and had the same number of BP measurements made, using either naive observers (Taylor et al. 1977; Irvine 1983) or random-zero sphygmomanometers (Benson et al. 1974; Patel and North 1975). Some investigators included psychotherapy (Taylor et al. 1977; Brauer et al. 1979; Bali 1979) or an exercise programme (Irvine 1983) as control procedures which matched relaxation treatment in expectation, complexity of schedules, elegance of biofeedback, elaborate psychophysiological measurements and the length and the frequency of home practice, and still showed greater reduction in BP.

The observed reduction is not likely to be due to increased compliance with concomitant antihypertensive drugs as has been suggested, because at least two studies showed significant reduction in BP in unmedicated patients (Bali 1979; Patel et al. 1981). A number of studies have now included a reasonable gap between the completion of relaxation training and follow-up and have reported persistence of reduced BP to a certain extent. If BP can remain low 4 years after the training in relaxation (Patel et al. 1985), it is unlikely to be due to non-specific placebo factors. It is possible that there are other modalities equally as effective as relaxation therapy (Waddon 1984), but it would be inappropriate to conclude from such observations that relaxation has no specific effect.

Mechanisms of Action

The question concerning the mechanisms through which relaxation therapy works is largely unanswered. Some investigators have shown that cardiovascular reactivity to experimental stress is reduced (Patel 1975 a; Jorgensen et al. 1981) and, therefore, assumed that such reduction in everyday life might be one of the underlying mechanisms, but others have failed to show any changes in reactivity (Goldstein et al. 1982). The latter researchers had not, however, shown any reduction in resting blood pressure either. Similarly, reduction in catecholamine and other stress hormones in either blood or urine have not been uniform. It has been shown that plasma renin activity (Stone and Deleo 1976; Patel et al. 1981) and plasma aldosterone are reduced in the short term but not in the long term (McGrady et al. 1981). The literature on hypertension is full of such biochemical controversies. Hence, conflicting results found by behaviour therapy investigators are hardly surprising. This may be partly due to heterogeneity of the hypertensive patients.

Several authors reported, at least during short-term follow-up, that those who stopped practising relaxation showed a rise in blood pressure. At 4-year follow up, however, Patel et al. (1985) found that only 14 out of 81 subjects admitted regular practice of relaxation and of these only three had practised it at least once a day in the previous week. A further 27 had practised relaxation at some time during the last 6 months. On the other hand, 63% said they sometimes and 20% said they often integrated brief relaxation during everyday situations, and 90% said they often, or sometimes, asked themselves to calm down under pressure. Those who practised relaxation regularly, as well as those who integrated brief relaxation practice in everyday life and cognitively changed their coping styles, showed greater reduction in blood pressure than those who did not.

It may be that the mechanisms responsible for short-term reduction in blood pressure are different from those responsible for their long-term persistence. It is a frequent experience of many clinicians that in many hypertensive patients treated with antihypertensive drugs, the control of BP becomes easier with time, and that when drugs are withdrawn, the BP may not start to rise for several months. This may be due to partial reversal of some of the factors normally responsible for maintaining or perpetuating hypertension.

The resetting of the baroreceptors and reversal of structural hypertrophy of resistance vessels have been demonstrated in both human and animal experiments (Folkow et al. 1973; Vaughan Williams et al. 1980). It is also the experience of some investigators of relaxation therapy that a considerable amount of relaxation practice is necessary before casual BP will consistently remain low initially (Patel 1975b; Richter-Heinrich et al. 1975). It may be that, in the long term, more subtle but pervasive changes in attitudes and beliefs, appraisals and subjective feelings, behavioural or cognitive coping styles, generated by early relaxation training, may be sufficient to maintain lower BP.

Implementation of Behaviour Therapy for Control of Hypertension in the Community

Before any therapy can be applied to a community at large it is necessary to have shown that:

1. The therapeutic effect is the direct result of the therapy.
2. The degree of effect is clinically meaningful as well as statistically significant.
3. The therapy is free from toxic side effects and preferably increases the quality of life.
4. The therapy is economically and technically feasible.
5. Clinicians or health care personnel other than investigators can be trained in applying the therapy.
6. The therapeutic effect should potentially decrease morbidity and mortality.

A number of controlled trials reviewed in this paper show that significant and clinically relevant reduction in BP is possible. The methods used may seem diverse, but close examination reveals some form of physical and mental relaxation at least initially and long-term changes in coping style of stress management. The relaxation and stress management therapy is remarkably free from side effects. There might, however, be danger if patients exclusively rely on relaxation taught by quasi-medical lay organizations or self-learnt and either omit or neglect medical advice. Behaviour therapy is not an alternative but a complement to antihypertensive drugs; it can be tried on its own at first and drugs added if an adequate response is not achieved.

The therapy can be cost effective. Patel et al. (1985) trained patients in groups of ten, thus reducing the total training time per patient to just 1 h. They used group biofeedback, which, according to Little et al. (1984), may be omitted, at least in the management of pregnancy hypertension, without losing the benefit. However, pregnancy hypertension is a self-limiting condition. Can the therapy be made cheaper still by eliminating the therapist? Brauer et al. (1979) found relaxation therapy conducted by home use of audio tapes no different from the training conducted by therapists at the end of a 10-week trial. However, at the follow-up at 6 months only the therapist-trained group showed significantly greater reduction in systolic BP. Thus, the presence of a therapist seems necessary. The potential saving in the cost of drugs, both in financial terms and in avoidance of side effects, and the increase in the sense of wellbeing (Peters et al. 1977 a) would still make this therapy cost effective. The reduction in BP in normotensive individuals (Peters et al. 1977 a; Patel et al. 1985) suggest the potential of the therapy in primary prevention of hypertension.

The investigators have, until now, developed their own programmes intuitively. It is necessary to standardise the therapy that is effective and to train other health care personnel in its use. A study in collaboration with some British general practitioners and nurses is to start shortly, and it would be interesting to see if consistent results amongst various therapists using the same training protocol can be obtained. At the present time it would be premature to recommend that this therapy be used on a wider scale, other than as part of larger scale evaluation procedures. In addition to supplying much needed morbidity data, such large, long-term clinical trials are the only way we can reliably identify potentially harmful effects.

Achieving the final proof will require considerable material and organizational commitments, but if the trend shown in the 4-year follow-up study (Patel et al. 1985) could be repeated, the financial and health care implications would be enormous. If behaviour modification - alone or judiciously combined with a small amount of antihypertensive drugs - can reduce blood pressure in the mild hypertensive group, as well as making some reduction in blood pressure in normotensive subjects who might otherwise be at risk, then it would seem that we could indeed have a mass strategy for primary prevention that is safe, cheap, effective and acceptable.

References

Alfredsson L, Ahlbom A (1983) Increasing incidence and mortality from myocardial infarction in Stockholm County. Br Med J 286: 1931-1933

Bali LR (1979) Long term effect of relaxation on blood pressure and anxiety levels in essential hypertensive males. A controlled study. Psychosom Med 41: 637-646

Benson H, Shapiro D, Tursky B, Schwartz G (1971) Decreased systolic blood pressure through operant conditioning techniques in patients with essential hypertension. Science 173: 740-742

Benson H, Rosner BA, Marzetta BR, Klemchuk BD (1974) Decreased blood pressure in pharmacologically treated hypertensive patients who regularly elicited the relaxation response. Lancet I: 289-291

Blackwell B, Bloomfield S, Gartside P, Robinson A, Hanenson I, Magenheim H, Nidich S, Zigler R (1976) Transcendental Meditation in hypertension. Lancet I: 223-226
Blanchard EB, Young LD, Haynes MR (1975) A simple feedback system for the treatment of elevated blood pressure. Behav Ther 6: 241-245
Brady JP, Luborsky L, Kron RE (1974) Blood pressure reduction in patients with essential hypertension through metronome-conditioned relaxation: a preliminary report. Behav Ther 5: 203-209
Brauer P, Horlick LF, Nelson B, Farquhar JW, Agras WS (1979) Relaxation therapy for essential hypertension. A Veterans Administration outpatients study. J Behav Med 2: 21-29
Buell P, Breslow L (1960) Mortality from coronary heart disease in Californian men who work long hours. J Chron Dis 2: 615-626
Christoph P, Luborsky L, Kron R, Fishman H (1978) Blood pressure, heart rate and respiratory responses to a single session of relaxation: a partial replication. J Psychosom Res 22: 493-501
Connolly MB (1976) Life events before myocardial infarction. J Human Stress 2: 3-17
Committee of Principal Investigators (1978) A co-operative trial in the primary prevention of ischaemic heart disease using clofibrate. Br Heart J 40: 1069-1118
Cottington EM, Matthews KA, Talbot E, Kuller LH (1980) Environmental events preceding sudden death in women. Psychosom Med 42: 567-573
Crowther JH (1983) Stress management training and relaxation imagery in the treatment of essential hypertension. J Behav Med 6: 169-187
Datey KK, Deshmukh SN, Dalvi CP, Vinekar MD (1969) "Shavasan", a yogic exercise in the management of hypertension. Angiology 20: 325-333
Deabler HL, Fidel E, Dillenkoffer RL, Elder ST (1973) The use of relaxation and hypnosis in lowering high blood pressure. Am J Clin Hypn 16, 2: 75-83
Doll R, Peto R (1976) Mortality of physicians from smoking: observations in male British doctors. Br Med J II: 1525-1536
Elder ST, Eustis NK (1975) Instrumental blood pressure conditioning of diastolic blood pressure in out-patient essential hypertension. Behav Res Ther 13: 185-188
Elder ST, Ruiz R, Deabler HL, Dillenkoffer RL (1973) Instrumental conditioning of diastolic blood pressure in essential hypertensive patients. J Appl Behav Anal 6: 377-382
Engel GL (1971) Sudden and rapid death during psychological stress. Folklore or folk wisdom. Ann Intern Med 74: 771-782
Folklow B, Hallback M, Lundgren Y, Sivertsson R, Weiss L (1973) Importance of adaptive changes in vascular design for establishment of primary hypertension. Studied in man and in spontaneously hypertensive rats. Circ Res [Suppl 1] 32, 33: 2-16
Frankel BL, Patel DJ, Horwitz D, Friedwald MT, Gaardner KP (1978) Treatment of hypertension with biofeedback and relaxation techniques. Psychosom Med 40: 276-293
Friedman EG, Hellerstein HK (1968) Occupational stress. Law school hierarchy and coronary artery disease in Cleveland attorneys. Psychosom Med 30: 72-86
Friedman H, Taub HA (1977) The use of hypnosis and biofeedback procedures for essential hypertension. Int J Clin Exp Hypn 25: 335-347
Friedman M, Rosenman R (1974) Type A behaviour and your heart. Knopf, New York
Glasgow MS, Gaardner KR, Engel BT (1982) Behavioural treatment of high blood pressure: II. Acute and sustained effects of relaxation and systolic blood pressure biofeedback. Psychosom Med 44: 155-171
Goldstein IB, Shapiro D, Thananopavarn C, Sambhi MP (1982) Comparison of drug and behavioural treatment of essential hypertension. Health Psychol I: 7-26
Gordon T (1957) Mortality experience among the Japanese in the United States, Hawaii and Japan. Public Health Report 72, Washington DC, pp 543-553
Harburg E, Blakelock EH, Roeper PJ (1979) Resentful and reflective coping with arbitrary authority and blood pressure. Detroit. Psychosom Med 3: 189-202
Havlik RJ, Feinleib M (eds) (1979) Proceedings of the conference on the decline in coronary heart disease mortality. US Department of Health, Education and Welfare. NIH publ. no. 79-1610
Hill JD, Hampton JR, Mitchell JRA (1976) A randomised trial of Home-versus-Hospital management for patients with suspected myocardial infarction. Br Med J II: 1035-1038
Hjiermann I, Home I, Byre KW, Leren P (1983) Effect of diet and smoking intervention on the incidence of coronary heart disease. Lancet II: 1301-1310

Hypertension Detection and Follow Up Program (1979) Co-operative Group. Five-year findings of the Hypertension Detection and Follow Up Program 1. Reduction in mortality of persons with high blood pressure, including mild hypertension. JAMA 242: 2562-2571
Intersociety Commission for Heart Disease Resources (1970) Primary prevention of the atherosclerotic diseases. Circulation 42, II: A55-A95
Irvine MJ (1983) A controlled study of relaxation and stress management in the treatment of essential hypertension. DPhil Thesis, Trinity College, Oxford University
Jacob RG, Kramer HG, Agras WS (1977) Relaxation therapy in the treatment of hypertension. Arch Gen Psych 34: 1417-1427
Jacobson E (1939) Variation of blood pressure with skeletal muscle tension and relaxation. Ann Intern Med 12: 1194-1212
Jorgensen RS, Housten BK, Zurawski RM (1981) Anxiety management training in the treatment of essential hypertension. Behav Res Ther 19: 467-474
Kallinke D, Kullick B, Heim P (1982) Behaviour analysis and treatment of essential hypertension. J Psychosom Res 26: 541-549
Kaplan BH, Cassel JC, Tyroler HA, Cornoni JC, Kleinbaum DG, Hames CG (1971) Occupational mobility and coronary heart disease. Arch Intern Med 128: 936-942
Karasek RA (1979) Job demands. Job decision latitude and mental strain: implications for job redesign. Am Sci Q 24: 285-308
Karasek RA, Schnall P, Schwartz J, Thorell T, Piper C (1981) Psychosocial characteristics of occupations in relation to prevalence of myocardial infarction: a study of two national random samples of American working men. Columbia University, New York
Klumbies G, Eberhardt G (1966) Results of autogenic training. In: Ibar JJ (ed) The treatment of hypertension. International Congress series 117. Excerpta Medica, Amsterdam, pp 46-47
Kobasa SC (1982) The hardy personality: towards a social psychology of stress and health. In: Suls J, Sanders (eds) The social psychology of health and illness. Erlbaum, Hillsdale
Kristt D, Engel BT (1975) Learned control of blood pressure in patients with high blood pressure. Circulation 51: 370-378
Lipid Research Clinics Trial Investigators (1984) Lipid Research Clinics Trials: primary prevention trial results. JAMA 251: 351-364
Little BE, Hayworth J, Benson P, Beard RW, Dewhurst J, Priest RG (1984) Treatment of hypertension in pregnancy by relaxation and biofeedback. Lancet I: 865-867
Luborsky L, Christoph P, Brady JP, Kron RE, Weiss T, Cohen M, Levy L (1982) Behavioural vs pharmacological treatment for essential hypertension: a needed comparison. Psychosom Med 44: 203-214
Luthe W (1969) Autogenic therapy, vols 1-6. Grune and Stratton, New York
Management Committee (1980) The Australian therapeutic trial in mild hypertension. Lancet I: 1261-1267
Marmot MG, Syme SL (1976) Acculturation and coronary heart disease in Japanese-Americans. Am J Epidemiol 104: 225-246
Marmot MG, Adelstein AM, Robinson N, Rose GA (1978) Changing social class distribution of heart disease. Br Med J II: 1109-1112
Marmot MG, Booth M, Beral V (1982) International trends in heart disease mortality. In: Gotto AM, Paoletti R (eds) Atherosclerosis reviews, vol 9. Raven, New York
Mather HG, Pearson NG, Reed KLQ (1971) Acute myocardial infarction. Home and hospital treatment. Br Med J 3: 334
Mather HG, Morgan DC, Pearson NG (1976) Myocardial infarction: a comparison between home and hospital care for patients. Br Med J I: 925-927
McGrady WV, Yonker R, Tan SY, Fine TH, Woewrner M (1981) The effect of biofeedback-assisted relaxation on blood pressure and selected biochemical parameters in patients with essential hypertension. Biofeedback Self Regul 6: 343-354
Medical Research Council Working Party (1985) MRC trial of treatment of mild hypertension: principal results. Br Med J 291: 97-104
Medical Research Council (1981) Report of the Working Party on Mild to Moderate Hypertension. Adverse reaction to bendrofluazide and propranolol in the treatment of mild hypertension. Lancet II: 536-543

Miller NE (1972) Postscript. In: Singh D, Morgan CT (eds) Current status of physiological psychology. Readings. Brooke/Cole, Monterey
Morris JN, Everitt MG, Pollard R, Change SPW Semmence AM (1980) Vigorous exercise in leisure time. Protection against coronary heart disease. Lancet I: 1207-1210
Multiple Risk Factor Intervention Trial Research Group (1982) Multiple Risk Factor Intervention Trial. Risk factor changes and mortality results. JAMA 248: 1465-1477
Oliver MF (1983) Should we not forget about mass control of coronary risk factors? Lancet II: 37-38
Parkes CM, Benjamin B, Fitzgerald RG (1969) Broken heart: a statistical study of increased mortality among widowers. Br Med J 1: 740-743
Patel C (1973) Yoga and biofeedback in the management of hypertension. Lancet II: 1053-1055
Patel C (1975 a) Yoga and biofeedback in the management of "stress" in hypertensive patients. Clin Sci Mol Med [Suppl] 48: 171s-174s
Patel C (1975 b) 12-month follow up of yoga and biofeedback in the management of hypertension. Lancet I: 62-65
Patel C, North WRS (1975) Randomised controlled trial of yoga and biofeedback in the management of hypertension. Lancet II: 93-95
Patel C, Marmot MG, Terry DJ (1981) Controlled trial of biofeedback-aided behavioural methods in reducing mild hypertension. Br Med J 282: 2005-2008
Patel C, Marmot MG, Terry DJ, Carruthers M, Hunt B, Patel M (1985) Trial of relaxation in reducing coronary risk: four year follow up. Br Med J 290: 1103-1106
Peters RK, Benson H, Peters D (1977 a) Daily relaxation response breaks in a working population: I. Effects on self-reported measures of health, performance and well-being. Am J Public Health 67: 946-953
Peters RK, Benson H, Peters JM (1977 b) Daily relaxation breaks in working population. II. Effects on blood pressure. Am J Public Health 67: 954-959
Pollack AA, Case DB, Weber MA, Laragh JH (1977) Limitation of transcendental meditation in the treatment of essential hypertension. Lancet I: 71-73
Puska P, Tuomilehto J, Salonon J (1979) Changes in coronary risk factors during comprehensive five-year community programme to control cardiovascular disease (North Karelia project). Br Med J II: 1173-1178
Reid D, Hamilton PJS, McCartney P, Rose G, Jarrett RS, Keen H (1976) Smoking and other risk factors for coronary heart disease in British civil servants. Lancet II: 979-984
Richter-Heinrich E, Knust V, Muller W, Schmidt KH, Sprung M (1975) Psychophysiological investigations in essential hypertensives. J Psychosom Res 19: 251-258
Richter-Heinrich E, Homouth B, Heinrich K, Schmidt H, Wiedermann R, Gohlke HR (1981) Long term application of behavioural treatment in essential hypertensives. Physiol Behav 26: 915-920
Rose GA (1975) The contribution of intensive coronary care. Br J Prev Soc Med 29: 147-150
Rose G (1981) Strategy for prevention: lessons from cardiovascular diseases. Br Med J 282: 1847-1851
Rose GA, Reid DD, Hamilton PJ, McCartney P, Keen H, Jarrett RJ (1977) Myocardial ischaemia, risk factors and death from coronary heart disease. Lancet I: 105-109
Russek HI, Zohman BL (1958) Relative significance of heredity, diet and occupational stress in coronary heart disease of young adults. Am J Med Sci 235: 266-277
Sales SM, House J (1971) Job dissatisfaction as a possible risk factor in coronary heart disease. J Chronic Dis 23: 861-873
Salonen JT, Puska P, Mustaniemi H (1979) Changes in morbidity and mortality during comprehensive community programme to control cardiovascular diseases during 1972-1977 in North Karelia. Br Med J 2: 1178-1183
Schwartz GE, Shapiro D (1973) Biofeedback and essential hypertension. Current findings and theoretical concerns. Semin Psychiatry 5: 495-503
Seer P, Raeburn JM (1980) Meditation training and essential hypertension: a methodological study. J Behav Med 3: 59-73
Shoemaker JE, Tasto DL (1975) The effect of muscle relaxation on blood pressure of essential hypertensives. Behav Res Ther 13: 29-43
Stone RA, De Leo J (1976) Psychotherapeutic control of hypertension. N Engl J Med 294: 80-84

Southam MA, Agras WS, Taylor CB, Kraemer HC (1982) Relaxation training: blood pressure during the working day. Arch Gen Psychiatry 39: 715–717

Surwit TS, Shapiro D, Good MI (1978) Comparison of cardiovascular biofeedback in the treatment of borderline hypertension. J Consult Clin Psychol 46: 252–263

Surwitt R, Shapiro D (1977) Biofeedback and meditation in the treatment of borderline hypertension. In: Beatty J, Legewie H (eds) Biofeedback and behaviour Plenum, New York

Syme SL (1975) Social and psychological risk factors in coronary heart disease. Modern Concepts Cardiovasc Dis 44, 4: 17–21

Syme SL, Hyman MM, Enterline PE (1964) Some social and cultural factors associated with the occurrence of coronary heart disease. J Chronic Dis 17: 277–289

Syme SL, Borhani NO, Buechley RW (1965) Cultural mobility and coronary heart disease in an urban area. Am J Epidemiol 82: 334–336

Taylor CB, Farquhar JW, Nelson E, Agras WS (1977) Relaxation therapy and high blood pressure. Arch Gen Psychiatry 34: 339–342

Theorell T, Floderus-Myrhed B (1977) Workload and risk of myocardial infarction. A prospective psychosocial analysis. Int J Epidemiol 6: 17–21

Tyroler HA, Cassel J (1964) Health consequences of cultural change. II. The effect of urbanisation on coronary heart mortality among rural residents. J Chronic Dis 17: 167–177

Vaughan Williams EM, Hassan MO, Floras JS, Sleight P, Jones VJ (1980) Adaptation of hypertensives to treatment with cardioselective and non-selective beta-blockers. Absence of correlation between bradycardia and blood pressure control and reduction in slope of QT/RR relation. Br Heart J 44: 437–487

Waddon TA (1984) Relaxation therapy for essential hypertension: specific or non-specific effects. J Psychosom Res 28: 53–61

Walsh P, Dale A, Anderson DE (1977) Comparison of biofeedback pulse wave velocity and progressive relaxation in essential hypertension. Percept Motor Skills 44: 839–843

WHO Collaborative Group (1983) Multifactorial trial in the prevention of coronary heart disease: III. Incidence and mortality results. Eur Heart J 4: 141–147

World Health Statistics Annual (1981) WHO, Geneva

How Does Relaxation Training Reduce Blood Pressure in Primary Hypertension?

D. W. JOHNSTON[1]

Introduction

There is now a growing body of evidence showing that training in relaxation techniques can reduce blood pressure in primary hypertension (see, for example, Johnston 1982). The following authors have all reported statistically reliable and clinically relevant reductions in casual blood pressure after some form of relaxation training in patients meeting conventional criteria for primary hypertension (Patel 1975a; Patel and North 1975; Taylor et al. 1977; Bali 1979; Brauer et al. 1979; Seer and Raeburn 1980; McGrady et al. 1981; Patel et al. 1981; Southam et al. 1982; Crowther 1983). Recently Little et al. (1984) reported that not only does relaxation training reduce blood pressure in pregnant hypertensive women, but it also decreases the frequency with which they have to be admitted to a hospital during their pregnancy. Reductions regularly obtained, particularly if patients start with pressures that are at least mildly elevated, can be substantial (see review by Jacobs et al. 1977). For example, Patel typically reports reductions from pre-treatment blood pressure levels of almost 170/100 mmHg to levels of at or below 140/90 mmHg; i.e. the average patient in such studies has well-controlled blood pressure at the end of treatment. The critical components of relaxation training with this group of patients have not been established, but most of the successful treatments include training, usually live, in some form of relaxation technique, regular practice in that technique, and training in the use of relaxation to cope with day-to-day stressors. Such an amalgam of techniques may perhaps be best regarded as a form of combined relaxation training and stress management. The occasional negative report, (e.g. Frankel et al. 1978; Surwit et al. 1978; Luborsky et al. 1982) has usually omitted one or more of these components and, in addition, may have studied patients with rather low blood pressure prior to treatment (e.g. Surwit et al. 1978). There are obviously many important questions about the efficacy of relaxation training in this context that are still both unasked and unanswered. It is probable that the most important of these is the extent to which the changes that are seen in casual clinic-measured blood pressures generalize to other situations (Southam et al. 1982). Nevertheless, the available data are sufficiently positive to suggest that it might be both interesting and fruitful to consider the mechanisms that might underlie these blood pressure reductions. Mechanism and efficacy are, of course, interrelated, and it would obviously aid the development and deployment of rationally based therapies if we knew how and in whom they worked.

There are many types of explanation possible in attempts to understand a complex psychological treatment. At this time it is probably best to consider all explana-

1 Department of Psychiatry, Oxford University, Warneford Hospital, Oxford OX3 7JX, UK

Biological and Psychological Factors
in Cardiovascular Disease
Ed. by T. H. Schmidt, T. M. Dembroski, and G. Blümchen

tions for which there are reasonable amounts of empirical data. This leads to the following types of answers to the problem we have posed:

The reduction in blood pressure produced by relaxation in patients with essential hypertension is:

1. An artefact
2. A non-specific effect
3. A simple direct effect
4. An effect on blood pressure reactivity
5. Caused by detectable neurogenic and hormonal changes.

After consideration of these explanations I shall then consider:

6. The paradoxical long-term effects of relaxation and, finally
7. How then does relaxation work?

Artefact

Many factors influence blood pressure and can be associated with its reduction, e.g. the passage of time, experience of blood pressure measurement, change in ambient temperature, altered drug compliance, alterations in weight or diet, systematic bias on the part of the measuring physician, etc. When not properly controlled for, such factors can seriously compromise the validity of clinical trials. Fortunately, most of the factors listed above have been dealt with satisfactorily in a reasonable number of studies. All the studies referenced above have included some form of control group so that one is able to exclude such low-level confounding variables as the passage of time or the patient's experience of blood pressure measurement. Furthermore, many studies (although, unfortunately, not all) have ensured either blind or automatic blood pressure measurement, and so a systematic bias is excluded (e.g. Patel and North 1975; Taylor et al. 1977; Brauer et al. 1979; Crowther 1983). Chesney and Black (in this volume) have reported that, in a substantial study, she found little difference in reductions in casual blood pressure between a variety of forms of relaxation-based treatments and blood pressure monitoring. Large, well-conducted studies of this kind are rare, and such a finding is obviously worrisome. However, it does appear that significant differences between monitoring and active treatment were obtained when the patients, or a subsample of them, were studied at their work place. Since blood pressure was higher at these times, this may well underscore the need to study patients with sufficiently elevated pressures for the effect of treatment to be detectable.

Most of the early studies examined patients who were already on hypertensive medication. Although the authors attempted to monitor patient use of medication, it is difficult in such studies to exclude the possibility of altered drug compliance selectively occurring in the active treatment group, which typically would be receiving more attention and interest. Fortunately, recent studies have shown that apparently equal effects can be obtained in unmedicated patients, in whom compliance is obviously not a relevant factor (e.g. Bali 1979; Patel et al. 1981). In a study that will be described below, we found little difference in response to treatment between medicated and unmedicated mild hypertensives (Irvine et al., in press). The other potentially confounding variables have been less rigorously examined. Irvine et al. found body weight to be quite unaltered by relaxation training, suggesting that at least in that study it was unlikely to be the basis of the observed reductions in pressure. Stone and DeLeo (1976) reported that sodium excretion stayed within the normal range in patients receiving relaxation training, thus suggesting that there were no significant changes in salt intake. It is perhaps somewhat unfortunate that body weight and diet do not appear to have been examined more often. While weight reduction or dietary change is not regularly incorporated as part of a relaxation programme, it is possible that in particularly health-conscious cultures or among health-conscious sections of the community, the decision to take part in a relaxation-based treatment may be associated with a decision to change to a healthier life-style. These problems are, however, relatively minor, and at present there is no reason to believe that the reductions in blood pressure produced by relaxation training are artefactual, and good reason to believe that they are genuine effects of some aspect of the treatment.

Non-specific Effects

Experience with other forms of behavioural treatment has shown that it is difficult to demonstrate convincingly that a specific therapeutic procedure is the main agent of behavioural change. It has even been claimed that comparatively effective treatments such as systematic desensitization, which have been exhaustively investigated, operate primarily through non-specific mechanisms (Kazdin and Wilcoxon 1976). There are clearly many potentially powerful non-specific aspects to relaxation training. If Patel's treatment approach is taken as prototypical, then the far from exhaustive list of such factors would include therapist contact, a plausible treatment rationale, training in a specific skill, practising such a skill and monitoring day-to-day events with a view to using these skills to alter one's response to them. These factors are not specific to relaxation training and stress management, and if the basis for the reductions in pressure observed is in these general factors, then other treatments that incorporate these features might be as effective, even if they do not incorporate relaxation or stress management and have no rational basis as a therapy for hypertension.

Two lines of evidence argue against the above possibility. The first, and weaker, evidence is the persistence of the blood pressure reductions after the patient has ceased to be in active therapy. Follow-up results from 6-15 months (e.g. Patel and North 1975; Patel 1977; Bali 1979; Patel et al. 1981; Crowther 1983) have been consistently good, and some have even reported greater blood pressure reduction 6 months after treatment (Brauer et al. 1979). This is certainly not what one would expect to occur if relaxation was operating primarily as a form of elaborate placebo, since, in that case, one might reasonably expect that the effects would diminish when the patient ceased to be in active therapy.

The second and more powerful source of evidence comes from controlled studies. At least three studies have incorporated a control group based primarily on some form of supportive psychotherapy. Taylor et al. (1977) and Brauer et al. (1979), using essentially the same control condition, showed that relaxation was superior to supportive psychotherapy, although in the Taylor et al. study, the effect was most pronounced immediately after treatment, while Brauer et al. found it much more pronounced 6 months later. Bali (1979), who added impressive physiological measurement to his version of supportive psychotherapy, also found relaxation to be more effective; indeed, he found that psychotherapy had no detectable effect on pressure. These results are encouraging, but one can reasonably doubt that psychotherapy is a totally appropriate control for all potentially significant aspects of relaxation training and stress management. It is doubtful if it is equally plausible to hypertensive patients, since it does not involve training in a specific skill or regular practice of that skill; nor do patients have to use that skill to cope with day-to-day events (although Bali did attempt, unsuccessfully, to get patients in psychotherapy to rest regularly). We (Irvine et al., in press) developed a control treatment that matched relaxation training more closely than supportive psychotherapy, with respect to what we believed were potentially critical non-specific ingredients. The relaxation training we took as our model was that described by Patel, as it incorporated many of the features common to other versions of relaxation training. It resembled, reasonably closely, our own use of relaxation training in clinical practice, and it has been shown to be at least as successful as any alternative. The control treatment consisted of mild mobility exercises (i.e., not vigorous aerobic exercise). Patients were given a rational explanation for these exercises, based on the argument that exercise would improve their circulation, and hence reduce blood pressure. The exercises were graded in complexity and in number of repetitions, and were learned over the same number of weeks as the relaxation technique by the "treatment" subjects. Patients practised these exercises both at home and throughout the day. During the day, mobility exercises were triggered by drowsiness, not by stress, as is the case in relaxation training. Since in Patel's form of relaxation subjects receive skin resistance feedback, exercise subjects also received such feedback; however, rather than attempting to increase skin resistance, they attempted to hold it constant throughout a session. These two procedures were compared in 32 hypertensive patients whose diastolic blood pressures fell between 90 and 109 mmHg and whose systolic blood pressure was below 200 mmHg. Half of the patients were receiving antihypertensive medication.

Before and after treatment, patients in both groups rated their expectation of, and satisfaction with, treatment as equal on a variety of rating scales. It therefore appears that we had produced a satisfactory control treatment, i.e. one that appeared to be very similar to the experimental treatment, both structurally and in its effect on patient expectancies. The design of the study included a 3-month initial baseline period, during which time all patients monitored their own blood pressure twice daily. Since patients entered the study with average blood pressures of 147/99 mmHg (average of six readings taken on two occasions), it is obvious from Fig. 1 that pressure had dropped without any specific intervention. Indeed, it dropped to a marked extent in medicated patients who were about to receive the control treatment. However, further reductions occurred only in subjects receiving relaxation training. At the end of the treatment period, the difference between the relaxation and the control condition was significant for diastolic pressure, and 3 months later for both systolic and diastolic pressure. This study, therefore, indicated that some aspect of the relaxation procedure did have a specific effect on blood pressure, an effect that was not produced by an equally plausible, equally complex,

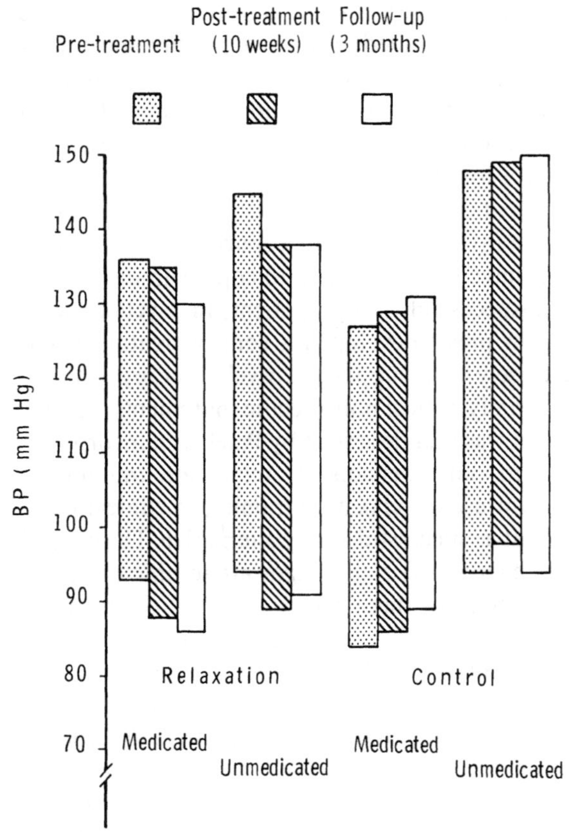

Fig. 1. Mean level of diastolic and systolic blood pressure before treatment, at the end of treatment, and 3 months later

and equally practised treatment, which did not include either relaxation, practice in relaxation, or the application of relaxation to deal with day-to-day stressors.

Two recent studies might appear to contradict the conclusion from the study of Irvine et al. Agras et al. (1982) examined the role of expectancy of therapeutic gain on blood pressure by the use of counterdemand instructions. Patients received three sessions of relaxation training on one day. Half of them were told that their blood pressure would drop immediately; the remaining patients were led to believe that they could expect little or no change that day. Systolic blood pressure dropped significantly more in patients told to expect an immediate drop. This finding does appear to indicate that expectancy of therapeutic gain may be important, but need not necessarily contradict the control trials described above. The latter were, in essence, attempts to hold expectancy constant while varying the treatment, while Agras et al. did the opposite. Taken in combination, the two types of evidence might suggest that a good therapeutic outcome is dependent on the appropriate expectancies being combined with the correct treatment. Further work is needed to explore this issue, both because expectancy and treatment have not been independently varied in the same study, and also because the Agras study was exclusively concerned with the immediate effects of relaxation on pressure. Moreover, it will be argued below that these may not be the same as the long-term effects of the practice of relaxation.

Wadden (1984) has recently questioned the specificity of relaxation training following a study in which he failed to find any difference between relaxation training and a form of cognitive therapy based on rational emotive therapy, which did not involve any form of relaxation. It is doubtful if Wadden's study should be regarded as a control study, since it is not clear what cognitive therapy is a control for. This study is best regarded as a comparison of two potentially active treatments which have an apparently different basis. It may tell us that blood pressure can be lowered by two different but specific psychological techniques, rather than that these two techniques share the same non-specific mechanism. There is, therefore, no reason to alter our earlier conclusion that the effects of relaxation training on blood pressure are specific to the three components we have identified.

Direct Effects of Relaxation

If it is accepted that relaxation has a specific effect on clinically measured blood pressure, then the simplest explanation of that effect would appear to be that relaxation has a direct effect on the blood pressure of those patients trained in relaxation techniques who practise these techniques regularly, and, as a result, lower their blood pressure. If relaxation works in this way, then the effect would be seen most clearly during, and immediately following relaxation practice. The evidence for this in studies of both hypertensives and normotensives is far from convincing.

In a small study of 15 hypertensive patients, Shoemaker and Tasto (1975) compared relaxation training with either blood pressure biofeedback or simply sitting, and claimed that relaxation was associated with a substantially greater reduction in diastolic pressure during five 60-min sessions. Cristoph et al. (1978) compared relaxation training and reading in a single session, within patients, in a study of hypertensives. While differences with respect to respiration rate and heart rate were obtained between reading and relaxation, no difference was observed in blood pressure. It can obviously be argued that subjects in this study received too little training for any possible effect to be detected. Glasgow et al. (1982) have reported on the self-recorded blood pressure of a large sample of hypertensive patients who were variously relaxing or using a form of blood pressure biofeedback. Relaxation was associated with a greater reduction in diastolic pressure than feedback of systolic blood pressure. No control condition was included in this study, and the bias introduced by subjects recording their own blood pressure is unknown. In the study described above, Irvine et al. (1985) measured blood pressure under identical conditions, before and after training, in both relaxation and exercise subjects. Blood pressure, averaged over the six sessions during which such measurements were taken, is shown in Fig. 2. No reductions in diastolic pressure were seen, but there was a slight drop in systolic blood pressure favouring the relaxation group. It must be remembered that, in this case, relaxation, involving predominantly passive procedures and meditation, was being compared with a mildly active procedure that included standing and moving gently. This failure to find a substantial difference is, therefore, dramatic testimony to the weakness of the immediate effects of relaxation training even in a study with a good clinical outcome. It should be pointed out that the necessity of ensuring that blood pressure was measured under similar condi-

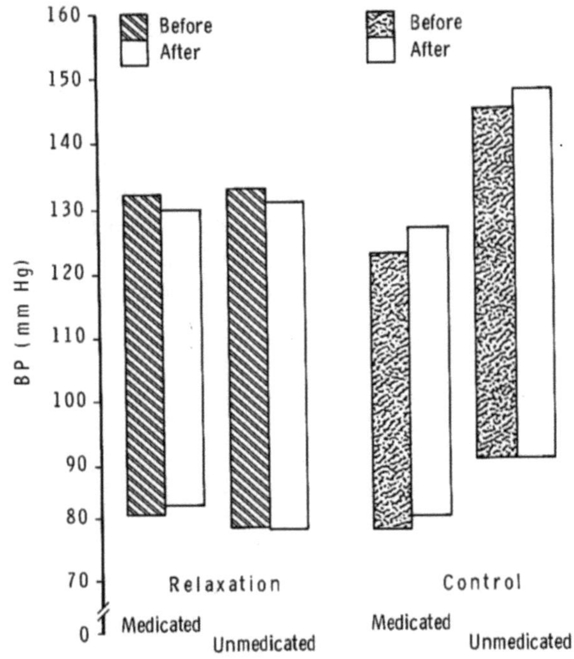

Fig. 2. Mean level of diastolic and systolic blood pressure immediately before and after treatment sessions

tions in both treatments meant that patients receiving relaxation training rose from the couch, on which such training was given, and sat at a table to have their pressure measured. This may have accounted for the lack of a significant drop in pressure despite lying or sitting passively for up to 30 min. However, it does not seriously weaken the comparison with the control condition, since it, at the very least, indicates that the effects of relaxation training are so fragile that they can be negated by taking several steps across a room.

An additional source of evidence that may be relevant to this issue is the relationship between the extent of relaxation practice and the reduction in blood pressure over a course of treatment. It can be suggested that if relaxation lowers blood pressure, patients who practise more should reduce their blood pressure by a greater amount. Taylor et al. (1983), using an ingenious automated method of recording relaxation practice by monitoring the use of a relaxation tape on a cassette player, found no relationship between such practice and outcome. Wadden (1983) relying on patients' own records of relaxation practice (which the Taylor et al. study suggests are reasonably accurate) found a mild positive relationship, while we (Irvine et al., in press) found a mildly negative relationship on some measures of blood pressure. Our finding that patients who practised more do slightly worse it, at first, paradoxical, but may well relate to the use of self-monitoring of blood pressure in our study. It is easy to see that patients whose blood pressure is not dropping may practise more, hence the causal link between pressure and practice may be opposite to the one predicted.

Since there is a comparative dearth of studies on the immediate effects of relaxation in hypertension, there is some justification for examining studies of BP reduction in normotensives. Tasto and Huebner (1976) following up the earlier study of Shoemaker and Tasto, compared quiet reading with three sessions of taped relaxation training. No difference was detected in the effectiveness of these two procedures. Steptoe and Ross (1982) found evidence of a very slight lengthening of pulse transit time (which is probably indicative of a reduction in systolic blood pressure, see Obrist et al. 1979; Marie et al. 1984) after a brief form of live relaxation training. This reduction was greater than that obtained in subjects quietly reading. Lo and Johnston (1984) found no difference between the effects of taped relaxation training and simply sitting, on either heart period or pulse transit time. These findings are, therefore, largely negative; however, it should be recalled that young normotensive volunteers have, by definition, low blood pressure, and it has already been pointed out that level of pressure may be an important determinant of outcome. In addition, two of the three studies described used taped relaxation, which may be inadequate (Brauer et al. 1979). On the other hand, there is not much evidence to support the proposition that relaxation has strong somatic effects. For example, Holmes (1984) has recently reviewed the literature on the somatic effects of meditation, a common component in the relaxation procedures used with hypertensives, and concludes that there is no convincing evidence that meditation has any greater effect than can be obtained from quietly resting. Earlier reviews by Borkovec and Sides (1979), King (1980) and Lehrer (1982) also suggest that the somatic effects of relaxation are not marked.

It would be inappropriate to conclude that relaxation has no specific effect on blood pressure; however, it is appropriate to suggest that there is no convincing body of evidence to suggest that it has. This is surely surprising and troubling in a widely used, and even more widely advocated treatment of demonstrable clinical effectiveness.

Effects of Relaxation on Cardiovascular Reactivity

The lack of evidence that relaxation lowers pressure acutely is disturbing, but it can be pointed out that most of the studies have been carried out on patients or subjects in a benign environment and in the presence of a therapist whom they knew well. These non-taxing settings may well be very different from the real world, in which the patient is being challenged or is challenging others, is rushing or is trying to encourage others to speed up. It may even be different from the normal context, in which blood pressure is measured by a busy clinician whom the patient may not know well and who may be about to make a significant decision about the patient's present or future health. Perhaps at times when the patient is aroused and the blood pressure is further elevated, relaxation comes into its own and a direct effect can be shown. Four studies of hypertensives have addressed this issue. In the first, Patel (1975b) examined the effects of relaxation and stress management on the pressor response to dynamic exercise (a version of the step test) and the cold pressor test. She found that patients reduced the systolic blood pressure response to exercise from 27 to 19 mmHg and the time to recover to a baseline value from 18 to 9 minutes. The control subjects dit not change. The systolic blood pressure response to the cold pressor test was reduced from 19 to 11 mmHg and recovery time from 11 to

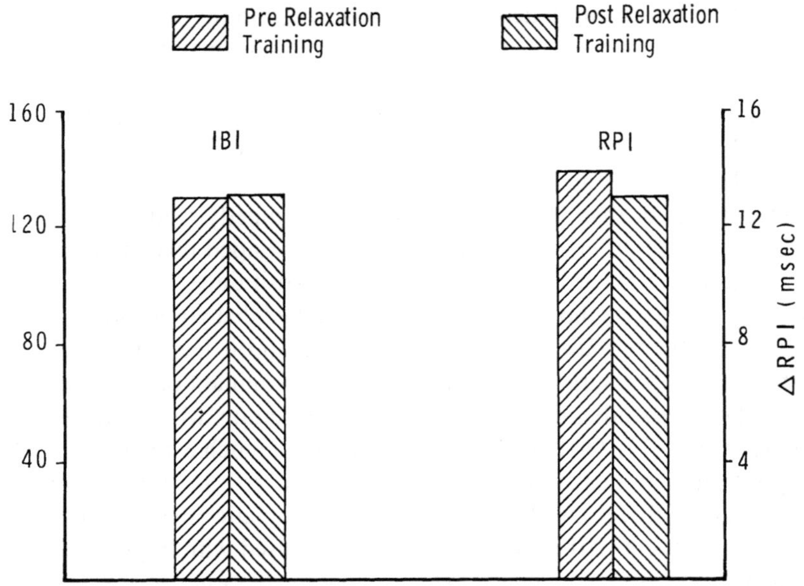

Fig. 3. Changes in interbeat interval *(IBI)* and pulse transit time *(RPI)* from pre-test baseline in patients doing mental arithmetic

6 minutes. Again the control subjects did not change. These very striking findings have not been confirmed in subsequent investigations. For example, Goldstein et al. (1982) reported, in summary form, that relaxation training did not reduce the cardiovascular response to a variety of laboratory stressors. However, the outcome of relaxation on clinically measured blood pressure was disappointing in this study, and so the findings may be aberrant. Jorgenson et al. (1981), using a version of anxiety management training that included relaxation, reported that treatment was associated with less of a reduction in systolic blood pressure on the Stroop task than was a wait list control. However, anxiety management did lower resting blood pressure. Irvine et al. (in press) examined the effects of relaxation and the control treatment (exercise) on the cardiovascular response to mental arithmetic, a continuous choice reaction time task and static exercise. There was no detectable effect of relaxation on the response to any of these stressors, despite the drop in pressure at post-treatment and follow-up. Figure 3 shows the change in heart period (IBI) and pulse transit time (RPI) during mental arithmetic, the most effective of the tasks we used. The similarity of the response before and after treatment is striking. Control subjects, who are not shown, did not reduce reactivity either.

The discrepancy between Patel's study and these others is puzzling, particularly as the therapy used by Irvine et al. was modelled very closely on that used by Patel. One possibly important difference between the studies is that it appears that Patel asked her patients to relax for 20 min prior to the stress tests and, presumably, suggested or implied that they should attempt to limit their response to the test. Subjects in the other studies were not so instructed; therefore, it is not known whether they did attempt to reduce their pressor response. Treatment, as carried out by Patel and ourselves, does include specific training in controlling the response to stress, but naturally concentrates on those stressors which the patient either was experiencing or was likely to experience. Artificial laboratory stressors were not discussed, and it might well be that the patient either did not attempt to control the response to such stressors, or that the situation was too novel for their training to operate. This issue needs further investigation.

The use of relaxation to reduce cardiovascular reactivity has been studied to a very limited extent in normotensives. The usual caveats about generalizing from such studies to hypertensive patients obviously apply. Steptoe and Ross (1982) failed to find any significant reduction in cardiovascular reactivity (IBI and RPI) to various cognitive tasks following relaxation training. Although in a subsidiary analysis they claimed that relaxation was associated with a reduction in those subjects who were most reactive initially. Lo and Johnston (1984) could find no effect of taped relaxation training on the cardiovascular response to dynamic exercise. Holmes (1984), in the review already mentioned, suggests that there is no convincing evidence that meditation has any specific effect on the somatic response to various stressors.

These studies suggest that the case that relaxation reduces the pressor response to stress is unconvincing. However, there are pointers that suggest this issue is far from closed. Two studies (Glasgow et al. 1982; Irvine et al. 1985) have, in addition to blood pressure recorded by professionals in a clinic, obtained self-recorded blood pressure at various times throughout the day, and both have found that relaxation or relaxation-like procedures were more effective on those occasions when pressure was highest. In the Glasgow et al. study this was seen in self-recorded pressure in the afternoon, while the Irvine et al. study found the professionally measured blood pressures were highest and showed treatment effects most clearly. These studies, therefore, suggest that not only is relaxation more effective in patients with the highest blood pressures (as Jacob et al. 1977 have shown), but also at those times when pressure is highest. Clearly this may simply be a statistical artefact, but it is also reasonable to consider why pressure is higher at some times than others. Stress is an obvious possibility. It is very likely that patients are more aroused in the afternoon at work than they are at home in the morning or evening, and having pressure measured in a clinic may well be a mildly stressful experience. This evidence is weak, since we lack any objective evidence that these patients were under stress. It does, however, suggest that further research, which attempts objectively to measure and manipulate stress and assess the effects of relaxation, is required. At the moment, however, only the weakest of cases can be made to support the proposition that relaxation reduces the pressor response to stress.

Subjective Effects of Relaxation

An alternative to the proposal that relaxation directly reduces blood pressure and the blood pressure response to stress, is to propose that relaxation produces subjective changes and that these changes lead to lower pressure. Perhaps patients can be made less anxious, depressed, or angry, and blood pressure drops as a consequence. Research that might bear on this hypothesis has been disappointingly limited. Bali (1979) showed that relaxation, but not supportive psychotherapy, was associated with significant reductions in anxiety, as assessed by the Taylor Manifest Anxiety

Scale (TMAS). These reductions in anxiety did not correlate with blood pressure reductions. Wadden (1984) has also shown that anxiety on the State-Trait Anxiety Inventory (STAI) and anxiety and depression on subscales of the Minnesota Multiphasic Personality Inventory (MMPI) dropped following relaxation training. Again these changes did not relate to the drop in pressure. Finally, Irvine et al. (1985) could find no evidence of reductions on the main scales of the Profile of Mood States (POMS) (McNair and Lorr 1964). Two points are worth making. It may not be damning for the underlying hypothesis that subjective change is uncorrelated with blood pressure reduction, since the mechanism linking the two is unclear and many independent factors must surely effect both. Until these independent factors can be assessed and considered, only the very strongest versions of the hypothesis are embarrassed by the failure to find a simple correlation between the two measures. Secondly, the choice of subjective states assessed in these studies may be unfortunate. There are few good reasons for believing that hypertensives are unduly anxious or depressed, and it was our experience that the patients started at far too low a level on the anxiety and depression scales of the POMS for change to be likely. The interest in the relationship between anger and its expression and hypertension (discussed by Chesney and Black and by Spielberger in this volume) may suggest that this is a more relevant subjective state, and studies of this variable may provide some support for a subjective change hypothesis.

Neurogenic and Hormonal Changes with Relaxation

Those authors who find a place for psychological factors in the aetiology of essential hypertension usually suggest that such factors operate through the sympathetic nervous system (SNS) (see reviews from a psychological perspective by Steptoe 1981 and Linden 1984, and from a physiological perspective by Folkow 1982 and Conway 1984). A corollary of this view is that most writers on the use of relaxation assume that it operates to reduce the SNS drive to the system or systems that are central to the production and maintenance of hypertension. This view has been stated most explicitly by Patel (1977).

Attempts to study the effects of relaxation on the SNS in hypertension can most conveniently be grouped by measure, which are either urinary or plasma measures of adrenaline and noradrenaline (or substances that relate to their production or breakdown; e.g. DBH and VMA) or hormones that are, in part, under SNS control and relate directly to alterations in pressure (e.g. renin and aldosterone).

Stone and DeLeo (1976), in an early and well-controlled study of a meditative form of relaxation, showed that such relaxation reduced standing but not supine plasma DBH, and that this reduction correlated with reductions in blood pressure. Brauer et al. (1979) failed to confirm either of these findings, but their subjects were supine when DBH was measured and they did not measure DBH at the time of maximum blood pressure reduction, which was 6 months after the end of treatment in their study. Two studies have examined the effect of relaxation on urinary catecholamines: McGrady et al. (1981) failed to demonstrate any reduction in total catecholamines or VMA and our recent study (Irvine et al. 1985) found that neither adrenaline or nor-adrenaline was reduced by relaxation. However, both of these studies did show reliable reductions in pressure.

The findings on alterations of plasma renin have also been quite variable. Pollack et al. (1977) failed to find any effect of meditation on either plasma renin or blood pressure; a result also obtained by Goldstein et al. (1982). Stone and DeLeo, in the study already mentioned, did not find any effect of relaxation on either standing or supine renin but did find a small reduction in furosemide-stimulated renin when upright. McGrady et al. (1981) found no reduction in plasma renin, but, rather puzzlingly, aldosterone, which is normally considered to be partly under the control of renin, did drop reliably. This may suggest that there was an undetected change in sodium or potassium intake in the relaxation patients. Patel et al. (1981), in a large study with a good clinical outcome, did find significant reductions in plasma renin and aldosterone after 8 weeks of treatment. Intriguingly, these effects were no longer significant 6 months later but the pressure reductions persisted. McGrady et al. also reported that urinary but not plasma cortisol was reduced by relaxation.

These results defy sensible summary; only aldosterone has been shown to respond to relaxation in more than one study, and even that finding is not reliably associated with the expected and probably causal changes in renin. These very mixed findings may relate to heterogeneity of the patients studied. The only common feature of all the subjects in these studies is that they all had mildly elevated blood pressure and were all prepared to carry out some form of relaxation training. Many of the patients were on medication (e.g. Pollack 1977; Brauer et al. 1979; McGrady et al. 1981), and the age range was enormous: The average age of Stone and DeLeo's patients was 28 years, while patients in the studies of Brauer et al., McGrady et al. and Pollack were well into their 50s. Few would suggest that hypertension is produced by one pathophysiological mechanism, and many would suggest that the mechanisms vary during the natural history of the condition. Goldstein (1983) has suggested that high levels of catecholamines are to be found most reliably in young established hypertensives, while Julius and Esler (Julius and Esler 1975; Esler et al. 1977) suggest that, although hypertensives can have elevated renin, substantial numbers have either normal or even depressed levels of renin. Given this heterogeneity, it is likely that interpretable results will be obtained only if homogeneous groups of patients with demonstrable abnormalities in the system of interest (i.e. high catecholamines, high renin) are studied. Of course, the finding that relaxation appears to be effective in many different types of patients at different stages in the condition, regardless of whether they are receiving medication, must diminish one's optimism that such changes are central to the effects of relaxation. However, studies of homogeneous groups are clearly needed and can hardly fail to be illuminating.

Findings in normotensives also suggest that relaxation does not have a reliable and simple effect on these measures of SNS activity. Relaxation has variously been shown to reduce plasma noradrenaline (Davidson et al. 1979), increase it (Lang et al. 1979), or leave it unchanged (Michaels et al. 1976). In one of the more careful studies on the topic, Hoffman et al. (1982) suggest that relaxation decreases the sensitivity of beta-adrenergic receptors; therefore, under some forms of challenge (which in their case was exercise) increased levels of noradrenaline will be found. This possibility raises the complexity of the issue considerably and suggests that measuring simple resting levels of circulating hormones or the by-products of neurotransmitters is unlikely to be adequate.

The Anomalous Long-Term Effects of Relaxation

Relaxation is a mildly time-consuming activity which requires a considerable degree of self-discipline and organization if it is to be practised regularly over months or years. It is widely held that hypertensives comply poorly with instructions to take medication (Sackett and Haynes 1976), and, as a result, blood pressure control with drugs is often inadequate. It is clear that the costs and benefits of relaxation compared with medication are very different, since relaxation requires considerable investment of time but is normally regarded as at least mildly pleasant, while drugs are simple to take but, occasionally, have nasty side effects. Nevertheless, it would be surprising if the long-term compliance with relaxation was markedly better than with medication. Actual data on the subject is notably lacking, but Libo and Arnold (1983), in a postal survey of relaxation practice in patients with a wide range of diagnoses, reported that only 15% of patients were practising daily 1-5 years after training, while 27% were practising once a week. This study did include hypertensives, but most of the patients suffered from conditions with troublesome and obvious symptoms (such as headache) which are likely to increase the frequency of practice. Thus, these figures are almost certainly overestimates of the practice of asymptomatic hypertensive patients. In our recent study (Irvine et al. 1985), 3 months after therapy, patients were practising approximately 5 times per week rather than the suggested 14, whereas during treatment it had been nearer 10. If compliance is as poor as these figures suggest (and clinical experience is in accordance with them), then one might expect that long-term blood pressure reductions following relaxation would be poor. In fact, they are strikingly good. A large number of studies have reported excellent blood pressure control 3-15 months after treatment (Patel 1975a; Patel and North 1975; Bali 1979; Patel et al. 1981; Southam et al. 1982; Irvine et al. 1985), and it has even been reported that control improves in the months following treatment (Brauer et al. 1979). Patel, in this volume, has reported good blood pressure control 4 years after treatment and has also found an associated reduction in cardiovascular morbidity. This latter finding must be treated with some caution given the small numbers involved, but it is highly suggestive and consistent with the blood pressure findings.

These findings are challenging. In the earlier sections of this paper it has been shown that the evidence that relaxation lowers blood pressure directly is very weak. Yet pressure does drop over time during treatment, and, while there is little reason to believe that people do continue to practise such relaxation, its effects persist for several years.

It is acknowledged that elevations in blood pressure are not as enduring as was once supposed. Indeed the recent finding of the Australian mild hypertension trial (Australian National Blood Pressure Study 1982) that 50% of untreated mild hypertensives normalize within 4 years, is powerful support for the use of a behavioural rather than a pharmacological treatment in such patients. However, the control studies of relaxation suggest that the positive findings do not simply reflect the natural history of untreated mild hypertension. However, these studies may well represent an important and interesting interaction between a behavioural treatment and the natural processes that normalize pressure. These long-term effects, taken in conjunction with the effects reported earlier, all suggest that relaxation is effective but that it does not operate through the mechanisms I have already identified.

How Then Does Relaxation Work?

In earlier sections of this paper the weakness of the evidence supporting existing theories on the role of relaxation in the treatment of hypertension has been documented. Obviously future research will alter and clarify these conclusions, which are tied to our present knowledge. However, it is probably most fruitful if the conclusions from these earlier sections are stated quite starkly and unduly dogmatically. It has been claimed that there is no reason to believe that relaxation has a specific direct effect on resting blood pressure, on blood pressure reactivity, or on emotional states which might mediate blood pressure reduction; nor has relaxation been shown to reliably reduce any of the conventional SNS markers. How then, does relaxation work? If these contentions are correct, the answer cannot lie in those factors which have already been studied, but must lie elsewhere. Two categories of evidence are strikingly missing from the six listed - behavioural and cognitive change accompanying and following relaxation. The description of relaxation treatments, such as the one used by Patel and ourselves, make it quite clear that relaxation and stress management are complex psychological treatments. Yet little is known about how they alter patients' behaviour (apart from how often patients set aside time to practise), and even less about how they effect patients' thinking. This is not because those aspects of human behaviour and experience are thought to be unimportant by theorists, either within the narrow confines of psychophysiology (e.g. the most influential psychological theory on the aetiology of hypertension, which stresses the role of behaviour and active coping; see Obrist et al. in this volume), nor in psychology in general, since the central concern of psychology for the last 70 years has been behaviour - and if behaviour is to be toppled from its pre-eminent position, then it will be by cognition. Nor are behaviour and cognitions regarded as peripheral by clinicians. I am sure that most practitioners in this field will agree that a great deal of therapeutic time is spent on getting people to monitor their behaviour, to search for subjective distress and arousal (on the assumption that it is associated with heightened blood pressure), and to persuade patients to deal with it, usually by relaxation. Despite this, there is no body of data on the use of such techniques, or their effects on day-to-day distress and elevations in pressure. If my contention that relaxation does not lower blood pressure directly is accepted, then the usefulness of relaxation is probably in the coping processes that are initiated by the complete treatment package. At its simplest, relaxation may be a readily available coping device which patients can use in difficult situations and which may serve as a distractor or perhaps alters the patient's ability to deal with the situation by making an alternative response available.

However, relaxation training is not confined to attempts to cope with distressing, arousing situations; therapy frequently involves some discussion of why certain situations are found distressing, and may even extend to questioning the necessity of getting involved in such troublesome situations at all. It has been my impression that relaxation training and stress management can induce a patient-initiated process of problem identification and solution that eventually leads to blood pressure reduction. It is surprising how often therapy seems to suggest to the patient, perhaps for the first time, that his or her blood pressure may be a response to their life situation and, more importantly, that they can do something about it. There is no reason to believe that this process is exclusive to relaxation. The recent report by Wadden (1984), suggesting that a cognitive therapy based on rational emotive therapy is as effective as relaxation, is perfectly compatible with this position. However, the lack of any form of control or placebo group in Wadden's study makes it difficult to determine if either treatment was, in fact, effective.

I, therefore, see relaxation training as one of a variety of socially, psychologically and professionally acceptable ways of initiating the patient's own processes of problem identification and solution. These speculations, stimulated by the disappointing support for other initially more plausible hypotheses, are based on clinical impressions gained in the treatment of hypertensives and other types of patients with relaxation-based therapies. Clearly, information on the actual behaviour of patients who have received relaxation training is vitally necessary. Do they monitor their own level of stress? Do they apply relaxation? Do they use other distraction techniques in addition to relaxation? Do they spontaneously generate other solutions to deal with their problems? Do they start to avoid difficult situations? Do they even work less or do less overtime etc., etc.? It is surprising and almost embarrassing that these questions have certainly not been answered and have scarcely been asked in the 15 years after the first good evidence that relaxation can lower blood pressure.

The cognitive changes induced by relaxation are harder to speculate on with any conviction. However, the long-term effects of relaxation suggest that some rather pervasive and self-maintaining change must occur, since I very much doubt if patients continue deliberately to practise whatever behavioural changes are induced by relaxation, year in and year out. It is my impression that, in some patients at least, subtle attitudinal changes occur as a result of relaxation training. This can be described in various ways, such as becoming more accepting of their life situation or more "laid back". In general, they appear to reduce their attempts to struggle with uncontrollable or nearly uncontrollable situations. These changes have not been documented and, even if they occur, may not relate directly to relaxation, but may be secondary to the behavioural changes discussed above. However, I am reluctant to believe that relaxation has no specific effect, and I would suggest that these attitudinal changes may relate to the regular practice of relaxation. At least, when patients are at the stage of having learned the technique, but have not become overfamiliar with it and bored, the immediate effect of relaxation is often described by patients as unusually pleasant. In other fields it is becoming clear that emotions such as depression and anxiety, which can be produced by temporary alterations in the patient's or subject's state, can alter the availability of certain cognitions; for example, depressive thoughts and memories become more available when in a depressed mood (see Bower 1981; Teasdale 1983). Therefore, it is possible that the subjective effect produced by the regular practice of relaxation can alter the availability of more adaptive cognitions and this can lead to attitudinal changes. These changes might be pervasive and persistent enough to explain the long-term effects of relaxation after the regular practice of the technique and/or of monitoring one's own behaviour have ceased or diminished drastically.

In proposing this possible cognitive role of relaxation I am uncomfortably aware that it is very easy to believe that a procedure that is used enthusiastically and extensively, particularly if one uses it oneself, must be having an effect. It may be salutory to recall that for a long time relaxation was assigned a critical role in desensitization, the once dominant form of behaviour therapy. However, research has shown that relaxation was quite an unnecessary part of desensitization, exposure to the feared situation being the active ingredient (Emmelkamp 1982). I am also aware that while there is now a widespread acceptance of the role of cognition in generating and maintaining behavioural change, the actual therapeutic procedures are still based on producing behavioural change first and then examining the changes in the supposedly causal cognitive processes; see Wilson's (1984) recent discussion of self-efficacy. This emphasis on cognition may, therefore, be both theoretically and therapeutically unhelpful. I would, most definitely, think it unfortunate if my discussion of a possible cognitive mechanism for part of the therapeutic effect of relaxation directed research away from the vital necessity of examining the actual behavioural changes induced by relaxation and stress management.

In summary, relaxation and stress management can lower blood pressure in mild primary hypertension, and the effects are unlikely to be artefactual and are due to some specific aspect of relaxation and stress management. However, there is no convincing evidence that relaxation either lowers blood pressure directly or reduces blood pressure reactivity, nor that it reduces dysphoric moods (in hypertensives). Furthermore, it has not been possible to demonstrate reliable effects of relaxation on conventional markers of SNS activity. It is suggested that future research should be extended to include a detailed study of both the immediate and enduring behavioural and cognitive effects of relaxation and stress management, since they may be, in part, the vehicle of therapeutic change.

Acknowledgement. The preparation of this paper was supported by a grant from the British Medical Research Council.

References

Agras WS, Horne M, Taylor CB (1982) Expectation and the blood-pressure-lowering effects of relaxation. Psychosom Med 44: 389-395

Australian National Blood Pressure Study (1982) Report of Management Committee. Untreated mild hypertension. Lancet I: 185-191

Bali LR (1979) Long term effect of relaxation on blood pressure and anxiety levels in essential hypertensive males: a controlled study. Psychosom Med 41: 637-646

Borkovec TD, Sides JK (1979) Critical procedural variables related to the physiological effects of progressive relaxation: a review. Behav Res Ther 17: 119-125

Bower GH (1981) Mood and memory. Am Psychol 36: 129-148

Brauer A, Horlick LF, Nelson B, Farquhar JU, Agras WS (1979) Relaxation therapy for essential hypertension: a Veterans Administration outpatient study. J Behav Med 2: 21-29

Christoph P, Luborsky L, Kron R, Fishman H (1978) Blood pressure, heart rate and respiratory responses to a single session of relaxation: a partial replication. J Psychosom Res 22: 493-501

Conway J (1984) Hemodynamic aspects of essential hypertension in humans. Physiol Rev 64: 617-660

Crowther JH (1983) Stress management training and relaxation imagery in the treatment of essential hypertension. J Behav Med 6: 169-187

Davidson DM, Winchester MA, Taylor CB, Alderman EA, Ingels NB (1979) Effects of relaxation therapy on cardiac performance and sympathetic activity in patients with organic heart disease. Psychosom Med 41: 303-309

Emmelkamp PMC (1982) Phobic and obsessive compulsive disorders: theory, research and practice. Plenum, New York

Esler M, Julius S, Zweifler A, Randall O, Harburg E, Gardiner H, DeQuattro V (1977) Mild high-renin essential hypertension: neurogenic human hypertension? N Engl J Med 296: 405-411

Folkow B (1982) Physiological aspects of primary hypertension. Physiol Rev 62: 347-504

Frankel BL, Patel DJ, Horwitz D, Friedwald MT, Gaardner KP (1978) Treatment of hypertension with biofeedback and relaxation techniques. Psychosom Med 40: 276-293

Glasgow MS, Gaardner KR, Engel BT (1982) Behavioral treatment of high blood pressure: II acute and sustained effects of relaxation and systolic blood pressure biofeedback. Psychosom Med 44: 155-171

Goldstein DS (1983) Plasma catecholamines and essential hypertension. An analytical review. Hypertension 5: 86-99

Goldstein IB, Shapiro D, Thananopavarn C, Sambhi MP (1982) Comparison of drug and behavioral treatments of essential hypertension. Health Psychol 1: 7-26

Hoffman JW, Benson H, Arns PA, Stainbrook GL, Landsberg L, Young JB, Gill A (1982) Reduced sympathetic nervous system responsivity associated with the relaxation response. Science 215: 190-192

Holmes DS (1984) Meditation and somatic arousal reduction: a review of the experimental evidence. Am Psychol 39: 1-10

Irvine J, Johnston DW, Jenner D, Marie GV (in press) Relaxation and stress management in the treatment of essential hypertension. J Psychosom Res

Jacob RG, Kramer HG, Agras WS (1977) Relaxation therapy in the treatment of hypertension. Arch Gen Psychiatry 34: 1417-1427

Johnston DW (1982) Behavioural treatment in the reduction of coronary risk factors: Type A behaviour and blood pressure. Br J Clin Psychol 21: 281-294

Jorgensen RS, Houston BK, Zurawski RM (1981) Anxiety management training in the treatment of essential hypertension. Behav Res Therapy 19: 467-474

Julius S, Esler M (1975) Autonomic nervous cardiovascular regulation in borderline hypertension. Am J Cardiol 36: 685-696

Kazdin AE, Wilcoxon L (1976) Systematic desensitization and non-specific treatment effects: a methodological evaluation. Psychol Bull 83: 729-758

King NJ (1980) The therapeutic utility of abbreviated progressive relaxation: a critical review with implications for clinical practice. In: In: Hersen M, Eisler RM, Miller PM (eds) Progress in behavior modification, vol 10. Academic, New York, pp 147-182

Lang R, DeHof KA, Meurer W, Kaufmann J (1979) Sympathetic activity and transcendental meditation. J Neural Transm 44: 117-135

Lehrer PM (1982) How to relax and how not to relax: a reevaluation of the work of Edmund Jacobsen-I. Behav Res Ther 20: 417-428

Libo LM, Arnold CE (1983) Relaxation practice after biofeedback therapy: a long-term follow-up study of utilization and effectiveness. Biofeedback Self Regul 8: 217-228

Linden W (1984) Psychological perspectives of essential hypertension. Karger, Basel

Little BE, Hayworth J, Benson P, Hall F, Beard RW, Dewhurst J, Priest RG (1984) Treatment of hypertension in pregnancy by relaxation and biofeedback. Lancet I: 865-867

Lo CR, Johnston DW (1984) The self-control of the cardiovascular response to exercise using feedback of the product of interbeat interval and pulse transit time. Psychosom Med 46: 115-125

Luborsky L, Crits-Cristeph P, Brady JP, Kron RE, Weiss T, Cohen M, Levy L (1982) Behavioral vs. pharmacological treatment for essential hypertension: a needed comparison. Psychosom Med 44: 203-214

Marie GV, Lo CR, Van Jones J, Johnston DW (1984) The relationship between arterial blood pressure and pulse transit time during dynamic and static exercise. Psychophysiology 21: 521-527

McGrady AV, Yonker R, Tan SY, Fine TH, Woerner M (1981) The effect of biofeedback-assisted relaxation on blood pressure and selected biochemical parameters in patients with essential hypertension. Biofeedback Self Regul 6: 343-354

McNair DM, Lorr M (1964) An analysis of mood in neurotics. J Abnorm Soc Psychol 69: 620-627

Michaels RR, Huber MJ, McCann DS (1976) Evaluation of transcendental meditation as a method of reducing stress. Science 192: 1242-1244

Obrist PA, Light KC, McCubbin JA, Hutcheson JS, Hoffer JL (1979) Pulse transit time: relationship to blood pressure and myocardial performance. Psychophysiology 16: 292-301
Patel C (1975a) Twelve month follow-up of yoga and biofeedback in the management of hypertension. Lancet I: 62-64
Patel C (1975b) Yoga and biofeedback in the management of "stress" in hypertensive patients. Clin Sci Mol Med 28 [Suppl]: 171-174
Patel C (1977) Biofeedback-aided relaxation and meditation in the management of hypertension. Biofeedback Self Regul 2: 1-41
Patel C, North WRS (1975) Randomized controlled trial of yoga and biofeedback in the management of hypertension. Lancet II: 93-95
Patel C, Marmot MG, Terry DJ (1981) Controlled trial of biofeedback-aided behavioural methods in reducing mild hypertension. Br Med J 282: 2005-2008
Pollack AA, Weber MA, Case DB, Laragh JH (1977) Limitations of transcendental meditation in the treatment of essential hypertension. Lancet I: 71-72
Sackett DL, Haynes RB (1976) Compliance with therapeutic regimes. John Hopkins University Press, Baltimore
Seer P, Raeburn JM (1980) Meditation training and essential hypertension: a methodological study. J Behav Med 3: 59-73
Shoemaker JE, Tasto DL (1975) The effects of muscle relaxation on blood pressure of essential hypertensives. Behav Res Ther 13: 29-43
Southam MA, Agras WS, Taylor CB, Kraemer HC (1982) Relaxation training: blood pressure during the working day. Arch Gen Psychiatry 39: 715-717
Steptoe A (1981) Psychological factors in cardiovascular disorders. Academic, London
Steptoe A, Ross A (1982) Voluntary control of cardiovascular reactions to demanding tasks. Biofeedback Self Regul 7: 149-166
Stone E, DeLeo J (1976) Psychotherapeutic control of hypertension. N Engl J Med 294: 80-84
Surwit TS, Shapiro D, Good MI (1978) Comparison of cardiovascular biofeedback, neuromuscular biofeedback and meditation in the treatment of borderline essential hypertension. J Consult Clin Psychol 46: 252-263
Tasto DL, Huebner LA (1976) The effects of muscle relaxation and stress on the blood pressure levels of normotensives. Behav Res Therapy 14: 89-91
Taylor CB, Farquhar JW, Nelson E, Agras WS (1977) Relaxation therapy and high blood pressure. Arch Gen Psychiatry 34: 339-342
Taylor CB, Agras WS, Schneider JA, Allen RA (1983) Adherence to instructions to practice relaxation exercises. J Consult Clin Psychol 51: 952-953
Teasdale JD (1983) Change in cognition during depression - psychopathological implications: discussion paper. J R Soc Med 76: 1038-1044
Wadden TA (1983) Predicting treatment response to relaxation therapy for essential hypertension. J Nerv Ment Dis 171: 683-689
Wadden TA (1984) Relaxation therapy for essential hypertension: specific or nonspecific effects. J Psychosom Res 28: 53-61
Wilson CT (1984) Fear reduction and the treatment of anxiety disorders. In: Wilson CT, Franks CM, Brownell KD, Kendall PC (eds) Annual review of behavior therapy, theory and practice, vol 9. Guildford, New York, pp 95-131

Hypertension: Biobehavioral Influences and Their Implications for Treatment

M. A. CHESNEY and G. W. BLACK[1]

Behavioral factors in essential hypertension have been investigated from two perspectives. Early studies focused on a search for dispositional characteristics that might constitute a "hypertensive personality." More recently, behavioral studies of hypertension have focused on its relationship to psychosocial stress. For the most part, these two lines of investigation have been pursued independently. In the first two sections of this paper, literature relevant to these two perspectives will be briefly reviewed. In the third section, preliminary data from a study of behavioral interventions for hypertension that suggest an integration of these two perspectives will be presented. Finally, implications of this model for biobehavioral approaches to blood pressure (BP) control will be discussed.

The Hypertensive Personality

Investigators throughout the twentieth century have described a cluster of attitudes or dispositions that characterize hypertensives. As with the early descriptions of behaviors related to coronary heart disease (Von Dusch 1868; Osler 1910), these proposed hypertensive attitudes were based on clinical observations rather than on empirical research. For example, in 1919, Moschowitz reported hypertensives as having a "restrained" type of personality. The first comprehensive account of the hypertensive personality was advanced by Alexander (1939, 1950). According to Alexander, hypertensives are caught in a central conflict between hostile impulses and passive-dependent needs. They characteristically fail to express anger; as a result, they experience tension, which leads to somatic changes and eventually to hypertension.

Relying on interview ratings, early investigations into the hypertensive personality drew conclusions consistent with Alexander's perspective. In three of these studies, hypertensives were found to be lower in assertive behavior and more obsessive-compulsive than psychiatric controls, and more depressed and anxious than medical/surgical patients (Gildea 1949; Gressel et al. 1949; Saslow et al. 1950). Wolf and Wolff (1946, 1951) observed a discrepancy between the overt behavior of hypertensives during interviews and clinical ratings of their unexpressed, underlying feelings. Specifically, the hypertensive individual was described as a person who presented a superficial affability to please others, while harboring suspicious attitudes and a desire to act aggressively. Similarly, Binger (1951) observed suppression of hostility in conjunction with passivity, dependence, and submissiveness. Al-

1 Department of Behavioral Medicine, SRI International (Stanford Research Institute), 333 Ravenswood Avenue, Menlo Park, CA 94025, USA

Biological and Psychological Factors in Cardiovascular Disease
Ed. by T. H. Schmidt, T. M. Dembroski, and G. Blümchen

though intriguingly consistent, these studies were not conducted in a double-blind fashion, and the findings therefore have to be interpreted with caution.

Later studies used standard personality inventories to assess characteristics of essential hypertensives. In one investigation (Pilowsky et al. 1973), the Edwards Personality Preferences Schedule (EPPS) and the Illinois Personality Assessment Test (IPAT) were given to unmedicated male hypertensives. The results indicated that the hypertensives were emotional, tense, unstable, and insecure. Of the subscales of these tests, The EPPS Deference and Abasement scales were directly correlated with BP. Using the Sixteen Personality Factor Questionnaire (16 PF; Catell et al. 1970), Harburg and his associates (Harburg et al. 1964) studied college men undergoing health examinations in which BP was examined in both home and school settings. Subjects with sustained elevated BP across settings were described as possessing "a self-image that may portray a basic conflict of wanting to assert oneself and yet being unable to do so" (Harburg et al. 1964).

To investigate personality characteristics of hypertensives, Baer et al. (1979) developed a brief self-report questionnaire from the behavior ratings of hypertensives listed by Harris and Singer (1967), and administered this scale to 335 normotensives and 332 essential hypertensives. The results indicated that hypertensives describe themselves as more hostile and tense or anxious than normotensives. The authors concluded that their findings were not consistent with the concept of anger suppression as prevalent in hypertensives. Their interpretation of suppression, however, was one of *denial* of anger. Rather than denial, the literature suggests that hypertensives experience as much hostility and anger as normotensives, or more, but that hypertensives express their anger outwardly or behave aggressively less often than normotensives. This distinction between hostile attitudes or feelings and hostile behaviors was reinforced by studies showing significant correlations of BP with feelings of hostility, but not with hostile or aggressive behavior (Esler et al. 1977; Whitehead et al. 1977).

More recently, Spielberger and his associates have examined anger expression and BP using the Anger Expression (AX) Scale (Spielberger 1985). In one of these studies, Johnson (1984) obtained systolic and diastolic measures for 1114 high school students and found significant *negative* correlations between the AX subscale that measures anger expression and BP for both males and females. Conversely, significant *positive* correlations were observed between BP and the AX subscale that assesses anger suppression. Thus, these findings support the concept of a relationship between BP and holding anger in. They also are consistent with the findings of an earlier study (Sullivan et al. 1981a, 1981b) that used the Anger-in/Anger-out Scale (Harburg et al. 1973) and reported a threefold greater prevalence rate of anger-in among adult, unmedicated hypertensives, compared with age-matched normotensives. Although the differences were not as marked, hypertensives were more anxious and depressed than normotensives. Differences in hostility were not found, suggesting that the relationship of anger and hostility to BP may be stronger for the *suppression* of these emotions.

There is evidence that inhibited anger may be especially characteristic of a subset of hypertensives, i.e., those who have high plasma renin activity (Esler et al. 1977). In a study of 31 patients with essential hypertension and 32 age-matched normotensives, significant differences in suppressed hostility as measured by the Anger-in/Anger-out Scale (Harburg et al. 1973) were found only between the normotensives and those hypertensive patients with high plasma renin activity. Esler and his colleagues (1977) wrote, "the patients with high-renin essential hypertension as a group were controlled, guilt-prone and submissive with a high level of unexpressed anger." Similarly, Perini et al. (1982) divided hypertension patients into two groups: those with high resting adrenaline and those with high resting noradrenaline. They observed the high-noradrenaline group to have more aggressive feelings, but to externalize them less often and to be less assertive than either the group with high adrenaline or a control group of normotensives. That the personality profiles of the high-noradrenaline and high-renin patients are similar may reflect the direct association between noradrenaline and renin. Taken together, these studies suggest that the relationship between BP and personality, if present, may be specific to a subgroup of hypertensives and may be mediated by neuroendocrine factors.

Some studies have failed to confirm the validity of a hypertensive personality of inhibited anger or aggression (see Lewinsohn 1956; Ostfeld and Lebovitz 1959; Cochrane 1969, 1973; Mann 1977). After finding no association between neuroticism and hypertension, Cochrane (1969) argued that prior findings may have reflected mood artificially influenced by medication. In support of this suggestion, Cochrane (1973) found no relationships between BP status and scores on the Maudsley Personality Inventory or on the Hostility and Direction of Hostility Questionnaire taken by volunteers in a heart disease prevention program. Similarly, Ostfeld and Lebovitz (1959) and Lewinsohn (1956) failed to distinguish between hypertensives and controls using the Minnesota Multiphasic Personality Inventory (MMPI). However, this scale is designed to measure more severe psychopathology than the others studied.

Despite negative findings, many studies of the hypertensive personality taken together point to suppressed anger or hostility as a prominent personality characteristic among individuals with essential hypertension. Beyond this summary statement, interpretations of etiological significance of these personality factors are difficult. The majority of studies are correlational and do not take into account the course of hypertension. That is, the studies do not distinguish between borderline and sustained hypertension conditions, which may have different psychological correlates. Little attention is paid to whether subjects are taking antihypertensive medications, many of which do have effects on mood states. In many of the early studies, the experimenter knew that the subjects had been diagnosed as having essential hypertension. The later studies using objective questionnaire techniques avoided this problem but remain correlational. Therefore, they may be revealing characteristics of individuals who are aware that they have been "labeled" hypertensive by the medical community. A study comparing hypertensive outpatients with normotensive outpatients suggests that "labeling" can have a significant impact on behavior and perhaps on BP. Specifically, Keane and his colleagues (Keane et al. 1982) found that a group of hypertensive patients responded less assertively than a nonpatient comparison group but similarly to a normotensive patient (medical/surgical) group. The authors suggested that the unassertive behavior displayed by both patient groups is a direct or indirect *effect* of chronic illness and the dramatic personality and behavioral changes that often accompany it. In contrast to this report, Sullivan and his colleagues (1981) found essential-hypertensive patients to be inwardly angry, anxious, and slightly depressed, whereas patients with secondary hypertension (pheochromocytoma), while also aware of their hypertension, did not share these characteristics.

One major research program that avoided some of these correlational and labeling pitfalls pointed again to suppressed anger and hostility as a personality variable relevant to hypertension. Harburg and his colleagues (Gentry et al. 1973; Harburg et al. 1973) proposed that suppressed hostility may be implicated in the greater prevalence of essential hypertension among black Americans. Suppressed hostility was assessed by presenting subjects with hypothetical provocative situations and obtaining self-reports about anger expression and about resultant guilt. The failure to express anger was found to be associated with elevated diastolic BP levels for all men, regardless of race. Labeling is not an issue because these BP levels, while elevated, were not necessarily in the hypertensive range, so only a small fraction of the subjects were "labeled" hypertensive. In subsequent analyses of this data set (Gentry et al. 1982), failure to express anger was also associated with elevated BP in women. An alternative style of handling anger provocation, referred to as "reflective coping," which involves keeping situations in perspective and responding in a constructive rather than an aggressive manner, was associated with lower BP levels (Harburg et al. 1979).

In a series of laboratory experiments, Hokanson and his associates directly investigated the effects of anger expression on BP in normotensive subjects. In one study, Hokanson observed that systolic BP increased when an experimenter harassed and frustrated subjects during an arithmetic computation. When subjects were given an opportunity to express their frustration or anger with counteraggression (delivering shocks to the experimenter), the BP tended to fall (Hokanson and Shetler 1961). A further study (Hokanson and Burgess 1962) revealed that counteraggression lowered BP only when the experimenter was presented as low in status (i.e., as a student), whereas counteraggression against a high-status experimenter (i.e., introduced as a professor) sustained the elevated BP. Although conducted with normotensive subjects, these studies again point to anger as a characteristic influencing BP. The prolonged BP elevation observed with the counteraggression against the high-status experimenter may have reflected the subjects' perception of the situation as one in which anger and hostility should be suppressed.

In addition to the cross-sectional research comparing personality characteristics of hypertensive subjects with those of other groups, and the laboratory research indicating a relationship between anger and its expression among normotensives, during the last decade longitudinal studies have provided additional support for the role of anger and suppressed hostility in hypertension. A 5-year prospective study of 10000 Israeli male civil service workers (Kahn et al. 1972) revealed that two of the nine significant predictors of incidence of hypertension were questionnaire items stating that workers would "restrain retaliation" and "brood" if hurt by a superior. McClelland (1979) observed that suppressed hostility, measured as "inhibited power motive" (a strong dispositional need for power in combination with a strong dispositional need to control overt aggressive expressions of this need) predicted elevated BP in a 20-year longitudinal study of 67 Harvard graduates. Most recently, a 25-year follow-up (Barefoot et al. 1983) of 255 medical students who had completed the MMPI while in medical school revealed that 13 of the 20 who developed hyper-

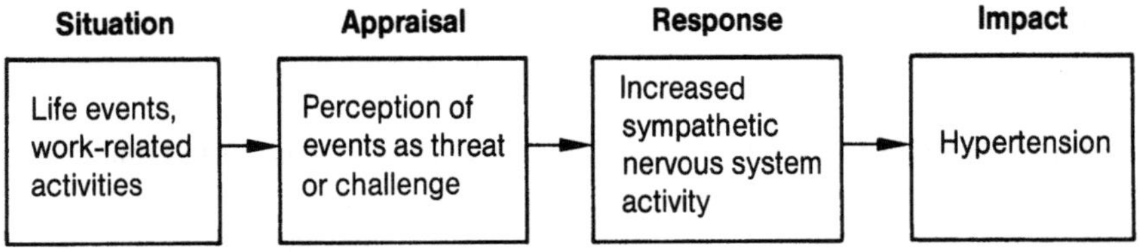

Fig. 1. Proposed model of the relationship of stress and hypertension

tension during the follow-up period had scores above the median on a hostility subscale (Cook and Medley 1954) of the MMPI.

In summary, as recent reviews of this literature conclude (Weiner 1977; Harrell 1980; Diamond 1982; Manuck et al. 1985), it is notable that the preponderance of available research suggests problems of anger or suppressed hostility as characteristics of some hypertensive patients.

Stress and Hypertension

Behavioral research in hypertension during recent years has focused on the relevance of psychosocial stress to the pathogenesis of hypertension. Evidence for a relationship between stress and hypertension is drawn from a number of epidemiological and observational studies. As reviewed by Kaplan (1978), at least 22 populations living in small, cohesive, protected societies have been found to have low BP levels that do not increase with age. In contrast, those who migrate to more western - and presumably more stressful - societies show BP levels that increase with age.

Certain work groups, such as air traffic controllers, who are known to be exposed to considerable stress in their work, have been shown to develop hypertension at rates significantly greater than those of comparison groups. For example, air traffic controllers were found to be five times as likely as nonprofessional pilots to develop hypertension (Cobb and Rose 1973). Other studies in the occupational setting have indicated that chronic or repeated exposure to an environmental stressor, industrial noise, is associated with increased prevalence of hypertension (Parvizpoor 1976; Jonsson and Hansson 1977; Andren et al. 1980). Animal models examining BP effects of chronic stress induced by avoidance conditioning and social crowding have confirmed the stress-hypertension association (Shapiro 1982).

The presumed pathway linking stress to BP, as shown in Fig. 1, involves environmental situations, such as life events or work-related activities, that the subject perceives as stressful, which in turn lead to increased sympathetic nervous system responses by one or more neurogenic pathways. The specific nature of this relationship and its integration with such factors as cardiac output, peripheral resistance, and the renin-angiotensin-aldosterone system in development and maintenance of hypertension remain elusive. As noted by Shapiro (1980), problems in quantifying behavioral stimuli, the retrospective or cross-sectional nature of most studies, and, in the majority of human research, a reliance on studies of acute stress are some of the reasons why these issues remain unresolved. Although studies of acute BP responses to stress do not necessarily apply to the development of this chronic condition, the research showing enhanced BP responses to certain psychological (see Drummond 1983) and physical stressors (see Hull et al. 1977) by normotensives and hypertensives often support the theory that excessive BP responses to stress may contribute to the development and maintenance of hypertension.

Confirmation of the hypothesis that enhanced cardiovascular responses to psychosocial stress is associated with increased risk of hypertension requires prospective studies. The only such studies have examined whether responses to the cold pressor test predict subsequent development of hypertension, and these yielded inconsistent results. This lack of convincing evidence has been attributed to the selection of the cold pressor task as an inappropriate stressor (Hastrup et al. 1982), perhaps because it involves alpha-adrenergic arousal. A potential alternative to prospective research designs involves the comparison of BP responses to stress in offspring of hypertensives and offspring of normotensives. Research relying on this design has reported significantly greater responses to stressors, such as reaction time (Hastrup et al. 1982) and mental arithmetic (Falkner et al. 1979), by offspring of hypertensives than by offspring of normotensives. These tasks are discussed in terms of their evoking beta-adrenergic reactivity and "active coping," in contrast to the cold pressor, which is perceived as involving "passive coping." Thus, as was the case with the literature on personality characteristics and hypertension, the relationship between stress and hypertension appears to be a complex one in which additional variables come into play, such as the type of stressor (e.g., beta-adrenergic vs. alpha-adrenergic). Additional variables, such as family history and the stage of hypertension (e.g., borderline or recently diagnosed mild hypertension as opposed to established moderate hypertension) are also likely to complicate any casual relationships between stress and hypertension.

Individual Characteristics: Mediating the Stress-Hypertension Relationship

The two behavioral factors in hypertension, i.e., personality and stress, have been studied in independent, parallel lines of research. Recent research suggests a model in which personality or behavioral characteristics, such as anger, mediate the relationship between stress and hypertension. This revised model, shown in Fig. 2, incorporates such behavioral or personality characteristics as hostility and unexpressed anger as factors that influence the appraisal of situations. Whether or not the excessive sympathetic arousal associated with stress is activated depends on whether these situations are appraised as stressors. For example, individuals who are high in hostility may more often perceive certain situations as stressors or challenging than individuals not high in hostility. Similarly, with individuals who suppress their feelings of hostility and do not effectively communicate their anger, these situations are more likely to remain unresolved, leading to sustained perceptions of stress and the resulting sympathetic arousal.

As yet, there is no direct evidence that anger and hostility mediate the relationship between stress and hypertension. However, support for the proposed model is contributed to by the research of Dembroski and his colleagues (Dembroski et al.

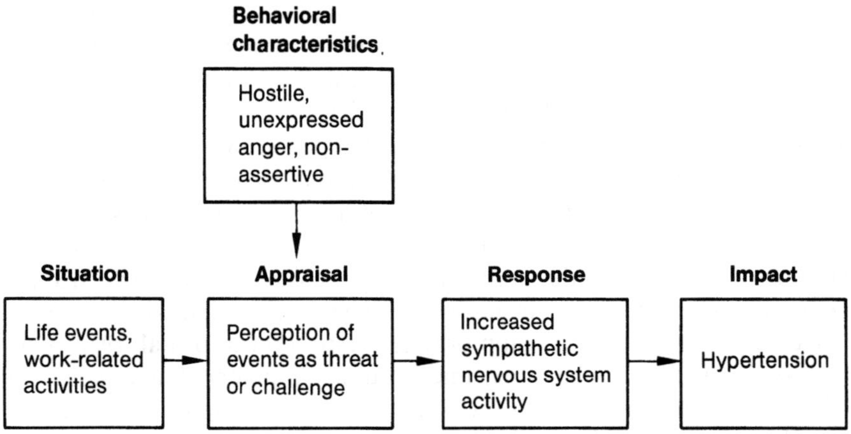

Fig. 2. Proposed model of the relationship of stress, behavior, and hypertension

1978; Dembroski et al. 1979). In a study of 50 male college students (Dembroski et al. 1978), subjects were presented with three tasks after being classified as Type A or Type B on the basis of the Type A structured interview (SI; Chesney et al. 1980). These tasks consisted of a choice reaction-time task in which instructions placed an emphasis on the importance of quick, accurate responding, a video "pong" game, and a series of difficult anagrams. As had been observed in other research discussed elsewhere in this volume, Type A subjects showed significantly greater cardiovascular arousal than Type B subjects in response to these tasks. Of particular interest here, the subjects' answers and speech stylistics during the SIs were rated for components of Type A behavior, including hostility. This permitted an examination of the influence of hostility on the relationship between the stressors and cardiovascular responses. The results clearly demonstrated that hostility was significantly related to systolic BP and heart rate responses to the stressors. Thus, hostility was found to influence cardiovascular reactivity to stress.

A subsequent study by these investigators (Dembroski et al. 1979) further confirms the influence of hostility on reactivity and provides support for another element in the proposed model, i.e., the role of hostility in the appraisal of situations as stressors. In this study, 84 male students were presented with the cold pressor test and a choice reaction-time task under both low challenge and high challenge conditions. The level of challenge in these tasks was varied by modifying the task instructions. The low-challenge instructions were delivered in a neutral tone of voice and implied that the task was routine and involved little difficulty. Conversely, the high-challenge tasks were presented with a crisp tone of voice and emphasized difficulty, i.e., the need for "will power" during the cold pressor task and the importance of speed and accuracy during the reaction-time task.

Subjects classified as Type A were found to respond to both the tasks with greater cardiovascular arousal than their Type B counterparts; a finding similar to that in the previous study (Dembroski et al. 1978). Also, as in the previous study, the subjects' SIs were rated for stylistic components, and a composite hostility/competitiveness score was obtained for each subject. The proposed model would predict that hostile/competitive subjects, tending to perceive a wider range of tasks as challenging, would appraise even the low-challenge situations as stressors and show greater cardiovascular responses to these conditions than subjects low in hostility/competitiveness. Consistent with this prediction, the more hostile/competitive subjects showed greater systolic and diastolic BP responses to the cold pressor test presented under low challenge, and greater systolic BP responses to the reaction-time task presented under low challenge than did their less hostile/competitive counterparts. In contrast to the differences in cardiovascular responses to the tasks under the low-challenge conditions that were observed between these two groups, there were no differences between the groups in response to the tasks under high challenge. This suggests that the more hostile subjects perceived even the milder challenges as stressors.

A related report of greater cardiovascular reactivity to laboratory stressors among normotensive individuals who are assessed to be high in anger was presented by Saab and her associates (Saab et al. 1983). In this study, subjects were classified as either high heart-rate reactors or low heart-rate reactors based on responses across three stressors: a competitive reaction-time task played with a harassing and deceitful confederate, a speech performance task with evaluation, and a mental arithmetic task presented under time pressure. Given the known intercorrelations among indices of cardiovascular arousal, it is not surprising that high heart-rate reactors tended also to show higher BP responses to the tasks than the low heart-rate reactors. However, of interest here, the subjects who showed the high heart rates in response to the tasks also scored significantly higher on the Trait Anger Scale (Spielberger 1985) than the subjects who showed the lower cardiovascular responses to the tasks. Thus, as in the studies by Dembroski and his associates (1978, 1979), anger or hostility was correlated with cardiovascular response to stress, a finding in support of the role of hostility as a mediator in the relationship between stress and sympathetic arousal.

While noting the significant results with regard to cardiovascular arousal and anger, as assessed by the Trait Anger Scale, the authors (Saab et al. 1983) cast doubt on their findings because parallel results were not observed with anger scores they obtained using the Novaco Anger Arousal Scale (Novaco 1975). Although both these scales purport to assess anger, there are differences between them that may have contributed to the observed incongruity. The Novaco Anger Arousal Scale instructs subjects to indicate the degree to which they would feel angered if confronted with various anger-provoking situations. This scale does not take into account how often subjects have in fact been confronted by these situations. The Trait Anger Scale, on the other hand, assesses the frequency with which subjects typically feel angry and may be a more direct measure of anger as a personality characteristic. In the context of the proposed model, which refers to subjects with high levels of hostile or angry feelings more readily perceiving and appraising situations as stressors than subjects with lower levels of these feelings, the Trait Anger Scale may be more appropriate.

The research discussed thus far in this section examined cardiovascular arousal in response to stressors in normotensive subjects. Sullivan and his associates (1981 a, b) conducted a similar, though small-sample, study comparing hypertensive and normotensive subjects. In their research, 15 essential-hypertensive patients and

13 normotensive volunteers (the number of normotensive subjects increased to 20 by the time of their second report; Sullivan et al. 1981 b) were given the Anger-in/Anger-out Scale (Harburg et al. 1973) and the Trait form of the State-Trait Anxiety Inventory (Spielberger et al. 1970). They were then presented with two stressors in the laboratory, a mental arithmetic task and an isometric hand-grip test. As reported earlier in this chapter, there was a significantly greater prevalence of subjects obtaining high scores on anger-in among the hypertensives than among the normotensives. However, the relationship between anger-in and BP and plasma noradrenaline response to the two stressors, although in the expected direction, was not significant.

Among the hypertensive patients, however, those with anxiety scores above the median had significantly larger increases in noradrenaline and systolic BP responses to mental stress and hand grip than the hypertensives with lower anxiety scores (Sullivan et al. 1981 b). Moreover, both hypertensive and normotensive subjects with the combination of higher anxiety scores and anger-in had an enhanced increase in systolic BP to hand grip. Noting that they observed a much smaller cardiovascular response across their subjects to the mental arithmetic task than that found by others, Sullivan and his colleagues concluded that their mental stressor was "inadequate." This task did differ from that used by others (see Saab et al. 1983) in that subjects were not under time pressure and were not interrupted and corrected when they committed errors in arithmetic. Another drawback of this study is the small sample size, a factor that often presents limitations when analyses involve interaction effects.

The research reviewed in this section, taken together, suggests that cardiovascular reactivity to potentially stressful situations is influenced by personality or behavioral variables such as anger, hostility, and perhaps anxiety. Thus, situations that are considered by some to present a challenge or stress may not necessarily evoke enhanced cardiovascular arousal in all subjects. The impact of these situations on the cardiovascular system appears to be determined, at least in part, by a dynamic relationship involving individual difference variables such as hostility and anger.

The literature reviewed in the first section of this chapter indicates that problems of anger or suppressed hostility may be characteristic of some hypertensive patients. The research just reviewed further indicates that these same characteristics are related to enhanced cardiovascular responses to stress, and one study (Dembroski et al. 1979) implies that these characteristics may influence the appraisal of situations as stressors. Thus, one mechanism by which personality or behavioral characteristics are associated with elevated BP and hypertension may be through their effect on the cognitive appraisal or perception of situations as stressful. This proposed model, by suggesting a dynamic interaction among stress, personality, and BP, has implications for the behavioral and pharmacological treatment of hypertension.

Implications for Behavioral and Pharmacological Approaches to Blood Pressure Control

There is increasing interest in the treatment of essential hypertension with behavioral or nonpharmacological treatments that might avoid or reduce the need for medication, or enhance BP control with medication. The biobehavioral model of stress, behavior, and hypertension proposed in the preceding section has implications for behavioral as well as pharmacological antihypertensive treatments. To date, behavioral approaches have included dietary sodium restriction, weight reduction, physical training, and, of relevance here, treatments based on relaxation or biofeedback training. The theoretical foundation for this training is that it offers skills that can be applied to reduce the impact of stress on hypertension. The efficacy of these treatments was demonstrated first in case studies and later in more systematic clinical investigations (for reviews see Johnston, this volume; Shapiro and Goldstein 1982; Shapiro and Jacob 1983). Although many of these studies were relatively small and inadequately controlled, they suggest that behavioral interventions based on relaxation and biofeedback result in modest declines in BP. For example, a number of studies (see Jorgensen et al. 1981; Southam et al. 1982; Crowther 1985) have found relaxation to be significantly more effective in lowering BP than no-treatment control conditions.

Despite these and other findings of clinical significance, the observed effectiveness of these treatments is not directly related or specific to the association between stress and hypertension. As Shapiro and Jacob (1983) noted in a recent review of behavioral approaches to hypertension, although these studies "force us to the conclusion that earlier work provided evidence for a specific effect of relaxation or biofeedback, indications for the importance of nonspecific "relationship" variables are also present. This should hardly surprise us, however, as nonspecific variables are also important for successful pharmacological therapy."

These observations, along with the studies attesting to the effectiveness of behavioral interventions, indicate the need for larger controlled studies and clinical trials. In a recent statement, the National Heart, Lung, and Blood Institute (1983) of the U. S. Department of Health and Human Services recognized the need to demonstrate the efficacy of these treatments in clinical trials but recommended that the treatment of mild essential hypertension be initiated with behavioral or other nonpharmacological interventions as long as these treatments were effective in maintaining BP control.

The biobehavioral model of stress, behavior, and hypertension proposed here implies that for some hypertensive patients, behavioral interventions might include a focus on anger. Specifically, attention could be paid to identifying situations that solicit or provoke anger, to patient attitudes and characteristics that influence their perceptions of these situations, and to patients' subsequent responses, including their feelings and behaviors as well as enhanced sympathetic arousal.

One possible behavioral approach to anger management might be similar to that proposed by Novaco (1975, 1979). In this approach, patients would be trained to attend to and monitor their feelings of anger and the situations in which these feelings are aroused. This monitoring would result in the identification of anger-provoking situations, some of which probably would occur frequently. The patients then would be trained to question their appraisal or perception of these situations as anger-provoking with the therapist serving as a model of alternative, less anger-provoking appraisals. For example, Novaco's treatment strategy teaches the patient "not to take things personally" (1979). Thus, patients who become angry while driving an automobile if slower-moving automobiles accelerate just when they begin to pass would be trained to question their habitual appraisal that the other drivers are doing this purposely to avoid being overtaken. Alternative appraisals would be considered such as that the other drivers accelerate because the act of being overtaken indicates to them that they are impeding traffic.

In the treatment approach developed by Novaco, patients would also be taught new, more adaptive skills for coping with or responding to anger-provoking situations. Among these skills, emphasis is given to training in effective, assertive communication. Novaco (1979) also teaches relaxation as one of these skills. Anger is accompanied by feelings of tension and arousal of the sympathetic nervous system. Moreover, relaxation skills provide patients with a strategy they can use to delay habitually quick responses to provocation. This delay is essential to permit patients to consider alternative appraisals and to recall newly acquired coping strategies. In the final and perhaps the most important phase of treatment, patients practice implementing their new, alternative appraisals of situations to avoid anger provocation, and their new skills for coping with and responding to these situations.

The application of treatment approaches such as that prosposed by Novaco in the treatment of hypertension is very new. Moon and Eisler (1983) reported significantly larger reductions in systolic BP in 20 normotensive subjects trained in either the procedure developed by Novaco (1979) or a related procedure emphasizing assertive communication skills than in 20 subjects in either a problem-solving or a no-treatment control group.

If data implicating anger in hypertension continue to be generated, there will be a need for systematic research in the development and evaluation of behavioral approaches to anger management. This research and these approaches will need to address several issues that could serve as barriers to the effectiveness of treatment (Chesney 1985). These barriers include the patient's perception (which in many cases may be accurate) that the social environment reinforces rather than discourages anger. A related barrier to anger modification is the perception that anger responses are not only adaptive but necessary for achieving personal goals. These issues are important determinants of what Bandura (1977) has termed "self-efficacy" - the patient's expectations about potential treatment outcomes (expectations that determine whether treatment is sought or initiated) and the extent of effort patients will expend on treatment. Therefore, if behavioral approaches to anger do not address these barriers, patients' self-efficacy about anger management is likely to be low, and treatment effectiveness will be impeded or blocked.

The proposed model of the relationships among stress, behavior, and hypertension also has implications for the pharmacological treatment of hypertension. Beta-adrenergic blocking drugs, a mainstay of antihypertensive therapy, have also been used in the treatment of anger and rage. As reviewed by Durel and Krantz (1985), propranolol has been shown to be effective in controlling explosive outbursts of rage among organic brain dysfunction patients (Elliot 1977; Williams et al. 1982). Durel and Krantz (1985) also point out that there is evidence from animal research that beta-adrenergic blockade reduces aggressive behavior and increases positive social contacts (see Jaekel 1982).

Beta-adrenergic blockage has recently been shown to modify anger or hostile behavior in Type A individuals. In a study of coronary heart disease patients given the Type A SI (Chesney et al. 1980), those patients taking propranolol were significantly lower in intensity of several components of Type A behavior than patients not taking this beta-blocking agent (Krantz et al. 1982). Although the content of responses to the SI was not different between these two groups, the patients taking propranolol were rated lower in potential for hostility and in the display of loud or explosive and rapid or accelerated speech stylistics.

More recently, Rüddel and his colleagues have reported changes in Type A behavior in hypertensives treated with beta-blocking agents (see Schmieder et al. 1983; Rüddel and Schmieder, this volume). In one study (Schmieder et al. 1983), hypertensive patients were randomly assigned to treatment with the beta-blocking agent atenolol or to treatment with diuretics. After 1.5–2 years of therapy, 5 of 11 patients in the beta-blockade group had changed their Type A behavior toward Type B behavior, whereas none of the 9 subjects in the diuretic group showed such a change. Of particular relevance here, ratings of hostility from the SI were significantly lower after therapy in the beta-blockade group than in the diuretic group.

The research documenting the effect of beta-adrenergic blocking agents on anger and hostility suggests that these medications might be particularly appropriate in the pharmacological treatment of hypertensive patients who experience high levels of anger and hostility. Moreover, these findings suggest that anger and hostility may be factors in the mechanism by which these pharmacological agents impact BP pressure and its control.

Conclusion

Research on behavioral factors in hypertension, as with the research on behavioral factors in coronary heart disease, has brought anger and hostility to the attention of the behavioral medicine community. Undoubtedly, future research on biobehavioral aspects of cardiovascular disease will include the study of anger and hostility. This research will need to address issues involved in the experience (frequency, duration, and intensity) of these emotions, their expression (anger-in, anger-out), and the physiological mechanisms by which these emotions exert their cardiovascular effects. It is important to note that this research in all likelihood will evolve into studies of components of anger in much the same manner as research on Type A behavior has evolved into identification of its coronary-prone components (Chesney et al. 1984).

Research on biobehavioral factors in hypertension should consider two points eloquently discussed by Groen (this volume). First, the role of biobehavioral factors in coronary heart disease and its risk factors, such as hypertension, is multifaceted. Not only are there behavior patterns or personality correlates, life situations or stresses and responses, but the interrelationships among these variables are dynamic. Humans observe, appraise, interact with, and change the environment, a process that, in turn, has an impact on their physiological responses and ultimate risk of cardiovascular disease. Therefore, caution must be exercised as we subdivide this dynamic system in models such as that proposed in this paper. Stressors cannot be studied without taking into account the individual's perceptions. Similarly, the emotion of anger cannot be studied in the absence of the contextual factors that provoke it.

Second, research on the treatment of anger, particularly suppressed anger, will undoubtedly be seen in the near future. Many might argue that such intervention research is premature until definitions of anger and hostility are clarified, instruments for their measurement are developed, and physiological mechanisms have been determined. However, as was the case with the clinical trial of behavioral treatments for hypertension reported here, intervention research can generate valuable data that can be analyzed to provide insight into definitions, measurement, and mechanisms. In this capacity, intervention serves as an experimental manipulation in much the same manner as does imposing stress in laboratory research. Responses to these manipulations, including changes in behavior patterns and cardiovascular and neuroendocrine correlates of these changes, can make significant contributions to our knowledge of biobehavioral factors in coronary heart disease. However, unlike stressors studied in laboratory research, for some individuals, anger interventions also have the potential to reduce BP and coronary heart disease risk.

References

Alexander F (1939) Emotional factors in essential hypertension. Psychosom Med 1: 173-179

Alexander F (1950) Psychosomatic medicine. Norton, New York

Andren L, Hansson L, Bjorkman M, Jonsson A (1980) Noise as a contributory factor in the development of elevated arterial pressure. Acta Med Scand 207: 493-498

Baer PE, Collins FH, Bourianoff GG, Ketchel MF (1979) Assessing personality factors in essential hypertension with a brief self-report instrument. Psychosom Med 41: 321-330

Bandura A (1977) Self-efficacy: towards a unifying theory of behavioral change. Psychol Rev 84: 191-215

Barefoot JC, Dahlstrom WG, Williams RB (1983) Hostility, CHD incidence, and total mortality: a 25-year follow-up study of 255 physicians. Psychosom Med 45: 59-63

Binger C (1951) On so-called psychogenic influences in essential hypertension. Psychosom Med 13: 273-277

Cattell RB, Eber HW, Tatsuoka M (1970) Handbook for the Sixteen Personality Factor Questionnaire. Institute for Personality and Ability Testing, Champaign

Chesney MA (1985) Anger and hostility: future implications for behavioral medicine. In: Chesney MA, Rosenman RH (eds) Anger and hostility in cardiovascular and behavioral disorders. Hemisphere, New York

Chesney MA, Eagleston JE, Rosenman RH (1980) The Type A structured interview: a behavioral assessment in the rough. J Behav Assessment 2: 255-272

Chesney MA, Hecker MHL, Black GW, Rosenman RH (1984) Behavioral factors in coronary heart disease. Proceedings of the American Psychological Association, 43

Cobb S, Rose RM (1973) Hypertension, peptic ulcer, and diabetes in air traffic controllers. JAMA 224: 489-492

Cochrane R (1969) Neuroticism and the discovery of high blood pressure. J Psychosom Res 13: 21-25

Cochrane R (1973) Hostility and neuroticism among unselected essential hypertensives. J Psychosom Res 17: 215-218

Cook WS, Medley DM (1954) Proposed hostility and pharisaic-virtue scales for the MMPI. J Appl Psychol 38: 414-418

Crowther JH (1985) Stress management training and relaxation imagery in the treatment of essential hypertension. J Behav Med (to be published)
Dembroski TM, MacDougall JM, Shields JL, Petitto J, Lushene R (1978) Components of the Type A coronary-prone behavior pattern and cardiovascular responses to psychomotor performance challenge. J Behav Med 1: 159-176
Dembroski TM, MacDougall JM, Herd JA, Shields JL (1979) Effect of level of challenge on pressor and heart rate responses in Type A and Type B subjects. J Appl Soc Psychol 9 (3): 209-228
Diamond EL (1982) The role of anger and hostility in essential hypertension and coronary heart disease. Psychol Bull 92 (2): 410-433
Drummond PD (1983) Cardiovascular reactivity in mild hypertension. J Psychosom Res 27: 291-297
Durel LS, Krantz DS (1985) The possible effects of beta-adrenergic blocking drugs on behavioral and psychological concomitants of anger. In: Chesney MA, Rosenman RH (eds) Anger and hostility in cardiovascular and behavioral disorders. Hemisphere, New York
Elliot F (1977) Propranolol for the control of the belligerent behavior following acute brain damage. Ann Neurol 1: 489-491
Esler M, Julius S, Zweifler A, Randall O, Harburg E, Gardiner H, DeQuattro V (1977) Mild high-renin essential hypertension: neurogenic human hypertension. N Engl J Med 296: 405-411
Falkner B, Onesti G, Angelakos ET, Fernandes M, Langman C (1979) Cardiovascular response to mental stress in normal adolescents with hypertensive parents. Hypertension 1: 23-30
Gentry WD, Harburg E, Hauenstein L (1973) Effects of anger expression/inhibition and guilt on elevated diastolic blood pressure in high/low stress and black/white females. Proc Am Psychol Assoc 115-116
Gentry WD, Chesney AP, Gary HE, Hall RP, Harburg E (1982) Habitual anger-coping styles: I. Effect on mean blood pressure and risk for essential hypertension. Psychosom Med 44: 195-202
Gildea E (1949) Special features of personality which are common to certain psychosomatic disorders. Psychosom Med 11: 273-281
Gressel GC, Shobe FO, Saslow G, DuBois M, Schroeder HA (1949) Personality factors in essential hypertension. JAMA 140: 265-272
Harburg E, Julius S, McGinn NF, McLeod J, Hoobler SW (1964) Personality traits and behavioral patterns associated with systolic blood pressure levels in college males. J Chronic Dis 17: 405-414
Harburg E, Hauenstein LS, Chape C, Schull WJ, Schork MA (1973) Social-ecological stress, suppressed hostility, skin color, and black-white male blood pressure: Detroit. Psychosom Med 35: 276-296
Harburg E, Blakelock EH, Roeper RJ (1979) Resentful and reflective coping with arbitrary authority and blood pressure: Detroit. Psychosom Med 41: 189-202
Harrell JP (1980) Psychological factors and hypertension: a status report. Psychol Bull 87: 482-501
Harris RE, Singer MT (1967) Interaction of personality and stress in the pathogenesis of essential hypertension. Hypertension 16: 104-114
Hastrup JL, Light KC, Obrist PA (1982) Parental hypertension and cardiovascular response to stress in healthy young adults. Psychophysiology 19: 615-622
Hokanson JE, Burgess M (1962) The effects of status, type of frustration and aggression on vascular processes. J Abnorm Soc Psychol 65: 232-237
Hokanson JE, Shetler S (1961) The effect of overt aggression on physiological arousal. J Abnorm Soc Psychol 63: 446-448
Hull DH, Wolthuis RA, Cortese T, Longo MR, Triebwasser JH (1977) Borderline hypertension versus normotension: differential response to orthostatic stress. Am Heart J 94: 414-420
Jaekel J (1982) Influence of selected beta-blockers on social interaction of rhesus monkeys. Activ Nerv Sup [Suppl 3]: 528 (abstract)
Johnson EH (1984) Anger and anxiety as determinants of elevated blood pressure in adolescents. Doctoral dissertation. University of South Florida, Tampa
Jonsson A, Hansson L (1977) Prolonged exposure to a stressful stimulus (noise) as a cause of raised blood pressure in man. Lancet I: 86-87
Jorgensen RS, Houston BK, Zurawski RM (1981) Anxiety management training in the treatment of essential hypertension. Behav Res Ther 19: 467-474

Kahn HA, Medalie JH, Neufeld HN, Riss E (1972) The incidence of hypertension and associated factors: the Israel ischemic heart disease study. Am Heart J 84: 171-182
Kaplan NM (1978) Stress, the sympathetic nervous system and hypertension. J Human Stress 4 (3): 29-34
Keane TM, Martin JE, Berler ES, Wooten LS, Fleece EL, Williams JG (1982) Are hypertensives less assertive? A controlled evaluation. J Consult Clin Psychol 50 (4): 499-508
Krantz DS, Durel LA, Davia JE, Shaffer RT, Arabian JM, Dembroski TM, MacDougall JM (1982) Propranolol medication among coronary patients: relationship to Type A behavior and cardiovascular response. J Human Stress 8: 4-12
Lewinsohn PM (1956) Personality correlates of duodenal ulcer and other psychosomatic reactions. J Clin Psychol 12: 296-298
Mann AH (1977) Psychiatric morbidity and hostility in hypertension. Psychol Med 7: 653-659
Manuck SB, Morrison RL, Bellack AS, Polefron JM (1985) Behavioral factors in hypertension: cardiovascular responsivity, anger, and social competence. In: Chesney MA, Rosenman RH (eds) Anger and hostility in cardiovascular and behavioral disorders. Hemisphere, New York
McClelland DC (1979) Inhibited power motivation and high blood pressure in men. J Abnorm Psychol 88, no 2: 182-190
Moon JR, Eisler RM (1983) Anger control: an experimental comparison of three behavioral treatments. Behav Ther 14: 493-505
Moschowitz E (1919) Hypertension: its significance, relation to arteriosclerosis and nephritis and etiology. Am J Med Sci 158: 668-684
National Heart, Lung, and Blood Institute (1983) Recommendations for treatment of mild hypertension. U.S. Public Health Service publication no 411-152. US Government Printing Office, Washington DC
Novaco RW (1975) Anger control: the development and evaluation of an experimental treatment. Lexington Books, Lexington
Novaco RW (1979) The cognitive regulation of anger and stress. In: Kendall PC, Hollon SD (eds) Cognitive-behavioral interventions: theory, research and procedures. Academic, New York, pp 241-285
Osler W (1910) Lumleian lectures. Lancet I: 687, 839, 973
Ostfeld AM, Lebovits BZ (1959) Personality factors and pressor mechanisms in renal and essential hypertension. Arch Intern Med 104: 497-502
Parvizpoor D (1976) Noise exposure and prevalence of high blood pressure among weavers in Iran. J Occup Med 18: 730-731
Perini C, Amann FW, Bolli P, Buhler FR (1982) Personality and adrenergic factors in essential hypertension. In: Brod J, Liebau H, Bahlmann J (eds) Contributions to nephrology. Karger, Basel
Pilowsky I, Spalding D, Shaw J, Korner PI (1973) Hypertension and personality. Psychosom Med 35: 50-56
Saab PG, Holroyd KA, Appel MA, Upole VK, Gorking L, Stauder LJ (1983) Cardiac hyperreactivity, psychological functioning, and essential hypertension. Paper presented at the Society of Behavioral Medicine, Baltimore, March, 1983
Saslow G, Gressel GC, Shobe FO, DuBois PH, Schroeder HA (1950) Possible etiological relevance of personality factors in arterial hypertension. Psychosom Med 12: 292-302
Schmieder R, Neus H, Friedrich G, Ruddel H (1983) Beta-blockers and Type A behavior: long-term effect and methodological problems. Psychophysiology 20: 470
Shapiro AP (1982) Stress and hypertension. In: Brunner HR, Gavras H (eds) Clinical hypertension and hypotension. Dekker, New York, pp 367-386
Shapiro AP, Jacob RG (1983) Nonpharmacologic approaches to the treatment of hypertension. Ann Rev Public Health 4: 285-310
Shapiro D, Goldstein IB (1982) Biobehavioral perspectives on hypertension. J Consult Clin Psychol 50: 841-858
Southam MA, Agras WS, Taylor CB, Kraemer JC (1982) Relaxation training: blood pressure lowering during the working day. Arch Gen Psychiatry 39: 715-717
Spielberger CD (1985) The experience and expression of anger. In: Chesney MA, Rosenman RH (eds) Anger and hostility in cardiovascular and behavioral disorders. Hemisphere, New York
Spielberger CD, Gorsuch RL, Lushene R (1970) The State-trait anxiety inventory. Consulting Psychologists Press, Palo Alto, California

Sullivan PA, Procci WR, DeQuattro V, Schoentgen S, Levine D, Van Der Meulen J, Bornheimer JF (1981a) Anger, anxiety, guilt and increased basal and stress-induced neurogenic tone: causes or effects in primary hypertension? Clin Sci 61: 389s-392s
Sullivan P, Schoentgen S, DeQuattro V, Procci W, Levine D, Van Der Meulen J, Borheimer J (1981b) Anxiety, anger and neurogenic tone at rest and in stress in patients with primary hypertension. Hypertension 3: II-119-II-123
Von Dusch T (1868) Lehrbuch der Herzkrankheit. Engleman, Leipzig
Weiner H (1977) Psychobiology and human disease. Elsevier, New York
Whitehead WE, Blackwell B, DeSilva H, Robinson A (1977) Anxiety and anger in hypertension. J Psychosom Res 21: 383
Williams DT, Mehl R, Yodofsky S, Adams D, Roseman B (1982) The effect of propranolol on uncontrolled outbursts in children and adolescents with organic brain dysfunction. J Am Psychiatry 21 (2): 129-135
Wolf GA, Wolff HG (1946) Studies on the nature of certain symptoms associated with cardiovascular disorders. Psychosom Med 8: 293-319
Wolf S, Wolff HG (1951) A summary of experimental evidence relating life stress to the pathogenesis of essential hypertension in man. In: Bell EG (ed) Hypertension. University of Minnesota Press, Minneapolis

Biobehavioral Effects of Antihypertensive Monotherapy: Oxprenolol and Nitrendipine

H. RÜDDEL, R. SCHMIEDER, J. NEUS, H. NEUS, H. OTTEN, W. LANGEWITZ, and A. W. VON EIFF[1]

Abstract

In order to decide whether beta-blockers or calcium antagonists are preferable as initial antihypertensive therapy, we investigated the efficacy of monotherapy with oxprenolol (160 mg once daily) and nitrendipine (20 mg once daily) in a single-blind randomized study. Only male civil servants with mild hypertension were included ($\bar{x}=43\pm6$ years of age; $n=92$). Clinical casual blood pressure (BP) was lowered equally in both groups, as was average BP at work, as assessed by ambulatory BP monitoring with Remler M2000 ($123\pm12/81\pm14$ vs. $129\pm17/80\pm10$ mmHg). This was done after casual BP had been within the normotensive range for 3 months. At equal levels of self-reported arousal and physical activity, systolic BP was lower in patients receiving oxprenolol. In the nitrendipine group, 24% discontinued therapy because of side effects, whereas only 12% receiving oxprenolol initially reported intolerable side effects. Patients on a regimen of oxprenolol reported less intense Type A characteristics in questionnaires administered after 3 months of therapy.

During chronic therapy, BP reactivity during mental arithmetic, cold pressor test, and 100-W ergometric exercise did not differ between the two groups, except for a greater increase in diastolic BP during mental challenge in patients whe were receiving oxprenolol (Δ DBP 17 ± 7 vs. 11 ± 3 mmHg, $P<0.05$). The hemodynamic pattern to mental stress was reversed during long-term therapy with beta-blocker (before therapy stroke volume increased: Δ SV $=+9\pm20\%$; after 6 months Δ SV $=-13\pm6\%$). The calcium antagonist did not alter the hemodynamic pattern during mental challenge. Both regimens were equally effective as initial antihypertensive monotherapy. However, the behavioral and hemodynamic effects of beta-blockade were different from those of the calcium antagonist. These differences may be important in deciding which of the two alternatives could best be used in patients with mild hypertension.

Introduction

Although it is now generally accepted that even patients with mild hypertension show greater morbidity than normotensives (Kannel et al. 1971) and that most of them would benefit from antihypertensive therapy (The Management Committee 1980), we urgently need more information on particular subpopulations, such as

1 Department of Medicine, University of Bonn, Sigmund-Freud-Straße 25, 5300 Bonn 1, Federal Republic of Germany (Correspondence should be addressed to the first author)

Biological and Psychological Factors
in Cardiovascular Disease
Ed. by T. H. Schmidt, T. M. Dembroski, and G. Blümchen

persons who do not benefit from therapy with diuretics (Hypertension Detection and Follow-Up Program Cooperative Group 1979) or borderline hypertensives who do not develop sustained hypertension (Julius 1978).

In an earlier study, we suggested that middle-aged men who were hypertensive and also exhibited the Type A behavior pattern should be treated with beta-blockers instead of diuretics, because atenolol not only effectively lowered casual BP, but also led to a change in behavior patterns towards Type B characteristics when patients were retested after 4-10 weeks (Schmieder et al. 1983a). In a long-term follow-up of these patients, the behavioral effects of the beta-blocker were still found after 1.5 years, although they were less pronounced (Schmieder et al. 1983b). These results are in agreement with the results published by Krantz et al., who found a lower incidence of Type A in patients with cardiac disease on beta-blockers compared with patients on diuretics (Krantz et al. 1982). Although we found that hemodynamic responses during the Type A interview were lower in patients taking atenolol compared with patients on diuretics, we were unable to attribute these results to the different drugs, as adaptation phenomena might have introduced a bias (Neus et al. 1981).

Beta-blockers have been shown to influence BP reactions to exercise and possibly to psychosocial interaction (Franz 1980; Neus et al. 1983; Schmieder et al. 1983a). In a group of previously untreated patients with essential hypertension, we examined whether a beta-blocker (oxprenolol), and a calcium antagonist (nitrendipine), were effective in lowering clinical casual BP and average BP at work assessed by ambulatory BP monitoring, and whether the hemodynamic response to mental and physical stress following therapy with these two drugs was similar or different. Because beta-blockade has been shown to affect behavior, we examined whether oxprenolol and nitrendipine equally influenced behavior patterns like Type A behavior, and finally, whether oxprenolol and nitrendipine differed in their side effects.

Methods

All employees in the departments of the West German Federal Government had been asked to participate in a BP screening at work. BP was taken in 11000 civil servants. Those with elevated BP (exceeding 140/90 mmHg), who were not using any medication and were free from any other disease, were also asked to have BP and heart rate (HR) measured at rest and while playing a video-game (Break Out; Atari) in a "stress booth" at the worksite. BP was measured with an automatic oscillometric device (Datascope). If resting BP prior to the video-game was also elevated, the patients had a complete clinical examination in the hospital, which included history and physical examination, fundoscopy, routine biochemical analyses, urinalyses, ECG, echocardiography, and several BP readings. Only patients with mild essential hypertension were included in this study. About 2 weeks later, all patients were subjected to psychophysiological testing in the laboratory.

If three out of four casual BP readings were elevated, antihypertensive therapy was started, with subjects randomly assigned to oxprenolol 160 mg (slow release) once daily and nitrendipine 20 mg once daily in a single-blind design. Oxprenolol

Table 1. Descriptive statistics[a] of the Type A questionnaires

	$\bar{x}$	S.D.	Kurtosis	Skewness
Framingham	0.65	0.10	-0.75	0.26
Thurstone	63.3	6.16	-0.40	-0.12

[a] Intercorrelation before therapy, $r=0.11$ (n.s.), $n=80$; after 3 months, $r=0.35$ ($P<0.05$), $n=45$; after 6 months, $r=0.35$ ($P<0.05$), $n=36$

and nitrendipine were chosen because both drugs can be given once a day, thus minimizing problems with compliance. Drugs were taken during breakfast, and at night (if necessary). After 4 weeks the dosages were doubled if BP was still higher than 140/90 mmHg. After 8 weeks, the study was continued as an open clinical trial. Only patients on effective monotherapy with beta-blockers or calcium antagonists were included in this report. The patients were seen every 2 weeks until normotensive BP readings were obtained and every 4 weeks thereafter. When they had been normotensive for 3 months, mental stress testing in the stress booth was repeated, followed by ambulatory BP monitoring with the Remler unit (Remler M2000) (Neus et al. 1984). Again, 3 months after ambulatory BP monitoring, psychophysiological testing in the laboratory was repeated. The results are based on 92 patients before therapy, 46 after 3 months, and 41 after 6 months of effective monotherapy (19 on oxprenolol and 22 on nitrendipine in the 6-month group).

Before therapy, the psychophysiological stress test consisted of mental arithmetic (adding one- and two-digit numbers, played over headphones at a speed of one number per second during a 3-min period while a counter-rhythmic beat of a metronome was also played), the cold pressor test (Hines and Brown 1936; Rüddel et al. 1984a), and a submaximal exercise test on the bicycle (Schulte et al. 1985) (work load: 100 W, recumbent). On retest, another mental arithmetic test was given, consisting of adding up one- and two-digit numbers from a screen without speaking aloud, while listening to affective noise of about 85 dB (A) over 5 minutes; at 1-min intervals the elapsed time was announced to avoid adaptation. The other tests were identical before and after therapy.

In the laboratory, BP was measured with a two-probe ultrasonic device every minute (Noffke and Schirmer 1981), HR was derived continuously by ECG recording, and SV was continuously assessed by impedance cardiography, which included an editing system which controlled for artifacts. Before therapy and twice during therapy (after 3 and 6 months with normotensive casual BP), all patients were asked to fill out a battery of questionnaires, including Type A scales. The descriptive statistics of the questionnaire scales and intercorrelations of the Type A scales are shown in Table 1.

Side effects of the antihypertensive regimen were assessed by clinical interviews asking for new "events," and by questionnaires asking for the incidence of many possible drug-related side effects and their relative importance for each individual patient. During ambulatory BP monitoring, the patients filled out diaries on level of physical activity and arousal prior to the BP readings.

All statistical analyses were calculated on the IBM computer of RHRZ Bonn with Fortran, SPSS, or SAS programs. In this paper, only descriptive statistics,

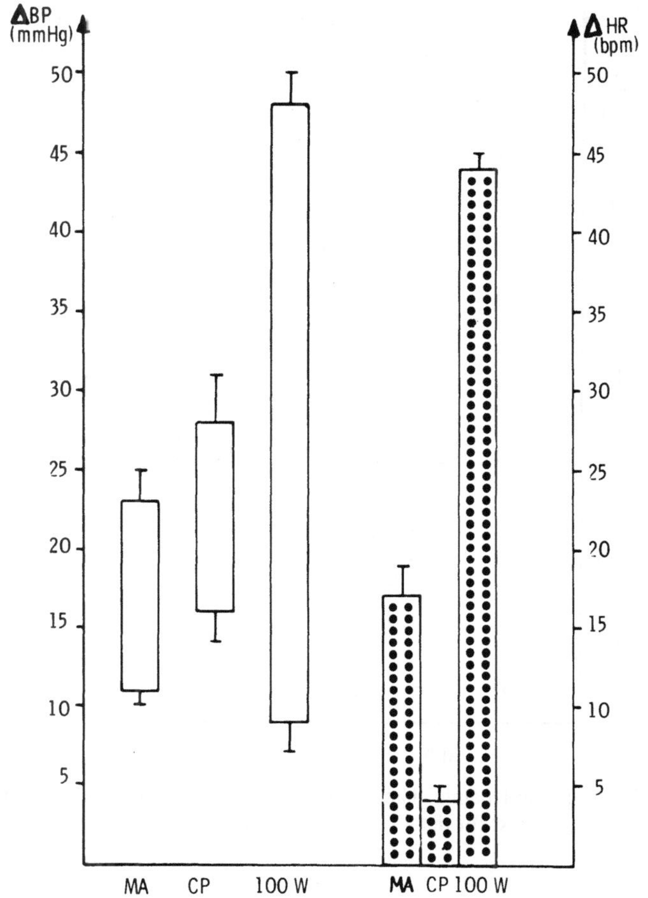

Fig. 1. Changes in BP and HR during mental arithmetic, the cold pressor test, and submaximal exercise testing (100 W) in patients with essential hypertension ($\bar{x} = 43 \pm 6$ years; $n = 89$) without therapy. *MA*, mental arithmetic; *CP*, cold pressor test; *W*, watt; *Δ BP*, increase of blood pressure from pretest baseline; *Δ HR*, increase of heart rate from pretest baseline *(right half)*

correlations, and *t*-tests (two-tailed) are reported. If not mentioned otherwise, means and standard errors of the mean are given in the figures, and means and standard deviations in the tables and in the Results section.

Informed consent to participate was obtained from each patient. All patients received copies of the reports that were sent out to their family physicians 8 weeks after beginning therapy, and after 6 and 9 months of follow-up.

Results

Hemodynamic Pattern Before Therapy

Before therapy, the patients treated with either oxprenolol or nitrendipine did not differ in age (43 ± 5 vs. 43 ± 6 years), weight (80 ± 8 vs. 82 ± 10 kg), screening BP ($153 \pm 11/98 \pm 11$ vs. $156 \pm 15/97 \pm 9$ mmHg), or lowest clinical casual BP after sitting for 5 min ($146 \pm 14/98 \pm 11$ vs. $146 \pm 14/98 \pm 11$ mmHg).

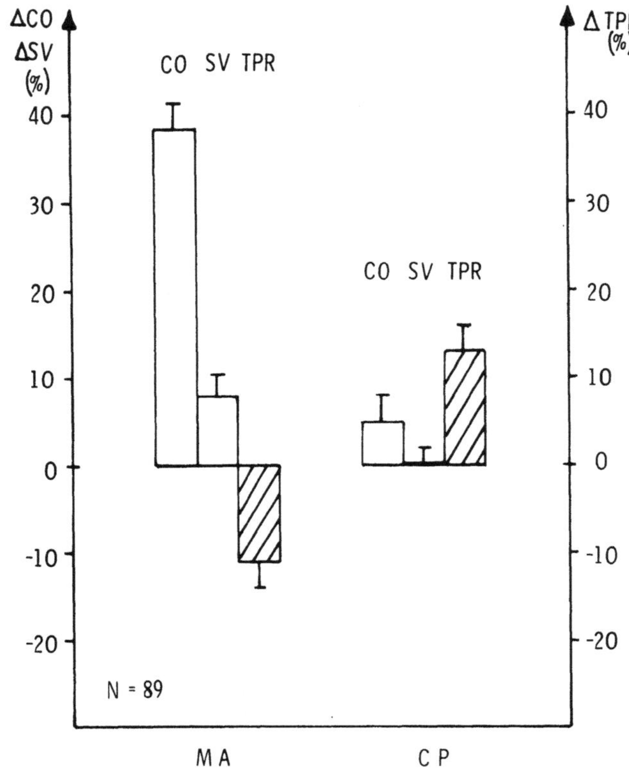

Fig. 2. Hemodynamic changes during mental arithmetic and the cold pressor test before therapy (n=89; see text for details). *CO*, cardiac output; *SV*, stroke volume; *TPR*, total peripheral resistance

During the mental arithmetic test, BP increased 23±11/11±5 mmHg, HR 18±11 bpm (see Fig. 1), with an increase of 9%±20% in SV. Total peripheral resistance (TPR) decreased 11±20% (see Fig. 2). The response to the cold pressor test was a BP increase of 28±12/16±8 mmHg and an increase of 4±6 bpm in HR; SV remained unchanged, and TPR increased 12±15% (see Figs. 1 and 2).

BP Response to Monotherapy with Oxprenolol and Nitrendipine

The two groups did not differ in their average response to antihypertensive therapy (for details see Rüddel et al. 1984b). When the patients had maintained normotensive casual BP for 3 months, they did not differ in BP during the video-game (142±7/92±6 vs. 146±10/96±10 mmHg). Resting BP prior to the video-game was somewhat higher in patients receiving the calcium antagonist (132±7/88±7 vs. 127±6/83±5 mmHg, $P<0.05$ for both systolic and diastolic BP). Resting HR was lower in those treated with oxprenolol (64±9 bpm), and in these patients HR did not increase during the video-game (65±8 bpm), whereas HR increased to 80±19 bpm in those patients treated with nitrendipine. Resting HR in the group on calcium antagonists was 72±12 bpm. Ambulatory BP monitoring revealed no differences in average systolic or diastolic BP at work (123±12/81±14 vs. 129±

Table 2. Systolic BP at different levels of self-reported physical activity and arousal in patients on nitrendipine and oxprenolol

	Self-reported physical activity				Self-reported arousal			
	1	2	3	4	1	2	3	4
Nitrendipine	129±2	127±3	135±5	144±5	128±2	129±2	133±3	147±11
Oxprenolol	120±1	123±2	130±3	130±4	118±1	125±2	130±3	131± 7
	$f(1{,}413)=8$; $P<0.001$				$f(1{,}374)=5$; $P<0.01$			

17/80±10 mmHg; for details see Schmieder et al. 1985). However, when all BP readings at the same level of self-reported physical activity and arousal were analyzed between the two regimens, those patients who were receiving oxprenolol had lower systolic BP than those receiving nitrendipine. Diastolic BP was not different between the two groups (see Table 2). Additionally, during the 1st hour of ambulatory BP recording, systolic BP was lower in those patients who were receiving oxprenolol (126±12 vs. 139±12 mmHg; $P<0.05$).

After 6 months of monotherapy the patients in both groups were not significantly different in any of the analyzed biochemical variables. Although patients receiving oxprenolol had slightly higher cholesterol levels (268±44 vs. 264±60 mg/dl), this difference was not statistically significant. The two groups did not differ in casual BP, either when measured after being seated for 5 min or when measured standing. Also, resting BP, obtained in the laboratory during the second psychophysiological examination, was not different between the two groups (124±12/82±8 vs. 125±13/83±7 mmHg). The BP responses to the second mental arithmetic test (23±11/16±6 vs. 21±9/11±3 mmHg) and the cold pressor test (31±18/19±7 vs. 23±13/15±8 mmHg) were not different between groups, except for the increase in diastolic BP during mental arithmetic, which was significantly greater in patients on beta-blockers ($t=2.82$; $P<0.05$). Also, hemodynamic patterns under mental challenge after long-term therapy were different between the two groups. During the first mental arithmetic test, patients receiving oxprenolol increased cardiac output (CO) by 5%±11%, while decreasing SV (−13%±6%), leading to an increase in TPR of 11%±8%. Those receiving nitrendipine increased CO by 42%±36% with an increase in SV (+2.5%±30%), resulting in a decrease of 9%±13% in TPR (the differences in CO, SV, and TPR all being significant at $P<0.05$). For further details see Schmieder et al. 1986 and Rüddel et al. 1986a.

Behavioral Aspects of Monotherapy with Oxprenolol and Nitrendipine

Although the Type A scales used in this study each assess different aspects of the Type A behavior pattern, patients on the oxprenolol regimen reported a significantly lower level of Type A characteristics in both questionnaires after 3 months: Framingham 0.58±0.12 vs. 0.67±0.07, $P<0.05$; Thurstone 60.6±4.8 vs. 65.5±6.0, $P<0.01$; see Fig. 3. After 6 months of therapy, however, the two groups differed only in the Framingham Type A score (0.60±0.12 vs. 0.67±0.07; $P<0.05$). (Details in Rüddel et al. 1986b).

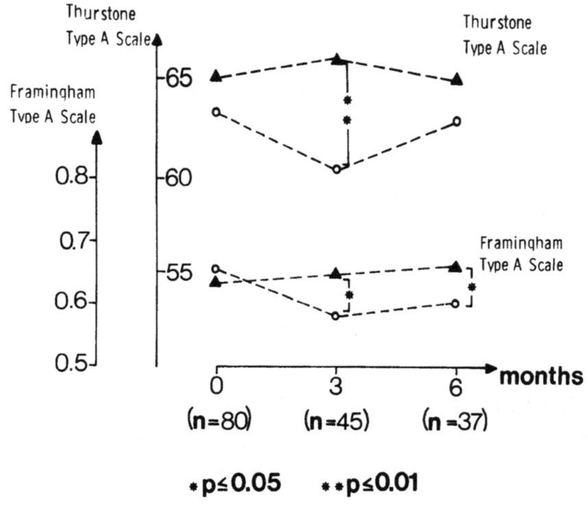

Fig. 3. Comparison of Type A questionnaire scores before and during therapy with beta-blockers (O---O) and calcium antagonists (▲---▲)

Side Effects of Oxprenolol and Nitrendipine

In this particular sample, patients reported a high incidence of subjective reactions before therapy, and 75% in each group reported some form of adverse reaction during the first 3 months of treatment. In the nitrendipine group, 24% of the patients discontinued treatment because of side effects, while in the oxprenolol group only 12% discontinued therapy.

Discussion

In this study we demonstrated that oxprenolol and nitrendipine effectively lowered clinical casual BP well into the normotensive range. This finding corroborated the results of a large number of studies (for summaries see: Taylor 1983; Deck et al. 1984; Julius 1984), and suggests that both drugs can effectively be used in an initial antihypertensive regimen. Also, it has been suggested that average BP at work is a better predictor of BP-related target organ damage than clinical BP (Perloff et al. 1983). Efficient initial antihypertensive drugs should also decrease BP at work. It is well documented that chronic treatment with oxprenolol decreases daytime BP without significantly influencing BP variability (Miller-Craig et al. 1983). Our results show that both drugs lower average BP at work equally well. A closer analysis of the results also confirms previous observations that the therapeutic effect of oxprenolol, which is a non-selective beta-blocking agent with both membrane-stabilizing and intrinsic sympathomimetic properties, is in excess of the plasma half-life of the drug. Although average BP at work and the BP between 10 a.m. and 5 p.m. was not different between the two groups, patients on the oxprenolol regimen had lower systolic BP during the first hour of ambulatory BP recording and lower BP at rest before the recording device was attached. This suggests that chronic treatment with oxprenolol results in a continuously lowered BP, independent of the time when the drug is taken, whereas BP decreases to stable levels within 1 h after nitrendipine is administered, even in long-term therapy. The clinical consequences of these observations are not yet clear. One might speculate that the central effect of chronic beta-blockade could explain these impacts on BP, HR, and HR variations, and these central effects of beta-blockers might also explain the behavioral effects of these drugs (Krantz 1984).

In this study we could corroborate our previous findings that beta-blockers alter Type A characteristics. However, it is not yet clear whether this effect is constant over time. In an earlier study with atenolol, we found an impact on Type A characteristics as assessed by the structured interview (SI), even after 1.5 years, whereas in this study the differences after 6 months of effective monotherapy between patients receiving oxprenolol and those receiving nitrendipine were no longer significant. In this study we administered Type A questionnaires instead of repeating the SI. The two methods assess different aspects of coronary-prone behavior (selected references: Dembroski et al. 1979; Matthews 1982; Steptoe 1984), which may be differentially effected by beta-blockade. These methodological problems in longitudinal studies have not yet been examined in detail. When the SI is given repeatedly over a relatively short time period, patients may be irritated when hearing the same questions again, and latency to the questions, voice stylistics, and the content of the answers will probably shift towards Type A characteristics.

One might have expected that the central effect of beta-blockade would also result in a reduced BP response to mental challenge, as is observed during submaximal exercise testing (Deck et al. 1984). However, the increase in systolic BP to mental challenge did not differ between the two groups in this study, and diastolic BP increased even more in those patients receiving oxprenolol. Also, during mental challenge, BP increases paralleled increases in TPR in patients receiving beta-blockers as long-term therapy. Lund-Johansen et al. have demonstrated during the last 15 years that TPR at rest rises after the initiation of therapy with propranolol or other beta-blockers. However, TPR at rest returns to pretreatment levels after several weeks of therapy (for example, see Lund-Johansen 1974; Man in t Veld and Schalenkamp 1982). Physiologically it is not surprising that the BP increase during mental challenge in patients on effective beta-blockade is predominantly the result of an increase in TPR, whereas the BP increase during mental challenge without medication is predominantly the result of an increase in CO. Most researchers found no attenuation of the BP response to mental challenge in hypertensives on beta-blockade (Neus et al. 1983). When BP responses during the mental arithmetic task before therapy, and during the modified mental arithmetic plus noise test after long-term monotherapy are compared with BP reactions of healthy normotensive males (von Eiff and Neus 1980; von Eiff et al. 1981), who show a smaller increase in BP, it seems obvious that at least systolic BP hyperreactivity to mental challenge, (which is a reproducible phenomenon and found mostly in early hypertension; Rüddel et al. 1984c; Schulte and Neus 1984), is not altered differently when oxprenolol is compared with nitrendipine.

Conclusion

In summary, we conclude that oxprenolol and nitrendipine could both be used as initial antihypertensive therapy. The rate of side effects leading to the withdrawal of the drug was high when the calcium antagonist was given, but only 12% when patients received the beta-blocker. If initial change of the Type A behavior pattern is desired, the beta-blocker would have advantages over the calcium antagonist. However, more information on the long-term impact of an increase in TPR during mental challenge (Eliot and Buell 1983) in patients on chronic beta-blockade is needed.

To help the clinician decide which drug to choose for antihypertensive therapy, we urgently need more long-term studies that also consider the time course of both the behavioral and the biological effects of the drugs, including the impact on the established risk factors for coronary heart disease such as cholesterol and Type A behavior patterns.

Acknowledgments. This research was supported by grants from Ciba-Geigy Co. and Bayer AG. The authors wish to give special thanks to Ulrike Pinger for support in organizing the hypertension clinic; to Gisela Schröder, Bettina Mahlow, Ulrike Pinger, and Hildegard Meller for excellent technical support; and to Brigitte Engels for never-ending help in preparing protocols and reports. Their thanks also go to Dr. Mckinney and Neva Burroughs for help in preparing this manuscript.

References

Dembroski TM, McDougall JM, Musante L (1979) The structured interview and questionnaire methods of assessing coronary-prone behavior in male and female college students. J Behav Med 2: 71-83

Eliot RS, Buell JC (1983) The role of the CNS in cardiovascular disorders. Hosp Pract 18: 189-199

Franz EW (1980) Differential antihypertensive effect of acebutolol and hydrochlorothiazide/amiloride hydrochloride combination on elevated exercise blood pressure in hypertensive patients. Am J Cardiol 46: 301-305

Hines EA, Brown GE (1936) The cold pressor test measuring the reactivity of the blood pressure: data concerning 571 normal and hypertensive subjects. Am Heart J 11: 1-9

Hypertension Detection and Follow Up Program Cooperative Group (1979) Five-year findings of the Hypertension Detection and Follow Up Program. I. Reduction in mortality of persons with high blood pressure, including mild hypertension. JAMA 242: 2572-2577

Julius S (1978) Borderline hypertension: clinical and pathophysiological significance. Adv Intern Med Pediatr 41: 51-84

Julius S (ed) (1984) Pharmamanual. A comprehensive guide to the therapeutic use of Trasicor®. Karger, Basel

Kannel WB, Gordon T, Schwartz MJ (1971) Systolic versus diastolic blood pressure and risk of coronary disease. Am J Cardiol 27: 335

Krantz D (1984) Behavioral effects of beta-blockers. In: Zanchetti A, Turner P (eds) Selected topics of cardiovascular drug therapy. Springer, Berlin Heidelberg New York Tokyo

Krantz DS, Durel LA, Davia JE, Shafter RT, Arabian JM, Dembroski TM, McDougall JM (1982) Propranolol among coronary patients: relationship to Type A behavior and cardiovascular response. J Human Stress 8: 4-12

Lund-Johansen P (1974) Hemodynamic changes at rest and during exercise in long-term beta-blocker therapy of essential hypertension. Acta Med Scand 195: 117-121

Man in t Veld AJ, Schalekamp MADH (1982) How intrinsic sympathomimetic activity modulates the haemodynamic responses to β-adrenoceptor antagonists. A clue to the nature of their antihypertensive mechanism. Br J Clin Pharmacol 13: 245S-257S

Matthews KA (1982) Psychological perspectives on the Type A behavior pattern. Psychol Bull 91: 293-329

Miller-Craig MW, Mann S, Bala Subramanian V, Altman DG, Raftery EB (1983) The effects of Oxprenolol on ambulatory intra-arterial blood pressure in essential hypertension. Eur J Clin Pharmacol 24: 713-721

Neus H, von Eiff AW, Friedrich G, Heusch G, Schulte W (1981) Das Problem der Adaptation in der klinisch-therapeutischen Hypertonieforschung. Dtsch Med Wochenschr 106: 622-624

Neus H, von Eiff AW, Friedrich G, Rüddel H, Schulte W (1983) The influence of beta-blockers and diuretics on blood pressure response. Z Kardiol 72: 617-621

Neus H, Gogolin E, Langewitz W, von Eiff AW (1984) Intermittent ambulatory blood pressure recordings in children. Methodological aspects and influence of family history on hypertension. Klin Wochenschr 62

Noffke H-U, Schirmer G (1981) Indirekte Blutdruckmessung mit einem Zwei-Sonden-Ultraschall-System. Biomed Tech 26: 162-167

Perloff D, Sokolow M, Cowan R (1983) The prognostic value of ambulatory blood pressures. JAMA 249: 2792-2798

Rüddel H, McKinney ME, Buell JC, Eliot RS (1984a) Reliabilität des cold pressor tests. Herzmedizin 7: 39-43

Rüddel H, Schmieder R, Langewitz W, Neus J, Wagner O, von Eiff AW (1984b) Efficacy of nitrendipine as baseline antihypertensive therapy. J Cardiovasc Pharmacol 6: 114-116

Rüddel H, Neus H, Langewitz W, Schulte W, von Eiff AW (1984c) Mental stress testing in the physician's office and in the field. In: Steptoe A, Rüddel H, Neus H (eds) Applied cardiovascular psychophysiology. Springer, Berlin Heidelberg New York Tokyo: 66-76

Rüddel H, Schmieder R, von Eift AW (1986a) Wirkung einer Langzeit-Monotherapie mit Nitrendipin auf hämodynamische Veränderungen unter psychischer Belastung. In: Distler A (Ed) Calciumantagonisten in der Hochdruck-Therapie. Schattauer Verlag, Stuttgart: 163-178

Rüddel H, Schmieder R, Langewitz W, Otten H (1986b) Effect of antihypertensive therapy with beta-blockers on type A behavior and hostility. Psychosom Med 48: 295 (abstract)

Schmieder R, Neus H, Friedrich G, Rüddel H, von Eiff AW (1983a) The influence of beta-blockers on cardiovascular reactivity and Type A behavior pattern in hypertensives. Psychosom Med 45: 417-423

Schmieder R, Neus H, Friedrich G, Rüddel H (1983b) β-blockers and Type A behavior. Long-term effect and methodological problems. Psychophysiology 20: 470 (abstract)

Schmieder R, Rüddel H, Langewitz W, Neus J, Wagner O, von Eiff AW (1985) The influence of monotherapy with Oxprenolol and Nitrendipine on ambulatory blood pressure in hypertensives. J Clin Exp Hypertension A7: 445-454

Schmieder RE, Rüddel H, Neus M, Messerli FH, von Eift AW (1986) Disparate hemodynamic response to mental challenge after antihypertensive therapy with beta blockers and calcium entry blockers. Am J Med (to be published)

Schulte W, Neus H (1984) Hemodynamics during emotional stress in borderline and mild hypertension. Eur Heart J 4: 803-809

Steptoe A (ed) (1984) Report of the discussion meeting on current research on the Type A behavior pattern in Europe. Concerted action "breakdown in human adaptation". Commission of the European Communities, Medical and Public Health Research Programme, Brussels

Stoepel K, Deck K, Ingram C, Corsing SH, Vanov SK (1984) Safety aspects of long term nitrendipine therapy. J Cardiovasc Pharmacol 6 (suppl 7): S 1072-1075

Taylor SH (1983) Oxprenolol in clinical practice. Am J Cardiol 52: 340-420

The Management Committee (1980) The Australian therapeutic trial in mild hypertension. Lancet I: 1261-1267

von Eiff AW, Neus H (1980) Verkehrslärm und Hypertonie-Risiko. Erste Mitteilung. MMW 122: 894-896

von Eiff AW, Friedrich G, Langewitz W, Neus H, Rüddel H, Schirmer G, Schulte W (1981) Verkehrslärm und Hypertonie-Risiko. Hypotholamus-Theorie der essentiellen Hypertonie. Zweite Mitteilung. MMW 123: 420-423

Type A, Social Context, and Adaptation to Serious Illness: A Longitudinal Investigation of the Role of the Family in Recovery from Myocardial Infarction

M. WALTZ[1]

Introduction

Over the last decade, numerous investigators have suggested the necessity for developing and testing multifactorial, biobehavioral models of the etiology of disease. These models have been envisaged as including groups of variables at the socioenvironmental, psychological, neuroendocrine, cardiovascular, and immunological levels. In a recent review article, Cohen (1980) notes the increasing interest in the role of psychosocial factors as one part of such a multifactorial model, but also criticizes the lack of specification of how such relationships are mediated psychologically and physiologically (see Herd and Weiss 1983). A growing body of research points to the important role of the family in a future biobehavioral model of the precipitation and prevention of physical illness. This research includes the family of origin and the family of adult life and the psychological and social factors linking these segments of the life history of the individual (see Groen, this volume). Speculation suggests that the individual's resources for coping with stress are dependent on certain characteristics of the family of origin and the family of adulthood (e.g., closeness to parents and marital intimacy). In general, the gratification of socioemotional needs in the family throughout the life span may be viewed as a pivotal factor influencing the development of a positive self-concept and the ability to cope at the psychological level with stressful life situations. For this reason, Solomon (1984) exhorts medical researchers to explore early childhood experiences to the same extent as is currently done by psychiatrists.

Solomon's suggestions should be extended to adult experiences in the marital dyad. Epidemiological studies have consistently found a relationship between marital status and mental health (e.e., Pearlin and Johnson 1977) and age-adjusted mortality. Marital status may be interpreted as a crude indicator of the health-protecting influence of marital intimacy, as well as for the stress of divorce and widowhood. The Israeli civil servant study (Medalie et al. 1973) is one of the few investigations to explore possible pathological and protective effects of different kinds of marital situations. The encouraging findings from this Israeli study suggest the need for a more penetrating exploration of pathogenic and salutogenic aspects of the marital bond. Possible avenues of future research might include biobehavioral mechanisms related to the following:

1. The gratification of socioemotional needs and the provision of a sense of social embeddedness in adequate spouse relations.

1 Oldenburg Cardiac Rehabilitation Study, University of Oldenburg, 2900 Oldenburg, Federal Republic of Germany

Biological and Psychological Factors
in Cardiovascular Disease
Ed. by T. H. Schmidt, T. M. Dembroski, and G. Blümchen

2. The contribution of marriage to coping with work-related and other stressors and to successful adaptation at the psychological level.

Envisaged here are the long-term behavioral, neuroendocrine, and physiological impacts of positive affective states arising from marital happiness and the sense of existential security the conjugal bond provides. Much research effort has been expended in studying the neuroendocrine markers of negative affect and stress, but little on their positive counterparts (i.e., the endocrine and immunological markers of happiness and positive affective states).

A second area of marital research should focus on the spouse relationship as a source of socioenvironmental stress and pathological influences. In comparison with the extensive research on work-related stressors, chronic marital problems have scarcely been investigated in relation to cardiovascular disease. The results to be reported on in this paper indicate an important inhibitory role of marital conflict in coping with stressful life situations. A life event, when superimposed on already existent stressors, which have become a fixture of a person's life, may easily exhaust the coping resources available to the individual. Unresolved problems-in-living in the marital sphere appear, in addition, to facilitate adaptation breakdown because of their impact on the individual's sense of self-worth and self-efficacy. Failure in the important area of marriage provides the individual with irrefutable evidence of his own incompetence and lack of control over the social environment. Mediated by psychological mechanisms related to the self-concept, chronic marital stressors may have an impact on life-style (e.g., smoking and alcohol consumption), as well as on pathological processes in various body systems (e.g., essential hypertension or immunosuppression).

In the Oldenburg Cardiac Rehabilitation Study the above-mentioned positive and negative dimensions of marital context were investigated relative to cognitive adaptation, the self-concept, psychological well-being, smoking behavior, and somatic outcomes. Serious illness and its sequelae were conceptualized as an adverse life-event. Processes of cognitive and emotional adaptation were explored in four marital contexts. Extreme Type-A individuals appeared to be disproportionately located in the conflictual marital context. The Jenkins Activity Scale (JAS) scores and marital context discriminated between patients doing well and doing poorly at 6 and 12 months after onset of illness; both influenced cognitive adaptation and health perceptions.

Role of the Family in a Multifactorial Model of Disease

Biobehavioral models of the stress/disease intermesh for guiding future empirical research should include putative mechanisms at the psychosocial, neuroendocrine, and cardiovascular levels. The major focus of such conceptual frameworks from the viewpoint of behavioral scientists is the identification of factors that influence how individuals cope with environmental stressors. Research on coping suggests mechanisms linking the social environment with the maintenance of health, as well as with the development of disease. A growing body of empirical findings allow speculation as to a central role of the family in the stress process. Successful coping at the psychological level is most probably facilitated if the family fulfills certain functions related to cognitive and emotional adaptation, which have been subsumed under the concept of *social support*.

At the cognitive level, the family influences how the individual perceives and interprets the stressful life situation confronting him. In a coherent, stable, and supportive family environment adverse life events, it may be postulated, will be perceived as less threatening and more controllable. A *sense of reliable alliance*, or the feeling that one has significant others who are always available in time of need, enhances feelings of mastery and self-efficacy. Secondly, the family may be viewed as a refuge, into which the individual can withdraw for psychological recuperation. Thirdly, cognitive processes of adaptation can be shared jointly through confiding, consolation, and reality reassurances. These cognitive supports provided by an adequate social environment would seem to play a pivotal role in how well the individual is able to restructure his assumptive world in the wake of a major life change. Individuals lacking such a family context do not receive the types of social supports discussed and may, therefore, arrive at an unrealistic appraisal of the stressors confronting them, i.e., extreme denial or pessimism.

At the level of emotional management, supportive families meet the increased needs of the individual for love, affection, and social embeddedness. Symbolic and object losses can be mourned together. Sustained by a sense of reliable alliance with significant others, the threats to the individual of an adverse life event are less menacing. Anxiety, and other forms of psychological distress are diminished because of the mere presence of others, but also through supportive social interaction, such as "getting things off one's chest." This emotional support afforded to the individual acts as a buffer against the emotional impact of the stressor and aids him in maintaining or regaining a reasonable emotional belance. An important psychological mechanism, in this respect, is the maintenance of a positive self-concept, including a sense of self-efficacy. Emotional support and maintenance of self-esteem, on the one hand, and a sense of reliable alliance, on the other, are provisions of close interpersonal relationships which would seem to bolster a positive view of the self. These mechanisms might be termed "love-based" and "efficacy-based" self-esteem. As Pearlin et al. (1981) have suggested, the maintenance of a positive self-concept plays an important role in the stress process. Feelings of worthlessness and loss of control are very probably precursors of adaptation breakdown caused by inadequate social support.

Background of the Study

Slightly over 1000 patients from 213 hospitals agreed to take part in the study. Male patients under the age of 60 years with a verified first myocardial infarction were selected. Data was gathered by means of written questionnaires at three points in time thus far:

T1: several weeks after the heart attack in the hospital
T2: 6-8 months after myocardial infarction
T3: approximately 1 year after onset of illness

Further data on process and outcome variables are to be collected at approximately annual intervals in the future. Data were also obtained from the spouse and physician.

Of the 1000 patients who began the study, 85% completed the second questionnaire, yielding a total of 841 respondents. An equally high rate of return was obtained for the third wave of the study, with a total sample of 604 patients. The attrition was to a small extent disproportionate among the self-employed. Other patient characteristics, including physical status, were investigated, and no noticeable differences in rate of attrition were found. The high motivation of the patients to participate in and continue in the study was not always shared by their spouse and family doctor. Among the former, 529 completed the extensive spouse questionnaire, and 470 family doctors returned the medical questionnaire at T3. The analysis presented in this paper includes only the 604 patients for whom we have longitudinal data from the three patient questionnaires and data on their medical status in the hospital.

The content of the patient and spouse questionnaires centered around four areas:

1. Perceptions of illness and its impact on major social roles
2. The family and work situation, especially chronic role strains and perceived social support in these areas
3. The impact of the illness on physical, psychological and social well-being, as well as on the patient's self-concept. (These variables were intended to monitor the recovery process and outcome.)
4. Experiences with medical treatment and the social bureaucracy

The information thus gained enabled us to observe how the physical impairment and disability experienced by the patient were related to his mental images of illness. The physical reality of the patient and the changing definition of his life situation could then be investigated relative to process variables, such as self-esteem, sense of mastery, and psychological distresss. An extensive list of outcome variables enabled us to observe how physical factors and social context influenced recovery.

A Conceptual Outline of the Stress Process following Serious Illness

Illness as a Source of Stress

A myocardial infarction entails for many patients, if not most, a profound change in their way of life, which is both undesirable and over which they have very little control. It can thus be conceived of as an "adverse life event," as this term has been used in stress research. A change in health status and, in particular, a decrease in functional capacity can have a wide-reaching impact on the individual's total life. It may force the individual to seek early retirement or to lower his career aspirations significantly. If work was an important part of his life and a source of personal reward, then the inability to continue as before can be a very undesirable life change. The same is true of leisure and social activities that were major aspects of the quality of life of the individual. Changes in social roles in the family (e. g., as head of household, breadwinner, and sexual partner) can form part of the impact of the illness on the total life space of the individual concerned. The loss of previous good health and functional capacity, as well as the forfeit of customary social roles and activities, are major characteristics of serious illness as a life event. These losses very often affect the emotional balance of the patient.

A second defining characteristic of serious illness as a life event is the threat it poses to the person and his psychological future. Cohen and Lazarus (1980) have described the threatening aspect of illness as follows: "Being ill can involve threats not only to life and physical well-being, but also to one's self-concept, belief systems, social and occupational functioning, values, commitments, and emotional equilibrium." Fears about cardiac death, a second infarction, and progression of the illness, are a source of stress and anxiety for most patients. Together with uncertainty about the future, they form a severe threat to the individual and his previous way of life.

Lazarus has defined the term "primary appraisal" as the individual's assessment of the loss and threat confronting him as the result of an aversive life event (Cohen and Lazarus 1980). This concept was operationalized in our study by a scale containing 18 items. These items cover various aspects of the illness:

Threats to life and fears of dying itself
Fears of progression of the illness
Permanent physical changes and the loss of functional capacity
Physical pain and negative symptoms of illness
Threats to personal independence and future plans
Threat to interpersonal relationships
Threat to future happiness

This 18-item scale measures important stresses associated with illness and is closely related to the patient's health perceptions and assessment of social disability. The variable *primary appraisal* was used to monitor processes of cognitive adaptation in the study.

The Social Context of Illness

The family and, especially, the patient's spouse are postulated to be critical factors influencing adaptation to myocardial infarction. The family is, for most patients, the most important source of moral encouragement, positive feedback, and esteem-bolstering interaction following their illness. The provisions of close interpersonal relationships, such as the marital dyad, have been termed "social support." Turner et al. (1983) defined the concept as follows: "Social support thus refers to the clarity or certainty with which the individual experiences being loved, valued, and able to count on others should the need arise." The experience of meaning very much to one's spouse or that she is genuinely involved with the patient and his illness provide the individual with a sense of social embeddedness and reliable alliance in an uncertain and incoherent world following the heart attack. These would seem to be critical characteristics of the social context in which recovery takes place. Social support has been shown to be an important resource of the individual in coping with the stress of serious illness.

The family may also be a source of chronic role strain to the individual. Social stress originating in an unsatisfying and conflict-ridden marital relationship may very possibly have been a contributory factor in the etiology of the cardiac condition, and can very well influence the patient's recovery following serious illness. Chronic role strains in the family, as in other areas of life, have been postulated by Pearlin et al. (1981) to lead to an erosion of the self-concept, influencing the development of feelings of low self-worth and lack of mastery over one's life. Pearlin et al. (1981) described this process as follows: "The enduring presence of noxious circumstances, precisely of the kind represented in role strains, apparently functions to strip away the insulation that otherwise protects the self against threats to it (Kaplan 1970). Persistent role strains can confront people with dogged evidence of their own failures . . . ." Such long-term stressors are fundamental factors in the life history of the patient, influencing his mental health and assessment of the supportiveness of his social environment at the outset of the stress process. They are also seen to be a critical factor influencing the provision of social support by the spouse and acceptance of it by the patient during the stress process. Pearlin et al. have studied chronic role strain in relation to the self-concept and vulnerability for neurotic disorders. This paper focuses on its effects on the primary appraisal of illness and on psychological well-being (Bradburn 1969).

Two types of chronic role strains will be studied - marital conflict and the emotional isolation of the patient. Marriage is viewed as the relationship in which most adults' needs for affection, intimacy, and belongingness are met. The gratification of these socioemotional needs is considered a major type of social support, emanating from everyday interaction in an emotionally close conjugal relationship. A lack of intimacy and genuine involvement in the marital dyad preclude the gratification of these needs and lead to feelings of emotional isolation. Chronic role strains, the provision of social support during the recovery process, and the quality of the marital relationship are thus postulated to be inseparable characteristics of the social context in which adaptation to illness takes place. Marital stress and social support should not be viewed as independent causal agents in our view. An emotionally satisfying relationship would seem to be characterized by the provision of adequate social support and a low level of chronic role strain. The opposite is the case in a marriage in which the patient is dissatisfied with his spouse. Instruments were developed to measure the quality of the marital relationship, conflict and other chronic role strains, and experienced social support during the recovery process. The first scale focuses on a negative assessment of the marriage and on dissatisfaction with the patient's marital relationship. The interrelation between these three groups of variables and their influence on psychological well-being will be analyzed.

Psychological Well-being

The term "psychological well-being," as developed by Bradburn (1969), is a malleable concept focusing on negative and positive aspects of everyday life. *Positive affect,* or the first dimension of psychological well-being, mirrors positive experiences in the family and other life areas. *Negative affect* reflects the problems, worries, and role strains of the individual. Serious illness and its sequelae change the life-style of

Table 1. Association of negative affect with measures of the emotional impact of illness at 1 year after infarction (T3)

Emotional Impact	Gamma coefficients
Feeling of uselessness	0.80
Loss of sense of coherence	0.77
Lonely	0.85
Sense of isolation	0.73
Troubled, worried	0.84
Tense	0.59
Gloomy, dejected	0.82
Bored	0.75
Social anomie	0.49
Loss of social prestige	0.70

$n=604$; $P \leqq 0.001$.

the individual and may considerably restrict his ability to experience success in daily activities and in positive interaction with others. This is the case if disability leads to a loss of major social roles and their corresponding social networks. Illness may also have an impact on the interpersonal relationships with significant others, either strengthening or weakening these social ties. Charmaz (1973) emphasizes the loss of positive daily experiences following serious illness and its impact on the individual's feeling of self-worth. At the same time, serious illness engenders feelings of uncertainty, uselessness, disorientation, anxiety, and powerlessness. Viney (1983) has termed this psychological impact "the images of illness."

Negative affect was found to have considerable overlap conceptually with negative images of illness, as shown in Table 1. These mental images of illness may be a direct result of the experience of physical impairment and disability or of its wider impact on the patient's life (e.g., forced retirement and loss of the work role). Social withdrawal and the forfeit of prized roles and activities are linked to social isolation, which is manifest in boredness, loneliness, and a sense of marginality.

The scale (five items) may, therefore, be viewed as a global indicator of the total emotional impact and psychological distress following serious illness. In our longitudinal study, negative affect may be considered to be tapping unsuccessful coping, and the development of cardiac invalidism, a form of adaptation breakdown. Positive affect, in contrast, may be viewed as mediating the successful psychosocial transition of the patient to his postinfarction situation in the long run. Individuals with high levels of positive affect have been able to restructure their lives in the family, in the world of work, or as a retired person, so as to have sufficiently happy experiences in everyday life. The Bradburn scales have been suggested as sensitive instruments for measuring the emotional aspect of quality of life (cf. Zautra 1983).

Major Variables and their Causal Ordering

Three groups of exogenous variables: medically-defined illness, social context, and the coronary-prone behavior pattern are posited as determinants of the two dimensions of psychological well-being. The cognitive processing of the life-event illness

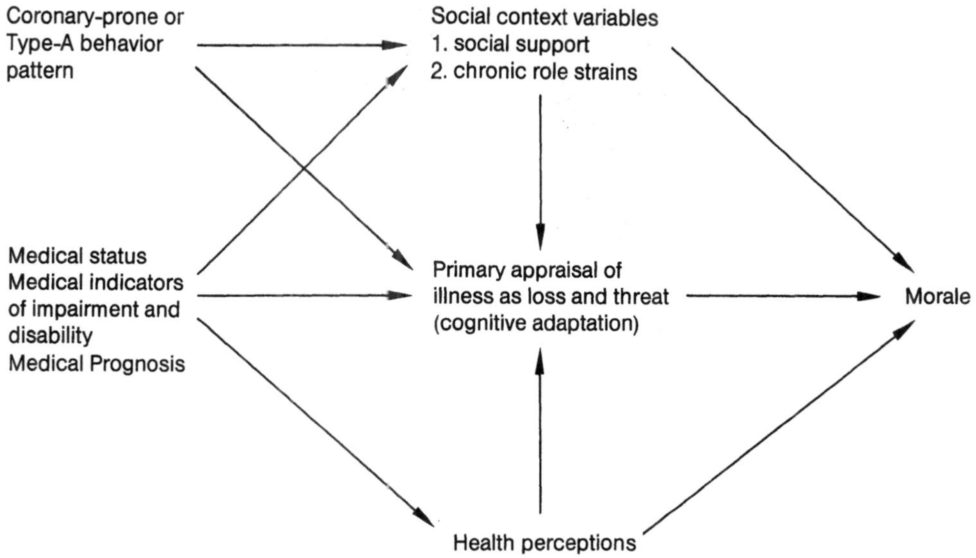

Fig. 1. An adaptation framework: prospective relationships among medical status, health perceptions, primary appraisal, social context, and morale

is influenced by these exogenous factors. As an intermediary variable, primary appraisal mediates the effect on positive and negative affect. In addition, social context has an important direct effect on the individual's feeling states. Quality of life is the balance between positive and negative affect.

Statistical Analyses

In the statistical analyses to be discussed in this section, the putative causal pathways linking exogenous and mediating factors with psychological well-being will be divided into the separate components of the conceptual model depicted in Fig. 1:

1. In a first set of analyses, the lower part of the model will be developed. It is postulated that the objective cardiac impairment of the patient and his own daily experiences with illness (subjective health) influence his primary appraisal of the stress of illness. Signals from his physician that he is seriously ill or the subjective experience of being sick and disabled will lead to a pessimistic definition of the situation (i.e., elevated scores on the *primary appraisal scale*). The subjective stress of illness, as assessed by the scale, will be high. This will lead to an elevation of dysphoric affect, as measured by the negative dimension of the Bradburn scale. The development of cardiac invalidism is mirrored by the scores of the patient on the *negative affect scale*. Medically defined and patient-defined health status, the perceived stress of illness, and psychological well-being form an important causal pathway linking disease and quality of life. These causal links, however, may be significantly modified by the social context in which the stress process takes place.

Table 2. Influence of subjective health perceptions on measures of cognitive and emotional adjustment at 1 year (T3) (gamma coefficients of association)

Measures of subjective health and perceived disability	Primary appraisal	Negative affect	Positive affect
Poor subjective health	0.78	0.56	−0.36
Cardiac symptoms	0.65	0.45	−0.23
Perceived impairment	0.63	0.37	NS
"Doing poorly"	0.81	0.72	−0.44
"Sickly and disabled"	0.73	0.58	−0.41
Sexual disability	0.59	0.46	−0.19
Disability in family role	0.55	0.49	NS
Loss of work role	0.42	0.25	NS
Disability in work role	0.47	0.34	NS

$n = 606$.

2. In a second step, salient dimensions of social context will be discussed and related to the patient's appraisal of his marital bond.
3. In a third step, the upper portion of the model will be developed, with particular focus on the negative impact of a conflictual and unsupportive social environment. Chronic marital stressors are postulated to overwhelm the coping resources of the individual relative to cognitive adaptation leading to a pessimistic definition of the situation. Adequate social support and the sense of reliable alliance it entails have the opposite effect. Cognitive adaptation as influenced by social context is a determinant of the level of positive and negative affective states, as assessed by the two Bradburn scales: Negative health perceptions are correlates of elevated negative affect; feelings of "returning to normal" are related to positive affect and high quality of life.
4. Finally, social context will be discussed as an independent determinant of the level of positive and negative emotions or quality of life of the patient. When people speak of quality of life, they often have their marital situation in mind (Zautra 1983).

Health Perceptions, Cognitive Adaptation, and Psychological Well-being

At the experiential level of the patient, illness manifests itself in physical discomfort, symptoms of angina pectoris and dyspnea, as well as in a perceived decrease in functional capacity. The individual becomes aware of a profound change in health status by no longer being able to engage in the tasks and activities he performed before his illness. Forced retirement is an important signal of this profound alteration. Impairment and disability influence health perceptions with a resulting impact on primary appraisal and affective states (see Table 2).

At T3, 1 year after their heart attack, a sizable portion of the patients still view themselves as sickly and unsure of themselves, whereas a similar proportion define themselves as "gradually returning to normal." These self-images discriminate between high and low scorers on the *primary appraisal scale*. The former are still experiencing high levels of existential threat caused by illness, resulting in extreme psychological distress and low quality of life. Patients who perceive themselves as

Table 3. Standard multiple regression analysis of Bradburn's morale measures at T3 on indicators of perceived recovery at T2 and medical status at T1

Predictors	Negative affect	Positive affect
Doing well/poorly	0.27	-0.12
Self-definition as sick and disabled	0.23	-0.15
Cardiac symptoms	0.14	-0.18
Medical status	NS	NS
R^2	0.27	0.14

$n = 604$; $P \leqq 0.01$.

Table 4. Standard multiple regression analysis of negative affect scores at 1 year (T3) on measures of primary appraisal and subjective health at 6 months (T2)

Measures of primary appraisal and subjective health (T2)	Beta coefficients
Primary appraisal (high stress of illness)	0.41[a]
Disability in family role	0.27[a]
Sexual disability	0.07[b]
Loss of work role	0.14[a]
Disability in work role	0.09[b]
Cardiac symptoms	0.08[b]
Medical status (T1)	NS

$n = 606$; adjusted $R^2 = 0.36$.
[a] $P < 0.01$.
[b] $P < 0.05$.

doing well have low scores on the *primary appraisal scale* and high scores on the *positive affect scale*. The latter appear to be adapting successfully to illness at the cognitive and emotional levels. These two patient groups are moving along quite different tangents of psychological recovery.

In the hospital at T1, 70% of the sample was distressed by fears concerning a drop in functional capacity. Marked changes in health perceptions occurred during the year. At T3, only 25% of the latter patients, but 86.5% of the former, saw their functional capacity as threatened. This shows how strongly physical aspects of recovery influence the morale of the patient (see Table 3). Successful adaptation has an impact on the positive dimension, continuing problems, and disability on the negative dimension of subjective well-being.

The patient's health perceptions are closely related to his definition of the situation (primary appraisal). Some patients view themselves at T3 as returning to normal. They perceive their present health status as good, whatever this may mean to them. Other patients still define themselves as sickly and disabled. Their health perceptions are less positive, as is their definition of their present life situation. Physical symptoms, a decrease in functional capacity, forced retirement, and other factors influence how the patient appraises his situation.

Table 5. Standard multiple regression analysis of quality of marital relationship (good/poor) on contextual measures of marital situation

Contextual variables	Standardized regression coefficients
Marital conflict	0.32[a]
Sexual rapport	-0.10[b]
Social support	-0.42[a]
Adequacy of support	-0.10[b]
"Perfect wife"	-0.17[a]
Good housekeeper	-0.09[b]
Warmhearted	-0.15[a]

Adjusted $R^2 = 0.62$.
[a] $P < 0.01$.
[b] $P < 0.05$.

Both health perceptions and primary appraisal are strongly associated with negative affect (see Table 4). The group of patients who view themselves as adjusting poorly have relatively high scores on the Bradburn scale both at 6 months and 1 year subsequent to their heart attack. This negative affect is related to feelings of uselessness, uncertainty about the future, helplessness, self-derogation and a low sense of self-efficacy, as described by Charmaz (1973) and Viney (1983). Other investigators have found poor health and disability to be a source of unhappiness, including Bradburn (1969). These perceptions of illness explain a large proportion of the variance in negative affect.

At the same time, positive affect also appears to be influenced by health perceptions, as Tables 2 and 3 show. That physical disability and the loss of social roles should lead to negative emotions is evident and supported by a large number of studies. A similar influence of health perceptions on positive affect may have several different causes. One is the sense of relief at having survived a life-threating illness and gradually "getting back to normal."

Social Context

Young (1983) has postulated that families can be evaluated in terms of how they affect illness. Major dimensions of close interpersonal relations were investigated in this respect. Some marriages are emotionally close. In others the social support provided by the spouse may very often be inadequate. Many patients feel themselves emotionally isolated in marriage and lacking a sense of social embeddedness. They do not feel that their wife is truly concerned about them and their heart attack. They lack a sense of reliable alliance with their marital partner, whom they cannot fall back on should the need arise. The marital relationship is very often a source of considerable stress, in addition to not fulfilling the emotional needs of the patient.

The *Quality of the Marital Relationship* scale (see Table 5) focuses on the patient's dissatisfaction with his spouse. The majority of our sample reported being satisfied with their marriages at all three time points of our study. In the hospital, 20% of the patients were worried about their marriage. Some patients reported a worsening of their relationship in the first 6 months after their infarction. At this time point, approximately 30% were not completely satisfied with their spouse and believed that they had chosen the wrong mate. One year after the infarction this proportion had dropped to 16% of the sample. Almost one-fifth of the patients considered their marital relationship a burden on them, and two-fifths sometimes thought they themselves were not the spouse they would like to be. These instruments do not allow much differentiation among good marriages. A patient's assessment of his relationship as above average, average, or below average only correlates weakly with the scale (0.54). The scale assessing quality of the marital relationship does correlate very strongly with items measuring emotional closeness, conflict, the adequacy of the social support received, and a lack of common interests between husband and wife. Characteristics of the spouse, such as warmheartedness or being a good housekeeper or "perfect wife" were strongly associated with the general appraisal of the relationship. Certain items which probed into the social support provided by the wife following the heart attack were particularly highly correlated with the scale. These included:

Clear signs of love and affection
The experience that the patient meant very much to his wife
The feeling that his spouse was always available to the patient (a sense of reliable alliance with the wife)
A feeling of genuine involvement and concern of the wife

The patient's appraisal of the quality of his marital relationship is viewed here as an empirical measure of the theoretical construct *family context*. It encompasses both negative and positive aspects of social context. There was a high degree of agreement between the patient and his spouse on how they viewed their marital relationship. Data from the spouse questionnaire at T3 corroborate the information provided by the patient at both T1 and T3. Marital dissension is strongly associated with a negative appraisal of the quality of the marriage. Experienced social support, or rather its absence, was also strongly associated with negative attitudes towards the spouse. The patient's perceptions of not receiving adequate emotional support following his illness may perhaps be interpreted as the "loneliness of emotional isolation," as Weiss has conceptualized this term (Weiss 1974). The social support scale would thus be tapping both the gratification of emotional needs and the individual's "pining for someone to be close to." The variables *warmheartedness* and a *perfect wife* may be tapping the same emotional climate in the marriage.

Different marital dyads can theoretically be located on a continuum ranging from emotionally close to emotionally isolated. Only a small group of patients considered their marital relationships as inadequate and distressing. Most of the instruments developed were therefore highly skewed and did not allow much discrimination between more or less emotionally close marriages. High interpersonal conflict and emotional isolation did appear to discriminate between different kinds of families. Patients living in such an inadequate social context did seem to have greater problems in cognitive and emotional adjustment, as will now be shown. The distinction between dissatisfaction and satisfaction with one's spouse may be the relevant distinction in the context of adaptation breakdown. Pearlin et al. (1981) point to the importance of chronic role strains in relation to feelings of self-worth and self-efficacy. Environmental stressors arising from poor interpersonal relationships appear to be major characteristics of the social context, which so far have not been sufficiently investigated. The nascent science of interpersonal relationships has focused on social support, intimacy, and the gratification of emotional needs, dimensions of context which may be difficult to measure. Future research on adaptation should focus more on negative aspects of social context and interpersonal bonds.

Influence of Social Context on Cognitive Adaptation

Cognitive processes of adjustment were assessed by the *primary appraisal scale*. This scale measures the somatic concerns and stress of illness. It has already been shown that primary appraisal is strongly associated with the health perceptions and perceived disability of the patient. High scores signify that the individual perceives his heart attack as a threat to his physical and psychological integrity. Poor subjective health and problems in adjustment are correlates of a pessimistic primary appraisal of the illness. It has been postulated that the social context of recovery in the family influences how the patient defines his situation. On the one hand, social support from family members is viewed as aiding the individual in restructuring his assumptive world. Cognitive processes of adaptation are facilitated if the social environment is perceived as secure, stable, and coherent. On the other hand, the family may be a source of chronic role strain. Marital conflict and a sense of emotional isolation may be additional environmental stressors encumbering cognitive adaptation by overwhelming the coping resources of the individual.

Marital status was not found to influence primary appraisal. The unmarried did not judge their illness and its impact on their lives to be more stressful than the married. Dissatisfaction with the spouse relationship, however, was associated with a pessimistic primary appraisal (see Table 6). Patients who perceived their marriage as poor prior to their illness (T1), or 1 year later (T3), had higher scores on the scale at T3. A lack of companionship, concern, or intimacy, as well as other indicators of emotional isolation, were associated with a negative definition of the situation. Reports of marital conflict or a worsening of the marriage during the year (T2, T3) were also strongly associated with pessimistic mental images of the patient's postinfarction situation. Marital dissension at both points of time was associated with high scores on the scale (gamma = 0.35; 0.37; $P \leqq 0.001$). Marital role strain at T1 and T3 also seemed to influence primary appraisal (gamma = 0.24; 0.26; $P \leqq 0.03$).

Three-quarters of the patients were satisfied with the social support they had received after returning home from the hospital. Most perceived that their spouse was genuinely involved in their recovery. They experienced love and affection or were able to confide in their spouses. They had a feeling that their wife was always "available to them and their problems." A minority of patients considered the social support and moral encouragement provided to them as inadequate. These perceptions were closely linked to variables measuring marital conflict and dissatisfaction. The provision of social support also appeared to influence cognitive processes of adaptation. High scores on the primary appraisal scale at T3 were associated with inadequate social support at T2 (0.24; $P \leqq 0.01$), as well as with a lack of concern

Table 6. Association of primary appraisal and negative affect at T3 with measures of social context in family (gamma coefficients)

Contextual variables	Primary appraisal	Negative affect
Marital status (married/unmarried)	NS	0.21[a]
Marital conflict T2	0.35	0.52
Marital conflict T3	0.37	0.50
Marital role strain T1	0.24[a]	0.49
Marital role strain T3	0.26[a]	0.68
Emotional support T2	-0.24[a]	-0.45
Adequacy of support T2	-0.24[a]	-0.52
Sense of reliable alliance with spouse		
at T2	-0.18[a]	-0.39
at T3	-0.32	-0.34

[a] $P \leq 0.05$; all others, $P \leq 0.01$.

(0.30; $P \leq 0.02$) and a lack of love and affection (0.24; $P \leq 0.01$). Patients who negated a sense of reliable alliance with their spouse at T3 defined their postinfarction situation more negatively than those who considered their wife as "always there for them and their problems" (0.32; $P \leq 0.001$).

Influence of Social Context on Emotional Adaptation

The same dimensions of social context that were shown to influence primary appraisal also appear to have an impact on the patient's morale. The degree of association between these variables and negative affect (see Table 6) is greater than the correlations with primary appraisal. Social context is viewed as influencing how the individual defines his life situation and cognitive processes of adjustment. Environmental stressors and the lack of emotional embeddedness in the family appear to handicap the patient in coping with the stress of illness, as reflected in primary appraisal. Social context thus influences morale indirectly. A sense of poor adjustment was shown to be an important determinant of negative affect, whereas successful coping was found associated with positive affect. Social context influences cognitive processes of adaptation and, via adjustment variables, subjective well-being. The social context is also posited as having a direct impact on well-being. Previous research by Lazarus and his co-workers has shown a high degree of association between "daily hassles" and negative affect (Kanner et al. 1981). Our study supports these findings. Marital conflict and the daily hassles encompassed in chronic role strains appear to be determinants of low morale. In addition, the nongratification of socioemotional needs also seems to have an impact on negative affect. Kanner et al. (1981) did not find such a relationship between "daily uplifts" and low morale. Hassles were associated with low morale, and uplifts with high morale. In a life crisis, such as myocardial infarction, inadequate social support appears to have a negative effect on subjective well-being. This may be due to the high interrelation between supportive interaction and the quality of the conjugal bond. Or it may be that the experience of not being loved, esteemed, and able to count on others in a crisis situation is a very pervasive type of environmental stressor.

Marital status was related to psychological well-being throughout the first year but especially in the first 6 months. At T1 and T2 approximately 50% of the unmarried patients had high scores on the negative affect scale. By the end of the first year (T3) the relation between marital status and well-being had weakened considerably. Positive affect appeared to be influenced by the status of being married somewhat more strongly than negative affect (gamma = 0.27; −0.21; $P \leqq 0.05$). The only really significant differences at T3 were between the unmarried and patients with an emotionally close relationship. Patients who reported a great deal of conflict in their marriages, moreover, had higher scores on negative affect than those without a spouse. "Normal" marriages and the unmarried did not even differ considerably in respect to negative affect. A rank ordering of patients relative to their level of psychological well-being is as follows:

Dissatisfied with marriage
Unmarried
Normal marriage
Emotionally close marriage

This variable correlated with both positive and negative affect (0.24; −0.29; $P \leqq 0.01$). Marital status appeared to be of greatest importance in the early stages of being a patient and to be overshadowed by marital stressors among the married after the patient had returned home from the hospital.

Adequate social support and emotional closeness influenced the patient's emotional balance throughout the whole period. Almost two-fifths of the patients reported a high level of intimacy in their marriage prior to their illness. Approximately a fifth appraised their relation as lacking this kind of emotional closeness at both T1 and T3. The high degree of association of these two variables with negative affect (−0.29; −0.40; $P \leqq 0.001$) may be interpreted as indicators of the emotional isolation of the patient. At the same time, spouse closeness is strongly associated with positive affect, as are other indicators of marital companionship and emotional support. Patients who viewed their marriage as characterized by a high degree of warmth and intimacy prior to the heart attack (T1) had high scores on positive affect at T3, 1 year later (0.32; $P \leqq 0.001$). The same is true of individuals who experienced that they meant very much to their spouse in the hospital (0.45; $P \leqq 0.001$). Experienced social support has been defined as the clarity and certainty with which one experiences being loved, esteemed, and able to rely on others. Indicators of love and affection experienced by the patient at T1 and T2 were good predictors of positive affect at T3 (0.39; 0.31; $P \leqq 0.001$). These findings would seem to provide evidence for an important role of social support relative to processes of emotional adjustment. More concrete types of social support with a moderate or high degree of association with positive affect at T3 included moral encouragement, social approval, and confiding. Encouragement and ego-bolstering interaction with the wife in the hospital, for example, was highly correlated with positive affect at T1 (0.44; $P \leqq 0.001$).

The same is true of social support from adult children, other relatives, and close friends. These results have been reported in Badura and Waltz (1984). Finlayson and McEwen (1977) also found that adult children were an important social resource in recovery from myocardial infarction. In our study, social support in the hospital was associated with higher scores on the scale measuring the positive dimension of subjective well-being. The perception of genuine concern and involvement or experiencing that he meant very much to his children apparently led to positive emotions in the patient. Just as with the spouse, this variable was strongly associated with a feeling of well-being (0.39; $P \leqq 0.001$). Moral encouragement was also related to positive affect (0.33; $P \leqq 0.01$). More general appraisals of the child-parent relationship include the level of intimacy and commitment in the filial social bond. Almost three-quarters of the patients were satisfied with their ability to confide in their children and with the aid and assistance they received following their heart attack. Confiding and a sense of reliable alliance were both associated with positive feeling states of the patient (0.43; $P \leqq 0.001$).

Coping with the Stress of Illness in Four Social Contexts

Adaptation to an adverse life event was studied in four different social contexts. Preliminary investigations identified interpersonal conflict and emotional closeness/social support as salient empirical dimensions of the spouse relationship and family context. A general conclusion from the analyses already discussed in the previous section is that individuals experiencing serious illness and its sequelae in a supportive environment are better equipped to cope with the stressors confronting them than other patients. The variables used to assess cognitive and emotional adjustment showed this quite clearly. The total sample was assigned to marital groups along two empirical dimensions based on the reports of both husband and wife: low vs. high marital conflict; emotional closeness vs. emotional isolation. Four crude categories reflecting various kinds of social environment resulted:

1. Group I: low marital conflict and high intimacy between the spouses
2. Group II: a residual category termed "normal marital context"
3. Group III: high marital conflict and low level of emotional closeness
4. Group IV: unmarried status

The curves depicted in Fig. 2 show that these social contexts discriminate between good and poor adaptation to myocardial infarction during the period so far studied. Patients in Group I reported relatively high levels of positive feeling states in the hospital and during the subsequent year. Approximately one-half of them had high scores on the positive affect scale, reflecting the emotional impact of an adequate spouse relationship. A relatively small proportion of this group had high scores on the negative affect scale which may have been due to the buffering effect of social support but also to low marital conflict. Social support was postulated as moderating the cognitive and emotional impact of environmental stressors and thus leading to low levels of negative affect. The sharp drop in the number of patients with high levels of dysphoric feelings from 49% to 35% between T2 and T3 supports this hypothesis. The conclusion may be drawn that patients in Group I are coping well with illness and gradually achieving a high level of quality of life. Extreme Type A individuals are underrepresented in Group I.

Groups III and IV appeared to be adjusting less well. Unmarried status and the conflictual marital context may be viewed as less favorable social environments for

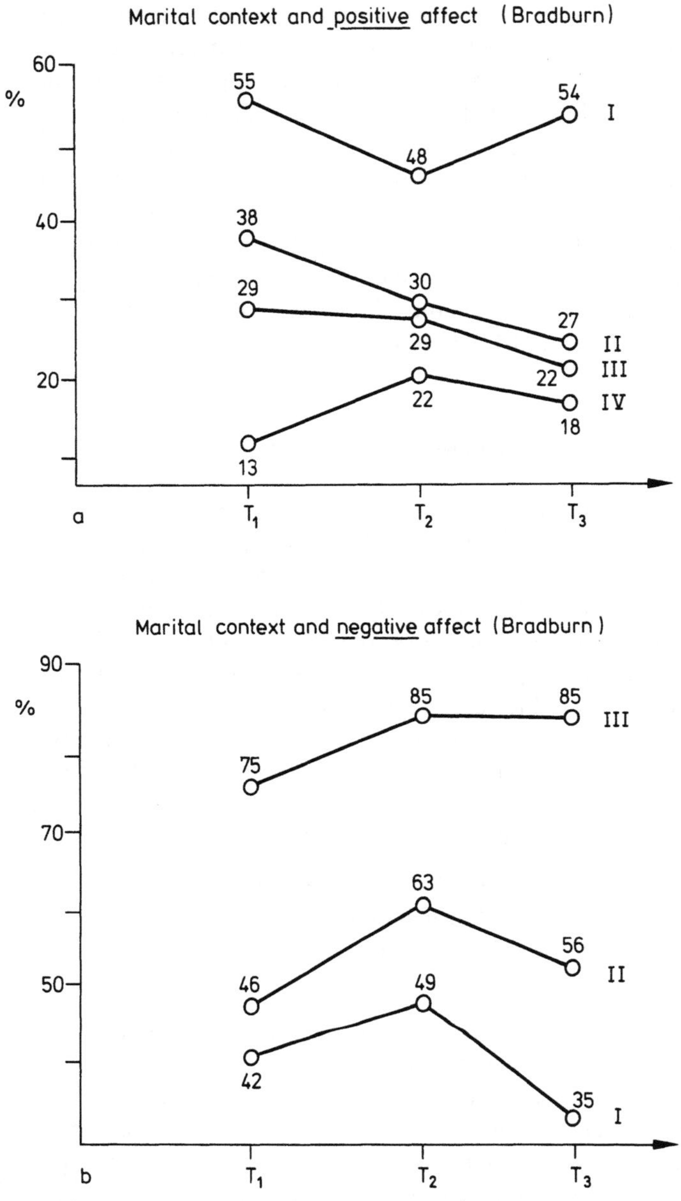

Fig. 2 a, b. Emotional adaptation in four marital contexts. **a** Proportion of patients in each group with high scores on the Bradburn positive affect scale. **b** Proportion of patients in each group with high scores on the Bradburn negative affect scale. (For details of marital context groups see text)

coping with a stressful life situation. The lack of social support as a buffer against the stress of illness, forced retirement, and other life changes in the wake of myocardial infarction is one reason suggested for a poorer psychological recovery. A second is the additional environmental stressors inherent in these two social contexts. In the hospital at T1 only 13% of the unmarried had high scores on the positive affect scale, and at T3 only about one-fifth of the patients in Groups III and IV reported high levels of positive affect. Lacking an intimate marital relationship, they were apparently not being provided with adequate social support and did not have the same opportunity as happily married individuals for gratifying social interaction in everyday life. Group III, the social context with high marital conflict, appeared to be characterized by psychological distress and the negative images of illness described in an earlier section. Most individuals in this group (75%–85%) reported elevated levels of negative feeling states throughout the study period. Marital conflict and a sense of emotional isolation is probably a major cause of this condition. In addition, the lack of social resources for coping with their physical and emotional problems can be viewed as hindering psychological recovery. Quality of life as the balance between positive and negative feeling states may be judged low in the conflictual marital context. Extreme Type A individuals were disproportionately located in this group.

Coronary-prone Behavior Pattern and Psychological Recovery

Serious illness may be conceptualized as a social experiment for investigating a putative causal influence of the coronary-prone behavior pattern on psychological adjustment. Based on the work of Glass (1983) and others, it is postulated that Type A and Type B individuals should differ relative to their degree of cognitive and emotional adaptation to the stress of myocardial infarction and its sequelae. The salient role of social context has already been discussed in this respect. Coronary-prone behavior was measured by a 17-item paper-and-pencil German version of the JAS devised by C.D. Jenkins and T.H. Schmidt. As a broad generalization, the group of patients located in the upper quartile of the JAS distribution defined themselves as "more sickly and unsure of themselves" than those individuals whose JAS scores were located in the lower quartile. This was particularly the case with Type A individuals who experienced high levels of physical disability or social impairment. This latter group reported the highest levels of emotional distress in the total sample at T2 and T3.

The *primary appraisal* scale was intended to assess the changing threat of myocardial infarction to the physical and psychological integrity of the individual. High scores on the scale at T1–T3 signify an elevated level of threat and subjective stress. Decreasing scores indicate successful adaptation; high scores may be viewed as an indicator of cardiac invalidism. Reports by husband and wife show that the scale discriminates well between good and poor adjustment. Approximately one-third of the sample appear to be having significant physical and psychological problems and to be recovering poorly 1 year after onset of illness. Extreme Type A individuals, especially those with notable health problems, are disproportionately located in this third of the sample. This group have primary appraisal scale scores of 25.0, 8 points above the sample mean, as compared to extreme Type B individuals with scores of 15.2 (T2) and 13.5 (T3). Eta as a measure of association was 0.28 ($P \leqq 0.01$) at T3. An analysis of variance with primary appraisal as the dependent variable and perceived disability, marital context, and the JAS scores as the explanatory variables showed significant main effects for all three of the latter:

Cardiac symptoms and social disability ($P \leqq 0.001$)
Poor marital context ($P \leqq 0.02$)
JAS scores ($P \leqq 0.01$)

A significant interaction effect between marital context and JAS was also noted ($P \leqq 0.04$). Health- and marriage-related problems appeared to be perceived as extremely distressing and threatening for Type A individuals relative to Type B.

The impact of the same variables on emotional adjustment during the first year, i. e., on positive and negative feeling states, as measured by the Bradburn scales, was also investigated. A significant interaction effect between perceived disability and JAS was discovered with negative affect as dependent variable. Angina pectoris, dyspnea, and perceived disability appear to lead to relatively greater dysphoric emotions in Type A individuals than in Type B. Analyses of variance using other measures of emotional impact at T3 (i. e., psychological distress, anxiety, and negative self-images) consistently substantiated this interaction term. It is tempting to speculate that the above-described adaptive processes at T1-T3 will be predictive of physical outcome in the next 2 years.

Discussion

The physical, social, and psychological sequelae of a myocardial infarction were investigated within an adaptation framework. Physical consequences of illness impinging on the total life of the individual included cardiac symptoms and a decrease in functional capacity. These had an impact on the activities and social roles of the individual in the marital-sexual sphere, in the family, on the job, etc. Forced retirement was a frequent consequence of serious cardiac impairment. Altogether, these sequelae of illness form a massive threat to the individual's sense of physical and psychological integrity.

In line with biobehavioral models of adaptation and disease, it was postulated that psychosocial factors influence coping outcomes and possibly neurobiological processes related to physical recovery. Social context and coronary-prone behavior were both found to be associated with cognitive coping processes. Extreme Type A individuals and individuals with a distressing or unsupportive marital relationship appraised their situation more negatively than other patients with the same degree of cardiac impairment. These patient groups experienced greater levels of threat and perceived stress in the wake of illness. Negative health perceptions and a high level of perceived threat were associated with dysphoric emotions as assessed at T1-T3 by the Bradburn negative affect scale. The same is true of problems-in- living in the marital role.

In contrast, positive health perceptions and "normalization" were correlates of positive feeling states. Social support was found to facilitate adjustment at the cognitive and emotional levels. Affection, confiding, esteem support, and a sense of reliable alliance with one's spouse were shown to influence the ability of the individual to cope effectively with the psychosocial sequelae of myocardial infarction. By reducing anxiety and the psychological distress of serious illness, a favorable social context should, therefore, have a positive impact on neuroendocrine processes and longevity. A conflictual marital context and the Type A behavioral pattern may be speculated as having the opposite effect (cf. Herd and Weiss 1983).

Future biobehavioral models of the stress-disease interface, it is suggested, should include data on social support, as well as on the social stress originating in inadequate interpersonal relationships. The further exploration of the relation of certain dimensions of the Type A construct to the types of social environments people have created for themselves also appears promising. This may be a pathway by which the former influences coping and pathophysiological processes. It is appealing to speculate that low marital intimacy and high interpersonal conflict are associated with Type A behavior. In-depth, rather than epidemiological, approaches are probably necessary for further advances in resolving this particular question. Since the present study is to be continued until 1986, some of these hypotheses can be investigated as further data becomes available on long-term psychosocial and somatic outcomes.

Acknowledgment. This research was supported by two grants from the West German Ministry of Research and Technology (BMFT). The principal investigator was Prof. Dr. Bernhard Badura (cf. Badura B et al. Leben mit dem Herzinfarkt. Springer, 1986).

References

Badura B, Waltz M (1984) Social support and the quality of life following myocardial infarction. Soc Indicators Res 14: 295-311

Badura B, Kaufhold G, Lehmann H, Pfaff H, Schott T, Waltz M (1986) Leben mit dem Herzinfarkt - eine sozialepidemiologische Studie. Springer, Berlin, Heidelberg, New York, Tokio

Bradburn N (1969) The structure of well-being. Aldine, Chicago

Charmaz K (1973) Time and identity, the shaping of selves of the chronically ill. Doctoral dissertation, University of California, San Francisco

Cohen F (1980) Personality, stress, and the development of physical illness. In: Stone G, Cohen F, Adler N (eds) Health psychology. Jossey-Bass, San Francisco

Cohen F, Lazarus R (1980) Coping with the stress of illness. In: Stone G, Cohen F, Adler N (eds) Health psychology. Jossey-Bass, San Francisco

Cohen M (1982) Psychosocial morbidity in cancer: a clinical perspective. In: Cohen J, Cullen J, Martin R (eds) Psychosocial aspects of cancer. Raven, New York

Finlayson A, McEwen J (1977) Coronary heart disease and patterns of living. Croom-Helm, London

Glass D (1983) Psychosocial influence and the pathogenesis of arterioslerosis. In: Herd JA, Weiss SM (eds) Behavior and arteriosclerosis. Plenum, New York

Herd A, Weiss S (eds) (1983) Behavior and arteriosclerosis. Plenum, New York

Kanner A, Coyne J, Schaefer C, Lazarus R (1981) Comparison of two modes of stress measurement: daily hassles and uplifts versus major life events. J Behav Med 4: 1-39

Kaplan H (1970) Self-derogation and adjustment to recent life experiences. Arch Gen Psychiatry 22: 324-331

Medalie J, Snyder M, Groen J, Neufeld H, Goldbourt U, Riss E (1973) Angina pectoris among 10000 men: 5-year incidence and univariate analysis. Am J Med 55: 583-594

Pearlin L, Johnson J (1977) Marital status, life strains, and depression. Am Sociol Rev 42: 704-715

Pearlin L, Lieberman M, Menaghan E, Mullan J (1981) The stress process. J Health Soc Behav 22: 337-356

Solomon G (1984) Emotions, immunity, and disease: an historical and philosophical perspective. In: Ballieux R (ed) Breakdown in human adaptation to stress. Nijhof, Boston

Turner J, Frankel G, Levin D (1983) Social support: Conceptualization, measurement and implications for mental health. Res Commun Ment Health 3: 67-111

Viney L (1983) Images of illness. Krieger, Malabar

Weiss R (1974) The provisions of social relationships. In: Rubin Z (ed) Doing unto others. Prentice Hall, Engelwood Cliffs

Young R (1983) The family-illness intermesh. Soc Sci Med 17: 395-398

Zautra A (1983) Social resources and the quality of life. Am J Commun Psychol 11: 275-289

Endurance Training and Its Importance in the Prevention of Degenerative Cardiovascular Diseases

W. HOLLMANN[1]

The topic addressed by this conference covers a wide spectrum of possibilities. The two main areas of modern sports medicine comprise preventive and rehabilitative medicine in conjunction with training and sports. In many cases, patients participating in a program of training also need medication. Therefore, I will limit myself to the following main topics: (a) the essential preventive effects of physical training in cardiology; (b) effects of drugs in connection with physical work and training.

Essential Preventive Effects of Training

The functional basis of a heart infarction is a disparity between the O_2 demand and the O_2 supply in the myocardium. How can physical training help prevent this situation? The quality of training must be evaluated on the basis of the five fundamental components of fitness: coordination, flexibility, strength, velocity, and endurance.

Coordination involves the interplay of the central nervous system and the skeletal musculature during a given movement. Exercise of given movements lowers the oxygen demand. This change becomes especially clear in sports with high demands for coordination, such as swimming. In some cases, a mere improvement of coordinative quality can reduce oxygen requirements by 50% for a given swimming speed. At the same time, the aerobic-anaerobic threshold increases, which is an expression of increased aerobic performance capacity.

With improving flexibility and strength, it is no longer possible to attain structural or functional adaptations of the internal organs that are of preventive importance, except possibly through isokinetic training. This can be proved directly and indirectly. Strength training of large muscle groups does not substantially change their maximal oxygen uptake. Top athletes in strength and power sports do not show a higher maximal oxygen uptake than that expected for normal untrained persons of the same body weight.

Velocity is also of no practical consequence to this type of conditioning. Because of its high load intensity and short duration, the work is performed anaerobically. High lactic acid levels and low pH values result, together with an intense increase in catecholamines. This enlarges the oxygen demand of the myocardium, but does not cause a desired functional or structural adaptation of the cardiopulmonary system.

What remains is the so-called general aerobic endurance. This involves the dynamic work of large muscle groups for at least 30-40 min, 3-4 times a week at the limit of the individual aerobic-anaerobic threshold, as determined by using the cri-

1 Institute for Cardiovascular Research and Sports Medicine, Deutsche Sporthochschule, 5000 Cologne 41, Federal Republic of Germany

Biological and Psychological Factors
in Cardiovascular Disease
Ed. by T. H. Schmidt, T. M. Dembroski, and G. Blümchen

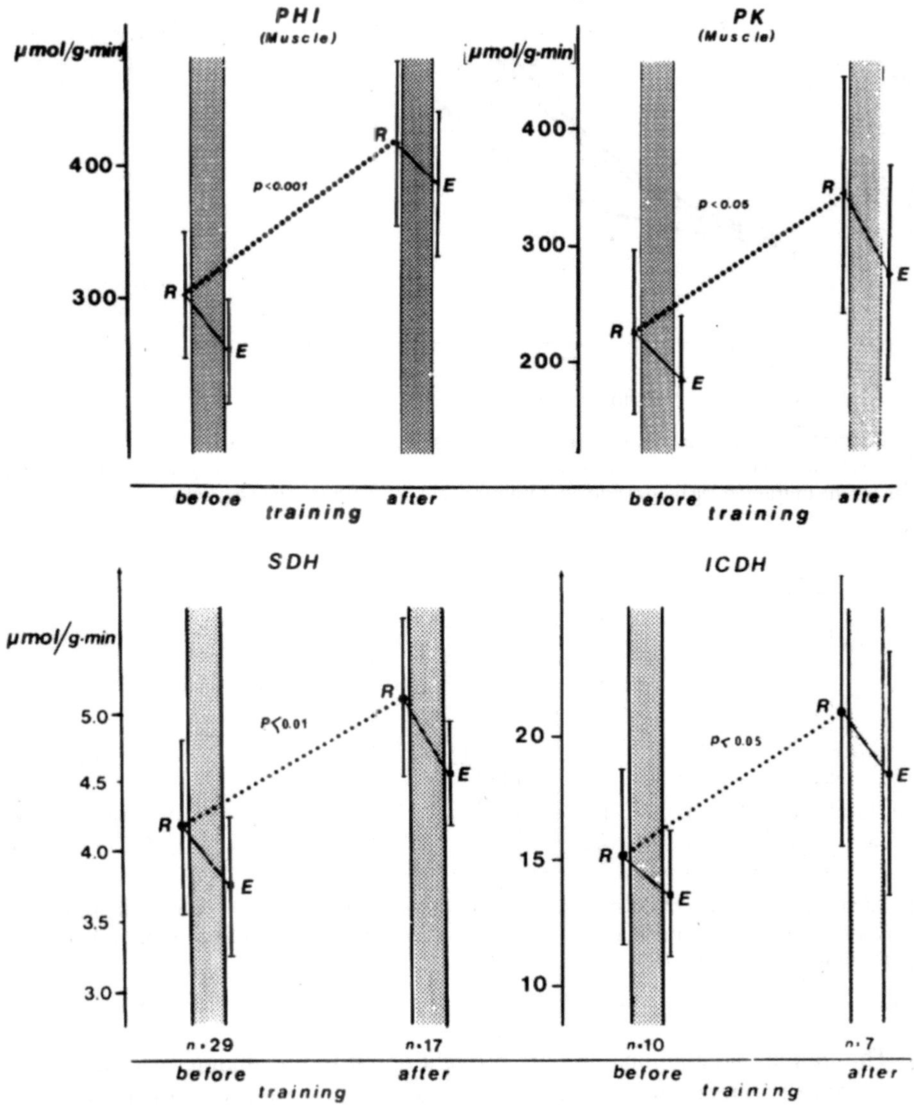

Fig. 1. Activity of the anaerobic enzymes phosphohexose isomerase *(PHI)* and pyruvate kinase *(PK)* and the aerobic enzymes sorbitol dehydrogenase *(SDH)* and isocitric dehydrogenase *(ICDH)* before and after a 12-week endurance training program for male persons aged between 56 and 70 years, as measured in the m. vastus lateralis

terion of 3 mmol/l lactic acid in the arterial blood. After 3 months or longer, this endurance training leads to a number of adaptations that are meaningful for the prevention of degenerative cardiovascular disease. In practice, pulse frequency should be between 130 bpm and 160 bpm in healthy males and females below the age of 50. In the case of healthy persons who are over 50, the following rule can be applied: 180 – age in years = pulse rate in training (Hollmann and Hettinger 1980).

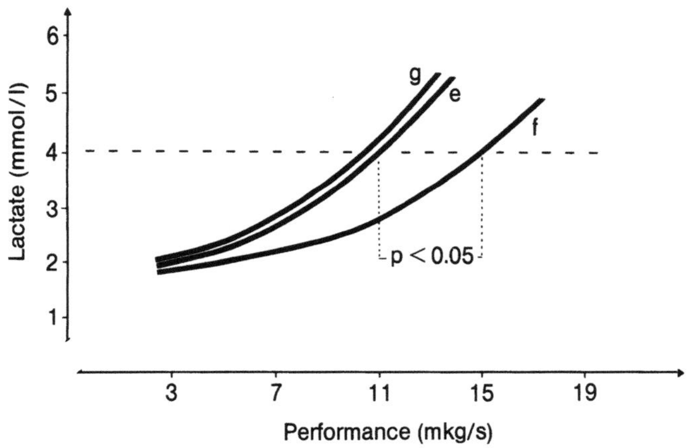

Fig. 2. Improvement in the aerobic-anaerobic threshold, as measured in the v. femoralis, after 12 weeks endurance training performed with one leg on a bicycle ergometer; *g* and *e* illustrate results for the untrained leg before and after training, *g* and *f* for the trained leg before and after training

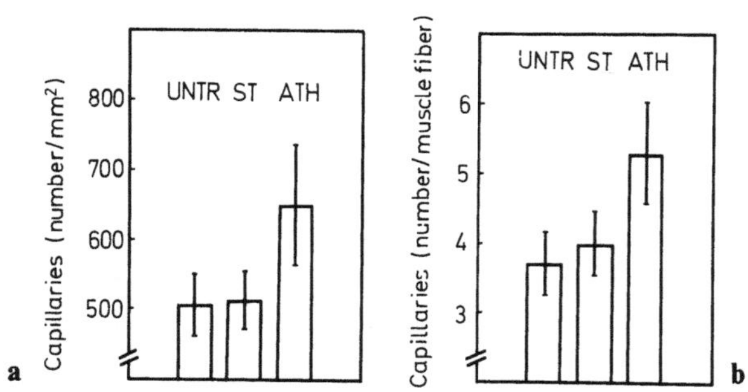

Fig. 3 a, b. Capillarization of the m. vastus lateralis of medical students (**a, b,** *bars at left*), sport students without endurance training (**a, b,** *middle bars*), and endurance-trained persons (**a, b,** *bars at right*). (From Schön et al. 1980)

The training adaptations that are brought about in this manner can be subdivided into peripheral and central mechanisms. In the case of peripheral mechanisms, we differentiate between metabolic and hemodynamic adaptations. The metabolic changes consist of an increase in the number and size of the mitochondria in the trained muscles as well as an augmentation in the activity of aerobic enzymes (Fig. 1), a rise in the aerobic-anaerobic threshold (Fig. 2), an increased hemoglobin content, and an augmentation in glycogen content.

Peripheral hemodynamic adaptation consists of improved capillarization. This involves the opening of rest capillaries, the lengthening and enlargement of existing capillaries, and the actual formation of new capillaries (Fig. 3). The result is an increase in capillary surface, which causes an improvement of the blood supply and thus in the supply of oxygen. In contrast to animal experiments, it has never been possible to establish the development of collaterals in men as a result of training.

Because of all these peripheral adaptations, peripheral aerobic performance capacity increases, and the sympathetic drive during rest and during a given submaxi-

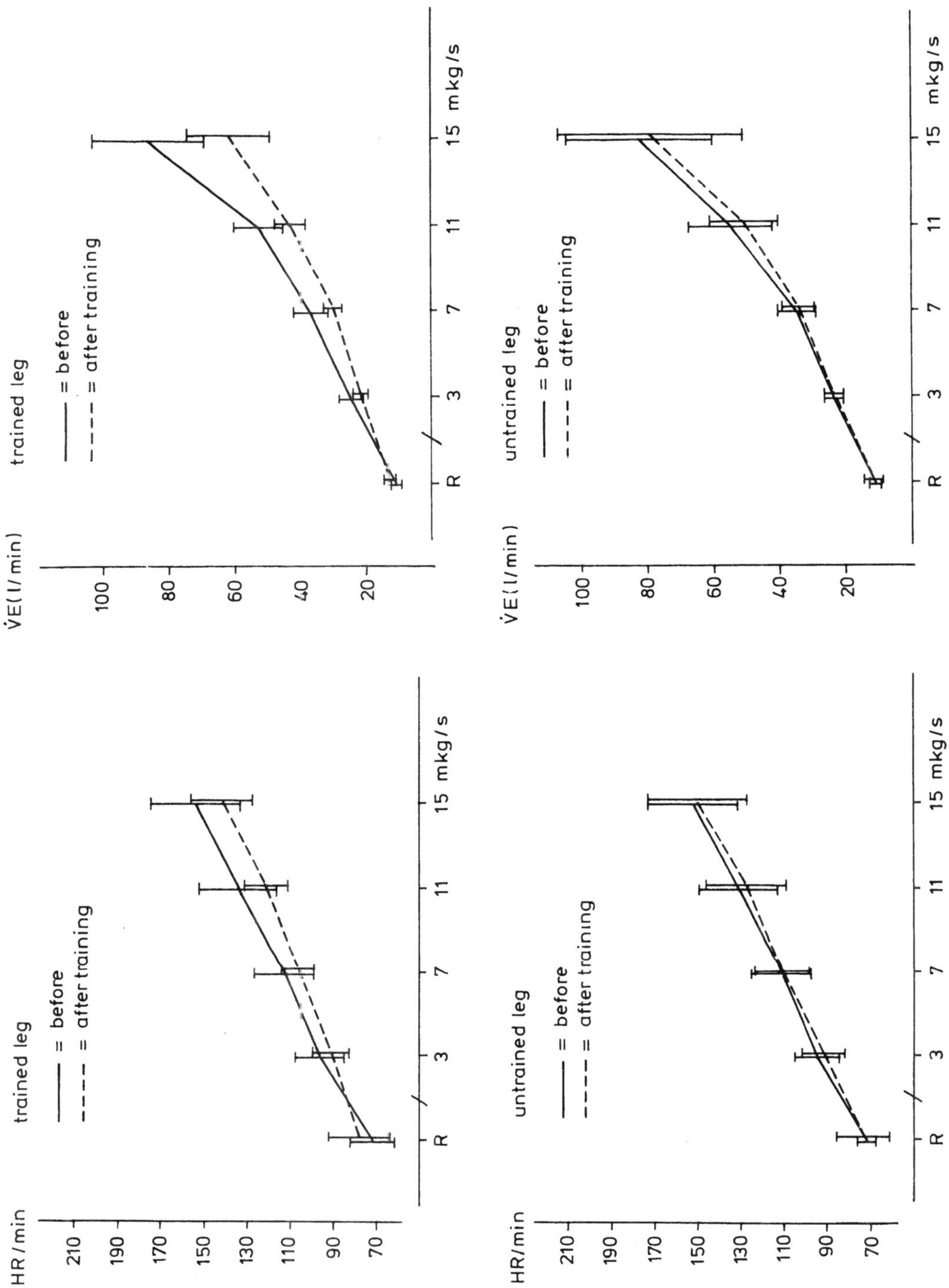

Fig. 4. Heart rate *(HR)* and ventilation *(V̇E)* before and after one-legged endurance training performed on bicycle ergometer

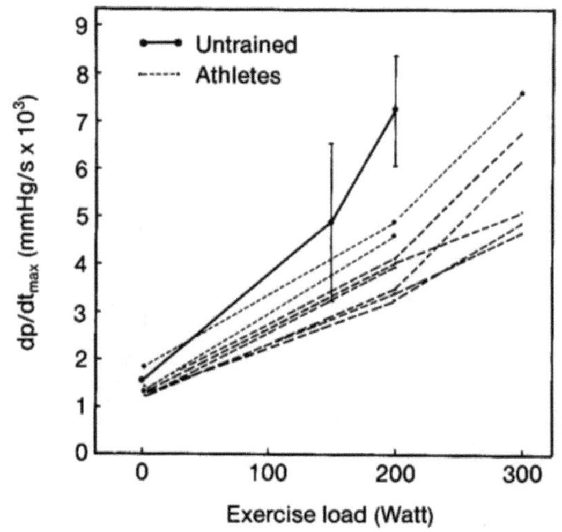

Fig. 5. Influence of training on the contractility of the heart muscle. (From Roskamm et al. 1971)

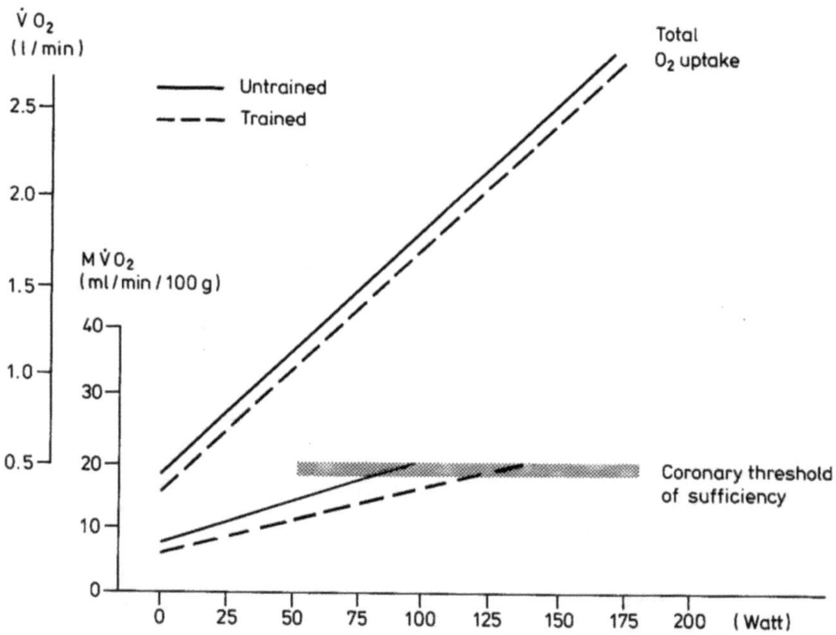

Fig. 6. Schematic representation of the effect of improved physical condition on the oxygen requirement of the heart muscle for given work loads. The *dark field* represents a zone of incipient coronary insufficiency. With improved physical condition, the patient attains a higher work load before reaching the danger zone

mal load decreases. This was demonstrated in our investigations on the influence of one-legged endurance training on a bicycle ergometer. When the endurance-trained leg is exercised, pulse frequency and respiratory minute value decrease significantly. Work with the untrained leg of the same person does not cause any significant alteration (Fig. 4).

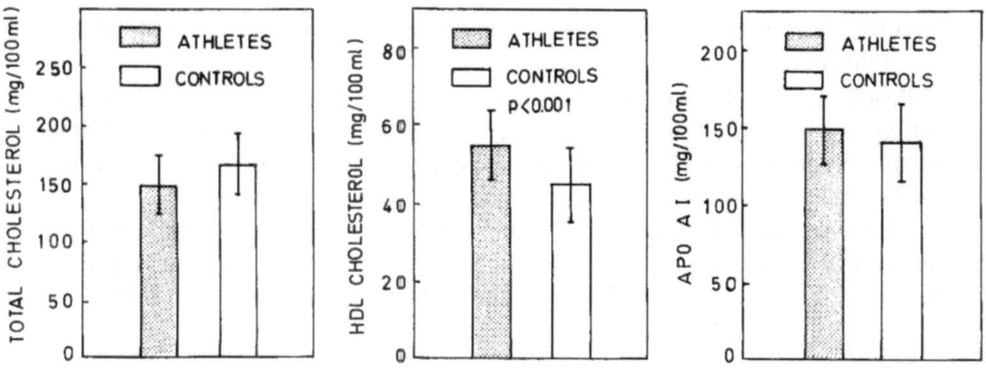

Fig. 7. Augmentation of the HDL and apolipoprotein A_1 fractions after 1 year of endurance training in 28 male persons between 40 and 60 years of age. (From Dufaux et al. 1979)

Central adaptations consist of: (a) a reduction in stroke frequency at rest and at given levels of work; (b) in some cases, a drop in systolic blood pressure during rest and work; (c) a prolongation of the diastolic phase; (d) a reduction in the contractility of the heart muscle (Fig. 5); (e) a reduction in the release of catecholamines at given levels of work. With the exception of the increase in the length of the diastole, all these mechanisms involve a reduction in the oxygen requirement of the myocardium. The prolongation of the diastole represents an extension of the crucial phase in which blood is supplied to the myocardium.

As a result of these adaptations, oxygen consumption of the myocardium drops at given levels of work (Fig. 6). In our opinion, these adaptations represent a very important result of training from the viewpoint of preventive cardiology in that they guard against a disparity between oxygen requirement and oxygen supply in the myocardium.

Another important factor is the influence of endurance training on the blood. The rigidity of the erythrocytes diminishes, allowing easier passage of erythrocytes through the capillaries. The adhesiveness and tendency of the platelets to aggregate are also reduced, effects which are potentially protective against the development of thrombosis. Although not proven, fibrinolytic activity at rest and during work may be higher in endurance-trained persons.

An important aspect of the effects of endurance training is their influence on lipoproteins. The low-density lipoproteins (LDH) fraction is reduced, and the high-density lipoproteins (HDL) and A1 apolipoprotein fractions are augmented (Fig. 7). Moreover, blood triglycerides are decreased, which protect against the development of atherosclerotic alterations. This effect was demonstrated in some very interesting investigations by Kramsch and coworkers (1981). Several groups of primates received an atherogenic diet. The animals were further divided into subgroups that lived under normal conditions in conjunction with this atherogenic diet and subgroups that engaged three times a week in jogging endurance training lasting 30–40 min per session. After 2–3 years, members of the untrained groups had developed several heart infarctions and typical atherosclerosis of the coronary vessels. Among the endurance-trained groups, there were no cases of heart infarction, and the coronary vessels showed a significantly bigger lumen and far fewer atherosclerotic lesions.

Based on this, we can understand the epidemiologic findings of Paffenbarger and coworkers in the USA (1978) and of Morris and coworkers in Great Britain (1980), who demonstrated a much lower incidence of heart infarction and heart disease mortality in groups of endurance-trained persons.

We believe that the decline of 28% in the incidence of heart infarction between 1968 and 1971 and the similar decrease of 31% during the 1970s in Japan represent multifactorial occurrences in which endurance training may also play a role.

Effects of Drugs During Work and Training

It is of practical importance to be familiar with the alterations in performance parameters produced by drugs. Among the most important medications are the beta blockers, which diminish heart rate (Fig. 8) and contractility, blood pressure, and

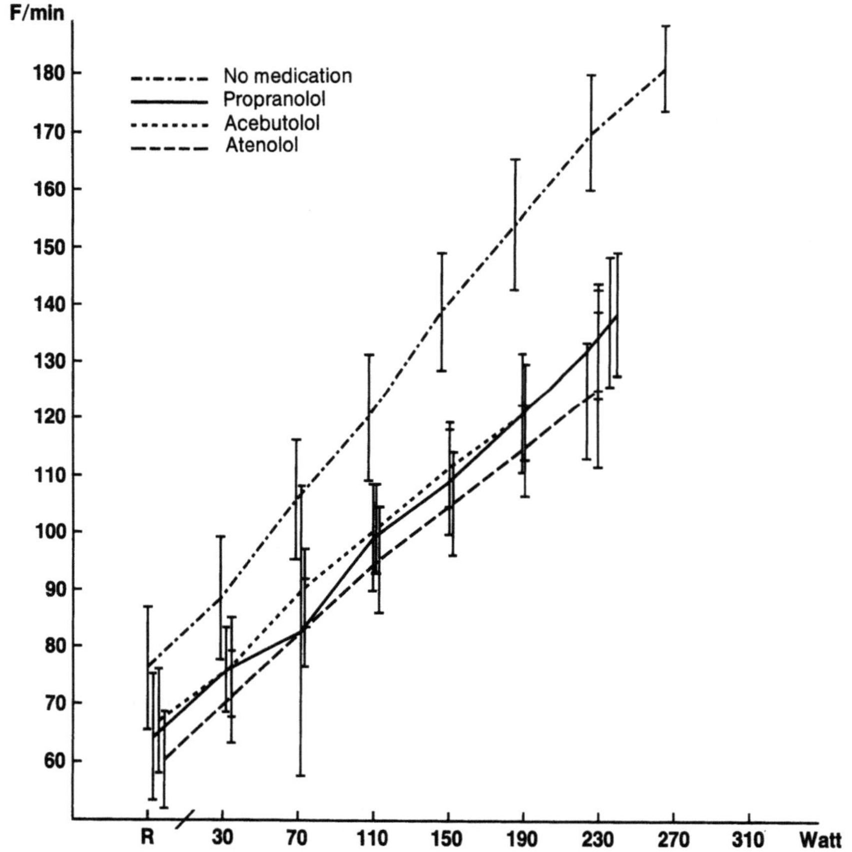

Fig. 8. Influence of different beta blockers on heart rate for given work loads on the bicycle ergometer

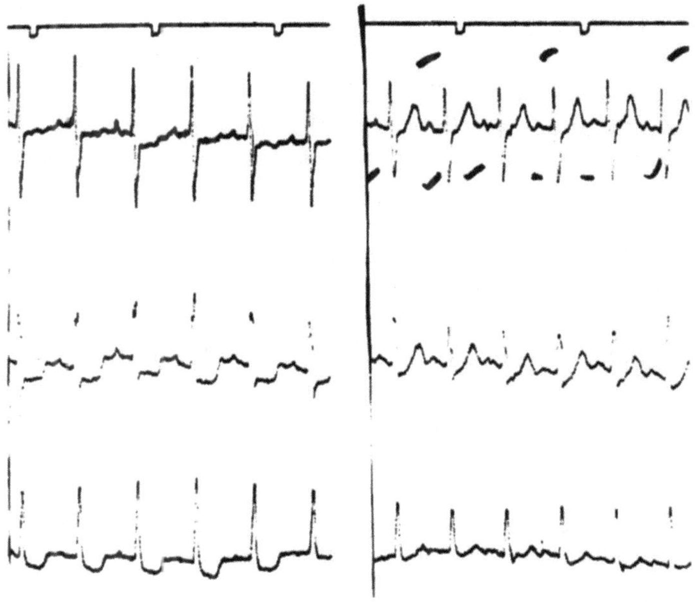

Fig. 9. ECG of a healthy person after administration of digitalis *(left)* and without digitalis *(right)* during exercise on a bicycle ergometer

other parameters related to myocardial oxygen requirements. Attention must be paid to the fact that beta$_1$-beta$_2$ receptor blockers can decrease the blood sugar level to the hypoglycemic range during long-lasting physical work. This effect on energy metabolism is especially important for young patients. Also affected are diabetics and persons who depend on full physical performance capacity and fitness to perform their jobs and enjoy their leisure-time pursuits. Therefore, a beta$_1$ receptor blocker should be given preference over beta$_1$-beta$_2$ blockers for diabetics who are involved in a physical training program.

The effect of beta blockers also depends on their dosage. Another point of view concerns their intrinsic sympathomimetic activity (ISA). The most intense effects are caused by drugs without ISA. Patients with a relatively low resting pulse rate should be given medication with an ISA effect.

An occasionally expressed fear that no training effect can be achieved during beta blockade could not be confirmed by our studies. In 1968, we investigated healthy sports students to whom 120 mg propranolol was administered daily for 6 weeks. The result showed statistically significant, but only slightly reduced, improvements in the performance parameters of the cardiopulmonary metabolic systems of the subjects as compared with a control group. However, maximum oxygen uptake during the administration of drugs such as propranolol and atenolol decreased by about 10%, while the anaerobic threshold was clearly less affected. This is due to the decreased production of lactic acid during beta blockade.

Nitro preparations are the classic medication used to reduce myocardial oxygen demand through a reduction in the amount of cardiac work. We were not able to observe any alterations in performance parameters during a given work load with nitro administration.

After administering digitalis, we found no significant difference at either a given submaximal work load or the borderline area of performance capacity. The training effect with digitalis was the same as that of the control group (Fig. 9).

However, the effects of digitalis combined with a beta blocker were identical to those induced with beta blockers alone. This holds true for both working conditions and training effects.

The third largest group of preparations used in treating coronary patients today are the calcium antagonists. In contrast to beta blockers, this group causes no impairment of physical performance capacity.

Postinfarction patients are often given anticoagulation treatment, which carries along with it the theoretical danger that undesired bleeding may occur, since it is a well-known fact that fibrinolytic activity is increased during muscular work. Indeed, we observed a few hematomas, and in two cases, bleeding into the lens of the eye occurred.

Diuretics also significantly reduce systolic and diastolic blood pressure at rest, but have little influence on blood pressure during exercise. This must be considered when patients perform physical training.

These findings can be summarized as follows: Endurance training in conjunction with an improvement in coordination is suitable as a measure of preventive cardiology. The altering effects of some drugs must be known in order to avoid inappropriate therapeutic decisions.

Summary

The essential preventive effects of physical training are described. Endurance training such as running, cycling, swimming, or cross-country skiing should be performed three to four times weekly, with each unit of training lasting 30-40 min, with a load intensity analogous to a pulse rate of 130-160 bpm for healthy persons under 50 years. Persons over 50 should use as a rule of thumb: 180 – age in years = pulse frequency during training. Peripheral and central training adaptations in hemodynamic and metabolic function can be observed, resulting in reduced oxygen demand by the heart muscle. This prevents a disparity between oxygen demand and oxygen supply to the heart muscle, which is the basis of ischemic heart disease. At the same time, blood flow properties are improved, and the tendency toward aggregation and the adhesiveness of platelets are reduced. The HDL level increases, while LDL and triglyceride levels decrease. All these alterations result in a relative degree of protection against acute hemodynamic and ischemic disasters.

Beta blockers alter hemodynamic and metabolic functions during work and training. $Beta_1$ and $beta_2$ blockers as well as beta blockers with and without ISA differ as to action and dose-effect relations. Nitro drugs and digitalis cause no significant changes in performance parameters during a given submaximal workload. The combination of a beta blocker with digitalis causes the same alterations as when the beta blocker is administered alone. In contrast to beta blockers, calcium antagonists do not lead to impairment of physical performance capacity. In some cases, the combination of training and anticoagulation treatment was associated with hematomas or bleeding into the lens of the eye. Diuretics reduce systolic and diastolic blood pressure at rest only, with no significant change during work.

References

Dufaux B, Liesen H, Rost R, Heck H, Hollmann W (1979) Über den Einfluß eines Ausdauertrainings auf die Serum-Lipoproteine unter besonderer Berücksichtigung der alpha-Lipoproteine (HDL) bei jungen und älteren Personen. Dtsch Z Sportmed 30: 123

Hollmann W, Hettinger TH (1980) Sportmedizin: Arbeits- und Trainingsgrundlagen. Schattauer, Stuttgart

Kramsch DM, Hspen AJ, Abramowitz BM, Kreimendahl T, Hood WD (1981) Reduction of coronary arteriosclerosis by moderate conditioning exercise in monkeys on an atherogenic diet. New Engl J Med 305 (25): 1483

Morris JN, Everitt MG, Pollard R, Chave SPW, Semmence AM (1980) Vigorous exercise in leisure-time: protection against coronary heart disease. Lancet II: 1207

Paffenbarger RS, Wing AL, Hyde RT (1978) Physical activity as an index on heart attack risk in college alumni. Am J Epidemiol 108: 161

Roskamm H (1971) Hämodynamik und Kontraktilität des gesunden und kranken Herzens bei körperlicher Belastung. Verh Dtsch Ges Herz Kreislaufforsch 37: 42

Schön FA, Hollmann W, Liesen H, Waterloh E (1980) Elektronenmikroskopische Befunde am M. vastus lateralis von Untrainierten und Marathonläufern sowie ihre Beziehung zur relativen maximalen Sauerstoffaufnahme und Laktatproduktion. Dtsch Z Sportmed 31 (12): 343

Subject Index

MIX
Papier aus verantwortungsvollen Quellen
Paper from responsible sources
FSC® C105338

FSC
www.fsc.org

If you have any concerns about our products,
you can contact us on
ProductSafety@springernature.com

In case Publisher is established outside the EU,
the EU authorized representative is:
Springer Nature Customer Service Center GmbH
Europaplatz 3, 69115 Heidelberg, Germany

Printed by Libri Plureos GmbH
in Hamburg, Germany